AF393351

Pathology Reviews • 1990

Pathology Reviews • 1990

Edited by

Emanuel Rubin, MD

Gonzalo Aponte Professor and Chairman
Department of Pathology and Cell Biology
Jefferson Medical College
Thomas Jefferson University
Philadelphia, Pennsylvania

and

Ivan Damjanov, MD

Professor
Department of Pathology and Cell Biology
Jefferson Medical College
Thomas Jefferson University
Philadelphia, Pennsylvania

米 Springer Science+Business Media, LLC

ISBN 978-1-4612-6783-6   ISBN 978-1-4612-0485-5 (eBook)
DOI 10.1007/978-1-4612-0485-5

Preface

The concept that human disease is a specialized branch of biology is universally accepted today, but in historical perspective, is actually of recent origin. At one time, the heliocentric theories of astronomy and the metallurgic transmutations of alchemy had their counterparts in magical and vitalistic approaches to human disease. Any relation between disease of humans and that of animals was not only unacceptable intellectually, but abhorrent theologically. Humans (and their diseases) were unique, and biology was the domain of those who studied animals and plants.

The unification of biology and the study of human disease, though begun some centuries ago, was conspicuously stimulated by the work of Darwin, and reached its full flower in this century. For example, the recognition that spontaneous diseases in animals often were similar to human disease led to the use of animal models in experiments with agents as diverse as bacteria and chemical carcinogens, and to the manipulation of cells in tissue culture. The trend toward accepting the importance of basic biological phenomena to elucidate the etiology and pathogenesis of disease became irreversible, and the visionary goal of interpreting morphologic observations on the basis of biochemical and physical events is being realized today. The change in emphasis in the study of disease was not revolutionary, as was, for example, the replacement of Newtonian mechanics by concepts based on the theories of Planck and Einstein. Rather, until the mid-20th century, the accretion of individual examples of the biological nature of disease processes provided the framework for an evolutionary change in thinking. The new psychological and philosophical milieu provided the basis for an unprecedented acceleration in the pace of biomedical research. It is clear that the biological revolution of the last 35 years was made possible not only by technological advances and innovative analytical methods, but also by an intellectual emphasis on the unity of biological processes. High school students are now aware that there is much to be learned about the human condition by studying bacterial DNA, the chloroplasts of green leaves, or the kinetics of enzymes in vitro.

This volume, one of an annual series, is derived from material published in *Laboratory Investigation,* and is devoted to exploring this interface of biology and disease. Techniques and experimental models, once considered esoteric or exotic, are now in the forefront of research directed toward a fuller understanding of human disease. The presentations of the various authors in this volume are not only expositions of scientific data, but also represent contributions to the continuing trend toward unifying all of science.

Emanuel Rubin
Ivan Damjanov

Contents

Section III: **TUMOR BIOLOGY**

Section I

CELL AND METABOLIC DISORDERS

Biology of Disease

Regulation of Liver Growth: Protooncogenes and Transforming Growth Factors

NELSON FAUSTO AND JANET E. MEAD

Department of Pathology and Laboratory Medicine, Division of Biology and Medicine, Brown University, Providence, RI

Liver Regeneration after Partial Hepatectomy
Protooncogene Expression During Liver Regeneration
Stages of Liver Regeneration: "Competence" and "Progression"
Growth Factors and Liver Regeneration
Role of Transforming Growth Factors α and β in Liver Regeneration: Positive and Negative Regulatory
  Loops
  TGF-β: negative control of hepatocyte replication
  TGF-α: autocrine stimulation of hepatocyte growth
Priming of Hepatocytes: Induction by Nutritional Changes
Hepatocyte Replication as A Response to Cell Death
The Existence of Stem Cells in Normal Liver
Summary and Update

After the fetal and postnatal growth of the liver, hepatocytes no longer proliferate actively. In adult humans and animals, hepatocytes have long life spans, ranging from 200 to 400 days or more (in the normal adult liver about 1 hepatocyte in 10,000 to 20,000 may be replicating at any one time), but it is a common observation that they divide in response to hepatic cell death or loss of liver tissue (7). Hepatocyte proliferation occurs in viral hepatitis, cirrhosis, hepatotoxic reactions, and massive liver necrosis as well as other conditions. It can be induced in experimental animals by partial hepatectomy or cell death caused by chemical agents such as carbon tetrachloride and dioxins (73, 83). In all of these cases, hepatic growth is a compensatory response to decreased liver mass or loss of cells but it is also possible to induce DNA synthesis and replication of normal liver hepatocytes. This adaptive response occurs in some types of nutritional changes and may be caused by agents such as hexachlorobenzene and organochlorine insecticides that cause minimal hepatocyte necrosis (8, 68, 72).

Hepatocyte growth responses are of particular interest because they take place *in vivo*, involve cells which are normally quiescent and, at least in the cases that have been well investigated, constitute highly regulated processes. The range of information which can be gathered in studies of liver growth is rather broad, but three important goals for these studies may be singled out: (a) the identification of external or intrahepatic signals which may trigger the growth response and make it stop at a fairly predictable point (b) the identification of

markers which correspond to the key events involved in the entry of hepatocytes into the cell cycle and progression to DNA synthesis and (c) the identification of the relationships between positive or negative growth signals and the major events of the replicative response (or, in other words, determining the connections between (a) and (b), above). Most of the information about the regulation of liver growth derives from studies of liver regeneration after partial hepatectomy in rats. Although the conclusions obtained from work with this system should be applicable to other hepatic non-neoplastic growth processes, liver regeneration after partial hepatectomy differs in some important ways from hepatic growth which follows cell injury. Moreover, since liver regeneration is often compared with liver carcinogenesis, it is well to keep in mind that during carcinogenesis there are drastic changes in the cellular composition of the liver which do not occur in the regenerating liver.

In this article, which is not comprehensive, we summarize recent research on the mechanisms of liver regeneration with emphasis on the expression of protooncogenes and growth factor effects. Using these data, we have attempted to construct a reasonably coherent picture of the regenerative process and formulate hypotheses to guide future work. We also briefly discuss the similarities and differences between liver regeneration after partial hepatectomy and hepatic growth occurring under other conditions and explore the important question of the existence of facultative stem cells in the normal liver.

LIVER REGENERATION AFTER PARTIAL HEPATECTOMY

The major features of liver regeneration after partial hepatectomy in rats are well known and have been the subject of detailed studies since Higgins and Anderson (34) described in 1931, a technique for the partial resection of rat liver (approximately 70% of the liver is removed in the standard procedure): (a) a minimum of 10 to 20% of the liver mass must be resected to trigger the growth response; (b) beyond this threshold, there is a reasonable proportionality between the extent of hepatocyte DNA synthesis and the amount of tissue removed (up to about a 75% deficit); (c) because the resection involves the removal of entire, intact hepatic lobes, no wound or exposed surface is created in the remaining tissue and none of the typical phenomena associated with wound healing (inflammatory exudate, granulation tissue, etc.) occur; (d) the growth response consists of the increase in size of the remaining hepatic lobes through cell hypertrophy and hyperplasia, but the lobes that have been removed do not grow back; (e) after 70% hepatectomy in young animals almost all hepatocytes replicate once and a fraction of the cells undergoes a second round of replication; (f) hepatocyte DNA synthesis is reasonably well synchronized and does not start until about 12 hours after the operation, reaching a peak at 24 hours; (g) nonparenchymal cells also replicate after partial hepatectomy but lag behind hepatocyte DNA synthesis by 1 to 3 days; (h) the regenerating liver doubles in weight by 48 to 72 hours after the operation and growth ceases in about 7 to 10 days when the liver mass reaches the original value of the intact liver ($\pm$ 10%) (7, 26, 33).

The synchronization of the response and its predictable end point make it clear that liver regeneration after partial hepatectomy is a strictly regulated nonautonomous growth process that must be controlled by the same factors that are responsible for the determination and maintenance of hepatic mass in the intact organism. Disruption of these regulatory mechanisms generates signals which cause hepatocytes to enter the cell cycle, progress to DNA synthesis and replicate, but only enough to restore organ mass. Since liver regeneration involves the whole liver tissue rather than hepatocytes alone, both parenchymal and nonparenchymal cells participate in the growth response. During this process, liver cells may respond to intra- or extrahepatic signals (paracrine and endocrine mechanisms) and may also be capable of synthesizing factors which promote their own growth (autocrine mechanisms).

PROTOONCOGENE EXPRESSION DURING LIVER REGENERATION

Shortly after it became known that viral oncogenes originate from counterparts present in the normal mammalian genome, we decided to investigate the expression of various cellular protooncogenes during liver regeneration. The intent of these studies was not only to learn whether or not these genes might be associated with *in vivo*, non-neoplastic growth processes, but also to determine whether the pattern of expression of protooncogenes might provide clues as to the regulatory mechanisms of liver regeneration. Our studies (30, 31, 78) showed that protooncogene expression during liver regeneration has three main characteristics: (a) it is specific, in that certain protooncogenes but not others are involved (transcripts of *fos*, *myc*, p53 and *ras* genes are elevated while *abl*, *mos*, *src* are not involved); (b) it is sequential, in that mRNAs from specific protooncogenes increase at well defined periods after partial hepatectomy, following the general order *fos*, *myc*, p53, *ras*; (c) it is transient in that increased transcripts for these various genes are found only during a period of a few hours (*fos*, *myc* and p53) or longer (about 30 hours for *ras*) during liver regeneration after which they return to their normal, basal level (Fig. 1).

Other studies have demonstrated a very rapid increase in *myc* transcripts in rat liver after partial hepatectomy or after cycloheximide injections (49), the expression of endogenous retrovirus-like sequences in regenerating rat liver at the time of DNA synthesis (37) and the increased expression of the *ets* gene in regenerating mouse liver (4). The pattern of protooncogene expression found during liver regeneration does not occur in renal compensatory growth (3), a process which involves mostly cellular hypertrophy rather than hyperplasia.

Protooncogene expression in hepatocytes in culture induced to undergo DNA synthesis by EGF, is similar to that observed during liver regeneration (42 and J. E. Mead and N. Fausto, unpublished observations). However, in culture, the length of the "windows" during which each protooncogene is expressed is longer than after partial hepatectomy (perhaps with the exception of *fos*), probably as a consequence of the better synchrony of DNA replication *in vivo* (J. E. Mead and N. Fausto, unpublished observations).

STAGES OF LIVER REGENERATION: "COMPETENCE" AND "PROGRESSION"

The highly regulated pattern of expression of protooncogenes in the regenerating liver is an indication that liver cells induced to replicate after partial hepatectomy progress to DNA synthesis in a stepwise fashion. Each step might represent the cell's response to a stimulus which makes its appearance at a particular point of the sequence. Alternatively the cell may synthesize receptors which make it capable to respond to an already existing stimulus. For more than 50 years investigators have been searching for a still elusive liver mitogenic factor(s), presumably of extrahepatic origin, capable of inducing hepatocyte DNA synthesis. Despite the progress which has occurred in the isolation and identification of such factors (25, 45, 55, 77), it seems unlikely that a single factor could be responsible for the whole sequence of events leading to hepatocyte replication. Thus, growth factors which by themselves may not induce DNA synthesis, might however be essential for the sequence of events which leads to DNA synthesis and might act only at specified points in the transit of hepatocytes from G0 to S (46). Based on these considerations, we formulated two hypotheses: (a) that the replicative response after

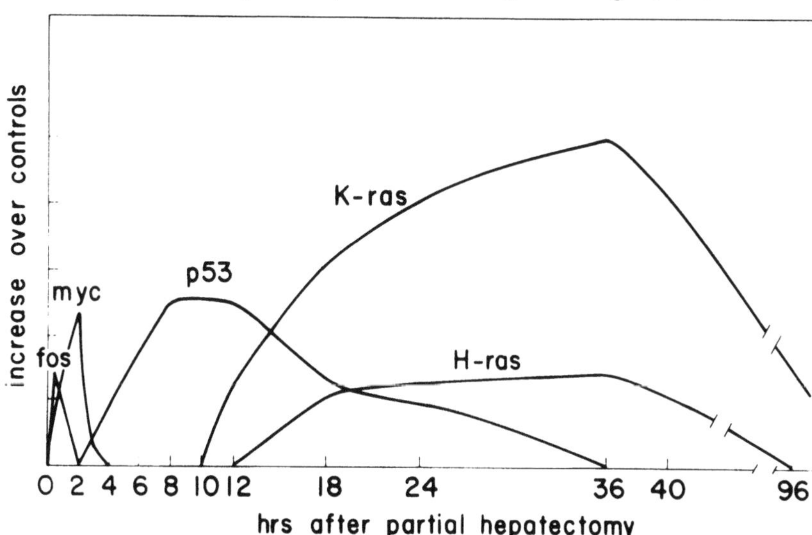

Fig. 1. Protooncogene expression during liver regeneration after partial hepatectomy in rats. The expression of 5 protooncogenes was measured by hybridization of liver polyadenylated RNA obtained at various times after partial hepatectomy (*abscissa*) with the ³²P-labeled cDNA probe specific for each gene. The amount of hybridization was determined by densitometry of the appropriate bands in Northern blots. The approximate sizes of the transcripts are: c-*fos*, 2.2 kb; c-*myc*, 2.2 kb; p53, 1.8 kb, c-Ha-*ras*, 1.2 kb, and c-ki-*ras*, 5.0 and 2.1 kb. Control levels (*ordinate*) represent the amount of each mRNA in the liver of sham-operated rats. A second peak of c-*fos* and c-*myc* expression which often occurs at 8 hours, has been omitted from the figure (21, 30, 31, 78).

partial hepatectomy can be divided into two phases, and (b) that the growth of the regenerating liver is controlled by its own cells, through the activation of intrahepatic autocrine and paracrine circuits that induce or terminate hepatocyte replication (21, 22).

We adopted the terms "competence" (or "priming") and "progression" used to identify stages of the cell cycle of fibroblasts in culture (61), to designate the two stages of the pre-replicative period of liver regeneration. "Competence," lasting for about 4 hours and characterized by an increase in *fos* and *myc* transcripts, may correspond to the passage of hepatocytes from G0 to G1, that is, their entry into the cell cycle. "Progression" (starting 4 hours after partial hepatectomy and lasting until about 14 to 16 hours) may involve the transit of hepatocytes from G1 to S, and is characterized mainly by an increase in p53 expression. The start of hepatocyte DNA synthesis and the major wave of cell division are associated with changes in the expression of *ras* genes.

The use of the terms "competence" and "progression" does not imply that similar growth factors are involved in the replication of hepatocytes *in vivo* and fibroblasts in culture and does not make less arbitrary the assignment of stages in a process which is probably a continuum (2). Nevertheless, if stages with their own markers exist in hepatocyte replication after partial hepatectomy, two predictions should follow: (a) it should be possible to identify and isolate hepatocytes which have been "primed" ("competent") to undergo DNA synthesis, and might differ from normal "unprimed" hepatocytes in their responses to growth factors; (b) it should be possible to identify autocrine or paracrine regulatory loops, that provide positive or negative signals which govern the progression of hepatocytes into DNA synthesis and replication.

GROWTH FACTORS AND LIVER REGENERATION

The serum of partially hepatectomized rats contains substances which are capable of stimulating hepatocyte DNA synthesis (25, 45, 55, 77). However, even though the existence of such factors seems well established, their site of origin (hepatic or extrahepatic) and identity remain largely unknown since they have not been purified to homogeneity and sequenced. Furthermore, the detection of growth factors in the serum of partially hepatectomized rats does not necessarily imply that such factors are responsible for triggering liver regeneration in the first place. It is conceivable that growth factors found in the serum of partially hepatectomized rats are produced and released by the regenerating liver, as a consequence of some initial event which induced hepatocytes to enter the cell cycle. In addition to undefined "serum factors," there are some known substances which are thought to play a role in hepatocyte DNA synthesis. They include norepinephrine, vasopressin, epidermal growth factor (EGF), insulin, and glucagon (reviewed in reference 52). Thyroid, parathyroid, and growth hormone levels can also influence the timing of DNA synthesis during liver regeneration (reviewed in reference 47). EGF (in conjunction with insulin) is the standard factor commonly used to induce DNA synthesis in primary hepatocyte cultures and can increase hepatic DNA synthesis when injected into normal rats (9, 51). This factor is not synthesized in rat liver but is efficiently taken up from the serum where it is present at relatively high concentration (15, 74). In the regenerating rat liver, the number of EGF receptors in hepatocytes decreases starting at about 12 hours after the operation (17), but it is not known if EGF is a physiologic ligand for the receptor.

Our own efforts have centered on the identification of growth factors involved in liver regeneration which have four characteristics: (a) they are synthesized in the liver; (b) their synthesis increases during liver regeneration; (c) they have an effect on DNA synthesis of hepatocytes in culture; (d) they have been purified to homogeneity, sequenced, and the respective genes cloned. Among the many factors which we have investigated in detail, two of them, the transforming growth factors α and β (TGF-α and TGF-β) fulfilled the specific requirements.

ROLE OF TRANSFORMING GROWTH FACTORS α AND β IN LIVER REGENERATION: POSITIVE AND NEGATIVE REGULATORY LOOPS

The transforming growth factors α and β share a similar name, but have entirely different structures, amino acid sequences, mRNA sizes, and cellular receptors. They were originally described, before their separate identification, as a single factor produced by tumor cells, capable of inducing anchorage-independent growth in non-neoplastic cells. Subsequent studies led to the purification to homogeneity of two distinct factors, the recognition that the factors can be produced by normal cells, that they may stimulate normal cell growth without inducing transformation and that TGF-β binds to cells through a specific receptor, whereas TGF-α binds to cells via the EGF receptor. A large amount of research has now shown that while TGF-α is generally mitogenic for a variety of cells, TGF-β can stimulate or inhibit cell growth, depending on the cell type involved and the presence of other factors. In addition, TGF-β has a multiplicity of effects (such as stimulation of angiogenesis *in vivo*, promotion of wound healing, effects on connective tissue proteins, *etc.*) that go far beyond its original description as a transforming growth factor (reviewed in references 29, 64).

TGF-β: NEGATIVE CONTROL OF HEPATOCYTE REPLICATION

TGF-β mRNA increases after partial hepatectomy reaching a maximum (8 to 10 times higher than normal) approximately 2 days after the major peak of DNA synthesis (6, 21). There is very little TGF-β mRNA in normal liver, in liver of sham-operated rats and in the regenerating liver in the first 2 to 3 hours after the operation. TGF-β mRNA becomes detectable (by conventional Northern blot hybridization techniques) at about 4 hours, stays at approximately the same levels until about 18 to 20 hours after the operation and rises to a peak value at 72 hours. It is most intriguing, however, that TGF-β turned out to be a very potent inhibitor of DNA synthesis of hepatocytes in culture (6, 10, 53, 56, 66, 76). TGF-β dose-response curves vary depending on the culture medium used, but generally as little as 100 pg/ml of TGF-β is usually sufficient to inhibit EGF-induced hepatocyte DNA synthesis by 80 to 90% (6).

If indeed TGF-β is an inhibitor of hepatocyte DNA synthesis *in vivo* as it is in culture, one faces the problem of explaining an apparent paradox, that is, why would a proliferation inhibitor increase in a tissue that is undergoing growth. Since we have postulated that autocrine or paracrine regulatory loops may control certain phases of growth in the regenerating liver, we wanted to know what cells in the liver contain TGF-β mRNA. The results showed, much to our surprise, that although hepatocytes have TGF-β receptors and respond to the factor, they do not synthesize it (at least as judged by the presence of TGF-β mRNA). The mRNA was instead found in nonparenchymal cells, primarily in liver nonparenchymal cell fractions enriched in endothelial cells (6).

It is possible that the increase in TGF-β mRNA and its synthesis in hepatic nonparenchymal cells have little to do with hepatocyte proliferation during liver regeneration. However, given the presence of TGF-β receptors in hepatocytes, the sensitivity of these cells to TGF-β in culture, the proximity of endothelial cells to hepatocytes, and the finding that TGF-β injections block hepatocyte DNA synthesis in regenerating rat liver *in vivo* (66a) it is plausible to assume that TGF-β has a role in controlling hepatocyte replication during liver regeneration. We have proposed that TGF-β is the effector of a paracrine regulatory circuit which is activated in the liver after partial hepatectomy and functions to prevent uncontrolled cell proliferation (Fig. 2). TGF-β would thus be part of the signaling mechanism which makes liver regeneration terminate at a predictable point (6, 21).

It might be a general characteristic of regulated growth processes that their triggering brings into play not only growth activators but also growth inhibitors which balance the positive stimuli. An interesting example is the drastic increase in TGF-β and its mRNA in lymphocytes stimulated to proliferate. It has been proposed that the increase in TGF-β, a potent inhibitor of lymphocyte DNA synthesis may prevent uncontrolled clonal expansion (41). In the case of the liver, it is logical to ask whether TGF-β keeps hepatocytes from replicating in normal adult livers and whether or not hepatocytes lose their sensitivity to the inhibitory effects of TGF-β during regeneration. It is unlikely that TGF-β maintains hepatocyte quiescence in normal livers, for at least two reasons: (a) there is very little TGF-β mRNA detectable in normal liver (although TGF-β is taken up from blood and rapidly metabolized in the liver, see reference 14); (b) normal hepatocytes do not undergo DNA synthesis

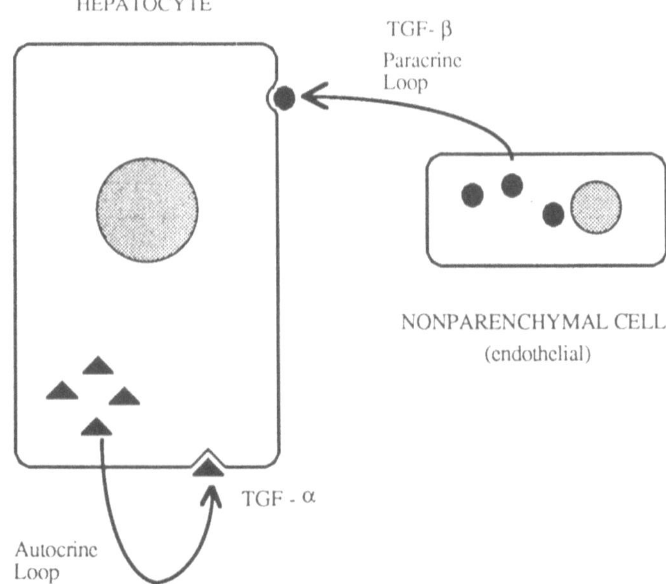

FIG. 2. Potential growth regulatory circuits during liver regeneration TGF-β may function as a negative effector in paracrine circuit involving hepatocytes and nonparenchymal (sinusoidal-lining) cells. TGF-α probably functions as a positive effector through an autocrine circuit which uses hepatocyte EGF receptors.

spontaneously in culture in the absence of TGF-β but require, instead, inducers such as EGF and insulin. As far as changes in the sensitivity of hepatocytes to TGF-β after partial hepatectomy, our own work indicates that, in culture, TGF-β inhibits DNA synthesis equally in hepatocytes from normal or regenerating liver (6). However, although there is general agreement that this is the case for hepatocytes obtained from regenerating livers 12 to 24 hours after partial hepatectomy, (76), there have been reports that hepatocytes from 3-hour regenerating livers (but not at other times) lose the capacity to bind TGF-β when maintained in culture for 3 to 4 days (12).

The observation that TGF-β inhibits EGF-induced DNA synthesis in hepatocytes in culture does not signify that TGF-β acts directly on a specific step in the sequence of events involved in DNA replication. Instead, it is conceivable that DNA synthesis inhibition is a consequence of TGF-β effects on other cellular functions. Since TGF-β increases the attachment of cells to extracellular matrices and enhances the synthesis of matrix components (38), one may envisage a scenario where TGF-β, secreted by nonparenchymal cells after the peak of hepatocyte DNA synthesis, acts to restore hepatocyte cell/cell or cell/matrix contacts which then leads to the eventual cessation of cell proliferation.

TGF-α: AUTOCRINE STIMULATION OF HEPATOCYTE GROWTH

In contrast to TGF-β, no inhibitory effect has been found for TGF-α in any tissue. Its effects involve stimulation of cell growth or transformation (29, 64). We measured the amount of TGF-α mRNA in the regenerating liver and found that it increases with a time course very similar to that of DNA synthesis. No TGF-α mRNA was detectable until approximately 12 hours after the operation; the maximum amount is found at 24 hours, coinciding with the peak of DNA synthesis (54a). TGF-α mRNA is present in hepatocytes and stimulates DNA synthesis of hepatocytes in culture (54a). An important consideration in gauging the physiologic importance of TGF-α during liver regeneration is that TGF-α binds to cells via the EGF receptor (although experiments to demonstrate this point in hepatocytes have not been done) (29, 64). Since the number of hepatocyte EGF receptors decreases in regenerating liver (17) but there are only small if any changes in serum EGF concentrations (15) and no synthesis of EGF in the liver, it is conceivable that the alteration in EGF receptor number might relate to the induction of TGF-α, another ligand which utilizes the EGF receptors (54a). If this view proves to be correct, one can postulate that TGF-α functions as an autocrine growth stimulator of hepatocytes during liver regeneration (Fig. 2).

In summary, mRNAs for the TGF-α and TGF-β increase during liver regeneration. The timing of TGF-α mRNA changes coincides with the major wave of DNA synthesis in the regenerating liver, whereas TGF-β mRNA reaches a maximum about 2 days later after the major wave of hepatocyte replication has passed. TGF-α may be the effector of an autocrine growth stimulatory mechanism for hepatocytes, whereas TGF-β, acting through a paracrine loop, might provide a stop signal to restrain hepatocyte replication (Fig. 2).

"PRIMING" OF HEPATOCYTES: INDUCTION BY NUTRITIONAL CHANGES

The regulatory circuits described above are unlikely to be involved in the events which determine the entry of hepatocytes into the cell cycle but are instead, mechanisms which operate in cells which are farther along the replicative sequence. Identification of the triggering events and the mediators which may put in motion the regenerative response are, obviously, of crucial importance. The changes in expression of the *fos* and *myc* protooncogenes after partial hepatectomy can be used as markers for the timing of early events and as indicators for the entry of hepatocytes into the cell cycle (G0→G1 transition). An examination of the expression of these two genes in the regenerating liver suggest that signals of whatever nature, capable of modulating gene expression are sensed by hepatocytes almost immediately after partial hepatectomy and that the G0→G1 transition may take about 4 hours or so. Similar conclusions regarding the rapidity of the response of hepatocytes to partial hepatectomy can be reached by examining the alterations in ornithine decarboxylase activity, ionic changes, and amino acid pools during the first 2 hours after partial hepatectomy (reviewed in reference 24). Given the time frame in which of these events occur, (*fos* transcripts are increased by 15 minutes after the operation) it is a good assumption that they are triggered by factors already present in the liver or blood or, alternatively, that they are synthesized almost immediately after partial hepatectomy. Hormones such as insulin, glucagon, nonepinephrine, and vasopressin fit into this category (16, 65). On the other hand, there is a real possibility that no single mediator, but rather, a constellation of changes brought about by the functional demands imposed on the regenerating liver, act to induce the entry of hepatocytes into the cell cycle. The remarkable functional adaptations of the regenerating liver are best illustrated by the lack of alteration in blood urea or ammonia after partial hepatectomy in rats, a demonstration that the liver remnant, with only a third of the original mass, efficiently and almost immediately, performs the metabolic tasks of the intact organ.

What type of functional deficits or adaptations may initiate events which could lead to DNA synthesis in quiescent hepatocytes of adult rat liver? An interesting way of studying this problem is to attempt to devise methods to induce DNA synthesis and hepatocyte replication in livers of intact animals. Using procedures which do not cause cell death, a functional deficit may be imposed on the liver in the absence of a decrease in tissue mass. One can then investigate if the imposed functional deficiency has an effect on hepatocyte DNA synthesis and mitosis.

An experimental model which has received considerable attention is the induction of hepatic DNA synthesis in rats given amino acid loads (8, 72). What is most remarkable in this model is that induction of liver DNA synthesis by amino acids occurs only in animals maintained for 2 to 3 days on a protein-free dietary regimen before receiving the amino acid load. Hepatocytes of normally fed or starved rats show no response to the amino acid solution (8). This experimental model can thus be divided into two stages: (a) a priming stage (the 2 to 3 day protein-free period) during which hepatocytes become capable of responding to growth stimuli but do not undergo DNA replication; (b) a second phase during which cells, primed in the protein-free period, respond to amino acid administration with a wave of DNA synthesis and mitosis.

If during the priming phase hepatocytes enter the cell cycle but do not fully progress to the S phase, "primed" hepatocytes should have patterns of gene expression similar to those of hepatocytes from regenerating livers before DNA replication. This is in fact the case for some protooncogenes; "primed" hepatocytes have high levels of *myc* and p53 mRNA's (21, 36 and J. E. Mead and N. Fausto, unpublished observations). Furthermore, such cells when placed in culture, respond much faster to EGF induction of DNA synthesis than cells from normal rats. It would also be expected that when "primed" hepatocytes are stimulated to undergo DNA synthesis, the peak of DNA synthesis would be reached in less than 24 hours (the time interval required for maximal DNA synthesis after partial hepatectomy). Indeed, when rats kept on protein-free regimens are given amino acids, the period of time between stimulus and the peak of DNA synthesis is 7 to 9 hours shorter than the corresponding length of time after partial hepatectomy (8 and J. E. Mead and N. Fausto, unpublished observations).

The work with this experimental model shows that: (a) functional alterations in hepatocytes caused by nutritional changes induce a "priming" stage in hepatocytes making them "competent" to undergo DNA synthesis; (b) "primed" hepatocytes are to some extent similar to hepatocytes of the regenerating liver; (c) "primed" hepatocytes do not enter DNA synthesis in the absence of further stimuli; (d) "primed" hepatocytes undergo DNA synthesis in response to stimuli which are ineffective for normal hepatocytes. However, we do not know by what mechanisms "primed" hepatocytes progress to DNA synthesis.

After partial hepatectomy, the complete chain of events from triggering to cell replication, automatically unfolds, but nutritional manipulation induces only the initial part of the sequence. In the nutritional model, DNA synthesis can be brought about by correcting (by the administration of amino acids) the functional alteration. Could a similar mechanism also operate during liver regeneration? We cannot answer this question because we are still ignorant about the nature of functional deficits (if any!) brought about by partial hepatectomy. Perhaps the replicative sequence after partial hepatectomy is triggered not as a consequence of a deficiency but, on the contrary, is caused by metabolic adaptations put in motion to prevent functional deficits. This is essentially a restatement of the "work load" theory of liver growth in more fashionable terms, with the suggestion that increased work load induces hepatocyte competence but not DNA synthesis.

HEPATOCYTE REPLICATION AS A RESPONSE TO CELL DEATH

Partial resection of the liver in humans elicits a surprisingly rapid regenerative response (40) which is likely to be regulated by mechanisms similar to those studied in the regenerating rat liver after partial hepatectomy. However, hepatocyte replication in the human liver occurs much more frequently as a response to hepatic injury caused by chemicals, viruses or anoxia. None of these conditions can be exactly reproduced in experimental models but a large number of chemicals, both necrogenic and non-necrogenic, cause hepatic injury and induce liver growth in laboratory animals. Most commonly used are necrogenic agents such as CCl_4 and galactosamine, but cell death is not a precondition for the growth response. For instance, many of the non-necrogenic agents that induce hepatic drug-metabolizing enzymes can cause liver hypertrophy and/or hyperplasia (68, 83).

Apparently, there is an intimate connection between liver growth and the hepatic response to cytotoxic drugs. One of the most interesting developments in this area is the finding that the expression of the multidrug-resistant gene (*mdr*) and of heat-shock genes increase after partial hepatectomy (11, 20, 79). As a result, cells of the regenerating liver exhibit a "multidrug-resistance" phenotype and are protected from the cytotoxic effect of many drugs. This phenotype has generally been considered to be associated with "initiated" hepatocytes during carcinogenesis but proliferating normal hepatocytes may exhibit a similar trait (13, 20, 79). Although the biologic significance of these findings is not yet fully understood, they indicate that non-neoplastic liver growth and resistance to cytotoxicity are closely linked processes.

The major difference between liver growth after surgical resection and chemical injury is that, after partial hepatectomy, liver regeneration starts in intact lobules and DNA synthesis occurs throughout the liver (although, initially, DNA synthesis is found mainly in hepatocytes adjacent to periportal areas, reference 62). In contrast, after chemical injury leading to cell death, regeneration takes place in damaged tissue. For reasons that are not entirely understood, the levels of serum alphafetoprotein (AFP) and of hepatic AFP mRNA are quite different in the two types of liver growth. Serum AFP (in human or experimental animals) and liver AFP mRNA (in rats or mice) increase little or not at all after partial hepatectomy. However, more substantial changes are detected in liver growth after carbon tetrachloride injury (in rats or mice) and in patients with acute or chronic hepatitis or massive liver necrosis, although, even in these cases, AFP levels are low in comparison to those found during liver development (1, 58–60,75, 82). One possible explanation for these findings is that in many types of liver injury, AFP may be found in proliferating liver epithelial cells (43) which are generally not seen in the regenerating liver after partial hepatectomy (see below).

Although regeneration induced by partial hepatectomy and cell injury may have different triggering events, it is conceivable that hepatocytes which have entered the cell cycle, progress to DNA synthesis through the same path in both processes. Indeed, the sequence of protooncogene expression after CCl₄ injury in rats (although not studied in great detail) is similar to that after partial hepatectomy. In both kinds of growth, increased expression of the *ras* genes coincides with the major wave of hepatocyte DNA synthesis, but the timing of these events differs (30, 31).

What mechanisms may initiate the growth response after hepatic cell death? In the absence of specific data, We can only speculate about this issue. As hepatocyte death and replication after chemical injury are mostly localized processes, confined to specific regions of the lobule and not occurring in all lobules (if we exclude massive hepatic necrosis), it is unlikely that hormones or functional deficits that have generalized effects throughout the liver might serve as major triggering agents. Instead, localized changes taking place in the areas of injury ought to be considered as potential stimuli. These changes may include alterations in cell/cell contact and cell/matrix interactions. It has been clearly demonstrated that the composition of the extracellular matrix can modulate hepatocyte gene expression in culture (63) and it would not be surprising if *in vivo*, the expression of some protooncogenes were modulated by similar influences. Acute CCl₄ injury is associated with changes in the composition of the liver matrix (deposition of fibronectin and collagen types I and IV) as well as with a partial uncoupling of hepatocytes as a consequence of the closure of gap junctions (50, 67). Loss of contact between hepatocytes and decreases in gap junction and hepatocyte cell adhesion proteins also occur after partial hepatectomy and may be important events associated with or necessary for hepatocyte replication (54, 57, 80).

THE EXISTENCE OF STEM CELLS IN NORMAL LIVER

No special replicative compartment is identifiable in the regenerating liver. Instead, the growth response involves (in young animals) the vast majority of hepatocytes. Why then be concerned about the existence of "stem cells" in the liver? The reasons are multiple and, indeed, research in this area has advanced considerably during the last few years (reviewed in references 23, 32, 48, 69): (a) after administration of some hepatotoxic agents (particularly galactosamine but also after carbon tetrachloride) liver epithelial cells containing AFP and with biochemical features of immature hepatocytes may proliferate (18, 43, 59, 60); (b) during the early stages of carcinogenesis induced by many chemical agents, epithelial cells containing AFP and other biochemical markers of immature hepatocytes proliferate actively and may constitute as many as 50% of the hepatic cells (23, 44); (c) even in the commonly used carcinogenic regimens involving 2-acetylaminofluorene in conjunction with partial hepatectomy or carbon tetrachloride injury there is a massive proliferation of liver epithelial cells (19, 28), and it has been shown by label transfer experiments that there is a precursor product relationship between the epithelial cells and hepatocytes (19); (d) liver epithelial cells transfected with an activated protooncogene or transformed *in vitro* by chemical carcinogens can pro-

duce hepatocellular carcinomas when inoculated into appropriate hosts (5, 81); (e) in embryonic mouse liver, hepatocytes and cells of intrahepatic bile ducts seem to derive from a common AFP-containing precursor cell type (71).

A large body of experimental work has thus established that epithelial cells with "stem cell" properties proliferate in many different conditions in the liver of humans and experimental animals. It is then logical to ask where these cells (or their precursors) are located in the normal liver and why they do not seem to proliferate actively in the regenerating liver after partial hepatectomy. It is important to first establish the point that the epithelial cells which proliferate in these various conditions constitute heterogeneous populations (23, 27, 35). What has been called "oval cell proliferation" during hepatocarcinogenesis is in reality the multiplication of many different cell types which include mature ductal cells, cells in transitional stages of development, less differentiated cells which function as "stem cells" as well as other, uncharacterized, cell types (23).

Why presumed stem cells do not seem to proliferate actively in the regenerating liver after partial hepatectomy and replenish the liver is not so puzzling if one accepts the proposition, well supported by experimental data, that these cells function as "facultative stem cells" and only proliferate when hepatocyte replication is inhibited (32, 39). When hepatocytes can replicate actively, as is the case after partial hepatectomy, there should been no need to activate a reserve cellular compartment. More difficult to establish is the localization of facultative stem cells in normal liver. Work using sensitive nucleic acid hybridization techniques has revealed that some nonparenchymal cells in normal adult rat liver contain the 2.3 kb AFP mRNA, but the cells that have this mRNA have not yet been identified (60 and J. Lemire and N. Fausto, unpublished observations). There are indications that "stem cells" might either be components of the ducts of Hering or are adjacent to them in portal spaces (70). However, despite the anatomical relationships with the biliary system, the presumed "stem cells," which are abundant at the early stages of carcinogenesis, do not seem to proliferate after bile duct ligation in rats.

In summary, even if after partial hepatectomy, hepatocytes replicate and replenish the tissue, livers of adult human and animals may contain cells which can function as facultative stem cells. Such cells proliferate and may differentiate into hepatocytes at the early stages or carcinogenesis induced by many chemicals. Similar cells are also seen in variable amounts after liver injury caused by some chemicals, but their role in these processes has not been investigated in detail. Although the facultative stem cells become conspicuous during carcinogenesis and some types of liver injury unrelated to neoplasia, they originate from cells which exist in normal liver. The identity of such cells is the subject of intense study at the moment.

SUMMARY AND UPDATE

Studies reviewed in this article show that protooncogenes are expressed in a sequential and regulated manner during liver regeneration. The expression of some of these genes can be used as markers for the entry of hepatocytes into the cell cycle and subsequent progression into DNA synthesis. While it is possible to mimic the early stages of the process ("priming") by manipulation of nutritional conditions in normal nonhepatectomized rats, the second stage ("progression") seems to be largely controlled within the liver through the activation of positive and negative regulatory loops involving the transforming growth factors α and β, respectively. As the details about specific hepatic autocrine and paracrine regulatory circuits are elucidated, it becomes evident that initiation and cessation of growth in the liver depend on interactions between the various components of hepatic tissue (hepatocytes, nonparenchymal cells, matrix) as well as on the metabolic adaptations of the liver in the whole animal.

Work conducted during the past year has shown that TGF-α may be a physiologic regulator of liver regeneration (54a). This growth factor is synthesized by hepatocytes and appears to act as an inducer of DNA synthesis after partial hepatectomy. Its stimulatory effects are balanced by the inhibitory action of TGF-β1(54a). A plausible hypothesis to explain liver growth after partial hepatectomy is that: (a) priming of hepatocytes is initiated by metabolic overload and/or by the action of any one of a number of substances (such as norepinephrine, vasopressin, angiotensin or gastrin) whose receptors are coupled to GTP-binding proteins; (b) the priming stage is associated with increased abundance of *fos* and *myc* transcripts; (c) the priming phase is followed by a progression step that includes the activation of an autocrine circuit involving TGF-α as a positive effector; (d) an inhibitory circuit in which TGF-β acts to prevent unrestrained cell proliferation. Most aspects of this hypothesis can now be tested experimentally.

Studies of drug-induced liver regeneration indicate that different triggering mechanisms of liver growth exist, but that the "progression" stages might be common, regardless of the initiating agent. Finally, despite the lack of participation of a "stem cell compartment" during liver regeneration, there is compelling evidence that the liver contains cells that function as "facultative stem cells" and proliferate after certain types of injury and in hepatocarcinogenesis.

Acknowledgments: We thank Joan Lemire for reading and discussing the manuscript, Drs. William E. Russell and A.J. Strain for sharing their data before publication and Jeanne Burke and Anna-Louise Baxter for their help in preparing the manuscript.

This work was supported by Grants CA23226 and CA35249 from the National Cancer Institute.

REFERENCES

1. Alpert E, Feller E: α-fetoprotein (AFP) in benign liver disease. Gastroenterology 74:856, 1978
2. Baserga R: The Biology of Cell Reproduction p 134. Cambridge, Harvard University Press, 1985
3. Beer DG, Zweifel KA, Simpson DP, Pitot HC: Specific gene expression during compensatory renal hypertrophy in the rat. J Cell Physiol 131:29, 1987
4. Bhat NK, Fisher RJ, Fujiwara S, Ascione R, Papas TS: Temporal and tissue-specific expression of mouse *ets* genes. Proc Natl Acad Sci USA 84:3161, 1987
5. Braun L, Goyette M, Yaswen P, Thompson NL, Fausto N: Growth in culture and tumorigenicity after transfection with the *ras* oncogene of liver epithelial cells from carcinogen-treated rats. Cancer Res 47:4116, 1987
6. Braun L, Mead JE, Panzica M, Mikumo R, Bell GI, Fausto N: Transforming growth factor β mRNA increases during liver regeneration: a possible paracrine mechanism of growth regulation. Proc Natl Acad Sci USA 85:1539, 1988
7. Bucher NLR, Malt RA: Regeneration of Liver and Kidney, pp 17-176. Boston, Little Brown Co., 1971
8. Bucher NLR, McGowan JA, Patel U: Hormonal regulation of liver growth. In Cell Reproduction, ICN/UCLA Symp on Molec Cell Biol, vol 12, edited by Dirksen ER, Prescott DM, Fox CF, pp 661-670. New York, Academic Press, 1978
9. Bucher NLR, Patel V, Cohen S: Hormonal factors concerned with liver regeneration. In Hepatotrophic Factors, Ciba Foundation Symposium 55 (new series), pp 95-107. Amsterdam, Elsevier, 1978
10. Carr BI, Hayashi I, Branum EL, Moses HL: Inhibition of DNA synthesis in rat hepatocytes by platelet-derived type β transforming growth factor. Cancer Res 46:2330, 1986
11. Carr BI, Huang TH, Buzin CH, Itakura K: Induction of heat shock gene expression without heat shock by hepatocarcinogens and during hepatic regeneration in rat liver. Cancer Res 46:5106, 1986
12. Carr BI, Thall A, Whitson RH, Itakura K: Transforming growth factor type β (TGF β) receptors decrease early in hepatic regeneration. Cell Biol 103:443a, 1986
13. Carr BI: Pleotropic drug resistance in hepatocytes induced by carcinogens administered to rats. Cancer Res 47:5577, 1987
14. Coffey RJ, Kost LJ, Lyons RM, Moses HL, La Russo NF: Hepatic processing of transforming growth factor β in the rat: uptake, metabolism and biliary expression. J Clin Invest 80:750, 1987
15. Cornell RP: Gut-derived endotoxin elicits hepatotrophic factor secretion for liver regeneration. Am J Physiol 249:551R, 1985
16. Cruise JL, Houck K, Michalopoulos GK: Induction of DNA synthesis in cultured rat hepatocytes through stimulation of α_1 adrenoreceptor by norepinephrine. Science 277:749, 1985
17. Earp HS, O'Keefe EJO: Epidermal growth factor receptor number decreases during rat liver regeneration. J Clin Invest 67:1580, 1981
18. Engelhardt NV, Baranov VN, Lazareva MN, Goussev AI: Ultrastructural localization of alpha-fetoprotein (AFP) in regenerating mouse liver poisoned with CCl₄. Histochemistry 80:401, 1984
19. Evarts RP, Nagy P, Marsden E, Thorgeirsson SS: A precursor-product relationship exists between oval cells and hepatocytes in rat liver. Carcinogenesis 8:1737, 1987
20. Fairchild CR, Ivy SP, Rushmore T, Lee G, Koo P, Goldsmith ME, Myers CE, Farber E, Cowan KH: Carcinogen-induced *mdr* overexpression is associated with xenobiotic resistance in rat preneoplastic liver nodules and hepatocellular carcinomas. Proc Natl Acad Sci USA 84:7701, 1987
21. Fausto N, Mead JE, Braun L, Thompson NL, Panzica M, Goyette M, Bell GI, Shank PR: Proto-oncogene expression and growth factors during liver regeneration. Symp. Fundament. Cancer Res 39:69, 1987
22. Fausto N, Shank PR: Analysis of proto-oncogene expression during liver regeneration and hepatocarcinogenesis. In Neoplasms of the Liver, edited by Okuda K, Ishak KG, pp 57-70. Tokyo, Springer-Verlag, 1987
23. Fausto N, Thompson NL, Braun L: Purification and culture of oval cells from rat liver. In Cell Separation: Methods and Selected Applications, vol 4, edited by Pretlow TGII, Pretlow TP, pp 45-77. Orlando, Academic Press, 1987
24. Fausto N: Liver regeneration. In Hepatology: A Textbook of Liver Disease, Ed. 2, edited by Zakim D, Boyer TD. Philadelphia, WB Saunders Co., in press
25. Francavilla A, Ove P, Polimeno L, Coetzee M, Makowa L, Rose J, Van Thiel DH, Starzl TE: Extraction and partial purification of a hepatic stimulatory substance in rats, mice and dogs. Cancer Res 47:5600, 1987
26. Gerhard H: A quantitative model of cellular regeneration in rat liver after partial hepatectomy. In Liver Regeneration After Experimental Injury, edited by Lesch R, Reutter W, pp 340-346. New York, Stratton International Medical Book Corporation, 1975
27. Germain L, Goyette R, Marceau N: Differential cytokeratin and α-fetoprotein expression in morphologically distinct epithelial cells emerging at the early stage of rat hepatocarcinogenesis. Cancer

Res 45:673, 1985

28. Ghoshal AK, Mullen B, Medline A, Farber E: Sequential analysis of hepatic carcinogenesis. Regeneration of liver after carbon tetrachloride-induced liver necrosis when hepatocyte proliferation is inhibited by 2-acetylaminofluorene. Lab Invest 48:224, 1983

29. Goustin AS, Leof EB, Shipley GD, Moses HL: Growth factors and cancer. Cancer Res 46:1015, 1986

30. Goyette M, Petropoulos CJ, Shank PR, Fausto N: Expression of a cellular oncogene during liver regeneration. Science 219:510, 1983

31. Goyette M, Petropoulos CJ, Shank PR, Fausto N: Regulated transcription of c-ki-*ras* and c-*myc* during compensatory growth of rat liver. Mol Cell Biol 4:1493, 1984

32. Grisham JW: Cell types in long-term propagable cultures of rat liver. Ann NY Acad Sci 349:128, 1980

33. Grisham JW: Morphologic study of deoxyribonucleic acid synthesis and cell proliferation in regenerating rat liver: autoradiography with thymidine H³. Cancer Res 22:842, 1962

34. Higgins GM, Anderson RM: Experimental pathology of the liver I: Restoration of the liver of the white rat following surgical removal. Arch Pathol 12:186, 1931

35. Hixon DC, Allison JP: Monoclonal antibodies recognizing oval cells induced in the liver of rats by N-2-fluorenylacetamide or ethionine in a choline-deficient diet. Cancer Res 45:3750, 1985

36. Horikawa S, Sakata K, Hatanaka M, Tsukada K: Expression of c-*myc* oncogene in rat liver by a dietary manipulation. Biochem Biophys Res Commun 140:574, 1986

37. Hsieh LL, Peraino C, Weinstein IB: Expression of endogenous retrovirus-like sequences and cellular oncogenes during phenobarbital treatment and regeneration in rat liver. Cancer Res 48:265, 1988

38. Ignotz RA, Massague J: Cell adhesion protein receptors as targets for transforming growth factor β action. Cell 51:189, 1987

39. Inaoka Y: Significance of the so-called oval cell proliferation during azodye hepatocarcinogenesis. Gann 58:355, 1967

40. Karran S, Eagles C: Regeneration. Park 1. Physical aspects. In Liver and Biliary Disease, edited by Wright R, Alberti KGMM, Karran S, Millward-Sadler, GH, pp 197–210. London, WB Saunders Co, 1979

41. Kehrl JH, Wakefield LM, Roberts AB, Jakowlew S, Alvarez-Mon M, Derynck R, Sporn MB, Fauci AS: Production of transforming growth factor-beta by human T lymphocytes and its potential role in the regulation of T cell growth. J Exp Med 163:1037, 1986

42. Kruijer W, Skelly H, Botteri F, van der Putten H, Barber JR, Verma IM, Leffert HL: Proto-oncogene expression in regenerating liver is simulated in cultures of primary adult hepatocytes. J Biol Chem 261:7929, 1986

43. Kuhlmann WD, Wurster K: Correlation of histology and alpha-fetoprotein resurgence in rat liver regeneration after experimental injury by galactosamine. Virchows Arch [A] 387:47, 1980

44. Kuhlmann WD: Localization of alpha-fetoprotein and DNA synthesis in liver cell populations during experimental hepatocarcinogenesis in rats. Int J Cancer 21:368, 1978

45. LaBrecque DR, Steele G, Fogerty S, Wilson M, Barton J: Purification and physical-chemical characterization of hepatic stimulator substance. Hepatology 7:100, 1987

46. Leffert HL, Koch KS, Lad PJ, Skelly H, de Hemptinne B: Hepatocyte growth factors. In Hepatology: A Text Book of Liver Disease, edited by Zakim D, Boyer TD, pp 64–75. Philadelphia, WB Saunders Co., 1982

47. Leffert HL, Koch KS, Moran T, Rubacalva B: Hormonal control of rat liver regeneration. Gastroenterology 76:1470, 1979

48. Lombardi B: On the mature, properties and significance of oval cells. In Recent Trends in Chemical Carcinogenesis, vol 1, edited by Pani P, Feo F, Columbano A, pp 36–56. Cagliari, ESA, 1982

49. Makino R, Hayashi K, Sugimura T: C-*myc* transcript is induced in rat liver at very early stage of regeneration or by cycloheximide treatment. Nature 310:697, 1984

50. Martinez-Hernández A: The hepatic extracellular matrix. II Electron immunohistochemical studies in rats with CCl₄-induced cirrhosis. Lab Invest 53:166, 1985

51. McGowan JA, Strain AJ, Bucher NLR: DNA synthesis in primary cultures of adult rat hepatocytes in a defined medium: effects of epidermal growth factor, insulin, glucagon and cyclic-AMP. J Cell Physiol 108:535, 1981

52. McGowan JA; Hepatocyte proliferation in culture. In Research in Isolated and Cultured Hepatocytes, edited by Guillouzo A, Guguen-Guillouzo C, pp 14–38, London, John Libbey Co., 1986

53. McMahon JB, Richards WL, delCampo AA, Song M-KH. Thorgeirsson SS: Differential effects of transforming growth factor-β on proliferation of normal and malignant rat liver epithelial cells in culture. Cancer Res 46:4665, 1985

54a. Mead JE, Fausto N: Transforming growth factor α (TGF-α) may be a physiological regulator of liver regeneration via an autocrine mechanism. Proc Natl Acad Sci USA, in press 1989

54. Meyer DJ, Yancey BS, Revel J-P: Intercellular communication in normal and regenerating rat liver: a quantitative analysis. J Cell Biol 91:505, 1981

55. Nakamura N, Teramoto H, Ichihara A; Purification and characterization of a growth factor from rat platelets for mature parenchymal hepatocytes in primary cultures. Proc Natl Acad Sci USA 83:6489, 1986

56. Nakamura T, Tomita Y, Hirai R, Yamaoka K, Kaji K, Ichihara A: Inhibitory effect of transforming growth factor-β on DNA synthesis of adult rat hepatocytes in primary culture. Biochem Biophys Res Commun 133:1042, 1985

57. Odin P, Öbrink B: Dynamic expression of the cell adhesion molecule cell-CAM 105 in fetal and regenerating rat liver. Exp Cell Res 164:103, 1986

58. Panduro A, Shalaby F, Weiner FR, Biempica L, Zern MA, Shafritz DA: Transcriptional switch from albumin to α-fetoprotein and changes in transcription of other genes during carbon tetrachloride induced liver regeneration. Biochemistry 25:1414, 1986

59. Petropoulos C, Andrews G, Tamaoki T, Fausto N: α-Fetoprotein and albumin mRNA levels in liver regeneration and carcinogenesis. J Cell Biol 258:4901, 1983

60. Petropoulos CJ, Yaswen P, Panzica M, Fausto N: Cell lineages in liver carcinogenesis: possible clues from studies of the distribution of α-fetoprotein sequences in cell populations isolated from normal, regenerating and preneoplastic rat livers. Cancer Res 45:5762, 1985

61. Pledger WJ, Stiles CD, Antoniades HN, Sher CD: Induction of DNA synthesis in BALB/c3T3 cells by serum components: reevaluation of the commitment process. Proc Natl Acad Sci USA 74:4481, 1977

62. Rabes HM, Tuczek HV, Wirsching R: Kinetics of hepatocellular proliferation after partial hepatectomy as a function of structural and biochemical heterogeneity of the rat liver. In Liver Regeneration After Experimental Injury, edited by Lesch R, Reutter W, pp 35–52. New York, Stratton International Medical Book Corporation, 1975

63. Reid LM, Narita M, Michiyasu F, Murray Z, Liverpool G, Rosenberg L: Matrix and hormonal regulation of differentiation in liver cultures. In Research in Isolated and Cultured Hepatocytes, edited by Guillouzo A, Guguen-Guillouzo CG, pp 225–258. London, John Libbey Co., 1986

64. Roberts AB, Sporn MB: Transforming growth factors. Cancer Surv 4:683, 1985

65. Russell WE, Bucher NLR: Vasopressin modulates liver regeneration in the Brattleboro rat. Am J Physiol 245:G321, 1983

66a. Russell WE, Coffey RJ, Ouellette AJ, Moses HL: Type β transforming growth factor reversibly inhibits the early proliferative response to partial hepatectomy in the rat. Proc Natl Acad Sci USA 85:5126, 1988

66. Russell WE: Transforming growth factor beta (TGF-β) inhibits hepatocyte DNA synthesis independently of EGF binding and EGF receptor autophosphorylation. J Cell Physiol, 135:253, 1988

67. Saez JC, Bennett MVL, Spray DG: Carbon tetrachloride at hepatototoxic levels blocks reversibly gap junctions between rat hepatocytes. Science 236:967, 1987

68. Schulte-Hermann R: Induction of liver growth by xenobiotic compounds and other stimuli: CRC Crit Rev Toxicol 3:97, 1974

69. Sell S, Leffert HL: An evaluation of cellular lineages in the pathogenesis of experimental hepatocellular carcinoma. Hepatology 2:77, 1982

70. Sell S, Salman J: Light and electron-microscopic autoradiographic analysis of proliferating cells during the early stages of chemical hepatocarcinogenesis in the rat induced by feeding N-2-fluorenylacetamide in a choline-deficient diet. Am J Pathol 114:287, 1984

71. Shiojiri N: Enzymo- and immunocytochemical analyses of the differentiation of liver cells in the prenatal mouse. J Embryol Exp Morph 62:139, 1981

72. Short J, Brown RF, Husakova JR, Gilbertson JR, Zemel R, Lieberman I: Induction of DNA synthesis in the liver of the intact animal. J Biol Chem 147:1757, 1972

73. Smuckler EA, James JL: Irreversible cell injury. Pharmacol Rev 36:77S, 1984

74. St. Hilaire RJ, Jones AL: Epidermal growth factor: its biological and metabolic effects with emphasis on the hepatocytes. Hepatology 2:601, 1982

75. Stillman D, Sell S: Models of chemical hepatocarcinogenesis and oncodevelopmental gene expression. Methods in Cancer Res 25:135, 1979

76. Strain AJ, Frazer A, Hill DJ, Milner RDG: Transforming growth factor β inhibits DNA synthesis in hepatocytes isolated from normal and regenerating rat liver. Biochem Biophys Res Commun 145:436, 1987

77. Thaler FJ, Michalopoulos GK: Hepatopoietin A: Partial characterization and trypsin activation of a hepatocyte growth factor. Cancer Res 45:2545, 1985

78. Thompson NL, Mead JE, Braun L, Goyette M, Shank PR, Fausto N: Sequential protooncogene expression during rat liver regeneration. Cancer Res 46:3111, 1986

79. Thorgeirsson SS, Huber BE, Sorrell S, Fojo A, Pastan I, Gottesman MM: Expression of the multidrug-resistant gene in hepato-carcinogenesis and regenerating rat liver. Science 236:1120, 1987

80. Traub O, Druge PM, Willecke K: Degradation and resynthesis of gap junction protein in plasma membranes of regenerating liver after partial hepatectomy or cholestasis. Proc Natl Acad Sci USA 80:755, 1983

81. Tsao M-S, Grisham JW: Hepatocarcinomas, cholangiocarcinomas and hepatoblastomas produced by chemically transformed cultured rat liver epithelial cells. A light and electron-microscope analysis. Am J Pathol 127:168, 1987

82. Watanabe A, Shiota T, Hayashi S, Nagashima H: Serum α-fetoprotein in fulminant hepatitis and hepatic regeneration following partial hepatectomy. Biochem Med 32:132, 1984

83. Zimmerman HJ: Chemical hepatic injury and its detection. In Toxicology of the liver, edited by Plaa GL, Hewitt WR, pp 1–45, New York, Raven Press, 1982

Biology of Disease

Mechanism of Mineral Formation in Bone

H. Clarke Anderson

*Department of Pathology and Oncology, University of Kansas Medical Center,
Kansas City, Kansas*

Abstract
Introduction
Mineralization Mechanism in Embryonic Bone
The Role of Phosphatase and Membrane Phospholipids in Vesicle Calcification
Matrix Vesicle Biogenesis
Discussion and Conclusions

ABSTRACT

The mechanism of mineral formation in bone is seen best where active new bone formation is occurring, *e.g.*, in newly forming subperiosteal bone of the embryo, in the growing bone of young animals, and in healing rickets where the calcification process in osteoid is reactivated. A large body of ultrastructural evidence, using conventional and anhydrous methods for tissue preparation, has shown convincingly that extracellular matrix vesicles are present at or near the mineralization front in all of the above, and that these vesicles are the initial site of apatite mineral deposition. Thus bone resembles growth plate cartilage, predentin, and turkey tendon in having calcification initiated by matrix vesicles. Once the calcification cascade is begun, matrix vesicles are no longer needed to support mineralization and are consumed by the advancing mineralization front in which performed crystals serve as nuclei for the formation of new crystals. The rate of crystal proliferation is promoted by the availability of Ca^{2+}, PO_4^{3-}, and the presence of collagen, and retarded by naturally occurring inhibitors of mineralization such as proteoglycans and several noncollagenous calcium-binding proteins of bone including bone-Gla protein (osteocalcin), phosphoproteins, osteonectin, and α-2HS-glycoproteins. New electron microscopic immunocytochemical findings in our laboratory suggest that the origin of alkaline phosphatase-positive bone matrix vesicles is polarized to the mineral-facing side of osteoblasts and may be concentrated near the intercellular junctions of human embryonic osteoblasts.

INTRODUCTION

There is a basic similarity to all forms of skeletal calcification. Because all of the elements of the calcification process are clearly seen by examination of calcification in growth plate cartilage, this tissue will be used at first to describe the process. Then comparable features of calcification will be illustrated in bone.

In the epiphyseal growth plate of long bones (Fig. 1), mineralization is restricted to the longitudinal septal cartilage matrix into which matrix vesicles are dispersed selectively as clusters. Matrix vesicles are cell-derived, membrane-invested particles, usually measuring 100 to 200 nM, into which the first calcium phosphate mineral is deposited (13, 28). The first mineral appears within these extracellular vesicles, often in close apposition to the inner leaflet of the vesicle membrane (Fig. 2). There are several important reasons why matrix vesicles are well suited to serve as the initial site of calcification including: (a) The presence of a high concentration of Ca-binding acidic phospholipids (57, 106, 131); (b) The presence in vesicle membranes of phosphatases (Table 1) with the ability to hydrolyze a variety of naturally occurring organic phosphoesters, *e.g.*, ATP, ADP, AMP, 5′-AMP, pyrophosphate, phosphoethanolamine, etc. (3, 5, 6, 67, 71, 90, 95, 97, 101, 120, 137, 138) yielding orthophosphate, (PO_4) for use in the formation of nascent $CaPO_4$ mineral; and (c) a membrane-invested internal microenvironment protecting the first mineral nuclei while they are in a more soluble precrystalline state before conversion to hydroxyapatite (HA).

After formation of the first mineral, crystals of HA begin to accumulate within the confines of the matrix vesicle membrane (Figs. 3 and 4). Figure 3 presents a very elegant demonstration of mineral accumulation within a vesicle of mouse growth plate which was processed by freeze-substitution, *i.e.*, the most advanced, state-of-the-art method of anhydrous tissue preparation for electron microscopy (generously contributed by Prof. Ozawa of Niigata University). Although some doubt has been raised concerning the existence of an association between matrix vesicles and solid phase mineral (81, 119), there now appears to be ample independent evidence of such an association as seen by different anhydrous tissue preservation techniques to substantiate the presence of mineral within matrix vesicles of cartilage, bone, predentin, and calcifying turkey tendon (Table 2).

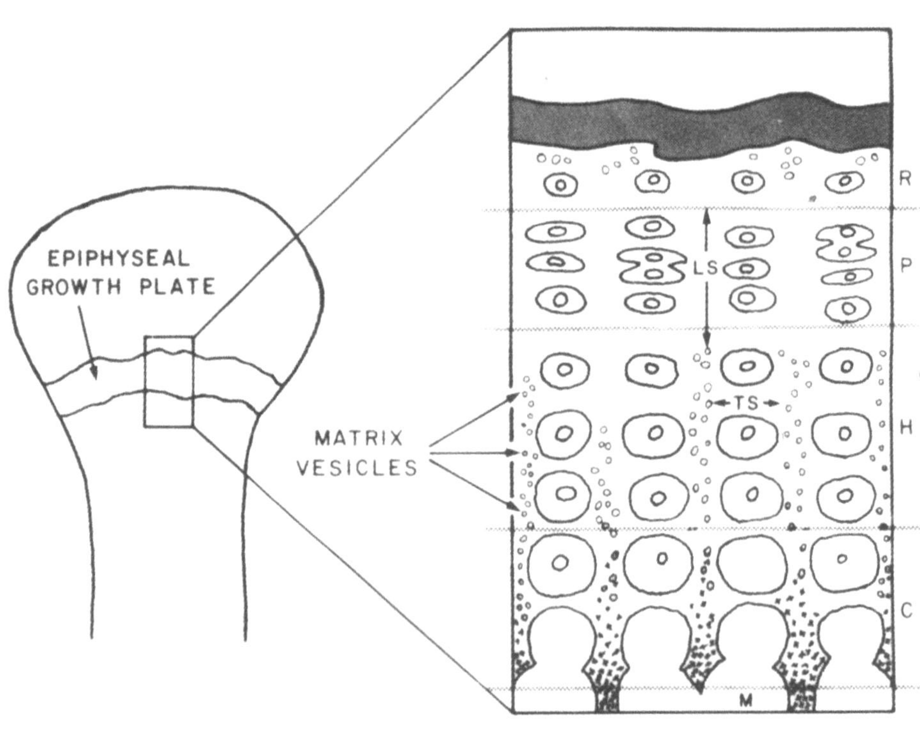

FIG. 1. Diagram of the epiphyseal growth plate of a long bone, the site at which growth in length occurs. The growth plate is subdivided into the following anatomical regions: The reserve zone (R), at the top of the growth plate, contains apparently inactive chondrocytes. The proliferative zone (P) is a zone of active cell division where cell columns first appear, thus allowing the matrix to be anatomically subdivided into transverse matrix septa (TS), separating cells within a column, and longitudinal septa (LS), separating adjacent cell columns. The hypertrophic zone (H) contains enlarging chondrocytes and many matrix vesicles, found in clusters in the longitudinal septa. The first mineral crystals arise within matrix vesicles of the hypertrophic zone (see Fig. 2). The calcifying zone (C) contains degenerating chondrocytes. This is the level at which proliferating mineral spreads from matrix vesicles radially outward to infiltrate the interstices of the longitudinal septal matrix. At the base of the growth plate lies the bony metaphysis (M) with small vessels which remove the uncalcified transverse matrix septa and degenerative cells, leaving calcified longitudinal septa upon which osteoblasts from the marrow will deposit new bone (the primary spongiosa). (Reprinted from "Calcium in Biological Systems", Plenum Press, NY, 1985).

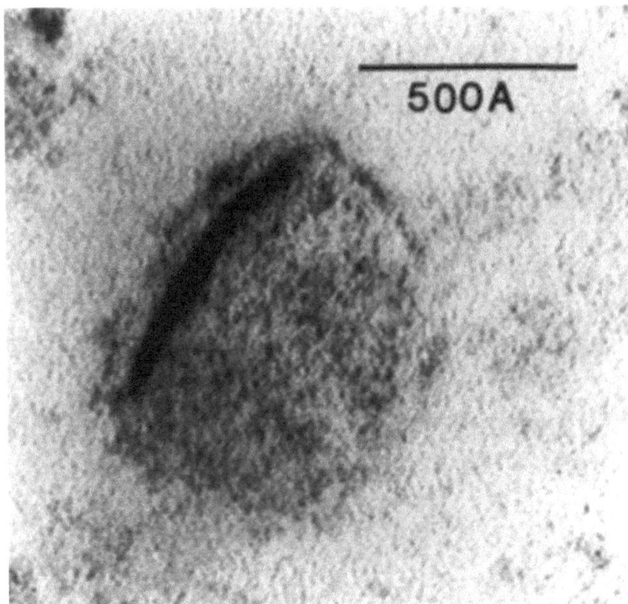

FIG. 2. Electron micrograph of a calcifying matrix vesicle in the hypertrophic zone of rat growth plate. The first electron microscopically observable crystalline apatite mineral is seen as a needle-like, electron-dense precipitate within the matrix vesicle, often in apposition to the inner leaflet of the vesicle membrane. Stained with lead and uranium, ×312,000. (Reprinted from "Endocrine Control of Bone and Calcium Metabolism", Vol. 8B, Excerpta Medica, Amsterdam, 1984).

The phase of extravesicular mineral proliferation (*phase 2*, Fig. 4) begins with the exposure of HA to the extracellular fluid. Figure 4 suggests that rigid HA crystals actually penetrate or perforate the vesicle lipid bi-

TABLE 1. PHOSPHATASES OF MATRIX VESICLE MEMBRANES

Alkaline phosphatase
ATPase (including Ca-ATPase)
p-NPPase (not inhibited by levamisole)
Nucleoside triphosphate pyrophosphohydrolase
Inorganic pyrophosphatase
5'-nucleotidase

layer. A good deal of electron microscopic evidence has suggested that such a perforation occurs. Recently, this supposition has been strengthened by the experimental work of Eanes and Hailer (46) in which HA is induced to form and to accumulate within artificially produced liposomes. In Eanes' experimental model, the intravesicular HA ultimately perforates its investing liposomal membrane. Exposure of HA to the extraliposomal fluid leads to a rapid proliferation of extravesicular HA, both *in vivo* and *in vitro* (13, 16, 20, 98).

After providing for the site-specific deposition of a few seed crystals between collagen fibrils of the matrix, the work of matrix vesicles is completed. Such "seed" crystals can then serve as templates for new crystal proliferation, given normal concentrations of Ca^{2+}, PO_4^{3-} and pH in cartilage matrix extracellular fluid (63). The phase of crystal proliferation (*phase 2*, Fig. 4), is essentially a physicochemical process, and its rate is governed by extracellular fluid components that accelerate the rate of crystal proliferation, *e.g.*, example sufficient Ca^{2+} and/or PO_4^{2-} and perhaps collagen (59, 134); or slow its rate, *e.g.*, low Ca^{2+} and/or PO_4^{3-} (16–18, 51, 98) in rickets plus calcium-binding, noncollagenous proteins of the matrix that inhibit crystal proliferation (Table 3). The latter inhibitory proteins include proteoglycans (35, 38, 40, 45,

100), bone Gla-protein known as "osteocalcin" (32, 92, 107, 111), phosphoproteins (42, 54, 92), osteonectin (92, 111, 127) and the α-2HS-glycoprotein of bone (127). For obvious reasons, it is very important to the host animal to confine and direct the mineralization process toward biologically useful deposition only. Therefore only certain strategically located cells are able to initiate mineralization through the elaboration and selective placement of active matrix vesicles. When it is uncontrolled, mineralization contributes materially to the morbidity associated with important calcific diseases (21) such as ath-erosclerosis (41, 104, 124–126), arteriosclerosis (74), heart valve calcifications (73, 74, 85, 116), arthritis (11, 12, 36, 43, 62, 78, 91, 112, 117, 128), cataracts (50), and tympanosclerosis leading to deafness (53, 88).

Phase 2 of progressive mineralization does not rely upon the intermediation of matrix vesicles. In fact, when the matrix becomes heavily mineralized, residual matrix vesicles are buried, fragmented, and essentially destroyed by the encroachment of proliferating mineral crystals (13, 110). Thus matrix vesicle numbers decline in the zone of provisional calcification of the growth plate (110), and have not been identified in the matrix of fully mineralized bone (80).

MINERALIZATION MECHANISM IN EMBRYONIC BONE

The first mineralization that occurs in embryonic long bones is found in a collar of osseous tissue that forms at the surfaces of the midshaft of the cartilaginous bone rudiment during days 5 through 8 (Hamilton-Hamburger Stages 18–22) of embryonic chick development (Fig. 5). During this period, mesenchymal cells form a fibrous periosteum with preosteoblastic cells closely apposed to the shaft of the cartilage rudiment. These cells acquire the features and synthetic activities of osteoblasts (15). Mature osteoblasts are situated toward the center of the bone shaft. They begin to secrete a bony matrix characterized by the presence of larger, type I collagen fibrils (130) as apposed to the characteristic type II collagen seen in cartilage (93). Regarding the timing of these events, at 6 days of embryonic development, the avian femur is composed almost entirely of noncalcified cartilage. At 7 days, the first collar of periosteal cells appears, and there is evidence of early osteoid deposition at the junction of cartilage and osteoblasts, but still no light microscopic evidence of calcification. At 8 days, the calcification of osteoid is well underway beneath the new layer of periosteal osteoblasts, but still no cartilage calcification has occurred.

Matrix vesicles are seen first within the osteoid matrix underlying centrally located osteoblasts (Fig. 6), and almost immediately intravesicular HA crystals are seen (Fig. 6). Thus, in structure and function, matrix vesicles of bone appear to be analogous to matrix vesicles of growth plate cartilage. However, the average diameter of bone matrix vesicles is smaller than that of cartilage

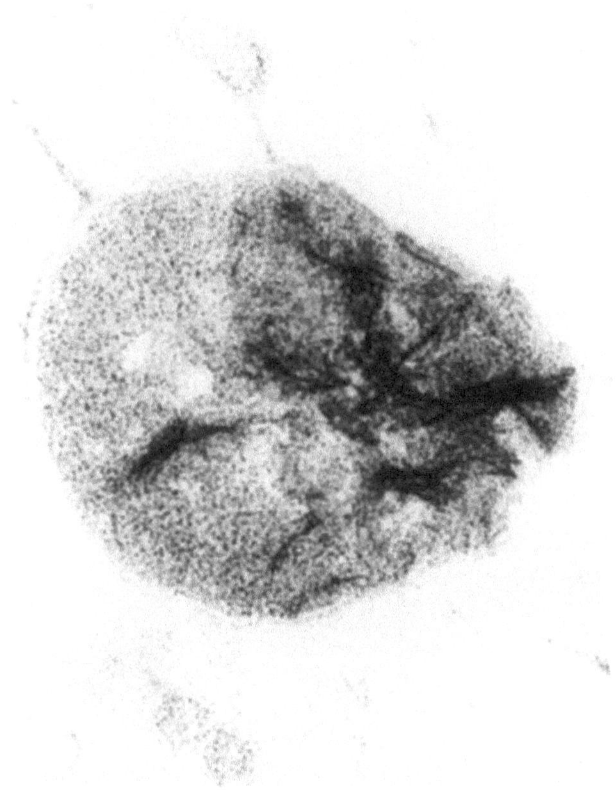

FIG. 3. Electron micrograph of calcifying matrix vesicle in growth plate cartilage prepared by freeze-substitution. Electron-dense needles of hydroxyapatite mineral accumulate within the confines of the vesicle membrane before proliferation at the surface of the vesicle and into the surrounding cartilage matrix. The faint droplets and linear interconnecting strands in the matrix are probably condensed proteoglycan. ×200,000. (Generously contributed by Prof. H. Ozawa, Niigata University, Japan; Jap J Oral Biol. 27:751, 774, 1985).

TABLE 2. OBSERVATIONS OF SOLID PHASE MINERAL WITHIN MATRIX VESICLES PREPARED BY ANHYDROUS TECHNIQUES

Investigators	Tissue studied	Techniques	References
Ali *et al.*	Growth plate, rabbit	Ultracryomicrotomy	8–10
Gay and Schraer	Embryonic bone, chick	Ultracryomicrotomy microincineration	55, 56
Barckhaus *et al.*	Growth plate, guinea pig	Freeze-dried nonaqueas embedment	25
Huntziker *et al.*	Growth plate	Freeze-substitution, nonaqueas embedment	68
Morris *et al.*	Growth plate rat	Ultracryomicrotomy freeze-substitution, nonaqueas embedment	94
Ozawa and Yamamoto	Growth plate osteoid predentin	Pyroantimonate fixation inert dehydration ultracryomicrotomy	102
Akisaka *et al.*	Growth plate chick bone	Rapid freeze, freeze-substitution	2, 4
Ozawa *et al.*	Growth plate	Rapid freeze, freeze substitution	103
Landis	Turkey tendon	Ultracryomicrotomy	82

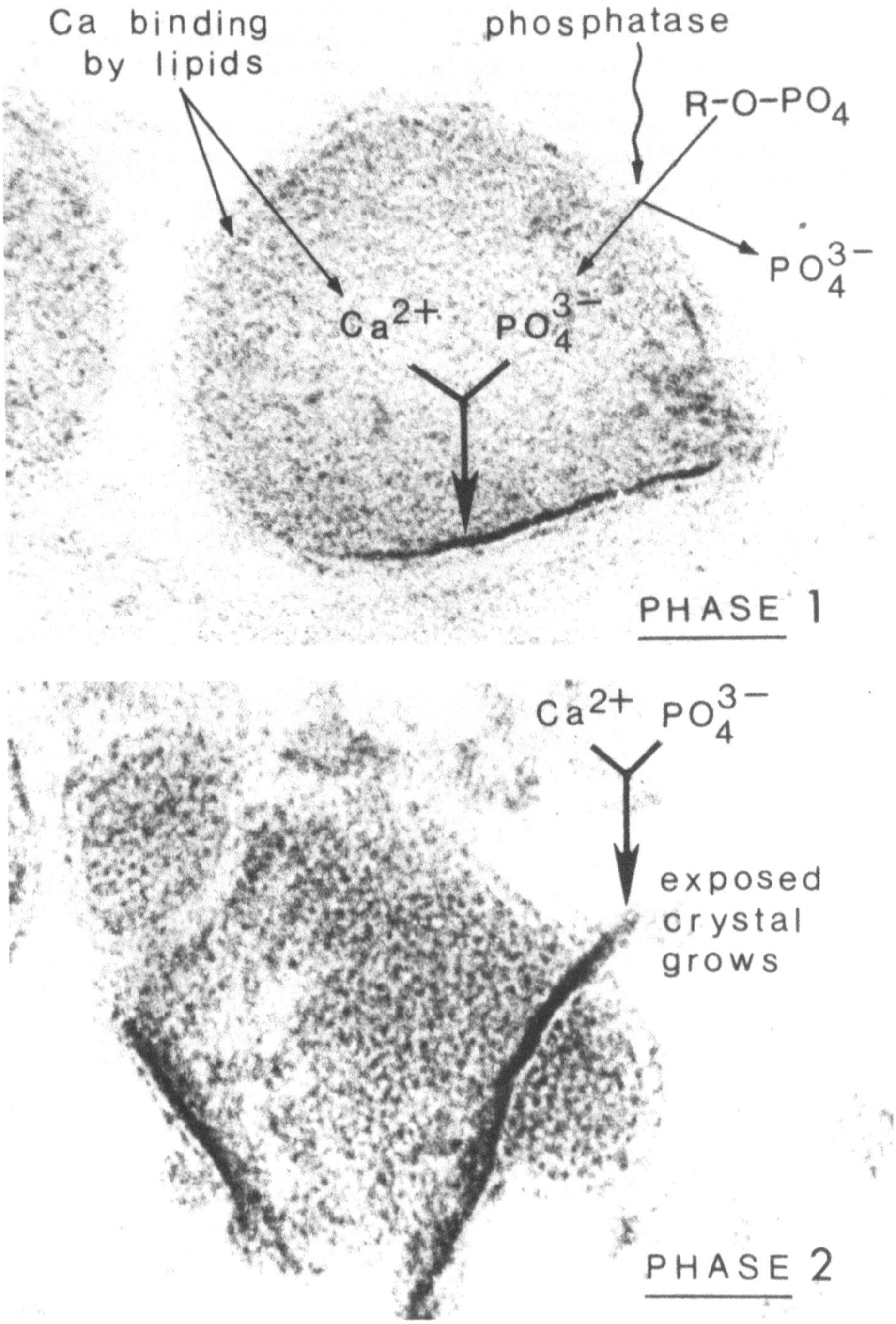

FIG. 4. Scheme for mineralization in matrix vesicles. During *phase 1*, intravesicular calcium concentration is increased by its affinity for lipids of the vesicle membrane interior. Phosphatase (*e.g.*, alkaline phosphatase, pryophosphatase, or adenosine triphosphatase) at the vesicle membrane acts upon ester phosphate of matrix or vesicle fluid to produce a local increase in PO_4 in the vicinity of the vesicle membrane. The intravesicular ionic product (Ca^{2+} × PO_4) is thereby raised, resulting in initial deposition of Ca and PO_4 near the membrane. With accumulation and growth, intravesicular crystals are exposed to the extravesicular environment. *Phase 2* begins with exposure of performed apatite crystals to extravesicular fluid, which in normal animals is supersaturated with respect to apatite, enabling further crystal proliferation. Matrix vesicles pictured are in rat growth plate cartilage. (From Anderson, Metab Bone Dis Relat Res 1:83, 1978).

TABLE 3. MOLECULES GOVERNING RATE OF MINERAL PROLIFERATION

Promoters		Inhibitors	
Ca^{2+}	PO_4^{3-}	Ca^{2+}	PO_4^{3-}
Ester phosphate (*e.g.*, AMP)		Polyphosphate (ATP, PP_i)	
Collagen		Bone Gla protein (osteocalcin)	
		Proteoglycan aggregates	

matrix vesicles, the number of matrix vesicles in bone is not as great as in cartilage where clusters of matrix vesicles are readily seen, and the time between vesicle formation and vesicle calcification appears to be very brief in bone as compared with cartilage. All of these factors tend to make it more difficult to find matrix vesicles of bone in early stages of calcification. However, careful electron microscopic inspection of active bone formation has usually revealed matrix vesicles in the newly formed osteoid (23, 26), and there are now numerous confirmatory reports (Table 4).

Some investigators have attempted to "catch" bone matrix vesicles of postfetal bone in a relatively unmineralized state by examining osteomalacic bone, either in spontaneously occurring osteomalacia (44), or as seen in some patients on renal dialysis (19), or in the induced osteomalacia of low phosphate rickets (20). In all instances, osteoid accumulates upon the surfaces of bone spicules because of impaired advancement of the mineralization front (19, 20, 44), and matrix vesicles accumulate in the osteoid, often with internal but no external

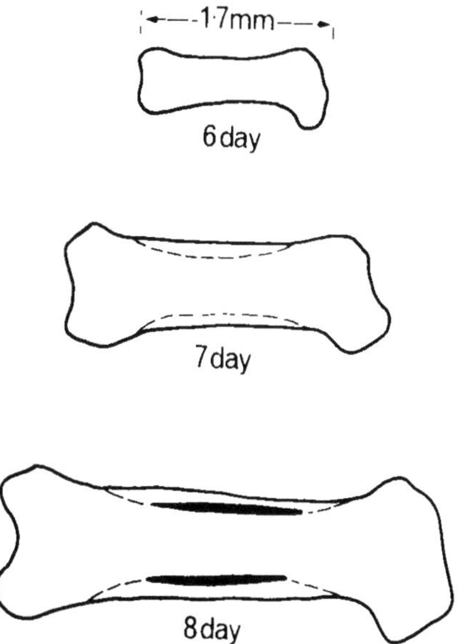

FIG. 5. Diagram of stages in the development of chick embryonic femur. At day 6 of gestation, the femur consists of an entirely cartilaginous rudiment. By day 7, a collar of periosteum has formed around the midshaft of the bone with rounded osteoblasts lining the cartilage surface. Between osteoblasts and cartilage, an osseous matrix is present which is composed primarily of collagen fibrils measuring about 40 nM in diameter. The bone matrix at this stage contains matrix vesicles (Fig. 6), and a number of these vesicles contain apatite. On day 8, a dense laminar deposition of apatite (appearing as a *dark line* in the figure) has formed at midshaft in the bone matrix near its junction with cartilage. This apatite layer is separated from adjacent osteoblasts by bone matrix containing numerous vesicles. Examination of the osteoblastic layer away from the central shaft region and nearer the bone ends reveals earlier stages of mineralization in which many matrix vesicles are visualized, but only a few have begun to accumulate apatite. It appears that mineral deposition begins centrally and spreads centripedally in a wavelike fashion.

mineral (Fig. 7). In one unpublished study of induced recalcification of experimental low phosphate osteomalacia in rats (T. F. Johnson, D. C. Morris, H. C. Anderson, submitted for publication), matrix vesicles were abundantly evident in osteoid before healing was induced by giving the animals a normal diet plus a phosphate injection. Within only 24 hours, these matrix vesicles were very quickly mineralized to form small radial clusters of HA. Simultaneously, the calcification front, *i.e.*, the mineral surface at the interface between mineralized bone and unmineralized osteoid, accumulated mineral and moved rapidly toward the osteoblastic cell layer, thus narrowing the average osteoid seam width from 7.3 ± 0.5 μm to 2.3 ± 0.7 μm within 48 hours. The advancing mineral front engulfed many of the small clusters of apatite which by this time had enveloped the matrix vesicles. These observations emphasized the early role of matrix vesicles in calcification of bone, and also showed that after a mineralization front is established in bone, it can spread into adjacent osteoid without the assistance of matrix vesicles given normal extracellular levels of Ca^{2+} and PO_4^{3-}. Thus matrix vesicles appear to be involved only in the initial or *phase I* mineral initiation, and it is not at all surprising that matrix vesicles are not evident in fully mineralized bone (80). In bone as in cartilage, progressive mineral deposition covers up the remains of matrix vesicles.

THE ROLE OF PHOSPHATASE AND MEMBRANE PHOSPHOLIPIDS IN VESICLE CALCIFICATION

There is a great deal of evidence indicating an important role for matrix vesicle alkaline phosphatase (ALP) and related enzymes such as alkaline inorganic pyrophosphatase in the normal mineralization of cartilage and bone. Some of the evidence is as follows. Chick bone matrix vesicle pyrophosphatase activity was required for the calcification of embryonic long-bone rudiments in

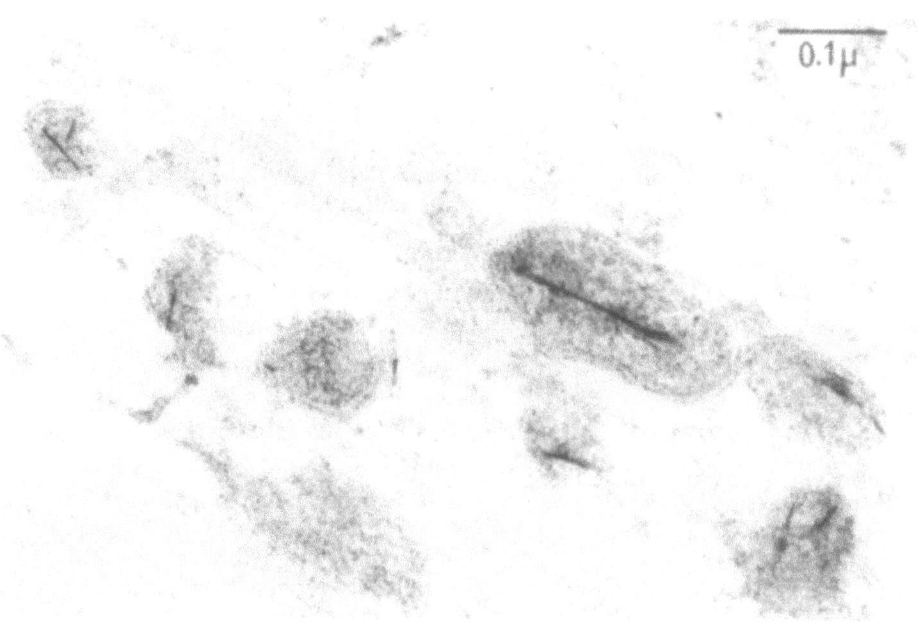

FIG. 6. Matrix vesicles containing needle-like profiles of apatite in the osseous matrix of 7-day chick femur, midshaft. The investing trilaminar membranes and the characteristic electron-dense contents of matrix vesicles are seen quite clearly. Stained with lead only. ×152,000. (Reprinted from Anderson and Reynolds, Dev Biol 34:211, 1973).

TABLE 4. CALCIFYING MATRIX VESICLES SIGHTED IN
POSTFETAL BONE

Tissue	Species	Reference
Bone repair	Dog	Schenk *et al.* 1970
Metaphysis, EHDP rickets	Rat	Schenk 1972
Avian medullary bone stimulated by estrogen	Pigeon	Bonucci and Gherardi 1975
Reparative alveolar bone	Rat	Sela *et al.* 1978
Normal alveolar bone	Rat	Bab *et al.* 1979
Woven bone	Rat	Martino *et al.* 1979
Osteomalacic bone of renal dialysis patients	Human	Anderson *et al.* 1980
Nutritional osteomalacia	Human	Dopping-Hepenstal *et al.* 1981
Metaphysis, healing rickets	Rat	Anderson *et al.* 1981

EHDP, ethane-1-hydroxy-1,1-diphosphonate.

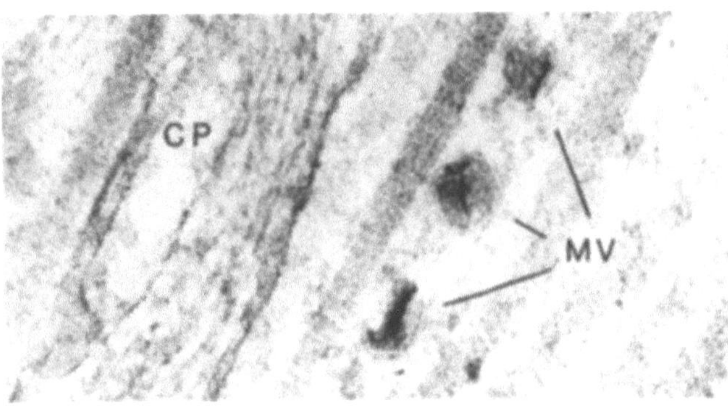

FIG. 7. Matrix vesicles in osteomalacic bone matrix of a patient with renal osteodystrophy. These vesicles are lying adjacent to an osteoblast, at the *left*, with its cell process (*CP*) traversing the field diagonally. The matrix vesicles are surrounded by faintly discernible membranes and contain single profiles of needle-like apatite mineral. The cell process is distinguished from matrix vesicles by a larger diameter and a less dense interior containing cytofilaments. ×142,900. (Reprinted from Anderson, *et al.*, Metab Bone Dis Relat Res 2S:79, 1980).

organ culture (15). Inhibitors of vesicle alkaline phosphatase activity such as heat, beryllium, levamisole and EHDP also inhibited calcification of matrix vesicles in tissue slices of rachitic rat growth plate cartilage (16–18, 22, 51), and the heat inactivation curve for isolated vesicle pyrophosphatase exactly paralleled the pattern of inhibition of calcification in growth plate tissue slices (22). The removal of phosphatase substrates such as AMP and β-glycerophosphate from calcifying solutions prevented calcification in growth plate tissue slices (18) and in isolated matrix vesicles (7, 64–66, 98), and, although solubilized ALP alone was not capable of initiating ^{45}CaPO$_4$ deposition (65), our studies have shown that when phosphatase is incorporated into the membranes of reconstituted vesicles, calcium deposition is restored (66).

Cytochemistry shows that most ALP, Ca-ATPase and pyrophosphatase activity resides in the matrix vesicle membrane (3, 5, 14, 27, 61, 71, 83, 84, 86, 90, 95, D. C. Morris, K. Masuhara, F. Takaoka, K. Ono, H. C. Anderson, submitted for publication, 101, 137, 138), and in the plasma membrane of adjacent hypertrophic chondro-

cytes (3, 5, 14, 86, 90, 95, 96) periosteal osteoblasts (27, 95, 99) and odontoblasts (83, 84, 101, 123) from which the membranes of matrix vesicles are apparently derived (2, 4, 37, 57, 58, 106, 122, 135). It is believed that a portion of the ALP molecule attaches to phosphatidylinositol of the matrix vesicle membrane.

ALP activation occurs just before the onset of matrix vesicle mineralization (2, 5, 90), and may well be the triggering event of the calcification cascade.

Evidence is strong for the involvement of lipids in membrane (vesicle) calcification. Isolated matrix vesicles were shown to be very enriched in acidic phospholipids (106, 131). Such lipids may serve as a nonenergy-requiring calcium trap during mineralization (39, 69, 106, 131, 132, 136). In fact, work by Wuthier *et al.* (132) indicates the presence of matrix vesicles of calcium-phospholipid-phosphate complexes (30, 31) which together with membrane-associated proteolipids are capable of initiating mineral *in vitro* (33, 34, 47–49), have been found in significant quantities in bone (30, 47) and in calcifying oral bacteria (33, 34, 48). The latter bacteria are associated with dental plaque and calculus formation. Any attempt to explain mineralization will have to take into account the role of lipids and particularly membrane phospholipids and proteolipids in the calcification mechanism. Matrix vesicles are notable depositories of Ca-binding phospholipids.

Extracted calcium-phospholipid-phosphate complex (Ca-PL-PO$_4$) from calcification sites is fully capable of initiating CaPO$_4$ deposition *in vitro* at physiologic levels of Ca^{2+} and PO$_4$$^{3-}$, with the formation of HA. These "complexed lipids" are speculated to exist within calcifiable membranes (30, 31, 34, 132). Thus, it is not theoretically necessary to invoke an additional enzymatic mechanism such as ALP to trigger calcification when eminently calcifiable Ca-PL-PO$_4$s are available in membranes at the calcification site. However, as detailed above, there seems to be good evidence for a role of ALP and related phosphatases in initiating calcification. In trying to account for this apparent duplication of calcification mechanisms, it is well to consider that in most studies, Ca-PL-PO$_4$ has been extracted from fully calcified tissues. Thus it is quite possible that there is a progressive formation of Ca-PL-PO$_4$ after mineral initiation by matrix vesicles and during subsequent progressive calcification. Mineral initiation by the matrix vesicle membrane may depend more upon phosphatase to concentrate PO$_4$$^{3-}$, while calcium-binding membrane phospholipids attract Ca^{2+} to the site of formation of nascent mineral (at the matrix vesicle membrane). The result would be the formation of the very first Ca-PL-PO$_4$ within or at the surfaces of membranes of the matrix vesicles.

MATRIX VESICLE BIOGENESIS

The process of matrix vesicle biogenesis in bone and cartilage appears to be mainly one of "pinching-off" from the plasma membrane of adjacent cells, to form noninverted vesicles (2, 4, 37, 58, 133). There are a number of biochemical similarities between plasma membranes and the membranes of matrix vesicles (Table 5) suggesting

TABLE 5. BIOCHEMICAL SIMILARITIES BETWEEN MATRIX VESICLE MEMBRANES AND PLASMA MEMBRANES

Presence of marker molecules
  5'-AMPase
  Sphyngomyelin
  Membrane-associated NTP-pyrophosphohydrolase
  H2 histocompatibility antigen

High levels of:
  Alkaline phosphatase
  Cholesterol
  Cholesterol: phospholipid
  Actin

Low levels of:
  Esterase (lysosomal marker)
  NADP-cytochrome C reductase (ER marker)

an origin of the latter from the former: (a) the plasma membrane marker enzyme 5'-AMPase is concentrated in matrix vesicles (6); (b) matrix vesicles have a high cholesterol-to-phospholipid ratio and are relatively enriched in phosphatidylserine as are plasma membranes (57, 106, 131); (c) the marker phospholipid sphyngomyelin is present in both plasma membranes and matrix vesicles (106, 131); (d) the H-2 histocompatibility antigen is detectable on the outer surfaces of both plasma membranes and matrix vesicle membranes (121); and (e) freeze-fracture studies of growth plate cartilage show a similar right-side-out distribution of intramembranous particles in the plasma membranes of chondrocytes, and in adjacent matrix vesicle membranes (37, 133). Also, a variety of electron microscopic approaches have produced images that are highly suggestive of chondrocyte and osteoblast budding including freeze-fracture studies (2, 4, 37, 102, 103, 122), high voltage examination of 1-μm sections of growth plate (58), and studies employing reconstruction of 3-dimensional images using serial thin sections (14, 28).

However, other modes of matrix vesicle formation may well occur, particularly cell break-up (28, 76, 77, 108, 124–126), and/or programmed individual cell disintegration, sometimes referred to as apoptosis (72). Either budding or cell breakup would tend to produce right-side-out, plasma membrane-derived vesicles (similar to matrix vesicles). Cellular disruption can account for some of the irregularity in size and shape that is often observed among matrix vesicles of cartilage (13). Furthermore, cell breakup is probably a major pathway for formation of the matrix vesicles that are involved in initial pathologic calcification of atherosclerotic plaques (124, 126), calcific stenosis of heart valves (73, 74), medial sclerosis of arteries (74), the calcification of bi-prosthetic heart valve implants (85, 116), and the calcification of nonskeletal neoplasms (1, 52, 75, 79, 87, 113). All of the above forms of extracellular calcification, are initially associated with the vesicular remains of broken cells.

The question arises as to whether there are specialized regions of the plasma membrane of skeletal cells that are predestined, by virtue of their selective composition, to be pinched-off to become matrix vesicles. Evidence in favor of this includes electron microsopic studies that indicate selective budding from the lateral edges of chondrocytes in the growth plate (109), and from the mineral-facing surfaces of osteoblasts (D. C. Morris, K. Masuhara, F. Takaoka, K. Ono, H. C. Anderson, submitted for publication, 105). Recent studies of Morris et al. (D. C. Morris, K. Masuhara, F. Takaoka, K. Ono, H. C. Anderson, submitted for publication) from our laboratory seem to indicate that the greatest concentration of ALP-positive matrix vesicles is near the intercellular junctions on the matrix-facing sides of human embryonic osteoblasts. Also, studies of the relative concentrations of various lipids and phospholipids in matrix vesicle membranes showed a selective concentration in vesicles of phosphatidylserine, sphyngomyelin, and cholesterol, greater than that present in the plasma membrane of the parent chondrocytes (57). This plus the well-documented higher specific activity of ALP in matrix vesicle membranes (6), suggested to Glaser and Conrad (57) that matrix vesicles bud from a selected region of the plasma membrane where these substituents are localized (i.e., a polarized membrane segment or domain).

The process of matrix vesicle biogenesis is just beginning to be studied in vitro. Several tissue culture systems have been developed in which cultivated cartilage or bone cells give rise to calcifiable matrix vesicles (57, 60, 129, 135). The additional synchrony and control over vesicle-generative events afforded by such culture systems will doubtless provide new insight into the effects of physiologic regulatory factors (hormones, etc.) and the possible temporal association, if any, between phases of the cell cycle and periods of matrix vesicle biogenesis.

DISCUSSION AND CONCLUSIONS

Mineralization of growing bone resembles that of growth plate cartilage in being initiated in association with submicroscopic, extracellular matrix vesicles. The matrix vesicles of bone differ from those of cartilage by being somewhat smaller and more rapidly calcified. However, in most respects, bone matrix vesicles closely resemble those of cartilage. In both cases, the matrix vesicles are extracellular and not connected to cells. Mineral develops first within matrix vesicles, and then accumulates as spherular aggregates upon the surfaces of the vesicles. The isolated matrix vesicles of the bone calcify as avidly as do those of cartilage in in vitro test systems.

The mechanism of matrix vesicle mineralization appears to reside in the vesicle membrane which, in turn, is probably derived from plasma membrane. Thus, the vesicle membrane carries with it into the matrix important cellular potentialities such as integral phosphatase activity and the special calcium affinity of its membrane phospholipids. Furthermore, being in the form of a vesicle allows the sealed-off membrane to create an enclosed and protective microenvironment for nascent mineral formation and preservation.

In the process of mineralizing, calcium-binding acidic phospholipids of the matrix vesicle membrane probably serve as a nonenergy-requiring calcium trap, localizing calcium in the vesicle membrane. As matrix vesicles approach the calcification front, their phosphatase activity is "turned on." There is much evidence, cited above, indicating a positive role for matrix vesicle alkaline and other phosphatases in mineral initiation. By the activity of these phosphatases, inorganic phosphate is provided at or within matrix vesicles at the site of formation of nascent calcium phosphate mineral. In order to initiate calcification, native matrix vesicles or reconstituted matrix vesicles require phosphatase to be an integral part of their membranes. Soluble ALP, alone, is incapable of initiating mineralization from solutions containing physiologic levels of Ca^{2+} and PO_4^{3-}, and must be bound into the membrane.

The process of matrix vesicle biogenesis in cartilage and bone is probably mostly one of "pinching-off" from the plasma membrane of adjacent cells to form noninverted vesicles. However, other modes of matrix vesicle formation may well occur, particularly cell breakup and sometimes programmed cell disintegration, referred to as "apoptosis." All of the above processes can yield a significant number of extracellular, right-side-out plasma-membrane derived matrix vesicles, however, cell disruption may account for some of the irregularity in size and shape that is often observed among subpopulations of matrix vesicles.

There is accumulating evidence to suggest that matrix vesicles are generated in a polarized fashion from skeletal cells, and are derived from chemically specialized domains of the plasma membrane where higher concentrations of calcium, acidic phospholipid, cholesterol, and/or phosphatase may assist the processes of vesiculation and calcification.

It is evident that new insight into the calcification mechanism has been gained through improvements in visualizing the process by electron microscopy. Such studies have shown that both normal and pathologic calcification often begins in an intimate relationship to exfoliated biologic membranes. Membrane-mediated calcification was not conceived of before it was actually possible to visualize the process in the electron microscope.

This work was supported by National Institutes of Health Grant DE05262 and a grant from the Kyocera Corporation, Inc.

Address reprint requests to: H. Clarke Anderson, M.D., Department of Pathology and Oncology, University of Kansas Medical Center, Kansas City, Kansas 66103.

REFERENCES

1. Ahmed A: Calcification in human breast carcinomas: ultrastructural observations. J Pathol 117:247, 1975
2. Akisaka T, Shigenaga Y: Ultrastructure of growing epiphyseal cartilage processed by rapid freezing and freeze-substitution. J Electron Microsc 32:305, 1983
3. Akisaka T, Gay CV: Ultrastructural localization of calcium-activated adenosine triphosphatase (Ca^+-ATPase) in growth plate cartilage. J Histochem Cytochem 33:925, 1985
4. Akisaka T, Subita GP, Shigenaga Y: Ultractural observations on chick bone processed by quick freezing and freeze-substitution. Cell Tissue Res 247:469, 1986
5. Akisaka T, Gay CV: Ultrastructural demonstration of p-nitrophenyl phosphatase (p-NPPase) activity in the epiphyseal growth plate. Acta Histochem Cytochem 19:21, 1986
6. Ali, SY, Sajdera SW, Anderson HC: Isolation and characterization of calcifying matrix vesicles from epiphyseal cartilage. Proc Natl Acad Sci USA 67:1513, 1970
7. Ali, SY, Evans L: The uptake of [^{45}Ca]calcium ions by matrix vesicles isolated from calcifying cartilage. Biochem J 134:647, 1973
8. Ali SY: Analysis of matrix vesicles and their role in the calcification of epiphyseal cartilage. Fed Proc 35:135, 1976
9. Ali SY, Gray JC, Wisby A, Phillips M: Preparation of thin cryosections for electron probe analysis of calcifying cartilage. J Microsc 111:65, 1977
10. Ali SY, Wisby A, Craig-Gray J: Electron probe analysis of cryosections of epiphyseal cartilage. Metab Bone Dis Relat Res 1:97, 1978
11. Ali SY, Griffiths S: Matrix vesicles and apatite deposition in osteoarthritis. In Proceedings of the Third International Conference on Matrix Vesicles, edited by Ascenzi, A, Bonucci, E, de Bernard, B, pp 241–247. Milano, Italy, Wichtig Editore,1981
12. Ali SY, Griffiths S: Formation of calcium phosphate crystals in normal and osteoarthritic cartilage. Ann Rheumat Dis 42 (Suppl):45, 1983
13. Anderson HC: Vesicles associated with calcification in the matrix of epiphyseal cartilage. J Cell Biol 41:59, 1969
14. Anderson, HC, Matsuzawa T, Sajdera SW and Ali SY: Membranous particles in calcifying cartilage matrix. Trans NY Acad Sci (Series II) 32:619, 1970
15. Anderson HC, Reynolds JJ: Pyrophosphate stimulation of calcium uptake into cultured embryonic bones: fine structure of matrix vesicles and their role in calcification. Dev Biol 34:211, 1973
16. Anderson HC, Cecil R, Sajdera SW: Calcification of rachitic rat cartilage by extracellular matrix vessels. Am J Pathol 79:237, 1975
17. Anderson HC, Sajdera SW: Calcification of rachitic cartilage to study matrix vesicle function. Fed Proc 35:148, 1976
18. Anderson HC, Hsu, HHT: A new method to measure ^{45}Ca accumulation by matrix vesicles in slices of rachitic growth plate cartilage. Metab Bone Dis Relat Res 1:193, 1978
19. Anderson HC, Johnson TF, Avramides A: Matrix vesicles in osteomalcic bone. Metab Bone Dis Relat Res 2S:79, 1980
20. Anderson HC, Hsu HHT, Johnson TF, Murphree SS, Stein RM: Matrix vesicles in rickets. In Proceedings of the Third International Conference on Matrix Vesicles, edited by Ascenzi A, Bonucci B, deBernard B, pp 223–227. Milano, Italy, Wichtig Editore, 1981
21. Anderson HC: Calcific diseases: a concept. Arch Pathol Lab Med 107:341, 1983
22. Anderson HC: Matrix vesicle calcification: review and update. In Bone and Mineral Research, edited by Peck WA, pp 109–149. Amsterdam, Elsevier Science Publishers, 1985
23. Ascenzi A, Bonucci E: Etude comparee au microcope electronique des phases initiales de la calcification de l'os et du cartilage. In Phosphate et Metabol Phosphocalcique, edited by Hioco AJ, pp 65–77. Paris, Sandoz, 1971
24. Bab IA, Muhlrad A, Sela J: Ultrastructural and biochemical study of extracellular matrix vesicles in normal alveolar bone of rat. Cell Tissue Res 202:1, 1979
25. Barckhaus RH, Krefting ER, Althoft J, Quint P, Hohling HJ: Electron microscopic microprobe analysis on the initial stages of mineral formation in the epiphyseal growth plate. Cell Tissue Res 217:661, 1981
26. Bernard GW, Pease DC: An electron microscopic study of initial intramembranous osteogenesis. Ann J Anat 125:271, 1969
27. Bernard GW: Ultrastructural localization of alkaline phosphatase in initial intramembranous ossification. Clin Orthop 135:218, 1978
28. Bonucci E: Fine structure and histochemistry of calcifying globules in epiphyseal cartilage. Z. Zellforsch Mikr Anat 103:192, 1970
29. Bonucci E, Gherardi G: Histochemical and electron microscope investigations on medullary bone. Cell Tiss Res 163:81, 1975
30. Boskey AL, Posner AS: In vitro nucleation of hydroxyapatite by bone calcium-phospholipid-phosphate complex. Calcif Tiss Res 22(s):197, 1977
31. Boskey AL, Posner AS, Lane JM, Goldberg MR, Cordella DM: Distribution of lipids associated with mineralization in the bovine epiphyseal growth plate. Arch Biochem Biophys 199:305, 1980
32. Boskey AL, Wians FH Jr, Hauschka PV: The effect of osteocalcin on in vitro lipid-induced hydroxy-apatite formation and seeded hydroxyapatite growth. Calcif Tiss Int 37:57, 1985
33. Boyan-Salyers BD, Boskey AL: Relationship between proteolipids

and calcium-phospholipid-phosphate complexes in *Bacterionema matruchotii* calcification. Calcif Tiss Int 30:167, 1980

34. Boyan BD, Landis WJ, Knight J, Dereszewski G, Zeagler J: Microbial hydroxyapatite formation as a mode of proteolipid-dependent membrane-mediated calcification. Scan Electron Microsc IV:1793, 1985

35. Campo RA, Betz RR: Loss of proteoglycans during decalcification of fresh metaphysis with disodium ethylenedraminetetraacetate (EDTA). Calcif Tiss Int 41:52, 1987

36. Caswell AM, Ali SY, Russell RGG: Nucleoside triphosphate pyrophosphatase of rabbit matrix vesicles, a mechanism for the generation of inorganic pyrophosphate in epiphyseal cartilage. Biochim Biophys Acta 924:276, 1987

37. Cecil RNA, Anderson HC: Freeze-fracture studies of matrix vesicle calcification in epiphyseal growth plate. Metab Bone Dis Relat Res 1:89, 1978

38. Chen CC, Boskey AL, Rosenberg L: The inhibitory effect of cartilage proteoglycans on hydroxyapatite growth. Calcif Tiss Intern 36:285, 1984

39. Cotmore JM, Nichols G JR, Wuthier RE: Phospholipid-calcium phosphate complex: enhanced calcium migration in the presence of phosphate. Science 172:1339, 1971

40. Cuervo LA, Pita JC, Howell DS: Inhibition of calcium phosphate mineral growth by proteoglycan aggregate fractions in a synthetic lymph. Calcif Tiss Res 13:1, 1973

41. Daoud AS, Frank AS, Jarmolych J, Franco WT, Fritz KE: Ultrastructural and elemental analysis of calcification of advanced aortic atherosclerosis. Exp Mol Pathol 43:337, 1985

42. DeSteno CV, Feagin FF: Effect of matrix bound phosphate and fluoride on mineralization of dentin. Calcif Tiss Res 17:151, 1975

43. Dieppe PA: Inflammation in osteoarthritis and the role of microcrystals. Semin Arthritis Rheum 11:121, 1981

44. Dopping-Hepenstal PJC, Ali SY, Stamp TCB: Matrix vesicles in the osteoid of human bone. In Proceedings of the thirty second International Conference on Matrix Vesicles, edited by Ascenzi A, Bonucci E, deBernard B, pp 229–234. Milano, Italy, Wichtig Editore, 1981

45. Dziewaitkowski DD, Majznerski LL: Role of proteoglycans in endochondral ossification: inhibition of calcification. Calcif Tiss Int 37:560, 1985

46. Eanes ED, Hailer AW: Liposome-mediated calcium phosphate formation in metastable solutions. Calcif Tiss Int 37:390, 1985

47. Ennever J, Boyan-Salyers B, Riggan LJ: Proteolipid and bone matrix calcification. J Dent Res 56:967, 1977

48. Ennever J, Riggan LJ, Vogel JJ, Boyan-Salyers B: Characterization of *Bacterionema malruchotii* calcification nucleator. J Dent Res 51:637, 1978

49. Ennever J, Vogel JJ, Riggan LJ: Calcification by proteolipid from atherosclerotic aorta. Atherosclerosis 35:209, 1980

50. Fagerholm P, Philipsborn B, Carlstrom D: Calcification in the human lens. Curr Eye Res 1:629, 1982

51. Fallon MD, Whyte, MP Teitlebaum SL: Stereospecific inhibition of alkaline-phosphatase by L-tetramisole prevents *in vitro* cartilage calcification. Lab Invest 43:489, 1980

52. Ferenczy A: Ultrastructural studies on the morphogenesis of psammoma bodies in ovarian serous neoplasia. Cancer 39:2451, 1977

53. Friedman I, Galey FR: Initiation and stages of mineralization in tympanosclerosis. J Laryngol Otol 94:1215, 1980

54. Fujisawa R, Kuboki Y, Sasaki S: Effects of dentin phosphophoryn on precipitation of calcium phosphate in gel *in vitro*. Calcif Tiss Int 41:44, 1987

55. Gay CV: The ultrastructure of the extracellular phase of bone as observed in frozen thin sections. Calcif Tiss Res 23:215, 1977

56. Gay CV, Schraer H, Hargest TE Jr: Ultrastructure of matrix vesicles and mineral in unfixed embryonic bone. Metab Bone Dis Relat Res 1:105, 1978

57. Glaser JH, Conrad HE: Formation of matrix vesicles by cultured chick embryo chondrocytes. J Biol Chem 256:2607, 1981

58. Glauert A, Mayo CR: The study of three dimensional structural relationships in connective tissues by high voltage electron microscopy. J Microsc 97:83, 1973

59. Glimcher MJH: Macromolecular aggregation states in relation to mineralization: the collagen hydroxyapatite system as studied *in vitro*. Proc Natl Acad Sci USA 43:860, 1957

60. Golub EE, Schattschneider SC, Berthold P, Burke A, Shapiro IM: Induction of chondrocyte vesiculation *in vitro*. J Biol Chem 258:616, 1983

61. Gothlin G, Ericsson JLE: Fine structural localization of alkaline phosphomonoesterase in the fracture callus of the rat. Isr J Med Sci 3:488, 1971

62. Halverson PB, Cheung HS, McCarty DJ, Garancis T, Mandel N: "Milwaukee shoulder" Association of microspheroids containing hydroxyapatite crystals, active collagenase, and neutral protease with rotator cuff defects. Arth Rheumat 24:474, 1981

63. Howell DS, Pita JC, Marquez JF, Madruga JE: Partition of calcium phosphate and protein in the fluid phase aspirated at calcifying sites in epiphyseal cartilage. J Clin Invest 47:1121, 1968

64. Hsu HHT, Anderson HC: A simple and defined method to study calcification by isolated matrix vesicles. Effect of ATP and vesicle phosphatase. Biochim Biophys Acta 500:162, 1977

65. Hsu HHT, Cecil RNA, Anderson HC: The role of adenosine triphosphatase, phospholipids and vesicular structure in the calcification of isolated and reconstituted matrix vesicles. Metab Bone Dis Relat Res 1:169, 1978

66. Hsu HHT, Anderson HC: Calcification of isolated matrix vesicles and reconstituted vesicles from fetal bovine cartilage. Proc Natl Acad Sci USA 75:3805, 1978

67. Hsu HHT: Purification and partial characterization of ATP-pyrophosphohydrolase from fetal bovine epiphyseal cartilage. J Biol Chem 258:3463, 1983

68. Huntziker EB, Hermann RK, Schenk RK, Marti T, Muller M, Moon H: Structural integration of matrix vesicles in calcifying cartilage after cryofixation and freeze-substitution. In Proceedings of the Third International Conference on Matrix Vesicles, edited by Ascenzi A, Bonucci E, deBernard B, pp 25–32. Milano, Wichtig Editore sre., 1981

69. Irving JT: The sudanophil material at sites of calcification. Arch Oral Biol 8:735, 1963

70. Deleted in proof.

71. Kanabe S, Hsu HHT, Cecil RNA, Anderson HC: Electron microscopic localization of adenosine triphosphate (ATP)-hydrolyzing activity in isolated matrix vesicles and reconstituted vesicles from calf cartilage. J Histochem Cytochem 31:462, 1983

72. Kardos TB, Hubbard MJ: Are matrix vesicles apoptotic bodies? In Factors and Mechanisms Influencing Bone Growth, pp 45–60. New York, Alan R Liss Inc, 1982

73. Kim KM, Huang SN: Ultrastructural study of dystrophic calcification of human aortic valve. Lab Invest 26:481, 1972

74. Kim KM: Calcification of matrix vesicles in human aortic valve and aortic media. Fed Proc 35:156, 1976

75. Kim KM: Neoplastic calcinosis. Fed Proc 41:919, 1982

76. Kim KM: Role of membranes in calcification. Surv Synth Pathol Res 2:215, 1983

77. Kim KM: Cell injury and calcification of rat aorta *in vitro*. Scan Elec Micr 4:1809, 1984

78. Kubota T, Sato K, Kawano H, Yamamoto S, Hirano A, Hashizumi Y: Ultrastructure of early calcification in cervical ossification of the posterior longitudinal ligament. J Neurosurg 61:131, 1984

79. Kubota T, Hirano A, Yamamoto S, Kajikawa K: The fine structure of psammoma bodies in meningocytic whorls. J Neuropathol Exp Neurol 43:37, 1984

80. Landis WJ, Paine MC, Glimcher MJ: Electron microscopic observations on bone tissue prepared anhydrously in organic solvents. J Ultrastruct Res 59:1, 1977

81. Landis WJ, Glimcher MJ: Electron optical and analytical observations of rat growth plate cartilage prepared by ultracryomicrotomy: the failure to defect a mineral phase in matrix vesicles and the identification of heterodispersed particles as the initial solid phase of calcium phosphate deposited in the extracellular matrix. J Ultrastruct Res 78:227, 1982

82. Landis WJ: A study of calcification in the leg tendons from the domestic turkey. J Ultrastr Molec Str Res 94:217, 1987

83. Larsson A: Studies on dentinogenesis in the rat. Ultrastructural observations on early dentin formation with special reference to "dentinal globules" and alkaline phosphatase activity. A Anat Entwickl Gesch 142:103, 1973

84. Larsson AK: Studies on dentinogenesis in the rat: the interaction between lead pyrophosphate solutions and dentinal globules. Calcif Tiss Res 16:93, 1974

85. Levy RJ, Schoen FJ, Levy JT, Nelson AC, Howard SL, Oshry LJ: Biologic determinants of dystrophic calcification and osteocalcin deposition in glutaraldehyde-preserved porcine aortic valve leaflets implanted subcutaneously in rats. Am J Pathol 113:143, 1983

86. Lewinson J, Toister Z, Silbermann M: Quantitative and distributional changes in the activity of alkaline phosphatase during the maturation of cartilage. J Histochem Cytochem 30:261, 1982

87. Lipper S, Dalzell JC, Watkins PJ: Ultrastructure of psammoma bodies of meningioma in tissue culture. Arch Pathol Lab Med 103:670,

88. Mann W, Riede VN, Jonas I, Beck C: The role of matrix vesicles in the pathogenesis of tympanosclerosis. Acta Oto-Laryngol (Stockholm) 89:43, 1980

89. Martino LJ, Yaeger VL, Taylor JJ: An ultrastructural study of the role of calcification nodules in the mineralization of woven bone. Calcif Tiss Int 27:57, 1979

90. Matsuzawa T, Anderson HC: Phosphatases of epiphyseal cartilage studied by electron microscopic cytochemical methods. J Histochem Cytochem 19:801, 1971

91. McCarty, DJ, Halverson PB, Carrera GF, Brewer BJ, Kozin F: "Milwaukee Shoulder" - association of microspheroids containing hydroxyapatite crystals, active collagenase and neutral protease with rotator cuff defects. Arthr Rheumat 24:464, 1981

92. Menanteau J, Neuman WF, Neuman MW: A study of bone proteins which can prevent hydroxyapatite formation. Metab Bone Dis Relat Res 4:157, 1982

93. Miller EJ, Matukas VJ: Chick cartilage collagen: a new type of alpha-1 chain not present in bone or skin of the species. Proc Natl Acad Sci USA 64:1264, 1969

94. Morris DC, Vaananen HK, Anderson HC: Matrix vesicle calcification in rat epiphyseal growth plate cartilage prepared anhydrously for electron microscopy. Metab Bone Dis Res 5:131, 1983

95. Morris DC, Vaananen HK, Munoz P, Anderson HC: Light and electron microscopic immunolocalization of alkaline phosphatase in bovine growth plate cartilage. In Cell Mediated Calcification and Matrix Vesicles, edited by Ali SY, pp 21–26. Amsterdam, Elsevier Science Publishers BV, 1986

96. Deleted in proof.

97. Muniz O, Pelletier JP, Martell-Pelletier J, Morales S, Howell DS: NTP pyrophosphohydrolase in human chondrocalcinotic and osteoarthritic cartilage. I. Some biochemical characteristics. Arthr Rheumat 27:186, 1984

98. Murphree S, Hsu HHT, Anderson HC: The in vitro formation of crystalline apatite by matrix vesicles isolated from rachitic rat epiphyseal cartilage. Calcif Tiss Int 34:52, 1982

99. Nakajima H, Mizuhira V, Oida S, Goseki M: Histochemistry of periosteum of membranous bone in ossification (ALPase). Acta Histochem Cytochem 19:396, 1986

100. Nemethcsoka M, Sarkozi A: The effect of proteoglycans of cartilage and oversulfated polysaccharides on the development of calcium-hydroxyapatite (CHA) crystal formation in vitro. Acta Biol Hung 33:407, 1982

101. Ozawa H, Najima T: Ultrastructure and cytochemistry of matrix vesicles in developing cartilage and tooth germ. In Fourth International Congress on Histochemistry and Cytochemistry, pp 311–312. Kyoto, 1972

102. Ozawa H, Yamamoto T: An application of energy-dispersive x-ray microanalysis for the study of biological calcification. J Histochem Cytochem 31:210, 1983

103. Ozawa HG, Yamamoto T, Takano Y, Ejiri S: Fine structure and elemental analysis of calcifying epiphyseal cartilage prepared by freeze-substitution methods at liquid helium temperature. In Proceedings of the Eight International Conference of Calcium Regulating Hormones, Vol B (workshops), pp 428–431. 1983

104. Paegle RD: Ultrastructure of calcium deposits in arteriosclerotic human aortas. J Ultrastruct Res 26:412, 1969

105. Palumbo, C: A three-dimensional ultrastructural study of osteoid-osteocytes in the tibia of chick embryos. Cell Tissue Res 246:125, 1986

106. Peress NS, Anderson HC, Sajdera SW: The lipids of matrix vesicles from bovine fetal epiphyseal cartilage. Calif Tiss Res 14:275, 1974

107. Price PA, Otsuka AS, Poser JP, Kristaponis J, Raman N: Characterization of a γ-carboxyglutamic acid-containing protein from bone. Proc Nat Acad Sci USA 73:1447, 1976

108. Rabinovitch AL, Anderson HC: Biogenesis of matrix vesicles in cartilage growth plates. Fed Proc 35:112, 1976

109. Ralphs JR, Ali SY: Histochemical localization of alkaline phosphatase in rabbit ulnar growth plate. In Cell Mediated Calcification and Matrix Vesicles edited by Ali SY, pp 69–74. Amsterdam, Elsevier Science Publishers BV, 1986

110. Reinholt FP, Hjerpe A, Jansson K, Engfeldt B: Sterological studies on the epiphyseal growth plate in low phosphate, vitamin D-deficiency, rickets with special reference to the distribution of matrix vesicles. Calcif Tiss Int 36:95, 1984

111. Romberg RW, Werness PG, Riggs BL, Mann KG: Inhibition of hydroxyapatite crystal growth by bone-specific and other calcium-binding proteins. Biochemistry 25:1176, 1986

112. Sarkar F, Uhthoff HK: Ultrastructural localization of calcium in calcifying tendonitis. Arch Pathol 102:266, 1978

113. Sato K, Kubota T, Yamamoto S, Ishikura A: An ultrastructural study of mineralization in craniopharyngiomas. J Neuropathol Exp Neurol 45:463, 1986

114. Schenk RK, Miller J, Zinkernagel R, Willenegger H: Ultrastructure of normal and abnormal bone repair. Calcif Tissue Res 41 (Suppl):110, 1970

115. Schenk RK: Remarks to the Santa Catalina colloquium on comparative molecular biology of extracellular matrices, edited by Slavkin HC, pp 226–231. New York, Academic Press, 1972

116. Schoen FJ, Levy RJ: Bioprosthetic heart valve failure: pathology and pathogenesis. Cardiol Clin 2:717, 1984

117. Schumacher HR, Gibilisco P, Reginato A, Cherian V: Implications of crystal deposition in osteoarthritis. J Rhematol (Suppl No 9): 40, 1983

118. Sela J, Bab IA, Muhlrad A: Ultrastructural and biochemical characterization of extracellular matrix vesicles in healing alveolar bone sockets: preliminary indications for the presence of contractile proteins. Metab Bone Dis Relat Res 1:185, 1978

119. Shepard N, Mitchell N: Ultrastructural modifications of proteoglycans coincident with mineralization in local regions of rat growth plate. J Bone Jt Surg 67A:455, 1985

120. Siegel SA, Hummel CF, Carty RP: The role of nucleoside triphosphate pyrophosphohydrolase in in vitro nucleoside triphosphate-dependent matrix vesicle calcification. J Biol Chem 258:8601, 1983

121. Slavkin HC, Trump GN, Mansour V, Matosian P, Mino WG: Localization of H-2 histocompatibility alloantigens on mouse embryonic tooth epithelial and mesenchymal cell surfaces. J Cell Biol 60:795, 1974

122. Spycher MA, Moor H, Ruettner JR: Electron microscopic investigations on aging and osteoarthritic human articular cartilage. II The fine structure of freeze-etched aging hip cartilage. Z Zellforsch Mikr Anat 98:512, 1969

123. Takano Y, Ozawa H, Crenshaw MA: Ca-ATPase and ALPase activities at the initial calcification sites of dentin and enamel in rat incisor. Cell Tiss Res 243:91, 1986

124. Tanimura A, McGregor DH, Anderson HC: Matrix vesicles in atherosclerotic calcification. Proc Soc Exp Biol Med 172:173, 1983

125. Tanimura A, McGregor DH, Anderson HC: Calcification in atherosclerosis. I. Human studies. J Exp Pathol 2:261, 1986

126. Tanimura A, McGregor DH, Anderson HC: Calcification in atherosclerosis. II. Animal studies. J Exp Pathol 2:275, 1986

127. Triffitt JT: Noncollagenous proteins of bone: potential functions and uses. In Cell Biology of Bone, Proceedings of the Joint Meeting of the Bone and Tooth Society and the British Connective Tissue Society, 1987

128. Uhthoff HK, Sarkar F: Calcifying tendonitis—its pathogenetic mechanism and a rationale for its treatment. Int Orthop 2:187, 193, 1978

129. Vaananen, HK, Morris, DC, Anderson, HC: Calcification of cartilage matrix in chondrocyte cultures derived from rachitic growth plate. Metab Bone Dis Relat Res 5:87, 1983

130. Vondermark K, Vondermark HGS: Study of differential collagen synthesis during development of chick embryo by immunofluorescence. 2. Localization of type 1 and type 2 collagen during long bone development. Dev Biol 53:153, 1976

131. Wuthier RE: Lipid composition of isolated cartilage cells, membranes and matrix vesicles. Biochim Biophys Acta 409:128, 1975

132. Wuthier RE, Gore ST: Partition of inorganic ions and phospholipids in isolated cell membrane and matrix vesicle fractions:

evidence for Ca-Pi-acidic phospholipid complexes. Calcif Tissue Res 24:163, 171, 1977

133. Wuthier RE, Linder, RE, Warner GP, Gore ST, Borg TK: Non-enzymatic isolation of matrix vesicles: characterization and initial studies on ^{45}Ca and ^{32}P-orthophosphate metabolism. Metab Bone Dis Relat Res 1:125, 1978

134. Wuthier RE: Calcification of vertebrate hard tissues. In Metal Ions in Biological Systems, Calcium and its Role in Biology, Vol 17, edited by Sigel H, pp 417-472. New York, New York, Marcell Dekker, 1984

135. Wuthier RE, Chin JE, Hale JE, Register TC, Hale LV, Ishikawa Y: Isolation and characterization of calcium-accumulating matrix vesicles from chondrocytes of chicken epiphyseal growth plate cartilage in primary culture. J Biol Chem 260:15972, 1985

136. Yaari, AM, Brown CE: Role of lipids in mineralization - an experimental model of membrane transport of calcium and inorganic phosphate. In Calcium in Biological Systems, edited by Rubin RP, Weiss GP, Putney JW Jr, pp 625-629. New York, Plenum Press, 1985

137. Yamada M: Ultrastructural and cytochemical studies on the calcification of the tendon bone joint. Arch Hist Jap 39:347, 1976

138. Yamada M, Ozawa H: Ultrastructural and cytochemical studies on the matrix vesicle calcification in the teeth of the killifish, oryzias latipes. Arch Hist Jap 41:309, 1978

Biology of Disease

Contractile Cells in Normal and Fibrotic Lung

KENNETH B. ADLER, ROBERT B. LOW, KEVIN O. LESLIE, JOHN MITCHELL, AND JOHN N. EVANS

Department of Anatomy, Physiological Sciences and Radiology, College of Veterinary Medicine, North Carolina State University, Raleigh, North Carolina; the Department of Physiology & Biophysics, College of Medicine, University of Vermont, Burlington, Vermont; and the Department of Pathology, College of Medicine, University of Vermont, Burlington, Vermont

INTRODUCTION

Interstitial pulmonary fibrosis represents a group of fibrosing lung diseases, often of unknown etiology, characterized by hypercellularity and deposition of connective tissue within the interstitium of the alveolar wall (32, 65). Increased "stiffness" of the lung leads to reduced lung volumes and lowered dynamic compliance (80). In interstitial fibrosis, as well as several other forms of lung injury, there is an apparent increase in smooth muscle (SM) cells organized into bundles within areas of the lung where these cells normally are present but difficult to detect, such as the alveolar duct (69, 89, 119). This increase in acinar SM can be quite prominent, and, in some cases, the degree of parenchymal SM hyperplasia is sufficiently excessive to be referred to as "muscular cirrhosis of the lung" (2, 7, 33, 110, 152).

A separate but related phenomenon often confused with smooth muscle hyperplasia occurs in parenchymal regions of fibrotic lungs in human patients and animal models of pulmonary fibrosis: in interstitial areas, associated with the connective tissue infiltrate, cells which share many morphologic characteristics of both fibroblasts and smooth muscle cells are observed in great numbers. These cells are very similar morphologically to the "myofibroblast" described extensively in the literature as a key cell in the general processes of wound healing and tissue remodeling (57, 96). Proliferation of cells with potential to contract and thereby generate force within the parenchyma could be a major contributor to the severely impaired, life-threatening lung function characterizing end stages of the disease.

This review will explore the spectrum of both muscle and nonmuscle contractile cells in the lung, their relationships to normal pulmonary structure and function, and their possible role in alterations related to development of pulmonary fibrosis. The similarities and differences in origin, proliferation and differentiation of contractile cells in pulmonary fibrosis and in a variety of other injured and remodeling tissues also will be discussed.

CONTRACTILE CELLS IN NORMAL LUNG

Although not considered a "muscular organ" the lung contains a substantial number of cells with contractile features. The most easily-recognizable are SM cells surrounding airways (bronchi and bronchioles) and large to medium-sized blood vessels. Airways have a substantial muscle coat that decreases in thickness with decreasing luminal diameter. The 3-dimensional arrangement of individual cells, as well as their cytoplasmic contractile proteins, is optimized to produce narrowing of the airway upon contraction, thereby regulating airflow into segmental, subsegmental, and acinar regions of the lung (92). Proximal to respiratory bronchioles, SM fibers are oriented in an annular fashion, but beyond this point they spiral around the airway out to the level of the alveolar sacs. This arrangement of SM fibers around the most peripheral air passages has been likened to a "geodesic network" and may be responsible for an additional proposed physiologic function at this site, namely sphincter-like contraction of alveolar openings that could modulate alveolar ventilation and wall tension (101).

Arteries and veins of the lung also are invested with a SM coat that attenuates as vessel diameter decreases. At the preacinar level, SM is disposed in a circular fashion, but this changes to a spiral configuration in immediate pre- and post-capillary regions (100). The delicate muscle coat of acinar vessels (not easily apparent by light microscopic examination) provides a mechanism for adjustments to blood flow within the lung down to the level of the alveolus. Pulmonary capillaries do not have an organized SM coat, but rather are associated with pericytes distributed along their length at regular intervals (100, 157). These cells are characterized by delicate cytoplasmic extensions which surround the capillary wall and provide a mechanism for perfusion adjustments at the level of the alveolar microenvironment.

The parenchyma of the normal lung possesses a contractile capability unusual for mammalian nonmuscle tissue (46, 47, 76). The bulk of parenchymal contractile cells reside distally at the level of the acinus and are configured as organized SM, functioning to regulate luminal diameter of airways and blood vessels. Additional SM cells associated with alveolar ducts presumably are capable of altering alveolar wall tension by contraction (7, 101).

A second type of contractile cell, the contractile interstitial cell (CIC), resides in the interstitium of the mammalian lung at the level of the alveolar wall (46, 76). These cells have been described only recently, as they are identifiable solely by the presence of cytoplasmic microfilament bundles revealed by electron microscopic or immunohistochemical techniques (3, 76, 129, 146). First described by Kapanci *et al.* (76–78) CIC share several ultrastructural characteristics of normal fibroblasts and of smooth muscle. They are located within the thick portion of the air-blood barrier. Although not surrounded by basal lamina, long pseudopodal projections of the cells extend between alveolar and capillary basement membranes, usually perpendicular to the alveolar basement membrane and tangential or oblique to the capillary basement membrane. Their cytoplasm contains compact bundles of parallel filaments of actin beneath the plasmalemma and obliquely inserted into it. At points where bundles of microfilaments join to the cell membrane, there often are dense zones, forming hemidesmosome-like complexes which also are seen where these interstitial cells contact fibrils of extracellular collagen or elastin. The cytoplasm of these cells contains abundant rough endoplasmic reticulum, many free ribosomes, prominent Golgi, and condensed mitochondria surrounding an indented nucleus. These ultrastructural features are quite similar to those of "myofibroblasts" which have been described in a number of pathologic lesions (see below), and the CIC can be classified as a subclass of myofibroblast present in normal peripheral lung tissue. Interestingly enough, freeze-fracture studies of human and other mammalian lungs have demonstrated the presence of communicating junctions between these cells, and it has been suggested they can behave as a functional syncytium (97).

The related "lipid interstitial cell" (LIC) described by Kaplan *et al.* (79) is found in the alveolar wall of rat, hamster and mouse lung in late fetal life. These cells are most abundant 5 to 10 days after birth and appear to decrease in frequency as the animal matures. The cytoplasm of LICs is replete with lipid droplets (containing primarily triglycerides) as well as prominent bundles of microfilaments (79). Relationships between the LIC and CIC remain somewhat unclear, but formation of alveoli postnatally is characterized by differentiation of interstitial fibroblasts into both "myofibroblasts" (CIC) and "lipid-filled" fibroblasts (LIC) at different levels of new alveolar buds (18). It is possible that these cells represent different subclasses of microfilament-containing interstitial cells (see below).

Another similar cell is the capillary pericyte. As they are positioned similarly to CIC within the interstitium of normal adult lung, it is difficult to distinguish CIC from pericytes in many planes of section, despite some subtle ultrastructural differences. Generally, pericytes have a clear cytoplasm and are surrounded by basement membrane of associated capillary endothelium. Microfilament bundles within the pericyte usually are oriented parallel to the capillary basement membrane (157).

There is no doubt that the contractile protein, actin, is a major constituent of microfilaments such as are found in CIC, LIC and capillary pericytes. This has been demonstrated by immunolocalization at the light and electron microscopic levels. Specifically with regard to lung, Kapanci *et al.* (78) have shown prominent staining of normal lung parenchyma, particularly alveolar walls, using antibodies to actin, a finding confirmed by others (3, 46, 146). Such actin filaments also decorate with heavy meromyosin to create characteristic arrowhead-like structures when viewed in the electron microscope (3). The prominent immunohistochemical and immunofluorescent staining in normal lung tissue reflects the high proportion of interstitial cells that contain substantial amounts of actin filaments. Using ultrastructural morphometry, Kapanci *et al.* (78) reported that 42% of total interstitial volume of the rat lung is occupied by CIC, which comprise 18% of all parenchymal cells, values somewhat higher than those reported by Adler, Callahan, and Evans (4). Relatedly, actin is the most prominent extractable protein of the lung (91). The vast majority of actin is localized in alveolar epithelium, endothelium, capillary pericytes, and CIC, a conclusion based on the volume contribution of these cells to peripheral lung (2) as well as the known high actin content of such cells (146). Low *et al.* (90, 91) have shown that more than 90% of lung actin is not of the smooth muscle type, although specific localization of cells containing these nonmuscle isoforms of actin has yet to be carried out.

CONTRACTILITY OF NORMAL PULMONARY PARENCHYMA

Kapanci *et al.* (76) originally demonstrated an *in vitro* contractile response of rat lungs to hypoxia and epinephrine that differed from the contractile response characteristic of smooth muscle associated with bronchi and pulmonary arteries. Results of more detailed studies by Evans and Adler (46) pointed toward a similar conclusion. Isolated parenchymal strips respond differently to histamine, acetylcholine and epinephrine than isolated airways and vessels of the same size as found within the strips. For example, strips contract with epinephrine, whereas airway preparations relax. The differences in contractile responses have been attributed to the presence of CICs within the strips (74, 76). Additional evidence for such conclusions has come from parallel studies of fibrotic lung (see below).

It has been hypothesized that CIC may play an important role in fine tuning of ventilation-perfusion matching. As an example, Kapanci *et al.* (76, 77) hypothesized that hypoxia, known to cause parenchymal strips to contract, would shut down capillary blood flow, causing a shunting of blood to normoxic regions of the lung. On a larger scale, contractile elements of the parenchyma could offer a mechanism for rapid changes in lung elastic recoil. Weibel and Gil (158) describe a pulmonary mechanical continuum consisting of: (a) peripheral elements of the pleura and its extensions which contribute passive (connective tissue) elements; (b) bronchovascular axial components which contribute passive (connective tissue) elements as well as active components made up of smooth muscle surrounding vessels and airways; (c) in between, parenchymatous alveolar septal elements contributing a passive component to the mechanical continuum due to connective tissue and surface tension forces. We have proposed that, as well, these parenchymatous elements contain an active component, the CIC, the contractility of which can be rapidly modulated by ambient conditions, such as oxygen tension or local concentrations of catecholamines (46).

Indeed, there are a number of reports in the literature indicating that rapid and reversible changes in elastic recoil and lung volume do occur. This is well-demonstrated in asthmatics (162). Rapid, repetitive, reversible changes in total lung capacity and compliance also have been described associated with exercise (70, 106) and in response to metaproterenol (70). Fenaterol, a β-2-antagonist, has been reported to cause a reduction in lung recoil pressure (37). Analagous studies in animal models have shown that increased elastic recoil and decreased lung volumes occur in dogs in response to hypoxia (136) and increases in elastic recoil pressure at lung volumes

above functional residual capacity have been reported in rats exposed to epinephrine (48).

CONTRACTILE CELLS IN PULMONARY FIBROSIS

HUMAN FIBROTIC LUNGS

Most inflammatory diseases of the lung result in some degree of fibrosis within the alveolar interstitium [5, 30, 31, 34, 53]. However, there are certain diseases in which interstitial fibrosis, presumably initiated by an inflammatory reaction within the alveolar wall, is paramount (36), but the etiology and pathogenesis are unknown. Hallmarks of the end-stage disease are the same in most instances, with parenchymal destruction and progressive fibrosis resulting in development of the so-called "honeycomb lung" (69). These elements expand and solidify the once delicate alveolar interstitium, resulting in progressive decreases in lung compliance and decreased lung volumes, leading to a net reduction in gas exchange.

Smooth Muscle Hyperplasia. Proliferation or hyperplasia of SM cells in fibrotic lungs is a lesion familiar to many pulmonary physicians. The concept is based on early descriptions of morphologically distinctive, hyperplastic SM in the parenchyma of individuals with a variety of chronic lung diseases. In its most severe forms, this morphologic finding was termed "muscular cirrhosis of the lung" [33, 110, 152]. Subsequent investigators have used this term to refer to a variety of pulmonary diseases in which prominent parenchymal SM is combined with variable fibrosis (2, 89). During the first half of this century, sporadic cases appeared in the literature and bona fide muscular cirrhosis of the lung was considered a rare disease. To emphasize this point, Davies *et al.* (35) described 5 patients with diffuse fibrosing alveolitis with "muscular cirrhosis". A survey conducted by these authors revealed only 25 additional cases in the world literature. In a review of the musculature of the lungs in pulmonary disease, Liebow, Loring, and Felton (89) described several patterns of SM hyperplasia which varied considerably in location and extent, depending on the nature of the lung injury. Limited by techniques available at that time, it was concluded that contractile elements likely play a secondary role in the schema of lung injury, and that when fibrosis and SM were found at the same site, the latter were entrapped by the former. Diseases of the lung in which SM hyperplasia is observed include emphysema, bronchiectasis, abscess and diffuse interstitial fibrosis (2, 89).

Lymphangiomyamatosis. Another form of SM hyperplasia in the lung has been described in the rare condition of lymphangiomyamatosis. This distinctive disease of SM first was characterized clinically by Cornog and Enterline (27) in 1966. The disease is confined to women in their reproductive years, presents with shortness of breath, and progresses to death from pulmonary compromise in 1 to 10 years. In the lung, irregular aggregates and nodular masses of SM are seen in the interstitium associated with lymphatic and vascular channels. SM proliferation also is attended by loss of lung parenchyma and eventual honeycombing (28). There has been intense speculation regarding the origin of SM cells in this disease, but no certain answer has been forthcoming.

"Nonmuscle" Contractile Cells in Fibrotic Lung Disease. Based upon preliminary electron microscopic observations by Dr. Arnold R. Brody at the University of Vermont during the mid 1970s, our group examined samples of fibrotic human lung (obtained from open lung biopsies) for the presence of interstitial cells with contractile morphology (*e.g.*, bundles of cytoplasmic microfilaments) (3). Initially, the specimens were examined by light microscopy after staining with Masson's trichrome, and graded for fibrosis using a scoring system of 0 to 4+, with 0 being no visible fibrosis (using interstitial connective tissue and cellularity as criteria) and 4+ being extensive fibrosis. The more fibrotic lungs appeared to contain increased amounts of actin in septal regions, as demonstrated by immunohistochemical studies utilizing the DNAase I—antiDNAase I technique to identify actin by immunofluorescence (154). Examination by electron microscopy revealed the interstitium of the fibrotic lungs to be filled with cells containing prominent bundles of cytoplasmic filaments composed of actin, as determined by heavy meromyosin staining after glycerination.

Evans *et al.* (49) examined a different set of human lung specimens recovered from open lung biopsy or pulmonary resection. Parenchymal strips approximately 5 × 5 × 10 mm were isolated from these samples and mounted on myographs. Contractile responses to K$^+$ depolarization and to graded dosages of histamine, acetylcholine and epinephrine were measured. Fibrosis in each strip, based on histologic appearance with Masson's trichrome stain of paraffin-embedded sections, was graded as described above.

The strips could be divided into three different groups, depending on the degree of fibrosis. The first group, scoring <1.5 on the fibrotic scale ($N = 10$) were called "mildly" fibrotic; the second group, "moderately" fibrotic (1.5 to 3.0; $N = 8$ strips); the third group, "severely" fibrotic, >3.0; $N = 4$ strips). Each of the severely fibrotic group had histochemically definable (positive trichrome stain) smooth muscle in parenchymal regions. All strips contracted with K$^+$ depolarization and in response to histamine. The more fibrotic strips generated significantly more force (contracted more) than the less fibrotic strips. However, responses to acetylcholine and epinephrine were more complex. Acetylcholine only contracted strips labeled as moderately and severely fibrotic. With epinephrine, mildly fibrotic strips did not respond at all, whereas moderately fibrotic strips contracted and severely fibrotic strips relaxed. Thus, contractile responses of human lung strips to pharmacologic stimulation appear altered in fibrotic lung tissue, seeming to depend on the degree of fibrosis and the presence or absence of parenchymal smooth muscle (49).

If one were to extrapolate these data on isolated parenchymal strips to the whole lung *in vivo*, it would appear that elements within fibrotic human lungs are capable of increased contraction, especially in response to local endogenous mediators of inflammation or humoral compounds (*e.g.*, histamine) that may be present in high concentration because of the underlying lung disease (67). Thus, elements within the parenchyma, if properly stimulated, could contract, adding to lung "stiffness" and reduced compliance already present and further compromising the ability of the fibrotic lung to function.

Other investigators have observed increased microfilament-containing cells in diseased human lungs. Large numbers of myofibroblast-like cells have been observed within alveolar interstitia of open lung biopsy specimens from patients with hypersensitivity pneumonitis (82, 116). Similar cells also have been observed in pulmonary interstitium of patients suffering from systemic scleroderma with pulmonary fibrosis (78).

ANIMAL MODELS OF FIBROSIS

Although studies with fibrotic human tissue are of obvious interest, the pathogenesis is difficult to study. Fibrosis usually is well-advanced before symptoms appear in patients. In addition, problems common to many studies with human tissues and cells, such as great variability in samples, lack of appropriate controls, differing environmental/occupational exposure and smoking and lung disease history, age and sex differences, difficulty in obtaining suitable samples, etc. add to the difficulties in generating interpretable data. Thus, a number of animal models of pulmonary fibrosis have been developed to better study the pathogenesis of the disease.

A popular model of pulmonary fibrosis is generated in rodents by instillation intratracheally with bleomycin sulfate, an antineoplastic drug which causes inflammation and pulmonary lesions greatly resembling fibrosis in humans. Models have been developed in hamsters (24–26, 131), rats (38, 107, 140, 141, 159), mice (1, 50, 108), rabbit (105), dog (17) and several other species.

We have carried out extensive studies using the bleomycin-instilled rat to address the question of altered contractility of the lung in pulmonary fibrosis. Evans *et al.* (47) isolated parenchymal strips from lungs of bleomycin-instilled Fischer 344 rats and from saline-instilled (control) animals 4 weeks after instillation. When mounted on myographs, strips from bleomycin rats generated approximately twice as much force as controls (force expressed as force/gram wet weight of tissue) in response to potassium depolarization and graded dosages of acetylcholine and epinephrine. Thus, increased force was generated in response to stimulation by: (a) receptor-dependent (acetylcholine, epinephrine) and; (b) receptor-independent (potassium depolarization) mechanisms. Therefore, it appeared that a basic change in contractile capability of the fibrotic tissue, rather than in receptor sensitivity, was involved in the increased contraction.

The strips did not contain significantly different amounts of airway or vascular smooth muscle, as determined by light microscopy and image analysis, suggesting alterations in smooth muscle were not responsible for increased contractile force generated by fibrotic strips. What was apparent, however, was a dramatic increase in myofibroblast-like cells throughout the fibrotic interstitium, as determined by electron microscopy, correlating with increased immunofluorescent staining of the interstitium with antibodies to myosin (47). Doane *et al.* (38) also demonstrated increased cells staining positively with antimyosin antibodies in parenchymal regions of bleomycin-fibrotic rat lungs.

If, indeed, the numbers of nonmuscle contractile cells are increased in lungs of these animals, this should be reflected in the amount of the contractile protein, actin, within the lung. Thus, Low *et al.* (90, 91) examined the actin content of peripheral lung of 28 day bleomycin rats *versus* saline-instilled controls. When the lungs were dissected free of major airways and vessels, it was found that approximately 10% of total sodium dodecyl sulfate-extractable protein in the lung was actin, an unusually high value for nonmuscle tissues. Surprisingly, the bleomycin lungs showed only a slight and statistically insignificant increase in total actin (although these findings did not preclude increases in actin content in focal areas of fibrosis). However, there was a significant increase in the polymerized "F" form of actin *versus* the unpolymerized or soluble "G" form ("F" actin appears as microfilaments in electron micrographs). These data were interpreted as indicating increased microfilaments within lung cells, or increased numbers of cells with microfilaments. Almost all (>90%) of the increased actin was of a nonmuscle isoform, precluding its origin from smooth muscle (90, 91). Paradoxically, Mitchell *et al.* (102) utilized a monoclonal antibody specific for α-smooth muscle actin to demonstrate an apparent increase in cells containing this smooth muscle-specific isoform of actin within the bleomycin-fibrotic rat parenchyma. Interestingly enough, these cells generally do not stain with antibodies specific for smooth muscle myosin (102) suggesting that, although they express a smooth muscle-specific isoform of actin, they are "non-muscle" cells, possibly of fibroblastic origin (see the "Discussion" section of reference 102). Further immunohistochemical and ultrastructural studies are now underway to characterize the cell types involved.

We also carried out an electron microscopic morphometric study to quantify alterations within parenchyma in bleomycin-fibrotic rats (2). Lungs were sampled 14 days postbleomycin instillation, a time when fibrotic alterations presumably are occurring, and at 28 days, a time when fibrotic changes are maximal. Myofibroblasts, identified by the presence of cytoplasmic bundles of microfilaments, increased dramatically at 28 days (the time of maximal fibrosis) almost 10-fold in number and 4-fold in volume, when compared with saline controls. At 14 days, the changes were along the same lines, but not as great in magnitude. Increased numbers and volumes of myofibroblasts correlated with increased fibrosis in each separate sample (20).

An increase in microfilament-containing cells also has been found in other forms of lung injury leading to fibrosis. Thet, Parra, and Shelburne (139) studied injury and repair after acute exposure of rats to high oxygen (100% oxygen for 60 hours) with recovery in ambient air. Total interstitial cell number and volume, interstitial thickness and collagen all were increased. The interstitium became filled with myofibroblasts during the first few days after injury, during the repair process, but

numbers of these cells returned to normal within a few days, correlating with a return to normal lung architecture. In contrast, animals exposed chronically to high oxygen (85% O_2 for 14 days) demonstrated persistent fibrotic changes, with the myofibroblast population doubling between 7 and 14 days of recovery (40).

Experimental treatment of rat lungs with the herbicide, paraquat, also results in development of a model of pulmonary fibrosis, both interstitial and intraalveolar (54). After the early inflammatory events, interstitial fibroblasts migrate across damaged epithelium into the alveolar regions, where they undergo "differentiation" into myofibroblast-like cells (54).

Thus, experimental evidence indicates an increase in myofibroblast-like cells in parenchyma of fibrotic lungs of both human patients and animal models. Increased numbers of cells which stain positively for the presence of the contractile proteins, actin (3, 47) and myosin (38, 147) characterize fibrotic parenchyma of humans and animal models. Both qualitative and quantitative electron microscopic examination of fibrotic lung tissue from human patients (3, 49) and animal models (2, 20, 40, 47, 54, 139) reveal increased cells with prominent bundles of cytoplasmic filaments within the fibrotic interstitium. Parenchymal strips isolated from lungs of human patients (49) and fibrotic rats (47) demonstrate increased contraction in response to a variety of pharmacologic stimuli. Biochemical studies reveal a significant increase in nonmuscle, filamentous actin in bleomycin-fibrotic rat lungs (90, 91).

PROLIFERATION OF FILAMENT-LADEN CELLS IN GRANULATION TISSUE

Pulmonary fibrosis often is referred to as "scarring of the lung," and, indeed, does seem to have much in common with the processes of injury, repair, and scarring as seen in other tissues and organs. Fibroblast proliferation and increased deposition of collagen are hallmarks of these processes in a variety of tissues (96, 116, 124).

Studies of wound healing, scarring, and development of granulation tissue have revealed extensive proliferation of apparent nonmuscle cells containing prominent bundles of cytoplasmic microfilaments, similar to observations of fibrotic lung. In 1972, Gabbiani *et al.* (58) described the "contracting scar" concept in granulation tissue. Using surgical scars as a model, they observed proliferation of cells with ultrastructural features of both fibroblasts and SM cells. The cells were named "myofibroblasts". Electron microscopic examination of myofibroblasts reveals bundles of microfilaments within the cytoplasm, with electron-opaque areas similar to dense bodies of muscle cells scattered within bundles close to the plasmalemma. The cells generally have elongated, serrated nuclei with one or more nucleoli, well-developed rough endoplasmic reticulum and Golgi areas, scattered mitochondria, and occasional pinocytotic vesicles. Some cell-cell junctions of the macula adherens and nexus type are observed, and the cells often are associated with partial basement membranes (55, 56, 58, 59, 122, 124). These cells stain positively with antibodies to actin, indicating the presence of polymerized, filamentous actin (61). These cells essentially are identical morphologically to proliferating filament-containing cells observed in fibrotic human and animal lungs.

The analogy between granulation tissue and fibrotic lung does not stop at morphologic similarities. Strips of granulation tissue contract in response to serotonin, epinephrine, prostaglandin (PG)Fl$_a$, angiotensin, vasopressin, and bradykinin, but at a slower rate than smooth muscle. The same strips relax in response to papaverine, PGE$_1$, and PGE$_2$ (58). Strips of fibrotic lung also contract in response to epinephrine, and show increased contractile responses to a number of stimuli (47, 49).

Granulation tissue has been called a "contractile organ or a "temporary muscle" (13). The cell type responsible for this phenomenon appears to be a modified form of fibroblast situated within the connective tissue matrix of the scar tissue and characterized by abundant actin-containing microfilaments. After the wound closes and re-epitheliazation occurs, the scar tissue retracts and myofibroblasts "disappear" (60, 113). Since pulmonary fibrosis in humans is a progressive disease, the analogy to scarring and granulation tissue does not seem to follow to this end-point; as opposed to single wounds, whatever stimulus provokes a fibrotic response and myofibroblast proliferation appears to persist within the lung or, conversely, to provoke a chronic response.

The literature is replete with other descriptions of proliferation of myofibroblast-like cells, usually associated with pathologic situations characterized by connective tissue retraction, hypertrophic scars, and tissue remodeling (124). Such cells, identified by electron microscopy or with immunofluorescently tagged antibodies to contractile proteins, are present in granulation tissue of healing skin and oral mucosal wounds (133). The same is true in human (12) and CCl$_4$-induced liver cirrhosis in the rat (73); focal nodular hyperplasia of the liver in the vicinity of proliferating bile ductules and in recesses between parenchymal cells (21); the fibrous capsule surrounding silicone breast implants in humans (that may cause contraction severe enough to become symptomatic) (114); atheromatous plaque (62); nodular fascitis (160); infantile digital fibromatosis (14); other fibramatosis (51, 60, 78, 135); around implanted dental materials in connective tissue capsules (81, 93); tenosynovitis (64); ischemic contracture of muscle (64); soft tissue ganglia (163); aortic intimal thickening (62); radiation-induced pseudosarcoma of skin (9); hypertrophic scars (75); pulmonary sarcoidosis (85); burn contractures (83); human anterior capsular cataract (104); villous stroma of human placenta (52); radial scars (8); avascular capsule surrounding free-floating intraperitoneal blood clots (22); chronic otitis media (11); in "pockets" formed around inserted pacemakers (115); leiomyomatosis peritonealis disseminata (109); fibrous tissue around torn semilunar cartilage (63); various granulomas (5, 44); and a number of neoplastic and quasi-neoplastic conditions (68, 116, 123, 153). Dupuytren's disease, or Dupuytren's contracture, is a disease of the hand characterized by progressive contraction of the palmar fascia. It has been shown that myofibroblast-like cells proliferate within nodules at the disease site, and it is these cells which generate the force that causes contraction of the palmar fascia and resultant flexion of digits (6, 41, 71, 74, 143, 149).

WHAT IS THE ORIGIN OF FILAMENT-LADEN CELLS IN REMODELING TISSUE?

Historically, actin microfilament-containing cells such as those described above have been labeled "myofibroblasts" (41, 58, 71, 96, 129, 130) and have been thought to derive from fibroblasts and therefore contain fibroblastic rather than SM determinants, such as nonmuscle actin isoforms. However, stromal cells of mammary carcinomas (129) as well as some parenchymal cells of bleomycin-induced pulmonary fibrosis (102) contain α-SM actin, an isoform of actin which allegedly is specific for smooth muscle cells (129). Our preliminary results indicate the same is true in human fibrosis of unknown etiology as well as oxygen-induced lung injury in the rat. A muscle-specific actin antibody also has been reported to stain other selected granulation tissues including microfilament-containing cells involved in Dupuytren's contracture and parenchymal tissue from some cases of advanced human pulmonary fibrosis (87). At the same time, some of these tissues (*e.g.*, Dupuytren's contracture) stain negatively with antibodies specific for smooth muscle myosin (41, 143), as does bleomycin-fibrotic pulmonary interstitium (102).

Eddy, Petro, and Tomasek (41), Tomasek *et al.* (143) and Skalli *et al.* (129, 130) propose that the term "myofibroblast" be reserved for granulation tissue cells that do not contain smooth muscle determinants. This would continue to include cells characteristic of the bulk of granulation tissues, but the existence of SM determinants in some fibrotic stromal reactions may define a new category of fibrotic response and suggest the possibility of unique contractile properties.

With this in mind, we propose the following classification scheme for parenchymal microfilament-containing cells of the lung: with regard to normal lung, SM cells of airways and blood vessels, together with their close "relatives", pericytes and septal cells, may make up one subclass. These cells express SM isoforms of actin (*e.g.*, α-SM actin) and SM myosin, and probably are closely related to SM. A second subclass consists of parenchymal cells, such as the CIC and LIC, which contain prominent microfilament bundles but do not appear to contain muscle-associated contractile proteins (129, 130). These cells would be classified as myofibroblasts according to criteria proposed by Tomasek *et al.* (143) and Skalli *et al.* (129, 130) as they contain abundant microfilaments but not SM determinants.

The situation becomes more complex in fibrotic lung, as some proliferating interstitial cells appear to contain a SM-associated isoform of actin (102). There appear to be at least three separate populations of proliferating filament-containing interstitial cells, with one population perhaps related to SM or pericytes, and thus expressing SM-associated isoforms of actin and SM myosin; the second population expressing α-SM-actin but nonmuscle myosin; and the third expressing nonmuscle isoforms of actin and myosin. It is probable that many of the proliferating myofibroblast-like cells within the fibrotic parenchyma begin to express a SM-related isoform of actin (α-SM actin) because of a stimulus related to the fibrotic process, similar to stromal cells of certain mammary carcinomas and certain myoepithelial cells (129, 130). Obviously, many more immunohistochemical and electron microscopic studies need to be done to address this question, as definitions of possible relationships between proliferating filament-laden cells and fibroblasts, myofibroblasts, CIC, pericytes, or SM cells require further elucidation.

WHAT ARE THE STIMULI FOR PROLIFERATION OF MICROFILAMENT-CONTAINING CELLS IN INJURED LUNG?

Our incomplete understanding of the origin of these cells places constraints on discussions of possible signal mechanisms responsible for their proliferation and reorganization. Nonetheless, the literature suggests several underlying mechanisms that provide focus for further research. These alternatives include roles for extracellular matrix, mechanical stress, and growth factors and mediators, and are outlined below.

The Role of Extracellular Matrix. Gabbiani (55, 59, 61) has pointed out that fibroblasts, when routinely cultured on plastic or glass substrata, assume a phenotype similar to the myofibroblast-like cell characteristic of granulation tissue and remodeling lung, and is distinctly different from the normal *in vivo* tissue fibroblast. These cells now stain intensely with antibodies to actin and myosin, particularly in structures referred to as stress fibers. Cultured fibroblasts develop an extensive cytoplasmic fibrillar system that can become interconnected in the form of gap junctions. Thus, they are metabolically coupled, a major difference from normal tissue fibroblasts. Such interconnected fibroblasts can contract *in vitro* in response to serotonin (56). These cells also form specific cell-matrix contacts that Singer *et al.* (127) have labeled the "fibronexus." It would appear, then, that stimuli related to the culture substratum provoke a number of changes within cells, including polymerization and reorganization of actin, that may provide the cells with contractile capability.

Culture systems which more nearly approximate the *in vivo* environment of the fibroblast, particularly its 3-dimensional association with extracellular matrix components, preserve fibroblast morphology (and presumably function) more like what is observed *in vivo*. Elsdale and Bard (45) developed a system in which cells could be cultured on a matrix of repolymerized Type I collagen fibers, a system which has been modified by others to permit cultivation within, as well as on the surface of, such hydrated collagen lattices. Tomasek *et al.* (142) demonstrated that fibroblasts plated within hydrated collagen gels adopt a morphology resembling that *in vivo* and distinctly different than the flattened, multipolar, stress fiber-containing cells observed on tissue culture plastic. These workers also have implicated actin and tubulin filaments in the acquisition of bipolarity and cell

elongation characteristic of fibroblasts within collagen gels (142).

In a series of papers, Schor *et al.* (120, 121) examined the behavior of normal and transformed cells of diverse lineages when plated on collagen gels. They noted that cells of mesenchymal origin (*e.g.*, fibroblasts and SM cells) migrate into the collagen gels, whereas epithelial cells, both normal and transformed, tend to remain on the surface. Once within the gels, the fibroblasts make multiple contacts with the collagen fibers. Some of these contacts, especially in the presence of fibronectin, ultrastructurally resemble the "fibronexus" described by Singer *et al.* (127).

It is apparent, then, that the organization and type of extracellular substratum can have a major influence on fibroblast morphology, possibly through effects on the cytoskeleton. More direct evidence for such effects has been observed with epithelial cells. For example, Sugrue and Hay (137) reported that addition of the extracellular matrix components, collagen, laminin, and fibronectin to floating cultures of corneal epithelium inhibit blebbing of the basal epithelial surface and reorientation of cortical actin filaments. The presence of a collagen matrix promotes proliferation and differentiation of corneal epithelial cells to a stratified epithelium similar to that observed *in vivo* (66). Whereas flattened corneal epithelial cells respond to fibroblast growth factor, collagen-supported columnar epithelial cells respond to epidermal growth factor, a more "normal" mitogenic response (66). Furthermore, Tseng *et al.* (145) demonstrated that when endothelial cells are grown on extracellular matrix, total collagen synthesis is lower but more efficient, with collagen deposited primarily into the cell layer.

Recently, Bissel *et al.* (15) have reviewed the data relating extracellular matrix, cytoskeleton and differentiated function, and proposed a model of interaction whereby native periodicities in the matrix influence synthesis and assembly of the cytoskeleton, which, in turn, affects gene expression, perhaps even feeding back on the matrix, leading to a "dynamic reciprocity" between the cell and its matrix. Ingber and Jamieson (72) have proposed a model of histodifferentiation in which cells act as "tenegrity structures" sensing and responding to physical forces transduced through extracellular matrix components via membrane contacts and cytoskeletal proteins.

Commensurate with the potential importance of matrix in modulating proliferation and differentiation of myofibroblast-like cells in the fibrotic lung and other reorganizing tissues is an extensive literature demonstrating matrix elements in involved areas. Obviously, the extracellular matrix is altered considerably in the disease state. There is increased and probably altered fibronectin (39, 111) collagen (26, 95, 134, 138) elastin (65, 134) and glycosaminoglycans (65, 80) in granulation tissue and in fibrotic lungs. Aberrant interactions between the extracellular matrix and pulmonary fibroblasts or other cells could be a key stimulus modulating both proliferation and differentiation of myofibroblast-like cells in the fibrotic lung.

Mechanical Stress. It has been appreciated for some

time that mechanical stress is an important factor regulating cell and tissue growth (112). Much of this work has focused on striated muscle (155) or cultured muscle cells (29) and has indicated a selective loss of differentiation-specific contractile proteins in tissues or cells whose capacity for spontaneous generation of tension has been inhibited. In addition, passive tension or stretch has been shown to affect tissue metabolism and induce collagen deposition in a number of organs (60).

Several studies have recently appeared in the literature in which tissue culture models have been applied to the problem of metabolic control by passive stretch. Seidel *et al.* (125) showed that smooth muscle cells from canine saphenous vein cultured and then stretched (10%, 1 Hz) on polyurethane membranes have a significant increase *versus* controls in protein/cell, while at the same time maintaining the same amount of actin and myosin/cell. They also observed the cells to realign perpendicular to the direction of strain. Further, Leung, Glagov, and Matthews (88) have shown that cyclic stretching (10% stretch, 52/minute, 2 days) of medial cells from rabbit aorta grown on purified elastin membranes results in a significant increase in precursor incorporation into a number of extracellular matrix constituents, including collagen (total, type I and type III), chondroitin sulfate, and hyaluronate.

Similarly, Vandenburg and Kauffman (150, 151) reported a series of ingenious experiments in which primary cultures of embryonic chick skeletal muscle were grown on silicone membranes and then subjected to passive stretch. Their initial report (150) provided evidence that a 10% stretch over a period of 18 hours leads to an increase in amino acid transport and synthesis of proteins, including myosin heavy chains. They were subsequently able to show a reduction in the rate of degradation of long-lived proteins (151).

The primary cultures utilized by these workers in their first series of experiments were mixed cultures of myotubes and connective tissue fibroblasts in which they observed that stretch also induced an apparent proliferative increase in the fibroblast population. Earle's L-strain fibroblasts cultivated in a similar fashion on a stretchable silicon rubber substratum will tend to orient with their long axis perpendicular to the direction of the stretch (19). However, few data are available on the metabolic consequences of passive stretch on fibroblasts, even though it might reasonably be anticipated that the connective tissue matrix should respond to external mechanical stresses placed upon an organ.

When cultured endothelial cells from bovine carotid artery are exposed to "shear stress" (liquid flow) *in vitro*, they undergo reorganization of their F-actin-containing cytoskeleton culminating in the formation of "stress fibers" similar to those observed in cultured fibroblasts, aligned in the direction of flow (23, 156). Squier (132) combined wounding and stretching in skin of hairless mice. Stretching by itself resulted in no evidence of inflammation, but provoked the development of myofibroblast-like cells in the tissue. The combination of stretching and wounding also stimulated proliferation of these cells, but wounding only did not provoke such a response. These results suggest that myofibroblast-like cells derive from a modulation of existing fibroblasts brought about by mechanical tension within the material (126, 133). Kolega (84) found similar effects in epidermal epithelium from fish skin in culture. In cells held under mechanical tension by micromanipulation or by locomotive activity of other cells within the epithelium, microfilaments were aligned parallel to the tension.

Obviously, cells within the fibrotic interstitium are subjected to significant alterations in physical and mechanical stresses as the lung undergoes remodeling during the laying down of excessive connective tissue. Clearly, this must be considered as a possible stimulus for altered proliferation and organization of microfilament-containing cells within the fibrotic parenchyma.

Epithelial Integrity. Chemical signals from damaged epithelium may be an important contributor to the increased numbers of filament-laden cells characterizing the fibrotic lung. It is known that a lesion which precedes proliferation of myofibroblast-like cells in interstitial areas of lungs of rodents instilled with bleomycin is epithelial damage and type II cell hyperplasia (4, 20). Vaccaro, Brody, and Snider (148) have shown large areas of bare basement membrane within alveolar regions in bleomycin-instilled hamsters, a lesion which precedes proliferation of interstitial cells. In granulation tissue, an important key to fibroblast-myofibroblast interconversion appears to be epithelial integrity (14) as closure of the wound by re-epitheliazation could be a signal for dissipation of the connective tissue matrix and myofibroblasts, and change in production of type III to type I collagen (14).

CONSEQUENCES OF PROLIFERATION OF MYOFIBROBLAST-LIKE CELLS IN THE FIBROTIC LUNG

It remains a central problem to determine the possible functions of the increased filament-laden cells in the interstitium of fibrotic lungs. Two areas of particular focus involve; (a) what matrix elements these cells synthesize, and; (b) whether or not they are indeed contractile.

MATRIX ELEMENTS PRODUCED BY MYOFIBROBLAST-LIKE CELLS

A primary activity of myofibroblast-like cells surely involves synthesis of new connective tissue, as their well-developed rough endoplasmic reticulum, Golgi, and endocytic vesicles reflect active protein synthesis. Experimental evidence from other related systems suggests these cells synthesize both collagen and elastin. In granulation tissue, collagen synthesis is active as wound closure proceeds (123). Collagen synthesized in granulation tissue initially, when filament-laden cells are present, consists of increased type III (55). Restoration of normal proportions of type I collagen coincides with "dedifferentiation" of these cells into normal appearing fibroblasts (13, 56). Myofibroblast-like cells in the aorta synthesize elastin, collagen, and matrix material (161). Proliferation of myofibroblast-like cells is associated with synthesis of collagen in tumors (123), and it is known that similar cells populating stromal regions in scirrhous mammary carcinoma can produce both collagen and elastin (98, 144) as they do in granulation tissue (13). Myofibroblasts isolated from baboon liver produce collagen and elastin in response to the ethanol breakdown products, acetaldehyde and lactate (118). Intracytoplasmic collagen is observed within myofibroblasts in granulation tissue near human cartilage tears (63).

Although direct evidence for production of connective tissue elements by pulmonary myofibroblast-like cells has not yet been provided, such cells in interstitial regions of bleomycin-fibrotic rat lung (47) and in lungs of rats exposed chronically to high oxygen (40) are associated intimately with collagen and elastin, as are myofibroblasts in developing lung (18, 142). It is possible that these cells can produce much of the connective tissue which infiltrates the fibrotic interstitium. Conversely, their presence in large numbers within the fibrotic interstitium (40, 41) does not appear at odds with the concept of interstitial cells producing the increased amounts of connective tissue characterizing fibrosis.

CONTRACTILE ACTIVITY

This is a question of obvious importance if there are increased numbers of myofibroblast-like cells in fibrotic lungs. Results of experiments suggesting such contractility have been considered above in some detail. Again, much relevant experimental evidence has been generated in other healing or remodeling tissues characterized by proliferation of similar cells. In rats given experimental skin wounds, myofibroblast-like cells in the granulation tissue develop gap junctions, allowing for cell-cell communication and perhaps synchronous contraction (57). Microfilament-containing cells in granulation tissue also develop cell-to-stroma connections, allowing for contraction at the same time collagen is laid down (55).

How is force developed within such cells transferred to the connective tissue matrix, allowing for contraction? Baur and Parks (10) describe "myofibroblast anchoring strands," extracellular structures that connect termini of actin bundles within myofibroblasts to collagen fascicles in the extracellular space of wound-healing tissues. These strands are comprised of fibrils of fibronectin. They may serve to translate contractile forces developed intracellularly to the collagen matrix for contraction of the wound, and also may be involved in alignment of collagen fibrils.

Fibronectin has been identified via immunohistochemistry in skin wounds induced in rabbits (111), and it has been theorized that fibronectin could be involved in the processes of cell contraction and migration. As mentioned above, Singer et al. (127) have described connections between myofibroblasts in granulation tissue and the extracellular matrix as a new organelle, the "fibronexus," a transmembrane association between intracellular actin and extracellular fibronectin fibers. Using double-label immunogold electron microscopy, fibronectin and actin were localized specifically on the respective external and internal components of myofibroblast fibronexuses (128). When biopsies of guinea pig skin wounds were examined by electron microscopy, fibronectin and actin fibers were co-localized at the myofibroblast surface along attenuated cellular processes which extended deeply into the extracellular matrix. The fibronexus appears to connect collagen fibrils to intracellular actin microfilaments, and thus could serve to transmit the collective forces generated by intracellular actin microfilaments throughout the granulation tissue.

If indeed myofibroblast-like cells are involved in wound contraction, then one should be able to alter wound contraction by inhibiting cell contraction. Wound contraction *in vivo* can be inhibited by Trocinate$^{®}$, a smooth muscle relaxant (94). Cytochalasin B, an inhibitor of microfilament formation (actin polymerization) relaxes granulation tissue *in vitro* (60) although cytochalasin B was reported ineffective *in vivo* in inhibiting contraction of granulation tissue (42). Adler *et al.* (4) have demonstrated that cytochalasin D inhibits contraction of isolated pulmonary parenchymal strips, as well as isolated pulmonary vessels, essentially a preparation of SM, so effects of these purported microfilament "inhibitors" on muscle and nonmuscle tissues must be interpreted carefully.

The fibrotic lung, as well as other inflamed and injured tissue, also contains increased amounts of circulating and local immune and inflammatory mediators, many of which may have severe effects on the contractile function of microfilament-containing cells that make up a significant percentage of the interstitial cell population (2, 40). For example, rats with bleomycin-induced fibrosis demonstrate a 10-fold increase in parenchymal mast cells, coincident with a 14-fold increase in lung histamine levels (67). Other inflammatory and immune mediators that may alter cellular contractility are present in increased amounts in the fibrotic lung. These can be products of mast cells, neutrophils, and mononuclear phagocytes, and include such potent bioactive substances as platelet-activating factor, serotonin, interferon, interleukins, tumor necrosis factor, growth factors, and various chemotactic factors. Relatedly, increases in eosinophils, lymphocytes, neutrophils, macrophages and monocytes (as well as increased release of various mediators by these cells) have been reported in fibrotic lungs (16, 24, 86).

Other potential mediators are metabolites of arachidonic acid. These potent bioactive compounds could be released by inflammatory cells attracted to sites of injury and inflammation. In hamsters with bleomycin-induced pulmonary fibrosis, increased production of PGE_2 by fibroblasts has been reported (25). Alveolar macrophages from bleomycin-fibrotic rats produce increased amounts of lipoxygenase metabolites of arachidonic acid (159), compounds also increased in the bleomycin-fibrotic mouse lung (108). Indeed, bleomycin-induced fibrosis can be inhibited in rodents by inhibitors of both cyclooxygenase and lipoxygenase enzyme systems (108, 140, 159) suggesting an important role in the fibrotic process for eicosinoids. Granulation tissue contracts in response to prostaglandins (103, 117), and wound contraction *in vitro* is affected by inhibitors of prostaglandin synthesis (99). Erlich and Wyler (43) postulate that PGE, shown to be released by fibroblasts grown in collagen lattices in response to macrophage-derived inflammatory mediators, may regulate cell contraction.

Contraction of the fibrotic mass in the lung and other organs due to development of contractile elements may be an important component of the wound-healing process. The proliferation of such cell types, however, also could lead to distortion of normal tissue architecture, and thus contribute to organ dysfunction which characterizes many pathologic fibroses (43). Contractility of microfilament-containing cells in pulmonary fibrosis can be expected to alter parenchymal mechanics leading to decreased compliance and reduced lung volumes (see above). It may also serve as a mechanism for reducing the volume of nonfunctional fibrotic tissue, thus preserving space for more functional alveolar regions.

CONCLUSIONS AND DIRECTIONS FOR FUTURE STUDIES

Since Kapanci *et al.* (76) first brought the concept of the lung as a contractile organ to the attention of the pulmonary community in 1974, our knowledge of the role played by contractile elements in the function of normal and diseased lung has grown, but only modestly. Obviously, contractile elements within the lung can be of major importance in modulating lung function under normal conditions, and may be involved in pulmonary alterations in a variety of disease states, especially fibrosis.

With regard to fibrotic lung, our group has demonstrated, utilizing correlative morphologic (immunostaining, qualitative and quantitative electron microscopy, image analysis, histochemistry); pharmacomechanical (myograph studies of isolated parenchymal strips); and biochemical (actin content, polymerization and isoform determinations) approaches, that contractile cells proliferate within the interstitium of fibrotic human and animal lungs, that fibrotic lungs contain increased amounts of contractile proteins, and that fibrotic lungs are capable of increased contraction. We suggest that this phenomenon occuring within fibrotic lungs is quite similar to proliferation of myofibroblast-like cells characterizing injury and repair in a variety of other tissues and organs, such as granulation tissue of skin.

There exists a continuum of filament-containing and probably contractile cell types within the injured lung, ranging from normal fibroblasts to well-defined smooth muscle cells, and including CICs, LICs, myofibroblasts, pericytes, and intermediate-type cells. Information about interrelationships, origins, proliferation, differentiation (or de-differentiation), functions, and contributions of these cells to lung function in patients with pulmonary fibrosis is needed to both increase our understanding of an important lesion in various forms of interstitial fibrosis, and to elucidate some aspects of the pathogenesis of the disease. Where do these cells come from; what do they do; and how do they contribute to altered lung function in fibrosis; are some obvious questions that should be addressed in future studies.

Acknowledgments: We are indebted to Dr. Giulio Gabbiani, Department of Pathology, University of Geneva, for his helpful advice, for allowing us use of a number of antibodies, and for providing guidance and direction for many of our studies described in this review. We thank Dr. John E. Craighead, Department of Pathology, University of Vermont College of Medicine, for helpful suggestions.

This work was supported by Public Health Service Grant 14214 (SCOR) from The National Heart, Lung and Blood Institute.

Dr. Adler and Dr. Evans are Established Investigators of the American Heart Association.

Address reprint requests to: Dr. Kenneth B. Adler, Department of Anatomy, Physiological Sciences and Radiology, North Carolina State University, College of Veterinary Medicine, 4700 Hillsborough St., Raleigh, NC 27606.

REFERENCES

1. Adamson IYR, Bowden DH: The pathogenesis of bleomycin-induced pulmonary fibrosis in mice. Am J Pathol 77:185, 1974
2. Adler KB, Callahan LM, Evans JN: Alterations in the cellular population of the alveolar wall in bleomycin-induced pulmonary fibrosis in rats: an ultrastructural morphometric study. Am Rev Respir Dis 133:1043, 1986
3. Adler KB, Craighead JE, Vallyathan NV, Evans JN: Actin-containing cells in human pulmonary fibrosis. Am J Pathol 102:427, 1981
4. Adler KB, Krill J, Alberghini TV, Evans JN: Effect of cytochalasin D on smooth muscle contraction. Cell Motil Cytoskeleton 3:545, 1983
5. Bachofen M, Weibel E: Basic patterns of tissue repair in human lungs following unspecific injury. Chest 65 (Suppl):45, 1974
6. Badalamente MA, Stern L, Hurst LC: The pathogenesis of Dupuytren's contracture: contractile mechanisms of the myofibroblasts. J Hand Surg [Am] 8:235, 1983
7. Baltisberger W: Glatte muskulatur der menschliche lung. Zschr Anat Entwickl-gesch 61:249, 1921
8. Battersby S, Anderson TJ: Myofibroblast activity of radial scars. J Pathol 147:33, 1985
9. Baur PS, Larson DL, Stacey TR: The observation of myofibroblasts in hypertrophic scars. Surg Gynecol Obstet 141:22, 1975
10. Baur PS Jr, Parks DH: The myofibroblast anchoring strand—the fibronectin connection in wound healing and the possible loci of collagen fibril assembly. J Trauma 23:853, 1983
11. Berlinger NT, Schachern P: Myofibroblasts in chronic otitis media. Laryngoscope 93:1566, 1983
12. Bhathal PS: Presence of modified fibroblasts in cirrhotic livers in man. Pathology 4:139, 1972
13. Bhawan J: The myofibroblast. Am J Dermatopathol 3:73, 1981
14. Bhawan J, Bacchetta C, Joris I, Majno G: A myofibroblastic tumor: infantile digital fibromatosis (recurrent digital fibrous tumor of childhood). Am J Pathol 94:19, 1979
15. Bissell HG, Hall HG, Parry G: How does the extracellular matrix direct gene expression? J Theor Biol 99:31, 1982
16. Bitterman PB, Adelberg S, Crystal RG: Mechanisms of pulmonary fibrosis. Spontaneous release of the alveolar macrophage-derived growth factors in the interstitial lung disorders. J Clin Invest 72:1801, 1983
17. Bray BA, Osman M, Ashtyani H, Mandl I, Turino GM: The fibronectin content of canine lungs is increased in bleomycin-induced fibrosis. Exp Mol Pathol 44:353, 1986
18. Brody JS, Vaccaro C: Postnatal formation of alveoli: interstitial events and physiologic consequences. Fed Proc 38:215, 1979
19. Buck RS: Reorientation response of cells to repeated stretch and recoil of the substratum. Exp Cell Res 127:470, 1980
20. Callahan LM, Evans JN, Adler KB: Alterations in the cellular population of the alveolar wall in an animal model of fibrosis. A morphometric study. Chest 89:188, 1986
21. Callea F, Mebis J, Desmet VJ: Myofibroblasts in focal nodular

hyperplasia of the liver. Virchows Arch [A] 396:155, 1982
22. Campbell GR, Ryan GB: Origin of myofibroblasts in the avascular capsule around free-floating intraperitoneal blood clots. Pathology 15:253, 1983
23. Cervera M, Dreyfuss G, Penman S: Messenger RNA is translated when associated with the cytoskeleton framework in normal and VSV-infected HeLa cells. Cell 23:113, 1980
24. Chandler DB, Hyde DM, Giri SN: Morphometric estimates of infiltrative cellular changes during the development of bleomycin-induced pulmonary fibrosis in hamsters. Am J Pathol 112:170, 1983
25. Clark JG, Kostal KM, Marino BA: Bleomycin-induced pulmonary fibrosis in hamsters. An alveolar macrophage product increases fibroblast prostaglandin E2 and cyclic adenosine monophosphate and suppresses fibroblast proliferation and collagen production. J Clin Invest 72:2082, 1983
26. Clark JG, Overton JE, Marino BA, Uitto J, Starcher BC: Collagen biosynthesis in bleomycin-induced pulmonary fibrosis in hamsters. J Lab Clin Med 96:943, 1980
27. Cornog JL Jr, Enterline HT: Lymphangiomyoma, a benign lesion of chyliferous lymphatics synonymous with lymphangiopericytoma. Cancer 19:1909, 1966
28. Corrin B, Liebow AA, Friedman PJ: Pulmonary lymphangiomyomatosis. A Review. Am J Pathol 79:348, 1975
29. Crisona NJ, Strohman RC: Inhibition of contraction of cultured muscle fibers results in increased turnover of myofibrillar proteins but not of intermediate-filament proteins. J Cell Biol 96:684, 1983
30. Crystal RG, Fulmer JD, Roberts WC, Moss ML, Line BR, Reynolds HY: Idiopathic pulmonary fibrosis. Clinical, histologic, radiographic, scintographic, cytologic and biochemical aspects. Ann Intern Med 85:769, 1976
31. Crystal RG, Fulmer JD, Baune BJ: Cells, collagen, and idiopathic pulmonary fibrosis. Lung 155:199, 1978
32. Crystal R, Gadek J, Ferrans V, Fulmer JD, Line BR, Hunninghake GW: Interstitial lung disease: current concepts of pathogenesis, staging and therapy. Am J Med 70:542, 1981
33. Davidson C: Uber muskulare lungencirrhose. Berl Klin Wchnschr 44:33, 1907
34. Davies D, Crowther JS, MacFarlane A: Idiopathic progressive pulmonary fibrosis. Thorax 30:316, 1975
35. Davies D, Macfarlane A, Darke CS, Dodge OG: Muscular hyperplasia ('cirrhosis') of the lung and bronchial dilatations as features of chronic diffuse fibrosing alveolitis. Thorax 21:272, 1966
36. DeRemee RA, Harrison EG, Anderson HA: The concept of classic interstitial pneumonitis-fibrosis (CIP-F) as a clinico-pathologic syndrome. Chest 61:213, 1972
37. DeTroyer A, Yernault JC, Roderstein D: Influence of beta-2 agonist aerosols on pressure-volume characteristics of the lungs. Am Rev Respir Dis 118:987, 1978
38. Doane K, McReynolds RA, Wilson FJ: Immunofluorescence localization of contractile proteins in the rat lung following bleomycin treatment. Histochem J 15:82, 1983
39. Dubaybo BA, Thet LA: Changes in lung tissue and lavage fibronectin after paraquat injury in rats. Res Commun Chem Pathol Pharmacol 51:211, 1986
40. Durr RA, Bubayo BA, Thet LA: Repair of chronic hyperoxic lung injury: Changes in lung ultrastructure and matrix. Exp Mol Pathol 47:219, 1987
41. Eddy RJ, Petro JA, Tomasek JJ: Evidence for the nonmuscle nature of the "myofibroblast" of granulation tissue and hypertrophic scar: an immunofluorescence study. Am J Pathol 130:252, 1988
42. Ehrlich HP, Grislis G, Hunt TK: Evidence for the involvement of microtubules in wound contraction. Am J Surg 133:706, 1977
43. Ehrlich HP, Wyler DJ: Fibroblast contraction of collagen lattices in vitro: inhibition by chronic inflammatory cell mediators. J Cell Physiol 116:345, 1983
44. El-Labban NG, Lee KW: Myofibroblasts in central giant cell granuloma of the jaws: an ultrastructural study. Histopathology 7:907, 1983
45. Elsdale TR, Bard JBL: Collagen substrata for studies on cell behavior. J Cell Biol 54:626, 1972
46. Evans JN, Adler KB: The lung strip: evaluation of a method to study contractility of pulmonary parenchyma. Exp Lung Res 2:187, 1981
47. Evans JN, Kelley J, Low RB, Adler KB: Increased contractility of isolated lung parenchyma in an animal model of pulmonary fibrosis induced by bleomycin. Am Rev Respir Dis 125:89, 1982
48. Evans JN, Krill J, Adler KB, Low RB, Kelley J: Active cellular control of alveolar compliance. Current Probs Clin Biochem 13:142, 1983
49. Evans JN, Low RB, Kelley J, Krill J, Adler KB: The myofibroblast in pulmonary fibrosis. Chest 83:97, 1983
50. Fasske E, Morgenroth K: Experimental bleomycin lung in mice. A contribution to the pathogenesis of pulmonary fibrosis. Lung 161:133, 1983
51. Feiner H, Kaye GI: Ultrastructural evidence of myofibroblasts in circumscribed fibromatosis. Arch Pathol Lab Med 100:265, 1976
52. Feller AC, Schneider H, Schmidt D, Parwaresch MR: Myofibroblast as a major cellular constituent of villous stroma in human placenta. Placenta 6:405, 1985
53. Fraire AE, Greenberg SD, O'Neal RM, Weg JG, Jenkins DE: Diffuse interstitial fibrosis of the lung. Am J Clin Pathol 59:636, 1973
54. Fukuda Y, Ferrans DJ, Schoenberger CI, Rennard SI, Crystal RG: Patterns of pulmonary structural remodeling after experimental paraquat toxicity. The morphogenesis of intraalveolar fibrosis. Am J Pathol 118:452, 1985
55. Gabbiani G: The role of contractile proteins in wound healing and fibrocontractive diseases. Methods Achiev Exp Pathol 9:187, 1979
56. Gabbiani G: The myofibroblast: a key cell for wound healing and fibrocontractive diseases. In Connective Tissue Research: Chemistry, Biology & Physiology, p 183. New York, Alan R Liss Inc, 1981
57. Gabbiani G, Chaponnier C, Huttner I: Cytoplasmic filaments and gap junctions in epithelial cells and myofibroblasts during wound healing. J Cell Biol 76:561, 1978
58. Gabbiani G, Hirschel BJ, Ryan GB, Statkov PR, Majno G: Granulation tissue as a contractile organ. A study of structure and function. J Exp Med 135:719, 1972
59. Gabbiani G, Kocher O: Cytocontractile and cytoskeletal elements in pathologic processes. Arch Pathol Lab Med 107:622, 1983
60. Gabbianni G, Majno G: Dupuytren's contracture. Fibroblast contracture? An ultrastructural study. Am J Pathol 66:131, 1972
61. Gabbiani G, Ryan GB, Lamelin J-P, Vassalli P, Majno G, Bouvier CA, Cruchaud A, Luscher EF: Human smooth muscle autoantibody. It's identification as antiactin antibody and a study of its binding to "nonmuscular" cells. Am J Pathol 72:473, 1973
62. Geer JL: Fine structure of human aortic intimal thickening and fatty streaks. Lab Invest 14:1764, 1965
63. Ghadially FN, Lalonde JMA, Yong NK: Myofibroblasts and intracellular collagen in torn semilunar cartilages. J Submicrosc Cytol 12:447, 1980
64. Ghadially FN, Mehta PN: Multifunctional mesenchymal smooth muscle cells in ganglia of the wrist. Ann Rheum Dis 30:31, 1971
65. Goldstein RH, Fine A: Fibrotic reactions in the lung: the activation of the lung fibroblast. Exp Lung Res 11:245, 1986
66. Gospodarowicz D, Greenburg G, Birdwell CR: Determination of cellular shape by the extracellular matrix. Correlation with the control of cellular growth. Cancer Res 38:4155, 1978
67. Goto T, Befus D, Low R, Bienenstock J: Mast cell heterogeneity and hyperplasia in bleomycin-induced pulmonary fibrosis of rats. Am Rev Respir Dis 130:797, 1984
68. Hashimoto K, Matsui K, Akeho M, Okamoto K, Yumoto T, Endo A: A tumor composed of myofibroblasts. An ultrastructural study. Acta Pathol Jpn 32:633, 1982
69. Heppleston AG: The pathology of honeycomb lung. Thorax 11:77, 1956
70. Hudgel DW, Cooper D, Souhrada J: Reversible restrictive lung disease. Ann Intern Med 85:328, 1976
71. Hurst LC, Badalamente MA, Makowski J: The pathobiology of Dupuytren's contracture: effects of prostaglandins on myofibroblasts. J Hand Surg 11:18, 1986
72. Ingber DE, Jamieson JD: Cells as tensegrity structures: architectural regulation of histodifferentiation by physical forces transduced over basement membrane. In Gene Expression During Normal and Malignant Differentiation, edited by Anderson LC, Gahmberg CG, Ekblom P, p 13. London, Academic Press, 1985
73. Irle C, Kocher O, Gabbiani G: Contractility of myofibroblasts during experimental liver cirrhosis. J Submicrosc Cytol 12:209,

1980

74. James WD, Odom RB: The role of the myofibroblast in Dupuytren's contracture. Arch Dermatol 116:807, 1980

75. Judd PA, Finnegan P, Curran RC: Pulmonary sarcoidosis: a clinicopathological study. J Pathol 115:191, 1975

76. Kapanci Y, Assimacopoulos A, Irle C, Zwahlen A, Gabbiani G: "Contractile interstitial cells" in pulmonary alveolar septa: a possible regulator of ventilation/perfusion ratio? J Cell Biol 60:375, 1974

77. Kapanci Y, Mo Costabella P, Gabbiani G: Location and function of contractile interstitial cells of the lungs. In Lung Cells in Disease, edited by Bouhys A, p 69. Elsevier North Holland, Biomedical Press, 1976

78. Kapanci Y, Mo Costabella P, Cerutti P, Assimacopoulos A: Distribution and function of cytoskeletal proteins in lung cells with particular reference to "contractile interstitial cells". Methods Achiev Exp Pathol 9:147, 1979

79. Kaplan NB, Grant MM, Brody JS: The lipid interstitial cell of the pulmonary alveolus. Age and species differences. Am Rev Respir Dis 132:1307, 1985

80. Karlinsky JB, Goldstein RH: Fibrotic lung disease—a perspective. J Lab Clin Med 96:939, 1980

81. Katenkamp D, Neupert G, Stiller D: Myofibroblasts in connective tissue capsules around implanted dental materials. Exp Pathol (Jena) 18:31, 1980

82. Kawanami O, Basset F, Barrios R, Lacronique JG, Ferrans VJ, Crystal RG: Hypersensitivity pneumonitis in man. Light and electron microscopic studies of 18 lung biopsies. Am J Pathol 110:275, 1983

83. Kiryu H, Tsuneyoshi M, Enjoji M: Myofibroblasts in fibromatoses. An electron microscopic study. Acta Pathol Jpn 35:533, 1985

84. Kolega J: Effects of mechanical tension on protrusive activity and microfilament and intermediate filament organization in an epidermal epithelium moving in culture. J Cell Biol 102:1400, 1986

85. Lawson DL, Baur P, Linares H, Willis B, Abston S, Lewis SR: Mechanisms of hypertrophic scar and contracture formation in burns. Burns 1:119, 1973

86. Leibovich SJ, Ross R: A macrophage-dependent factor that stimulates the proliferation of fibroblasts in vitro. Am J Pathol 84:501, 1976

87. Leslie KO, Woodcock-Mitchell J, Mitchell J, Adler KB, Low R, Skalli O, Gabbianni G: Alpha smooth muscle actin distribution in developing and adult lung (abstr). J Cell Biol 105:25, 1987

88. Leung DYM, Glagov S, Matthews MB: Cyclic stretching stimulates synthesis of matrix components by arterial smooth muscle cells in vitro. Science 191:475, 1976

89. Liebow AA, Loring WE, Felton WL: The musculature of the lungs in chronic pulmonary disease. Am J Pathol 29:885, 1953

90. Low RB, Woodcock-Mitchell J, Absher PM, Evans JN, Adler KB: Contractile proteins of the lung. Current Probs Clin Biochem 13:149, 1983

91. Low RB, Woodcock-Mitchell J, Evans JN, Adler KB: Actin content of normal and of bleomycin-fibrotic rat lung. Am Rev Respir Dis 129:311, 1984

92. Macklin CC: The musculature of the bronchi and lungs. Physiol Rev 9:1, 1929

93. Madden JW: On "the contractile fibroblast". Plast Reconstr Surg, 52:291, 1973

94. Madden JW, Morton D, Jr., Peacock EE, Jr.: Contraction of experimental wounds: I. Inhibiting wound contraction by using a topical smooth muscle antagonist. Surgery 76:8, 1974

95. Madri JA, Furthmayr H: Collagen polymorphism in the lung. An immunochemical study of pulmonary fibrosis. Human Pathol 11:353, 1980

96. Majno G: The story of the myofibroblasts. Am J Surg Pathol 3:535, 1979

97. Martels H: Freeze-fracture demonstration of communicating junctions between interstitial cells of the pulmonary interalveolar septa. Am J Anat 155:125, 1979

98. Martinez-Hernandez A, Francis DJ, Silverberg SG: Elastosis and other stromal reactions in benign and malignant breast tissue. Cancer 40:700, 1977

99. McGrath MH: The effect of prostaglandin inhibitors on wound contraction and the myofibroblast. Plast Reconstr Surg 69:74, 1982

100. Meyrick B, Reid L: The alveolar wall. Br J Dis Chest 64:121, 1970

101. Miller WS: The musculature of the finer divisions of the bronchial tree and its relation to certain pathological conditions. Am Rev TB 5:689, 1921

102. Mitchell J, Woodcock-Mitchell J, Reynolds S, Low RB, Leslie KO, Adler KB, Gabbiani G, Skalli O: α-Smooth muscle actin in parenchymal cells of bleomycin-injured rat lung. Lab Invest, in press 1989

103. Montandon D, Gabbiani G, Ryan GB, Majno G. The contractile myofibroblast: its relevance in plastic surgery. Plast Reconstr Surg 52:286, 1973

104. Novotny GE, Paul H: Myofibroblast-like cells in human anterior capsular cataract. Virchows Arch [A] 404:393, 1984

105. O'Connor CM, O'Brien AO, Sweeney EC, FitzGerald MX: Progress of bleomycin-induced lung fibrosis in rabbits. Br J Exp Pathol 67:461, 1986

106. Peress L, Sybrecht G, Macklem PT: The mechanism of increase in total lung capacity during acute asthma. Am J Med 61:165, 1976

107. Phan SE, Varani J, Smith D: Rat lung fibroblast collagen metabolism in bleomycin-induced pulmonary fibrosis. J Clin Invest 76:241, 1985

108. Phan SH, Kunkel SL: Inhibition of bleomycin-induced pulmonary fibrosis by nordihydroguiaretic acid. The role of alveolar macrophage activation and mediator production. Am J Pathol 124:343, 1986

109. Pieslor PC, Orenstein JM, Hogan DL, Breslow A: Ultrastructure of myofibroblasts and decidualized cells in leiomyomatosis peritonealis disseminata. Am J Clin Pathol 72:875, 1979

110. Reisseisen FD: Uber den bau der lungen. Berlin, A. Rucker, 1822

111. Repesh LA, Fitzgerald TJ, Furcht LT: Fibronectin involvement in granulation tissue and wound healing in rabbits. J Histochem Cytochem 30:351, 1982

112. Rodbard S: Negative feedback mechanisms in the architecture and function of the connective and cardiovascular tissues. Perspect Biol Med 13:507, 1970

113. Rudolph R, Guber S, Suzuki M, Woodward M: The life cycle of the myofibroblast. Surg Gynecol Obstet 145:389, 1977

114. Rudolph R, Abraham J, Vecchione T, Guber S, Woodward M: Myofibroblasts and free silicon around breast implants. Plast Reconstr Surg 62:185, 1978

115. Rudolph R, Utley JR, Woodward M: Contractile fibroblasts (myofibroblasts) in a painful pacemaker pocket. Ann Thorac Surg 31:373, 1981

116. Rungger-Brandle E, Gabbiani G: The role of cytoskeletal and cytocontractile elements in pathologic processes. Am J Pathol 110:360, 1983

117. Ryan GB, Cliff WJ, Gabbiani G, Irle C, Montandon D, Statkov PR, Majno G: Myofibroblasts in human granulation tissue. Hum Pathol 5:55, 1974

118. Savolainen ER, Leo MA, Timpl R, Lieber CS: Acetaldehyde and lactate stimulate collagen synthesis of cultured baboon liver myofibroblasts. Gastroenterology 87:777, 1984

119. Scadding JG, Hinson KFW: Diffuse fibrosing alveolitis (diffuse interstitial fibrosis of the lungs). Thorax 22:291, 1967

120. Schor SL: Cell proliferation and migration on collagen substrate in vitro. J Cell Sci 41:159, 1980

121. Schor SL, Allen TD, Harrison CJ: Cell migration through three dimensional gels of native collagen fibres: collagenolytic activity is not required for the migration of two permanent cell lines. J Cell Sci 46:171, 1980

122. Schurch W, Seemayer TA, Lagace R, Gabbiani G: The intermediate filament cytoskeleton of myofibroblasts: an immunofluorescence and ultrastructural study. Virchows Arch [A] 403:323, 1984

123. Seemayer TA, Schurch W, Lagace R, Tremblay G: Myofibroblasts in the stroma of invasive and metastatic carcinoma. A possible host response to neoplasia. Am J Surg Pathol 3:525, 1979

124. Seemayer TA, Lagace R, Schurch W, Thelmo WL: The myofibroblast: biologic, pathologic, and theoretical considerations. Pathol Annu 15:443, 1980

125. Seidel CL, Ives CL, Vu B, Eskin SL: The effect of strain on vascular smooth muscle cells in culture. Physiologist 27:236, 1984

126. Shields B, Blobel G: Cell-free synthesis of fish preproinsulin, and processing by heterologous mammalian microsomal membranes. Proc Nat Acad Sci USA 74:2059, 1977

127. Singer II, Kawka DW, Kazazis DM, Clark RAF: In vivo codistri-

bution of fibronectin and actin fibers in granulation tissue: immunofluorescence and electron microscope studies of the fibronexus at the myofibroblast surface. J Cell Biol 98:2091, 1984

128. Singer II, Kazazis DM, Kawka DW: Localization of the fibronexus at the surface of granulation tissue myofibroblasts using double-label immunogold electron microscopy on ultrathin frozen sections. Eur J Cell Biol 38:94, 1985

129. Skalli O, Ropraz P, Trzeciak A, Benzonana G, Gillessen D, Gabbiani G: A monoclonal antibody against alpha-smooth muscle actin: A new probe for smooth muscle differentiation. J Cell Biol 103:2787, 1986

130. Skalli O, Vandekerckhove J, Gabbiani G: Actin-isoform pattern as a marker of normal or pathological smooth-muscle and fibroblastic tissues. Differentiation 33:232, 1987

131. Snider GL, Hayes JA, Korthy AL: Chronic interstitial pulmonary fibrosis produced in hamsters by endotracheal bleomycin. Pathology and stereology. Am Rev Respir Dis 117:1099, 1978

132. Squier CA: The effect of stretching on formation of myofibroblasts in mouse skin. Cell Tissue Res, 220:325, 1981

133. Squier CA, Leranth CS, Ghoneim S, Kremenak CR: Electron microscopic immunochemical localization of actin in fibroblasts in healing skin and palate wounds of beagle dog. Histochemistry 78:513, 1983

134. Starcher BC, Kuhn C, Overton JE: Increased elastin and collagen content in the lungs of hamsters receiving an intratracheal injection of bleomycin. Am Rev Respir Dis 117:299, 1978

135. Stiller D, Katenkemp D: Cellular features in desmoid fibromatosis and well-differentiated fibrosarcomas: an electron microscopic study. Virchows Arch [A] 369:155, 1975

136. Streider DJ, Laguarda R, Stigol LC, Wohl ME: Increased lung recoil during acute hypoxia in dogs. Respir Physiol 21:193, 1974

137. Sugrue SP, Hay ED: Response of basal epithelial cell surface and cytoskeleton to solubilized extracellular matrix molecules. J Cell Biol 91:45, 1981

138. Takiya C, Peyrol S, Cordier J-F, Grimaud J-A: Connective matrix organization in human pulmonary fibrosis. Collagen polymorphism analysis in fibrotic deposits by immunohistological methods. Virchows Arch [B] 44:223, 1983

139. Thet LA, Parra SC, Shelburne JD: Sequential changes in lung morphology during the repair of acute oxygen-induced lung injury in adult rats. Exp Lung Res 11:209, 1986

140. Thrall RS, Barton RW, D'Amato DA, Sulavik SB: Differential cellular analysis of bronchoalveolar lavage fluid obtained at various stages during the development of bleomycin-induced pulmonary fibrosis in the rat. Am Rev Respir Dis 126:488, 1982

141. Thrall RS, McCormick JR, Jack RM, McReynolds RA, Ward PA: Bleomycin-induced pulmonary fibrosis in the rat. Inhibition by indomethacin. Am J Pathol 95:117, 1979

142. Tomasek JJ, Hay ED: Analysis of the role of microfilaments and microtubules in acquisition of bipolarity and elongation of fibroblasts in hydrated collagen gels. J Cell Biol 99:536, 1984

143. Tomasek JJ, Schultz RJ, Episalla CW, Newman SA: The cytoskeleton and extracellular matrix of the Dupuytren's disease "myofibroblast": an immunofluorescence study of a nonmuscle cell type. J Hand Surgery 11A:365, 1986

144. Tremblay G: Stromal aspects of breast carcinoma. Exp Mol Pathol 31:248, 1979

145. Tseng SCG, Savion N, Gospodarowicz D, Stern R: Modulation of collagen synthesis by a growth factor and by the extracellular matrix: comparison of cellular response to two different stimuli. J Cell Biol 97:803, 1983

146. Tsilibary EC, Williams MC: Actin in peripheral rat lung: S1 labeling and structural changes induced by cytochalasin. J Histochem Cytochem 31:1289, 1983

147. Vaccaro C, Brody JS: Ultrastrucuture of developing alveoli. The role of the interstitial fibroblasts. Anat Rec 192:467, 1978

148. Vaccaro C, Brody JS, Snider GL: Alveolar wall basement membranes in bleomycin-induced pulmonary fibrosis. Am Rev Respir Dis 132:905, 1985

149. Vande Berg JS, Gelberman RH, Rudolph R, Johnson D, Sicurello P: Dupuytren's disease: comparative growth dynamics and morphology between cultured myofibroblasts (nodule) and fibroblasts (cord). J Orthop Res 2:247, 1984

150. Vandenburg H, Kaufman S: In vitro model for stretch-induced hypertrophy of smooth muscle. Science 203:265, 1979

151. Vandenburg H, Kaufman S: Protein degradation in embryonic skeletal muscle. Effect of medium, cell type, inhibitors and passive stretch. J Biol Chem 255:5826, 1980

152. Von Stossel E: Uber muskulare cirrhose der lunge. Beitr z Klin d Tuberk 90:432, 1937

153. Wakanishi I, Kajikawa K, Okada Y, Eguchi K: Myofibroblasts in fibrous tumors and fibrosis in various organs. Acta Pathol Jpn 31:423, 1981

154. Wang E, Goldberg AR: Binding of deoxyribonuclease I to actin: a new way to visualize microfilament bundles in nonmuscle cells. J Histochem Cytochem 26:745, 1978

155. Waterlow JC, Garlick PJ, Milkward DJ: In Protein Turnover in Mammalian Tissues and in the Whole Body, Oxford, North-Holland Publishing Co., 1978

156. Wechezak AR, Viggers RF, Sauvage LR: Fibronectin and F-actin redistribution in cultured endothelial cells exposed to shear stress. Lab Invest 53:639, 1985

157. Weibel ER: On pericytes, particularly their existence on lung capillaries. Microvasc Res 8:218, 1974

158. Weibel ER, Gil J: Structure-function relationships at the alveolar level. In Bioengineering Aspects of the Lung, edited by West JB, p 1. New York/Basel, Dekker, 1977

159. Wesselius LJ, Catanzaro A, Wasserman SI: Neutrophil chemotactic activity generation by alveolar macrophages after bleomycin injury. Am Rev Respir Dis 129:485, 1984

160. Wiseman JA: Nodular fascitis, a lesion of myofibroblasts: an ultrastructural study. Cancer 38:2378, 1976

161. Wissler RW: The arterial medial cell, smooth muscle or multifunctional mesenchyme? Circulation 36:1, 1967

162. Woolcock AJ, Read J: The static elastic properties of the lungs in asthma. Am Rev Respir Dis 98:788, 1968

163. Woyke S, Domagala W, Olszewski W, Korabiec M: Pseudocarcinoma of the skin. An electron microscopic study and comparison with fine structure of the spindle-cell variant of squamous cell carcinoma. Cancer 33:970, 1974

From: *Pathology Reviews • 1990* Edited by: E. Rubin and I. Damjanov Copyright © 1990 The Humana Press Inc., Clifton, NJ

Biology of Disease

Role of Folate Binding Proteins in Folate Metabolism

MADELEINE A. KANE AND SAMUEL WAXMAN

Medical Oncology and Hematology Sections, Denver Veterans Administration Medical Center and University of Colorado Health Sciences Center, Denver, Colorado, and Chemotherapy Foundation Laboratory, Department of Medicine, Mount Sinai Medical Center, New York, New York

ABSTRACT

The essential role of folates in cellular biochemistry is well established, but the nature of the participation by folate-binding proteins has been disputed. This review will define folate-binding proteins and distinguish them from low-affinity, nonspecific folate binders and folate-dependent intracellular enzymes. We outline changes in plasma folate-binding proteins in various clinical states, review their postulated functions, detail the biochemistry of mammalian soluble folate-binding proteins and their membrane-bound immunologically cross-reactive possible precursors, and present evidence that the latter proteins may function as the physiologic folate receptors and intracellular regulators of folate coenzyme availability.

INTRODUCTION

The essential role of folates in cellular biochemistry is well-established, but the nature of the participation by folate-binding proteins, previously reviewed, (11, 18, 39, 47, 57, 59, 79, 80, 94, 112, 113, 119) has been disputed. Plasma-binding proteins for the transport of small molecules such as vitamin B12, iron, and thyroid hormone may protect their ligands from proteolytic degradation and target them to appropriate effector cells. Specific high affinity plasma folate-binding proteins (FBPs), levels of which vary in certain normal and disease states, may perform a similar function for the physiologic form of folate in human circulation, N-5-methyltetrahydrofolate ($CH_3H_4PteGlu$). This review will define FBPs and distinguish them from low-affinity nonspecific folate binders and folate-dependent intracellular enzymes, out-

line changes in plasma FBPs in various clinical states, review their postulated functions, detail the biochemistry of mammalian soluble FBPs and their membrane-bound immunologically cross-reactive possible precursors, and present evidence that the latter proteins may function as the physiologic folate receptors and intracellular regulators of folate coenzyme availability.

FOLATE-BINDING PROTEIN: A DEFINITION

The term folate-binding protein has been applied to (a) enzymes utilizing folate coenzymes (13–15, 112, 120–122), (b) low affinity binders such as albumin (105) and hemoglobins (8, 42), and (c) specific high affinity FBPs, for which this term is reserved (51–54). FBPs have affinity constants (K_a's) for folic acid (PteGlu) in the range 10^9 to 10^{10} M^{-1} (See Table 1) and are a family of immunologically cross-reactive glycoproteins which exist in two physical forms. Soluble FBPs have been identified in serum (28, 115), milk (34, 48, 93, 110), neutrophils (20, 85), saliva (81), urine (41), cerebrospinal fluid (65), tumor tissue (102), and conditioned tissue culture medium (67). Particulate FBPs requiring detergent for solubilization have been found in milk (4, 113), serum of alcoholic patients with folate deficiency and liver disease (115), and in cell membranes (4, 5, 71, 77, 97, 106). Although PteGlu is the most studied folate ligand, FBPs exhibit a similar high affinity for the principal plasma folate, $CH_3H_4PteGlu$, as well. The specificity of FBPs is reflected by their relative affinities for the most commonly studied folate analogs: PteGlu $\geq$ $CH_3H_4PteGlu$ $>>>$ N-5-formyltetrahydrofolate ($CHOH_4PteGlu$) $\geq$ methotrexate (4, 5, 27, 119). Some FBPs exhibit a higher affinity for the naturally occurring 1-isomer of

TABLE 1. MAMMALIAN SOURCES OF FOLATE-BINDING PROTEINS

Source	Form	Mol wt	K_a	Purified	Reference
Rat intestine					
brush border	Particulate	16–24,000	2.5×10^4	No	71
brush border	Vesicles		2.4×10^6	No	100
Human placenta	Particulate	38,500	3.5×10^9	Yes	5
Hog choroid plexus	Particulate	51,000		Yes	108
Human choroid plexus	Particulate	45–60,000		Partial	109
Human milk	Particulate	35,000	1×10^9	Yes	4
Rat kidney	Particulate	30,000	7×10^9	Yes	96
Human KB cell	Particulate	40,000	2×10^9	Yes	27, 67, 74
Rabbit choroid plexus	Particulate	360–400,000	10^9	No	106
Human liver	Particulate	30,000	2×10^9	No	21
Rat renal cortex	Particulate	40–160,000	3×10^{10}	No	16
Human erythrocyte	Particulate	160,000		No	2
Human mononuclear cells	Particulate	160,000	ND[a]	No	Unpublished observation
Human HL60	Particulate	160,000	ND	No	Unpublished observation
Hog kidney	Soluble	38,500	5×10^{12}	Yes	64
Human umbilical	Soluble	40,000	9×10^{10}	Yes	62
Goat milk	Soluble	30,000		Yes	87
Human CML cells	Soluble	44,000	10^9	Yes	31
Human leukocytes	Soluble	25,000	2×10^{10}	No	55
Cow milk	Soluble		10^{10}	Yes	40, 117
Human cerebrospinal fluid	Soluble	25,000	10^{10}	No	44
Human milk	Soluble	30,000	10^9	Yes	4, 117
Human KB cell	Soluble	40,000		Yes	67
Human serum	Soluble	30,000		No	115
Hog intestinal					
brush border	Soluble	25,000		No	26
Human urine	Soluble	35,000	3×10^9	No	41
Human spleen	Soluble			No	22
Human mononuclear cells	Soluble	40,000		No	Unpublished observation

[a] ND, Not determined.

$CH_3H_4PteGlu$ (*e.g.*, porcine serum FBP), whereas others bind both diastereomers equally well (milk FBP) (56, 78, 101, 118). In addition, FBPs are relatively stable to oxidation and pH extremes. Sulfhydryl protectors do not enhance folate binding. FBPs release bound folates when exposed to low pH (~3). Folyl polyglutamates bind more tightly than the monoglutamates to milk FBPs (101), but no better than the monoglutamates to purified FBP from hog serum (97), hog kidney (64), or human leukemia cells (89). Methotrexate polyglutamates bound much more tightly to KB cell FBPs than the monoglutamates (27, 68).

CLINICAL ASPECTS OF FOLATE-BINDING PROTEINS

Plasma soluble FBPs have been quantified by radioactive PteGlu binding assays (115). Since these FBPs exist in both the apo and holo forms, endogenous folate removal is necessary before total FBP measurement by binding assay (see below) (83). Elevated levels of FBP may accompany folate deficiency states (115). Severe liver disease (19, 115) and oral contraceptives also elevated FBP. Significantly elevated levels of FBP were found in the third trimester of pregnancy in one study (17), but significantly lower total and unsaturated FBP levels were found in all pregnant women although plasma folate levels did not change (123). The folate binding ability of placental membranes from growth-retarded rat fetuses whose dams were exposed to chronic high doses of ethanol was significantly decreased, although endogenous folate was not removed or measured before binding assays (32). Soluble FBP levels were lower in estrogen-receptor-positive breast cancers, and higher in estrogen-receptor-negative ones (84).

Several clinical conditions may arise from defective folate transport, possibly a defective membrane-associated FBP. FBPs have not been measured in patients with Fragile X Syndrome. However, treatment of those individuals with pharmacologic doses of folates predictably results in clinical improvement in most cases (72). The possibility of a defect in folate transport remains to be investigated, and the significance of these reports is not clear (69). Severe megaloblastic anemia and mental retardation associated with an apparent inherited defect in intestinal folate absorption could be treated with high doses of folates (70–73). The macrocytosis associated with dilantin therapy appears to be due to interference with folate absorption, but the molecular mechanism has not been elucidated (7). Supplemental folate can overcome this hematologic side effect.

The major clinical application of FBPs at present is as laboratory reagents in the competitive radioligand binding assay for serum and red blood cell folate content. Although this assay approach avoids the expense, time and some of the pitfalls of the microbiologic assays, the commercially available kits use FBPs from different sources as well as different assay conditions which make them not directly comparable (101) with each other or the microbiologic assay. Also, folyl polyglutamates within the erythrocyte may bind differently to the FBP depending on its source, compared with the monoglutamates in serum. Thus, careful standardization is necessary. Nevertheless, the convenience and reproducibility of these assays make them useful for the clinical laboratory (118).

FOLATE-BINDING PROTEIN: A PHYSIOLOGIC SATURABLE MEMBRANE TRANSPORT SYSTEM FOR FOLATES

The transport mechanism and systems involved in the folate uptake by cells are controversial. This may be the result of folate transport studies using cells grown in the usual culture media, which contain 2 to 4 $\times$ 10^{-6} M PteGlu, a nonphysiologic folate level 100-fold higher than the normal plasma folate concentration. Based upon studies using cells grown in nonphysiologic media, a folate uptake system with specificity for reduced folates and K_t's about 10^{-6} M (Table 2) has been proposed as the relevant physiologic folate transport system (9, 36, 37, 47, 103). That these transport constants are two to three orders of magnitude lower than those reported for other recognized membrane receptors has been largely ignored, as has the fact that the observed uptake occurs in a concentration range 100 times higher than the folate concentration in human plasma, which is 10 to 50 nM. This system has an extremely low affinity for PteGlu, but similar K_t's for $CH_3H_4PteGlu$, $CHOH_4PteGlu$, and methotrexate (45, 57). Transport is inhibited by inorganic anions and enhanced by sulfhydryl protectors (45). This system appears to be the major mechanism of reduced folate uptake in some cultured mammalian cells (46, 57), and perhaps human erythrocytes as well, even though they contain small amounts of functional, and larger amounts of immunoassayable, high affinity FBPs (2).

In contrast, the membrane-associated FBP possesses properties which make it a logical candidate for the physiologic folate transport protein in cells and tissues where it is found. Not only is the affinity of FBPs for PteGlu in the range of other receptors for their ligands, but it is also high for $CH_3H_4PteGlu$ (3–5, 108, 109, 118). At normal plasma folate concentrations, unlike the putative reduced folate transport system, FBPs would be saturated with endogenous ligand. Endogenous folate occupies most folate-binding sites in milk (5, 88), serum (115), choroid plexus (106, 108), kidney (16, 96), placenta (4), and cells in tissue culture (67, 77) and must be removed by exposure of tissues to low pH conditions followed by dialysis or charcoal treatment before quantitation by binding assays. FBPs appear to be integral membrane proteins which have been identified on the surfaces of cells (e.g., human erythrocytes (2, 4), human KB cells (3), myeloblasts (114)). Thus membrane-associated FBPs have physiologic ligand affinity in the proper range, exist predominantly saturated with endogenous ligand under physiologic conditions, and are in the proper location to function as folate transport proteins. Some cells, however, such as human (K562, HL-60) and murine (L1210) leukemia cells in culture contain little to no high affinity FBPs as measured by binding assay or radioimmunoassay. Since they are routinely cultured in media containing very high folate levels (57–59, 103, 104), they may have permanently down regulated their FBP (46).

Experimental data that support a transport function for FBP have been obtained from several systems (35, 92). Saturable high affinity transport of $CH_3H_4PteGlu$ into the cerebrospinal fluid occurred against a concentration gradient in choroid plexus from human, hog, and rabbit, with transport constants (K_t's) of 12 nM (61), 90 nM (10) and 18 nM (106), respectively. High affinity FBPs have been detergent solubilized from the choroid plexus of rabbit (106, 107) and human (109), and purified to homogeneity from hog choroid plexus (108). The effects of anti-FBP antiserum on folate transport by choroid plexus have not been reported.

A membrane-associated FBP was solubilized with detergent and purified from rat kidney, and a specific antiserum to it was raised (96). Cross-reactive immunofluorescence was localized in the luminal border (brush border) of the tubular epithelial cells. In addition, intense cross-reactive immunofluorescence was observed in the rat choroid plexus. Inorganic anions ($Cl^- > Br^- > I^- > SO_4^{-2} > HEPES^{-1}$) enhanced $CH_3H_4PteGlu$ binding to the purified FBP, as was also observed in particulate brush border membrane preparations from rat kidney (97).

In subcellular preparations from rat kidney, particulate brush border membrane suspensions contained four-to-five times higher levels of a membrane-associated FBP (which required detergent for its solubilization) than particulate suspensions of the basolateral membranes, again demonstrating localization of the FBP to the luminal surface (16). The localization of the FBP to the luminal membrane of the tubule cells and the enhancement of folate binding by Cl^-, an abundant ion in urine, supports the role of the FBP in the reabsorption of folates from the urine. Urinary clearance studies demonstrated that the rate of clearance of a particular folate by the kidney was inversely proportional to its affinity constant (95). Microinfusion studies supported rapid carrier-mediated internalization of folic acid by renal tu-

TABLE 2. A COMPARISON OF THE PROPOSED FOLATE TRANSPORT SYSTEMS

	Reduced folate transport system	Folate-binding protein transport system
Substrates	N-5-Methyltetrahydrofolate	Folic acid
	N-5-Formyltetrahydrofolate	N-5-Methyltetrahydrofolate
	Methotrexate	
K_a (M^{-1})	10^6	10^9–10^{10}
Inorganic anions	Inhibit	No effect
Folic acid	Low affinity	High affinity
SH protectors	Protect	No effect
Purified protein	Not yet	Milk, placenta, choroid plexus, spleen, kidney, KB cells, leukemia cells, cord serum

bules with reappearance of folate binding sites on the luminal surface (98). A soluble FBP has also been found in the urine (41) and may arise from proteolytic cleavage of the membrane-associated FBP or be filtered from the serum.

Cultured monkey kidney (MA104) cells possessed high affinity specific binding sites for $CH_3H_4PteGlu$ (K_d = 3 nM at 4°C) (63). The folate binding was inhibited in a dose-dependent manner by monospecific rabbit anti-porcine FBP antiserum but increased as cellular folate content fell when cells were cultured in low folate medium. These results suggested folate binding was due to a specific membrane-associated FBP, and the number of available binding sites was influenced by the cellular folate content.

Human placenta contained large amounts of two membrane-associated FBPs which could be solubilized with Triton X-100 (4). Specific antiserum to purified placental FBP cross-reacted with purified FBPs from human milk (5), human KB cells (66, 67), murine melanoma cells (66), human and murine mammary tumor cells (66), normal human erythrocytes (1, 2) and inhibited folate binding to human erythrocyte ghosts (4), human KB cells (3), and monkey MA104 cells (63). This antiserum also inhibited uptake of PteGlu, $CH_3H_4PteGlu$, and methotrexate by human KB cells in a dose-dependent manner (3, 68).

Soluble serum FBP levels were elevated 3- to 4-fold in pregnant women (6, 29, 49), and 5- to 10-fold in premature infants and in cord blood (30, 38, 50) compared with nongravid women or older children, respectively. The purified soluble FBP from umbilical cord blood appeared to have a higher affinity for $CH_3H_4PteGlu$ than the folate-binding protein of maternal blood, suggesting the possibility that folate is accumulated by the fetus at the expense of the mother. The origins of the maternal and fetal soluble FBPs are currently not known, but placental membrane-associated FBP could be a precursor. The membrane-associated placental FBP might facilitate the directional transport of folate to the fetus.

Particulate FBPs (*i.e.*, proteins which can be sedimented by high-speed centrifugation or removed by Millipore filtration) have been identified in human, bovine, and goat milk (119) and purified from human milk after detergent treatment (5). This milk FBP is secreted in a membrane-bound form since it is a particulate protein and the bound folates are mainly polyglutamates (96). In this essentially accellular fluid, the FBP cannot serve a cellular transport function, but may function as a folate carrier to deliver large amounts of folate to the infant.

Two FBPs were found in a cell line derived from human epidermoid carcinoma (KB) cells: a soluble FBP, which they released into their growth medium, but which was not present in the cells, and a cellular FBP with the characteristics of an integral membrane protein (27, 66, 67). Large amounts of membrane-associated FBP compared with some other human cells were present in KB cells after they were adapted to and maintained in medium containing near physiologic folate levels (≤ 10 nM) (77). In these experiments, after 5 or 6 passes through low folate medium, the folate content of KB cells fell to 4 pmole/10^6 cells, their doubling time increased, cells

became megaloblastic, and their [^{3}H]thymidine incorporation was not normally suppressed by deoxyuridine (abnormal dU suppression test). After 12 to 15 passes in this medium, their growth rate and their morphology returned to "normal" and remained so for more than 50 passes, although folate content of these cells remained 1 pmol/10^6 cells or less (66, 68). Specific folate uptake by intact KB cells which were "adapted" to physiologic folate levels in their medium increased 10-fold for [^{3}H] PteGlu, and more than 40-fold for [^{14}C]$CH_3H_4PteGlu$; the K_t's for uptake were 5 nM and 12 nM, respectively (3). Folate uptake was inhibited in a dose-dependent manner by anti-human placental FBP antiserum, but not control serum (both sera were exhaustively dialyzed to remove free folate), indicating that an immunologically cross-reactive FBP was involved in the uptake (3). Normal human bone marrow cells in culture became megaloblastic and grew more slowly when antiserum to the human placental FBP was added to their medium. The addition of high levels of folates could overcome these effects (1). [^{3}H]Methotrexate uptake was also increased in KB cells grown in physiologic levels of folate and was also inhibited by specific antiserum to the human placental FBP (68).

Uptake studies could not distinguish between increases in unoccupied binding sites alone or increases in levels of folate transport protein in the KB cells adapted to growth in the medium with physiologic folate levels. When the levels of both the membrane-associated and soluble FBPs were measured, a 4-fold increase in both FBPs was observed in KB cells adapted to physiologic folate when measured by either [^{3}H]PteGlu binding after endogenous folate removal or by radioimmunoassay (66). The lower the folate content in the medium, the faster the increases in FBP took place. Reduced folates or PteGlu added to the medium prevented or reversed these changes. Similar results occurred in human and murine breast carcinoma cells. In addition, increased cell surface fluorescence by FACS for FBP was observed in folate-deficient HL-60 cells compared with folate-replete HL-60 cells incubated with fluorescein-tagged antiserum to the human placental folate receptor (A. C. Antony and C. Chitambar, personal communication). However, immunoreactive FBP was not detectable by radioimmunoassay (66) in HL-60 cells or K562 cells grown in either standard or low folate media (M. A. Kane and S. Waxman, unpublished observation). Thus, extracellular folate concentration influences intracellular folate concentration which appears to regulate FBP levels.

The biochemical properties of the two KB cell FBPs were very similar to the properties of the soluble and particulate FBPs purified from human milk, as assessed by gel filtration chromatography, polyacrylamide gel electrophoresis, and competitive binding assays (27, 67). Sucrose density gradient ultracentrifugation in H_2O and D_2O revealed that the KB cell membrane-associated FBP, like the particulate milk FBP, bound large amounts of Triton X-100, consistent with the hydrophobicity of its membrane location (5, 67). A covalently linked fatty acid moiety accounted for at least part of the hydrophobicity (74). The membrane-associated FBP contained 7 moles of fatty acid/mole of protein, and the soluble FBP contained only 0.05 moles of fatty acid/mole of protein. These two KB cell FBPs had the identical *N*-terminal 18 amino acid sequence. Several species of soluble and membrane-associated FBPs in KB cells could be identified by ion exchange chromatography (75). Fifty percent of the total cell-associated FBP was released intact from the cell surface by trypsin treatment of intact KB cells; the remainder was associated with intracellular membranes (3).

Intestinal folate absorption is a saturable, pH-dependent, energy-dependent, carrier-mediated process (94, 99). Transport constants in everted intestinal sacs have been reported in the micromolar range, but binding constants of isolated intestinal brush border membranes have indicated the presence of a high affinity binder (82), but none has been purified from intestinal tissue so far. The folate binding properties are distinguishable from the intestinal pteroylpolyglutamate hydrolase activity (82). The soluble FBP in milk may play a role in folate absorption (12), but the specific mechanism remains to be elucidated.

SOLUBLE FOLATE-BINDING PROTEIN

Soluble FBPs were first identified in milk (34) and comprise a heterogeneous group of homologous proteins with molecular weight = 30,000 to 40,000 (Table 1), which may originate from different sources and perform different functions (Table 3). Extracellular soluble FBPs may direct the transfer of absorbed or released folates to target cells (87), scavenge inactive forms of folate and carry them to the liver for metabolic conversion to $CH_3H_4PteGlu$ (88), trap folates in fetal circulation for fetal growth (5, 62), or in milk for neonate nutrition (12), control the composition of the intestinal flora by impairing absorption of folates by certain microbes (33), facilitate folate absorption in the intestine (12, 60, 91), and facilitate efflux of oxidized or inactive folates from cells which cannot metabolize them (119). Intracellular soluble FBPs have been reported in the cytosol and in organelles. The cytosolic FBPs in human chronic myelogenous leukemia cells were postulated to possess a storage function (86) and to facilitate transfer of folates to the nucleus (25), possibly exerting a control on DNA synthesis (25). Soluble FBPs were identified in the specific granules of normal human neutrophils and were released during an early step in degranulation (11), as are B_{12} binding proteins (11). These binding proteins have been postulated to exert a bacteriostatic activity by impairment of microbial folate absorption (33). The explanation for the wide variation in neutrophil folate binding levels in normal adults remains unclear.

THE BIOCHEMICAL INTERRELATIONSHIP OF THE SOLUBLE AND MEMBRANE-ASSOCIATED FOLATE BINDING PROTEINS

The immunologic cross-reactivity of the two forms of FBPs indicates a close structural homology between them. In KB cells, one group has reported identical amino acid compositions as expressed by mole percent for the two proteins (74) although another group reported different compositions (27). This had led to the specu-

TABLE 3. PROPOSED FUNCTIONS FOR FOLATE BINDING PROTEINS

Form	Location	Source	Proposed functions
Particulate	Extracellular	Milk (4)	Facilitate folate absorption
	Plasma membrane	Placenta (5)	Folate uptake (?Efflux)
		Choroid plexus (61, 106, 107)	
		Kidney (16, 64, 96)	
		Erythrocytes (2, 5)	
		KB cells (3, 77)	
	?Golgi ?Organelles	KB cells (3, 77)	Folate storage; folate coenzyme regulation
Soluble	Extracellular	Serum (29, 62, 114)	Folate transfer Folate "trap"
		Milk (4, 12, 33, 60, 116)	Facilitate folate absorption; impair intestinal microbe folate absorption
		KB cell medium (67)	?Folate efflux
	Intracellular cytosol	CML cells (23, 25, 86)	Folate storage; folate transfer to nucleus; control DNA synthesis
		Breast cancer (84)	
	Organelle	Neutrophil (11, 114) (Specific granule)	Impairment of microbial folate absorption

lation that soluble FBPs arise by specific proteolytic cleavage of the membrane-associated FBP precursor (5, 86) or that the particulate FBPs may consist of subunits of the soluble FBPs (5, 67). The subunit relationship was initially supported by the observations that a "large" and a "small" FBP could be identified in many tissues (*e.g.*, milk, serum, placenta) (113). In the presence of Triton X-100, the "large" FBP had a molecular weight ~160,000, and the "small" FBP a molecular weight ~40,000 (4, 5, 27, 67); however, on sodium dodecyl sulfate-polyacrylamide gel electrophoresis, both had molecular weight ~40,000 (5, 67). When the degree of detergent binding was determined based on sedimentation by sucrose density gradient ultracentrifugation in water and in deuterium oxide, 75% of the molecular weight of the "large" FBP was due to bound Triton X-100 (5, 67). In addition, detergent has been observed to enhance folate binding. The FBP purified from cow's whey exhibited a 5- to 10-fold increase in [^{3}H]PteGlu binding in the presence of the detergents Triton X-100 (40) or cetyltrimethylammonium bromide (5 to 10 mM) or in serum (43). Although this FBP was purified without detergent present and had a molecular weight = 29,800 by sedimentation equilibrium, this "activation" by detergent suggests that it may be predominantly the "particulate" form.

The molecular weights calculated from the amino acid compositions of the purified proteins are shown in Table

4 (soluble FBPs) and Table 5 (particulate FBPs). The calculated molecular weights for the purified soluble milk FBPs are all very similar (~30,000) and consistently a bit lower than the calculated molecular weights for the purified particulate FBPs (except for rat kidney). This supports the hypothesis that the particulate FBP is anchored in the cell membrane by a hydrophobic "tail." This "tail" consists, in part, of fatty acid moieties (74). The extracellular portion may be cleaved, with the folate-binding site intact, to produce the soluble FBP. For example, the soluble serum FBP in adult serum may arise from a hepatic (or other tissues) membrane-associated folate binder; fetal serum FBP may primarily arise from the placental folate receptor; urine FBP may arise from that found in the renal tubule brush border membrane, and soluble folate binder in cerebrospinal fluid may arise from the choroid plexus FBP. When the proteolytic digestion fragments of the purified soluble and particulate FBPs of human milk were analyzed by sodium dodecyl sulfate-polyacrylamide gel electrophoresis and visualized by Coomassie brilliant blue staining only, identical patterns were observed for each, again demon-

TABLE 4. AMINO ACID COMPOSITION OF SOLUBLE FOLATE-BINDING PROTEIN

Amino acid	Human milk[a] (111)	Cow milk[a] (111)	Human milk[a] (4)	Goat milk[a] (87)	Human spleen[a] (89)	KB cell[a] (27)	KB Cell (mol %) (27)	KB Cell (mol %) (74)
Aspartic acid	25	23	21	26	24	19	10	14.0
Threonine	12	10	8	12	10	13	6.8	5.2
Serine	16	17	13	21	8	17	8.9	7.2
Glutamic acid	30	24	24	24	28	26	13.6	15.2
Proline	17	16	12	22	22	12	6.3	ND
Glycine	13	11	10	29	18	16	8.4	6.0
Alanine	18	13	15	22	17	15	7.9	9.6
1/2-cystine	15	11	ND[b]	4	16	ND	ND	ND
Valine	10	8	7	16	7	10	5.2	5.6
Methionine	4	3	4	3	4	3	1.6	2.1
Isoleucine	6	7	5	10	6	5	2.6	2.6
Leucine	11	10	9	15	15	11	5.8	5.2
Tyrosine	13	9	7	7	8	6	3.1	4.4
Phenylalanine	16	8	14	7	8	10	5.2	4.4
Histidine	16	8	14	9	8	7	3.7	4.4
Lysine	15	13	8	12	15	12	6.3	7.2
Arginine	14	14	12	17	15	9	4.7	6.8
Tryptophan	ND	9	ND	ND	ND	ND	ND	ND
(Calculated mol wt)	(30,000)	(25,700)	(29,000)	(30,000)	(~42,000)	(24,200)		

[a] Moles of amino acid/mole of folate-binding protein.

[b] ND, Not determined.

TABLE 5. AMINO ACID COMPOSITION OF PARTICULATE FOLATE-BINDING PROTEINS

Amino acid	Rat kidney[a] (96)	Hog choroid plexus[a] (108)	Human placenta[a] (5)	Human milk[a] (4)	KB cell[a] (27)	KB cell (mol %) (27)	KB cell (mol %) (74)
Aspartic acid	19	27	32	38	29	6.2	13.0
Threonine	8	40	17	14	26	5.6	4.9
Serine	12	56	31	24	30	6.5	8.5
Glutamic acid	21	24	12	45	46	9.9	14.6
Proline	10	27	13	20	38	8.2	ND
Glycine	10	29	20	18	48	10.3	9.7
Alanine	9	21	20	25	37	8.0	9.3
1/2-cystine	6	10	12	ND	ND	ND	ND
Valine	7	28	32	12	36	7.7	4.9
Methionine	3	33	4	8	6	1.3	1.7
Isoleucine	5	11	6	13	23	4.9	2.6
Leucine	10	24	17	21	41	8.8	5.7
Tyrosine	8	12	10	13	19	4.1	4.4
Phenylalanine	7	10	10	22	26	5.6	4.0
Histidine	5	4	16	18	11	2.4	4.0
Lysine	15	21	19	24	28	6.0	6.1
Arginine	8	10	17	16	21	4.5	6.5
Tryptophan	6	4	ND	ND	ND	ND	ND
(Calculated mol wt)	(30,000)	(51,000)	(38,500)	(38,500)	(45,214)		(~42,000)

[a] Moles of amino acid/mole of folate-binding protein.

[b] ND, Not determined.

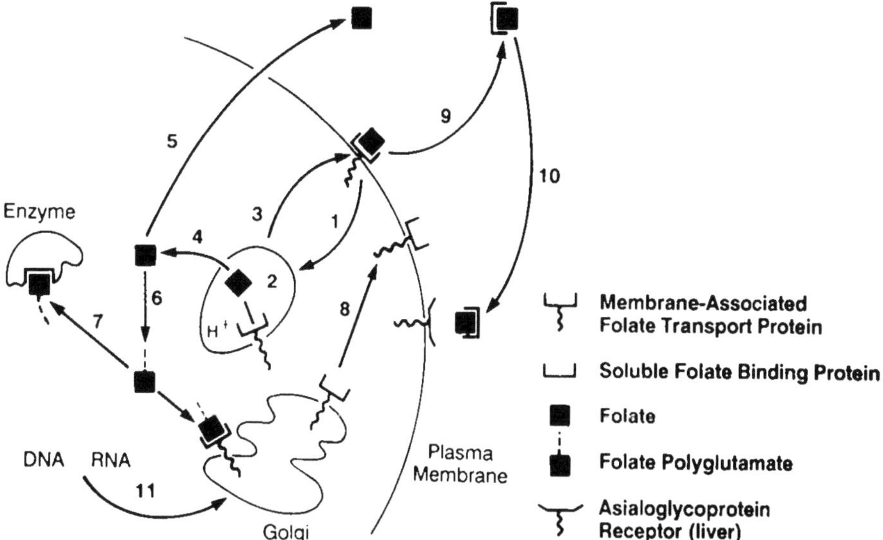

FIG. 1. Known and postulated properties of the folate-binding proteins. *1*, Folate ligands bind to membrane-associated folate transport protein on surface of cell. Internalization of the ligand-protein complex in an endosome is postulated. *2*, Acidification of the endosome vesicle is postulated, with resultant release of the bound folate. *3*, Folate transport in the endosome membrane recycles FBP to the plasma membrane (postulated). *4*, Freed intracellular folate diffuses throughout the cytosolic compartment. *5*, Free folate monoglutamate effluxes from the cell. *6*, Free folate monoglutamate is converted to the polyglutamate by the addition of 1-6 glutamic acid residues by the action of folyl polyglutamate synthetase. Folate polyglutamates do not readily efflux from the cell. *7*, Folate polyglutamates undergo metabolic conversions. The appropriate folate derivatives bind to specific enzymes involved in one-carbon transfers which require folate coenzymes or bind to intracellular FBP. *8*, Folate transport protein presumably undergoes specific glycosylations in the Golgi and then moves to the plasma membrane. A significant portion of membrane-associated folate-binding protein appears to be associated with intracellular membranes (24). *9*, The membrane-associated folate transport protein is the precursor for the soluble folate-binding protein. A membrane-associated protease presumably specifically cleaves the transport protein, with preservation of the binding site on the soluble product. The fate of the membrane-anchoring "tail," which apparently contains fatty acids, is unknown. *10*, Internalization of the soluble folate-binding protein with or without bound folate occurs in the liver via the asialoglycoprotein receptor. *11*, The amount of folate transport protein and its soluble product are increased in cells with a lowered folate content. The site of this regulation has not been characterized as yet.

strating an extremely close primary structure (M. A. Kane and J. F. Kolhouse, unpublished data). Presumably this staining technique did not provide high enough sensitivity to visualize the extra fragment from the particulate FBP.

The observation that KB cells grown in tissue culture release soluble FBP into their medium, but the membrane-associated FBP is the only cell-associated one, provided a convenient model system for studying the biochemical relationship of the two proteins. Pulse-chase studies in which KB cell FBPs were endogenously labeled with [^{35}S]methionine, purified, and their specific activities determined at various times after the pulse, produced results consistent with a precursor-product relationship (67). In these pulse-chase experiments, when cycloheximide was added to inhibit *de novo* synthesis after the pulse, the soluble FBP behaved as if it arose from an already synthesized pool of protein precursor (67).

SUMMARY

FBPs, which possess high affinity for PteGlu and CH$_3$H$_4$PteGlu, the major extracellular physiologic folate, exist in two immunologically related forms: (a) soluble extracellular, cytosolic and vesicular proteins, and (b) particulate integral membrane proteins. A model for the roles of FBPs in folate metabolism is illustrated in Figure 1. The membrane-associated FBPs are probably involved in folate translocation across cell membranes, and may control the availability of folate coenzymes inside the cell as well. The soluble FBPs appear to be a heterogeneous group with diverse functions. Current evidence suggests that the two FBPs in human KB cells and human milk are related in a precursor-product manner. Extracellular folate concentration regulates the levels of both the soluble and membrane-associated FBPs in human KB cells, but the metabolic level at which this regulation occurs requires further study. Serum folate concentration and hormone levels *in vivo* appear to affect circulating levels of soluble FBP. FBPs in milk appear to facilitate folate absorption in the intestine, which appears to proceed via a carrier-mediated system different from that studied in other tissues.

Acknowledgments: We greatly appreciate the excellent secretarial assistance of Jaclyn Silverman, Janice Evanish, and Joan Cole in the preparation of this manuscript.

This work was supported by the Chemotherapy Foundation, the Herman Goldman Foundation, and the Samuel Waxman Cancer Research Foundation (S.W.) and The Revson Foundation and National Institutes of Health Grant AM07300-01 (M.K.)

Address reprint requests to: Samuel Waxman, M.D., Division of Medical Oncology, Box 1178, Mount Sinai Medical Center, One, Gustave L. Levy Place, New York, NY 10029.

REFERENCES

1. Antony AC, Bruno E, Briddell RA, Brandt JE, Verma RS, Hoffman R: Effect of perturbation of specific folate receptors during erythropoiesis. J Clin Invest 80:1617, 1987
2. Antony AC, Kane MA, Kolhouse JF: Identification and characterization of a human erythrocyte membrane folate receptor (abstr). Clin Res 33:33, 1985

3. Antony AC, Kane MA, Portillo RM, Elwood PC, Kolhouse JF: Studies of the role of a particulate folate-binding protein in the uptake of 5-methyltetrahydrofolate by cultured human KB cells. J Biol Chem 260:14911, 1985

4. Antony AC, Utley CS, Marcell PD, Kolhouse JF: Isolation, characterization and comparison of the solubilized particulate and soluble folate binding proteins from human milk. J Biol Chem 257:10081, 1982

5. Antony AC, Utley CS, Van Horne KC, Kolhouse JF: Isolation and characterization of a folate receptor from human placenta. J Biol Chem 256:9684, 1981

6. Areelkul S, Yamarat P, Vongyuthithum M: Folic acid and folate binding protein in pregnancy. J Nutr Sci Vitaminol 23:447, 1977

7. Beck WS: Megaloblastic anemias II. Folic acid deficiency. In Hematology, edited by Beck WS, p 101. Cambridge, MA, MIT Press, 1977

8. Benesch R, Waxman S, Benesch R, Baugh C: The binding of folyl polyglutamates by hemoglobin. Biochem Biophys Res Commun 106:1359, 1982

9. Chabner BA: Methotrexate. In Pharmacologic Principles of Cancer Treatment, edited by Chabner B, p 229. Philadelphia, W B Saunders, 1982

10. Chen C, Wagner C: Folate transport in the choroid plexus. Life Sci 16:1571, 1975

11. Colman N, Herbert V: Folate binding proteins. Annu Rev Med 31:433, 1980

12. Colman N, Hettiarachchy N, Herbert V: Detection of a milk factor that facilitates folate uptake by intestinal cells. Science 211:1427, 1981

13. Cook RJ, Wagner C: Measurement of a folate binding protein from rat liver cytosol by radioimmunoassay. Arch Biochem Biophys 208:358, 1981

14. Cook RJ, Wagner C: Purification and partial characterization of rat liver folate binding protein. Biochemistry 21:4427, 1982

15. Cook RJ, Wagner C: Glycine N-methyltransferase is a folate binding protein of rat liver cytosol. Proc Natl Acad Sci USA 81:3631, 1984

16. Corrocher R, Abramson RG, King VK, Schreiber C, Dikman S, Waxman S: Differential binding of rat renal cortex brush border and basolateral membrane preparations. Proc Soc Exp Biol med 178:73, 1985

17. Corrocher R, Bambara LM, Pachor ML, Biasi D, Stanzial A, De Sandre G: Serum folate binding capacity in leukemias, liver diseases and pregnancy. Acta Haematol (Basel) 61:203, 1979

18. Corrocher R, Bambara LM, Pachor ML, De Sandre G: Folate binding proteins. Recenti Prog Med 66:361, 1979b

19. Corrocher R, Bambara LM, Pachor ML, Stanzial AM, Biasi D: Different binding proteins for folic acid in serum of patients with acute hepatitis. Acta Haematol (Basel) 64:281, 1980

20. Corrocher R, Pachor ML, Bambara LM, Ambrosetti A, De Sandre G: Folic acid binding protein in chronic granulocytic leukemia: The effect of methotrexate. Acta Haematol (Basel) 670:341, 1978

21. Corrocher R, Pachor ML, Bambara LM, De Sandre G: Evidence for a folic acid binding protein in human cell membrane. Acta Haematol (Basel) 66:202, 1981

22. da Costa M, Fischer C: Immunologic heterogeneity of the folate-binding proteins from chronic myelogenous leukemia cells and myelofibrosis spleen. J Lab Clin Med 98:956, 1981

23. da Costa M, Rothenberg SP: Studies with the folate binding protein in chronic granulocytic leukemia cells. I. Synthesis and release of binder by cells in short-term culture. Br J Haematol 34:581, 1976

24. da Costa M, Rothenberg SP, Beckman SJ: Rat liver nuclei contain receptors for a folate binding protein. Proc Soc Exp Biol Med 174:350, 1983

25. da Costa M, Sharon M: The synthesis of folate binding protein in lymphocytes during transformation. Br J Haematol 46:575, 1980

26. Elsborg L, Hansen SI, Skovbjerg H, Holm J, Lyngbye J: Chromatographic isolation and characterization of folate binding proteins in porcine intestinal epithelial brush border membrane. Int J Vitam Nutr Res 50:267, 1980

27. Elwood PC, Kane MA, Portillo RM, Kolhouse JF: The isolation, characterization and comparison of the membrane-associated and soluble folate-binding proteins from human KB cells. J Biol Chem 261:15416, 1986

28. Fernandes-Costa F, Metz J: Binding of methylfolate and pteroylglutamic acid by the specific serum folate binder. J Lab Clin Med 93:181, 1979

29. Fernandes-Costa F, Metz J: Role of serum folate binders in the delivery of folate to tissues and to the fetus. Br J Haematol 48:335, 1979

30. Fernandes-Costa F, Metz J: The specific folate-binding capacity of serum. Evidence that levels are not directly related to folate nutrition but influenced by hormonal status. J Lab Clin Med 98:119, 1981

31. Fischer CD, da Costa M, Rothenberg SP: Properties of purified folate binding proteins from chronic myelogenous leukemia cells. Biochim Biophys Acta 543:328, 1978

32. Fisher SE, Inselman LS, Duffy L, Atkinson M, Spencer H, Chang B: Ethanol and fetal nutrition: Effect of chronic ethanol exposure on rate placental growth and membrane-associated folic acid receptor binding activity. J Pediatr Gastroenterol Nutr 4:645, 1985

33. Ford JE: Some observations on the possible nutritional significance of vitamin B12 and folate binding proteins in milk. Br J Nutr 31:243, 1974

34. Ghitis J: The folate binding protein in milk. Am J Clin Nutr 20:1, 1967

35. Goldman ID: The characteristics of membrane transport of amethopterin and the naturally occurring folates. Ann NY Acad Aci 186:400, 1971

36. Goldman ID: A model for the study of heteroexchange diffusion: Methotrexate-folate interactions in L1210 leukemia and Ehrlich ascites tumor cells. Biochim Biophys Acta 233:635, 1976

37. Gregory JF: Denaturation of the folacin-binding protein in pasteurized milk products. J Nutr 113, 1329, 1982

38. Gross S, Kamen B, Fanaroff A, Caston D: Folate compartments during gestational maturation. J Pediatr 96:842, 1980

39. Halsted CH: The intestinal absorption of folates. Am J Clin Nutr 32:846, 1979

40. Hansen SI, Holm J, Lyngbye J: Change in binding properties of folate binding protein in cow's whey due to removal of a cofactor during affinity chromatographic purification. Biochim Biophys Acta 579:479, 1979

41. Hansen SI, Holm J, Lyngbye J: High-affinity protein binding of folate in urine. IRCS Med Sci 8:846, 1980

42. Hansen SI, Holm J, Lyngbye J: Evidence that the low-affinity folate binding protein in erythrocyte hemolysate is identical to hemoglobin. Clin Chem 27:1247, 1981

43. Hansen SI, Holm J, Lyngbye J: Detergent activation of the binding protein in the folate radioassay. Clin Chem 28:117, 1982

44. Hansen SI, Holm J, Lyngbye J: A high affinity folate binding protein in human cerebrospinal fluid. Acta Neurol Scand 71:133, 1985

45. Henderson GB, Grzelakowska-Sztabert B, Zevely EM, Huennekens FM: Binding properties of the 5-methyltetrahydrofolate methotrexate transport system in L1210 cells. Arch Biochem Biophys 202:144, 1980

46. Henderson GB, Tsuji JM, Kumar HP: Mediated uptake of polate by a high-affinity binding protein in sublines of L1210 cells adapted to nanomolar concentrations of polate. J Membrane Biol 101:247, 1988

47. Herbert V, Colman N: Release of vitamin binding proteins from granulocytes by lithium: vitamin B12 and folate binding proteins. Adv Exp Med Biol 127:61, 1980

48. Holm J, Hansen SI, Lyngbye J: Cofactor in serum for high affinity folate binding in milk. Clin Chem 26:1591, 1980

49. Holm J, Hansen SI, Lyngbye J: High and low affinity binding of folate to proteins in serum of pregnant women. Biochim Biophys Acta 629:539, 1980

50. Holm J, Hansen SI, Lyngbye J: A high affinity folate binding protein in umbilical cord serum. Scan J Clin Lab Invest 40:523, 1980

51. Holm J, Hansen SI, Lyngbye J: Characteristics of high-affinity folate binding in serum of a patient with chronic myelogenous leukemia. Clin Chim Acta 105:383, 1980

52. Holm J, Hansen SI, Lyngbye J: High affinity binding of folate to a serum protein in chronic myelogenous leukemia. Effect of binder concentration, pH, and temperature. Clin Chem 27:316, 1981

53. Holm J, Hansen SI, Lyngbye J: High affinity folate binding in chronic myelogenous leukaemia serum: relationship of binding characteristics to activity of disease and binder concentration. Scand J Haematol 26:153, 1981

54. Holm J, Hansen SI, Lyngbye J: High-affinity folate binding in leukocyte lysate from normal subjects: effect of concentration of binding protein, temperature and pH. Acta Haematol (Basel) 70:269, 1983

55. Holm J, Hansen SI, Lyngbye J: A high-affinity folate binding protein in normal human leucocytes: Ligand binding characteristics, ionic charge and molecular size. Biosci Rep 5:683, 1985

56. Horne DW, Briggs WT, Wagner C: Enzymic synthesis of (d)-L-5-methyltetrahydropteroylglutamate of high specific radioactivity. Methods Enzymol 66:545, 1980

57. Huennekens FM: Transport of folate compounds, pterins and adenine in L1210 mouse leukemia cells. Adv Enzyme Regul 20:389, 1981

58. Huennekens FM, Suresh MR, Grinishaw CE: In Chemistry and Biology of Pteridines, edited by Blair JA, p 1. New York, Walter de Gruyter & Co, 1983

59. Huennekens FM, Vitols KS, Henderson GB: Transport of folate compounds in bacterial and mammalian cells. Adv Enzymol 47:313, 1978

60. Izhak G, Galewski K, Rachmilewitz M, Grossowicz N: The absorption of milk-bound pteroylglutamic acid from small intestine segments. Proc Soc Exp Biol Med 140:248, 1972

61. Jensen ON, Olesen OV: Human choroid plexus transport of folates. Acta Psychol Scand 47:206, 1971

62. Kamen BA, Caston JD: Purification of folate binding factor in normal umbilical cord serum. Proc Nat Acad Sci USA 72:4261, 1975

63. Kamen BA, Capdevila A: Receptor-mediated folate accumulation is regulated by the cellular folate content. Proc Natl Acad Sci USA 83:5983, 1986

64. Kamen BA, Caston JD: Properties of a folate binding protein (FBP) isolated from porcine kidney. Biochem Pharmacol 35:2323, 1986

65. Kamen BA, Gross S, Caston JD: Role of cerebrospinal fluid binder in the uptake of folate by lymphoblasts. Methods Enzymol 66:678, 1980

66. Kane MA, Elwood PC, Portillo RM, Antony AC, Najfeld V, Finley A, Waxman S, Kolhouse JF: Influence on immunoreactive folate binding proteins of extracellular folate concentration in cultured human cells. J Clin Invest 81:2398, 1988

67. Kane MA, Elwood PC, Portillo RM, Antony AC, Kolhouse JF: The interrelationship of the soluble and membrane-associated folate binding proteins in human KB cells. J Biol Chem 261:15625, 1986

68. Kane MA, Portillo RM, Elwood PC, Antony Ac, Kolhouse JF: The influence of extracellular folate concentration on methotrexate uptake by human KB cells. Partial characterization of a membrane-associated methotrexate binding protein. J Biol Chem 261:44, 1986

69. Kesavan V, Noronha JM: Noninvolvement of a rat intestinal folate binding protein in physiological folate absorption. Experientia 40:8030, 1984

70. Lanzkowski P, Erlandson ME, Bezan AI: Isolated defect of folic acid absorption associated with mental retardation and cerebral calcification. Blood 34:452, 1969

71. Leslie GI, Rowe PB: Folate binding by the brush border membrane proteins of small intestinal epithelial cells. Biochemistry 11:1696, 1972

72. Levitas A, Braden M, Van Norman K, Hagerman R, McBogg P: Treatment and prevention. In The Fragile X Syndrome, edited by Hagerman RJ & McBogg PM, pp 201–228. Dillon, CO, Spectra Publishing Co, 1983

73. Luhby AL, Eagle FJ, Roth E, Cooperman J: Relapsing megaloblastic anemia in an infant due to a specific defect in gastrointestinal absorption of folic acid. Am J Dis Child 102:94, 1961

74. Luhrs CA, Pitiranggon P, da Costa M, Rothenberg SP, Slomiany BL, Brink L, Guillermo IT, Stein S: Purified membrane and soluble folate binding proteins from cultured KB cells have similar amino acid compositions and molecular weights, but differ in fatty acid acylation. Proc Natl Acad Sci USA 84:6546, 1987

75. Luhrs CA, Sadavisan E, da Costa M, Rothenberg SP: The isola-
tion and properties of multiple forms of folate binding protein in cultured KB cells. Arch Biochem Biophys 250:94, 1986

76. Lyngbye J, Hansen SI, Holm J: Kinetics of folate-protein binding. Methods Enzymol 66:694, 1980

77. McHugh M, Cheng YC: Demonstration of a high affinity folate binder in human cell membranes and its characterization in cultured human KB cells. J Biol Chem 254:11312, 1979

78. Nixon PF, Bertino JR: Enzymic preparations of radiolabeled +−L-5-methyltetrahydrofolate and +−L-formyltetrahydrofolate. Methods Enzymol 66:547, 1980

79. Nutrition Review: Serum folate binders are not correlated to folate nutritional status. Nutr Rev 40:234, 1982

80. Nutrition Review: Folate binder in milk may facilitate folate absorption. Nutr Rev 40:90, 1982

81. Pristoupilova K, Slavikova V: Specific folic acid binding protein in human saliva. Cas Lek Cesk 119:1103, 1980

82. Reisenauer AM, Chandler CJ, Halsted CH: Folate binding and hydrolysis by pig intestinal brush-border membranes. Am J Physiol 251:G481, 1986

83. Retief FP, Heyns AP, Oosthuizen M, et al: Comparison between the unsaturated plasma folate binder and in vivo labeled plasma folate binder. Acta Haematol (Basel) 60:296, 1978

84. Rochman H, Selhub J, Karrison T: Folate binding protein and the estrogen receptor in breast cancer. Cancer Detect Prev 8:71, 1985

85. Rothenberg SP, da Costa M: Further observations on the folate-binding factor in some leukemic cells. J Clin Invest 50:719, 1971

86. Rothenberg SP, Fischer CD, da Costa M: Binding of N^5,N^{10}-methylene tetrahydrofolate and the inhibition of thymidylate synthesis by a folate binding protein. Biochim Biophys Acta 543:340, 1978

87. Rubinoff M, Schreiber C, Waxman S: The isolation and characterization of the folate binding protein from goat milk. FEBS Lett 75:244, 1977

88. Rubinoff M, Abramson R, Schreiber C, Waxman S: Effect of a folate-binding protein on the plasma transport and tissue distribution of folic acid. Acta Haematol (Basel) 65:145, 1981

89. Sadavisan E, Rothenberg SP, da Costa M, Brink L: Characterization of multiple forms of folate-binding protein from human leukemia cells. Biochim Biophys Acta 882:311, 1986

90. Sadavisan E, Rothenberg SP: Isolation of the cDNA clone for a human folate binding protein (FBP) (abstr.) FASEB J 46:1004, 1987

91. Said HM, Horne DW, Wagner C: Effect of human milk folate binding protein on folate intestinal transport. Arch Biochem Biophys 251:114, 1986

92. Said HM, Strum WB: Cyclic AMP-3′,5-monophosphate and folate transport in rat jejunum. Biochem Biophys Res Commun 115:756, 1983

93. Selhub J, Arnold R, Smith AM, Picciano MF: Milk folate binding protein (FBP): A secretory protein for folate? Nutr Res 4:181, 1984

94. Selhub J, Dhar GJ, Rosenberg IH: Gastrointestinal absorption of folates and antifolates. Pharmacol Ther 20:397, 1983

95. Selhub J, Emmanouel D, Stavropoulos, Arnold R: Renal folate absorption and the kidney folate binding protein. I. urinary clearance studies. Am J Physiol 252:F750, 1986

96. Selhub J, Franklin WA: The folate binding protein of rat kidney. Purification, properties, and cellular distribution. J Biol Chem 259:6601, 1984

97. Selhub J, Gay AC, Rosenberg IH: Effect of anions on folate binding by isolated brush border membranes from rat kidney. Biochim Biophys Acta 557:372, 1979

98. Selhub J, Nakamura S, Carone FA: Renal folate absorption and the kidney folate binding protein. II. microinfusion studies. Am J Physiol 252:F757, 1986

99. Selhub J, Powell GM, Rosenberg IH: Intestinal transport of 5-methyltetrahydrofolate. Am J Physiol 246:G515–G520

100. Selhub J, Rosenberg IH: Folate transport in isolated brush border membrane vesicles from rat intestine. J Biol Chem 236:4489, 1981

101. Shane B, Tamura T, Stokstad ELR: Folate assay: A comparison of radioassay and microbiological methods. Clin Chim Acta 100:13, 1980

102. Sheppard K, Bradbury DA, Davies JM, Ryrie DR: Cobalamin and folate binding proteins in human tumour tissue. J Clin Pathol

37:1336, 1984

103. Sirotnak FM: Correlates of folate analog transport, pharmacokinetics and selective antitumor action. Pharmacol Ther 8:71, 1980

104. Sirotnak FM, Goutas LJ, Jacobsen DM, Mines LS, Barrueco JR, Gaumont Y, Gaumont Y, Kisliuk R: Carrier-mediated transport of folate compounds on L1210 cells. Biochem Pharmacol 36:1659, 1987

105. Soliman HA, Olesen H: Folic acid binding by human plasma albumin. Scan J Clin Lab Invest 36:299, 1976

106. Spector R: Identification of folate binding macromolecule in rabbit choroid plexus. J Biol Chem 252:3364, 1977

107. Spector R: Affinity of folic acid for the folate binding protein of choroid plexus. Arch Biochem Biophys 194:632, 1979

108. Suleiman SA, Spector R: Purification and characterization of a folate binding protein from porcine choroid plexus. Arch Biochem Biophys 208:87, 1981

109. Suleiman SA, Spector R, Cancilla P: Partial purification and characterization of a folate binding protein from human choroid plexus. Neurochem Res 6:333, 1981

110. Svendsen I, Hansen SI, Holm J, Lyngbye J: Isolation and characterization of the folate-binding protein from cow's milk. Carlsberg Res Commun 44:89, 1979

111. Svendsen I, Hansen SI, Holm J, Lyngbye J: The complete amino acid sequence of the folate-binding protein from cow's milk. Carlsberg Res Commun 49:123, 1984

112. Wagner C: Folate-binding proteins. Nutr Rev 43:293, 1985

113. Waxman S: Folate binding proteins. Br J Haematol 29:23, 1975

114. Waxman S: Studies on the origin of serum folate binding protein. In Chemistry and Biology of the Pteridines, edited by Kisliuk GM, Brown GM, P 619. North Holland, Elsevier, 1979

115. Waxman S, Schreiber C: Characteristics of folic-acid binding protein in folate-deficient serum. Blood 42:291, 1973

116. Waxman S, Schreiber C: The role of folic acid binding proteins (FABP) in the cellular uptake of folates. Proc Soc Exp Biol Med 147:760, 1974

117. Waxman S, Schreiber C: The purification and characterization of the low molecular weight human folate binding protein using affinity chromatography. Biochemistry 14:5422, 1975

118. Waxman S, Schreiber C: Determination of folate by use of radioactive folate and binding proteins. Methods Enzymol 66:468, 1980

119. Waxman S, Schreiber C, Rubinoff M: The significance of folate binding proteins in folate metabolism. Adv Nutr Res 1:55, 1977

120. Wittwer AJ, Wagner C: Identification of folate binding protein of mitochondria as dimethylglycine dehydrogenase. Proc Natl Acad Sci USA 77:4484, 1980

121. Wittwer AJ, Wagner C: Identification of folate-binding proteins of rat liver mitrochondria as dimethylglycine dehydrogenase and sarcosine dehydrogenase. Purification and folate-binding characteristics. J Biol Chem 256:4102, 1981

122. Wittwer AJ, Wagner C: Identification of the folate binding proteins of rat liver mitochondria as dimethylglycine dehydrogenase and sarcosine dehydrogenase. Flavo protein nature and enzymatic properties of the purified proteins. J Biol Chem 256:4109, 1981

123. Zamarano AF, Arnalick F, Sanchez Casas E, Sicilia A, Solis C, Vazquez JJ, Gasalla R: Levels of iron, vitamin B_{12}, folic acid and their binding proteins during pregnancy. Acta Haemat 74:92, 1985.

Biology of Disease

New Insights into "The Riddle of the Mast Cells": Microenvironmental Regulation of Mast Cell Development and Phenotypic Heterogeneity

STEPHEN J. GALLI

Departments of Pathology, Beth Israel Hospital and Harvard Medical School; and the Charles A. Dana Research Institute, Beth Israel Hospital, Boston, Massachusetts

Introduction
Origin, Distribution and Characteristics of Basophils and Mast Cells
  Introduction
  Origin and distribution of basophils
  Origin and distribution of mast cells
  Relationship between basophils and mast cells
Mast Cell Heterogeneity
  Introduction
  Evidence for heterogeneity of mast cell phenotypic characteristics *in vivo*
    Mast cell heterogeneity in rats and mice
    Mast cell heterogeneity in man
    Conclusions
  Alternative mechanisms which might account for mast cell heterogeneity
    Distinct mast cell lineages
    Cellular maturation/differentiation
    Changes associated with functional activation, including "born again immature mast cells"
    Acquisition of molecules derived from other cell types
  Microenvironmental regulation of mast cell development and phenotype
    Introduction
    Cytokine-dependent regulation of mast cell proliferation and maturation/differentiation
    Use of mast cells generated *in vitro* to demonstrate unidirectional changes in mast cell phenotype
    Demonstration of multiple, bidirectional changes in mast cell phenotype
    Conclusions
An *In Vivo* Model for Evaluating the Roles of Mast Cells of Distinct Phenotype in Health and Disease
Conclusions and Directions for Future Study

INTRODUCTION

At no time in recent memory has it been so difficult to offer succint generalizations about the biology of the mast cell, or its role in health and disease. This situation is something of a paradox, since there have been significant recent advances in experimental approaches for analyzing mast cell development, biochemistry and function, and the application of these methods has already generated much important new data. However, some of these findings have required that certain widely held beliefs about the mast cell be reevaluated. Indeed, in virtually every facet of the cell's natural history, from its differentiation and maturation to its biochemistry and function, recent work has revealed considerably more complexity than had previously been suspected to exist.

To those involved in mast cell research, this exciting progress has raised hopes that "the riddle of the mast cells" (223), *i.e.*, their specific roles in health and disease, might soon be solved. But to those whose acquaintance with the mast cell is more casual, the rapidly accumulating mass of new information may have caused no small amount of confusion.

The concept of "mast cell heterogeneity" has represented a focal point in recent discussions of mast cell biology (10, 80). In its most general sense, this concept simply serves to emphasize that different mast cell populations exhibit significant variation in multiple potentially important aspects of their phenotype. However, data demonstrating the existence of mast cell phenotypic heterogeneity have been interpreted differently by different investigators, and not all of these interpretations are mutually compatible. As a result, the perception that the discussion about mast cell heterogeneity may be generating as much heat as light is, at least in part, correct.

On the other hand, the appreciation that different mast cell populations can express significant variation in mediator content, responses to cytokines influencing proliferation or maturation, patterns of reactivity to potential stimuli of mediator release, and response to drugs affecting mast cell function has significantly enhanced our ability to propose and test critically hypotheses concerning the unique contributions of specific mast cell populations to particular disease processes or host defense mechanisms. Put differently, part of the problem in solving "the riddle of the mast cells" may have been the mistaken belief that information derived from the analysis of a single mast cell population could be used to generate sweeping generalizations about all mast cells. When viewed in this context, the complexities introduced into the understanding of mast cell biology by the evolving information about mast cell heterogeneity represent a rich source of insight into how different mast cell populations might perform different biologic roles.

The purpose of this review is not to catalogue every example of mast cell phenotypic variation. Much of this information is of interest primarily to investigators working in the mast cell field, many of whom have published their own views about mast cell heterogeneity (7, 15, 35, 36, 65–67, 135, 146, 204, 205, 238). Instead, I will focus primarily on the major generalizations about mast cell heterogeneity that are best supported by currently available information, and will point out what I believe are some of the critical gaps in our knowledge. In particular, I will consider the rapidly growing body of evidence indicating that much of mast cell phenotypic heterogeneity is regulated by local microenvironmental factors.

But before dealing with the significant differences in phenotype among different populations of mast cells, we should first briefly review the distinctions between mast cells and basophils. While identifying the unique contributions of mast cells to individual biologic responses or disease processes is difficult, this task can be even harder if it is not realized that a distinct cell population, the basophil, may be able to perform some functions quite similar to those of the mast cell.

ORIGIN, DISTRIBUTION, AND CHARACTERISTICS OF BASOPHILS AND MAST CELLS

INTRODUCTION

Ehrlich (62) identified mast cells in human connective tissues on the basis of the metachromatic staining properties of their prominent cytoplasmic granules. Ehrlich also described the basophil, a circulating leukocyte containing cytoplasmic granules similar in staining properties to those of mast cells (63). Later work established that mast cells and basophils share several notable features besides staining properties. Both cell types represent a major source of histamine and other potent chem-

ical mediators implicated in a wide variety of inflammatory and immunologic processes (reviewed in 84, 86, 117, 179, 239, 249). And in all mammalian species yet analyzed, both mast cells and basophils express plasma membrane receptors (Fc$_\epsilon$RI) that specifically bind, with high affinity, the Fc portion of IgE antibody (18, 127, 180, 183, 244).

After active or passive sensitization with IgE, exposure to specific multivalent antigen triggers both cell types to undergo an integrated, noncytolytic series of biochemical (127, 180, 239) and ultrastructural (51, 86, 156, 227) alterations, often referred to as anaphylactic degranulation or exocytosis, that results in the exposure of the matrices of the cytoplasmic granules to the external medium. These events are associated with the release of both preformed mediators stored in the cytoplasmic granules (such as histamine, heparin or other sulfated proteoglycans, and certain proteases) and the *de novo* synthesis and release of such mediators as prostaglandins and/or leukotrienes. A similar sequence of events may be initiated by antibodies to IgE or to the plasma membrane Fc$_\epsilon$RI (reviewed in 127, 180, 239). Basophils and mast cells thus represent critical effector cells in disorders of IgE-dependent immediate hypersensitivity, and in all probability perform important roles in protective immune responses involving IgE as well (9, 27, 79, 84, 127, 160, 171, 179, 190, 191, 239, 267, 268).

Degranulation of basophils and mast cells also may be induced in response to any of a long (and growing) list of immunologically nonspecific agents including certain complement fragments, lymphokines and cytokines, many naturally occurring or synthetic basic peptides, lectins, and some neuropeptides and neurotransmitters (84, 117, 179, 239). While sensitivity to many of these stimuli varies strikingly according to species and cell type, the fact that a wide range of stimuli other than IgE and antigen can induce basophil and/or mast cell mediator release has provided great scope for speculation concerning the potential roles of these cells in a variety of biologic responses and diseases not involving IgE (reviewed in 78, 90).

ORIGIN AND DISTRIBUTION OF BASOPHILS

Despite their many remarkable similarities, mammalian mast cells and basophils are clearly not identical. Basophils differentiate and mature in the bone marrow, circulate in the blood, and are not primarily found in connective tissues. In humans, the basophil in the least common blood granulocyte, with a prevalence of ~0.5% of total leukocytes and ~0.3% of nucleated marrow cells (81, 93, 136). Both cytogenetic evidence (201, 245) and recent *in vitro* studies (47, 129, 197) indicate that basophils share a common precursor with other granulocytes and monocytes. In addition, human basophils appear to exhibit kinetics of production and peripheral circulation similar to that of eosinophils (188, 198). The latter observations and other findings suggest that basophils may share more similarities with eosinophils than with neutrophils (47, 246).

Basophils can be recruited into the tissues during certain IgE-dependent reactions and in association with a variety of other inflammatory, immunologic, and pathologic responses (79, 86). However, basophils that infiltrate peripheral tissues can still readily be identified as basophils in appropriately fixed and processed specimens; no morphologic evidence of transition of these cells to mast cells has ever been reported.

ORIGIN AND DISTRIBUTION OF MAST CELLS

In contrast to basophils, mast cells are ordinarily distributed throughout normal connective tissue, where they are often situated adjacent to blood and lymphatic vessels, near or within nerves, and beneath epithelial surfaces, such as those of the respiratory and gastrointestinal systems and the skin, that are exposed to environmental antigens (16, 86, 179, 241, 249). Mast cells also represent a numerically minor component of normal bone marrow and lymphoid tissues. Under certain circumstances, mast cells also can appear within epithelia of the gastrointestinal, respiratory, or urinary tract, and in some species may normally occur in these sites (65–67, 113, 182, 241). Some species also have numerous mast cells in the fibrous capsules of internal organs or in physiologic transudates such as peritoneal fluid. Although the density of mast cells in various anatomical sites in individual species exhibits considerable variation, mature mammalian mast cells, unlike basophils, do not normally circulate in the blood.

It appears likely that mammalian mast cells are derived from precursors which originate in the bone marrow. This point was conclusively established in the mouse by Kitamura *et al.* (147–150) in an elegant series of experiments exploiting genetically mast cell-deficient mutant mice and their congenic normal (+/+) littermates. A double dose of mutant genes at either the *W* or *Sl* locus of the mouse produces the pleiotropic effects of macrocytic anemia, sterility, and lack of hair pigmentation (103, 230). Kitamura *et al.* (147, 148) found that WBB6F$_1$-*W/W^v* (*W/W^v*) and WCB6F$_1$-*Sl/Sl^d* (*SL/SL^d*) mice also express a profound deficiency of mast cells. Table 1 summarizes some of the characteristics of *W/W^v* and *Sl/Sl^d* mice, with particular emphasis on those features with a bearing on the mast cell deficiency. Additional information is provided in recent reviews (83, 146, 149, 195).

One critical observation was that adult WBB6F$_1$-*W/W^v* mice can develop tissue mast cell populations if they receive bone marrow cells derived either from the normal littermates (WBB6F$_1$-+/+ mice), or from semisyngeneic C57BL/6-*bg/bg* ("beige") mice (148). Because mast cells derived from beige mice contain giant cytoplasmic granules (34, 108), the mast cells which develop in WBB6F$_1$-*W/W^v* mice transplanted with C57BL/6-*bg/bg* bone marrow cells can be identified unambiguously as of donor origin (148). This approach was used to establish that mouse mast cells develop from circulating, bone marrow-derived precursors (148), and that a common precursor cell (similar or identical with the CFU-S) can give rise to both mast cells and granulocytes (151). In contrast to the WBB6F$_1$-*W/W^v* mouse, the genetically mast cell deficient WCB6F$_1$-*Sl/Sl^d* mouse fails to develop recognizable mast cells after either systemic or local injection

TABLE 1. CHARACTERISTICS OF GENETICALLY MAST CELL-DEFICIENT WBB6F$_1$-*W/W^v* OR WCB6F$_1$-*Sl/Sl^d* MICE[a]

Characteristic	WBB6F$_1$-*W/W^v*	WCB6F$_1$-*Sl/Sl^d*
Genetic background	WB/Re-*W*/+ x C57BL/6-*W^v*/+[b]	WC/Re-*Sl*/+ x C57BL/6-*Sl^d*/+[b]
Mutations	Chromosome 5 (*c-kit*)[c]	Chromosome 10[c]
Defect resulting in mast cell deficiency	Stem cells/mast cell lineage itself	Tissue microenvironment
Repair of mast cell deficiency with congenic +/+ bone marrow cells or mast cells	Yes	No
Mast cells (% of +/+ level in adult, disease-free mice)	<1%[d]	<1%[d]
Mast cells develop in skin at sites of chronic idiopathic or PMA-induced dermatitis	Yes[e]	No[e]

[a] Both WBB6F$_1$-*W/W^v* and WCB6F$_1$-*Sl/Sl^d* mice also have a macrocytic anemia, lack hair pigmentation, and are sterile (103, 230).

[b] The four possible genotypes of the F$_1$ mice (*W/W^v*, *W*/+, *W^v*/+, +/+, or *Sl/Sl^d*, *Sl*/+, *Sl^d*/+, +/+) can be distinguished according to coat color. The *W/W^v* and *Sl/Sl^d* mice are white with black eyes, the congenic +/+ mice are black, the various heterozygotes can be distinguished by the pattern of spotting.

[c] The gene product of the *W* locus of the mouse would appear to be the putative tyrosine kinase receptor *c-kit* (33, 91). The gene product(s) encoded by the *Sl* locus have not yet been identified.

[d] The skin of adult *W/W^v* or *Sl/Sl^d* mice contains rare mast cells (~0.3% the number present in congenic +/+ mice). No mast cells at all have been observed in the following organs/sites: bone marrow, spleen, thymus, brain, heart, lung, kidney, urinary bladder, liver, stomach, ileum, cecum, mesentery, peritoneal cavity, hindlimb skeletal muscle, uterus.

[e] See references 85 and 101.

of congenic +/+ cells containing mast cell precursors (148, 195). Remarkably, however, intravenous injection of *Sl/Sl^d* mouse bone marrow cells into *W/W^v* mice cures the anemia of these mice, and also repairs their mast cell deficiency (147). In aggregate, these findings demonstrate that the mast cell deficiency of the *W/W^v* mouse reflects an abnormality in the mast cell lineage itself, whereas the mast cell deficiency of the *Sl/Sl^d* mouse reflects an abnormality of tissue factors regulating mast cell development (147, 149, 195).

Very recent work indicates that the *W* locus is closely linked to (33) and actually encodes (91) the putative tyrosine kinase receptor *c-kit*, that has significant homology to the receptors for colony stimulating factor-1 (CSF-1) and platelet-derived growth factor (PDGF) (33, 91). The finding that the *W* locus encodes a putative tyrosine kinase receptor, taken together with the results of both the bone marrow transplantation studies mentioned above and *in vitro* analyses of various mixtures of hematopoietic and stromal cells derived from the mutant and normal mice (see below and 133, 146, 149), raises the possibility that the mast cell deficiency and other phenotypic abnormalities of the *Sl/Sl^d* mouse may reflect the effect of mutations involving the gene encoding the ligand for *c-kit* (33, 91). The identity of this ligand has not yet been established, however, nor has the possibility been excluded that mutations at *Sl* involve a gene other than that encoding the *c-kit* ligand. The elucidation of the gene encoded at the *W* locus also suggests possible explanations for previous observations that mature mast cells developed locally in the dermis at sites of chronic idiopathic (85) or phorbol 12-myristate 13-acetate- (PMA-) induced (101) dermatitis in W/W^v but not Sl/Sl^d mice. For example, sites of dermatitis may have increased levels of the ligand for *c-kit*, that can interact with an abnormal receptor expressed by immature W/W^v cells in the mast cell lineage, or may provide signals that mimic or bypass those generated by the interaction of *c-kit* with its ligand.

But whatever the precise nature of their mutations at the molecular level, genetically mast cell-deficient mice already have provided important biological information about the natural history of the mast cell. Such work indicates that the circulating mouse mast cell precursor is present in normal blood in small numers ($\sim$1-2/10^5 nucleated cells) and cannot be identified as a mast cell by morphology (195). It also seems unlikely that basophils represent mast cell precursors in the mouse. Mouse peripheral blood basophils have not yet been purified, but they appear to exhibit light (263) and electron (58, 122) microscopic features similar to those of the basophils of other mammalian species. And while the number of basophils in the circulation of normal mice is quite low (263) (the number of circulating basophils in WBB6F$_1$-W/W^v and congenic +/+ mice is $\sim$2-3–10^3 nucleated cells, ref. 132), this number is substantially greater than the apparent number of circulating mast cell precursors.

In vitro studies have confirmed the hematopoietic origin of mouse mast cells. In 1980, Hasthorpe reported that cells with several phenotypic characteristics of mast cells could be grown from the spleen cells of a mouse previously injected with the cell-free supernatant from Friend-virus producing erythroleukemia cells (114). The growth of these mast cells was promoted by factor(s) present in the supernatants of pokeweed mitogen-stimulated spleen cells. However, the mast cells contained c-type virus particles by electron microscopy.

In 1981, several groups discovered that apparently pure populations of cells with many of the features of mast cells could be generated by culturing normal mouse hematopoietic cells in media derived from mitogen-activated T cells, cloned Ly1$^+$2$^-$ inducer T cells, or WEHI-3B tumor cells (189, 192, 214, 236, 261). While several different designations initially were proposed for these cells (189, 192, 214, 236, 261), the currently available evidence supports the view that they are most appropriately regarded as immature mast cells (88, 189, 280). These cells can be grown in large quantities compared to the numbers of mast cells that can be isolated directly from mice. And while the growth of the primary populations of mast cells generated *in vitro* typically is limited, it is possible to isolate long-term growth factor-dependent mast cell lines (189, 264, 279) or clones (88, 189) from such populations. IL-3-dependent mast cell lines can be routinely established from hematopoietic cells

infected with Harvey sarcoma virus either *in vitro* or *in vivo* (219). Colonies of growth factor-dependent mouse mast cells can also be generated from single progenitor cells in semi-solid methylcellulose cultures (194), a system particularly well-suited for *in vitro* studies of the relationship of mast cells to other hematopoietic lineages (194, 206, 207).

Growth factor-independent mast cell lines can arise spontaneously from growth factor-dependent populations (279), can be produced by infection of growth factor-dependent mast cell populations with Abelson-murine leukemia virus (Ab-MuLV) (208) *in vitro* or by injecting mice with Ab-MuLV (8), or can be derived by co-culturing mouse hematopoietic cells with fibroblasts producing the Kirstein murine sarcoma virus (KiSV) (222). Some of the KiSV-immortalized mast cell lines (KiSV-MC) more closely resemble in their phenotypic characteristics mature peritoneal mast cells than do classical growth factor-dependent mouse mast cells (222). As a result, they may facilitate the isolation of cDNA encoding products characteristic of mature mast cells (222, 254). On the other hand, the KiSV-MC are tumorigenic *in vivo* (222) and may exhibit other differences from normal mature mast cells.

RELATIONSHIP BETWEEN BASOPHILS AND MAST CELLS

The many similarities between basophils and mast cells have encouraged some to speculate that one of these cells might in some way give rise to the other. I believe that this notion is unlikely to be correct. Mammalian basophils and mast cells express several differences in natural history, as summarized in Table 2, but these two cell types are distinct in other respects as well. Morpho-

TABLE 2. NATURAL HISTORY OF MAMMALIAN BASOPHILS AND MAST CELLS[a]

Characteristic	Basophils	Mast cells
Origin of precursor cells	Bone marrow	Bone marrow[b]
Site of maturation	Bone marrow	Connective tissues; serosal cavities (some species)
Mature cells in the circulation	Yes	No
Mature cells recruited into tissues from circulation	Yes (during immunologic, inflammatory responses)	No
Mature cells normally residing in connective tissues	No (not detectable by microscopy)	Yes
Proliferative ability of morphologically mature cells	None reported	Yes (under certain circumstances)
Life span	Days (like other granulocytes)	Weeks to months[c]

Reproduced with permission, from (84).

[a] Note: Most data for basophils are derived from studies in humans and guinea pigs, as there have been very few studies of basophils in mice (see text).

[b] Established with certainty only in the mouse (see text).

[c] Based on studies in murine rodents.

logic differences between mature basophils and mast cells have been appreciated in all mammalian species which have been carefully investigated (50, 86). The most extensive studies have been performed with human cells (49–52, 55–57, 59–61, 109, 143, 283), the results of which are summarized in Table 3. Figure 1 is an electron micrograph illustrating the morphological differences between a mature human basophil and a mature mast cell observed in the same tissue. Mature basophils and mast cells also differ in mediator production and response to corticosteroids and other drugs (reviewed in 9, 36, 84, 234, 235), and express differences in histochemistry (201) and in reactivity with various antibodies (20, 221, 224).

On the other hand, one might argue that the many phenotypic differences between basophils and mast cells may be analogous to those distinguishing circulating monocytes and their derivatives (*e.g.* macrophages) residing in the tissues. While this possibility has not formally been rejected, it is difficult to reconcile with a number of findings. For example, no evidence has been presented, in any species, indicating that mature circulating basophils are capable either of mitosis or of differentiation into mast cells. The rare reports of patients with hereditary or acquired abnormalities affecting basophil numbers or morphology indicate that eosinophils

may also be affected in these disorders, but not mast cells (137, 184, 262). Finally, morphologically identifiable mast cells clearly can exhibit mitotic activity (55), indicating that this cell lineage is capable of replication independently of a stage resembling that of the circulating basophil. Taken together, these observations favor the view that mature basophils represent terminally differentiated granulocytes, not circulating mast cell precursors.

MAST CELL HETEROGENEITY

INTRODUCTION

Before beginning a detailed analysis of mast cell heterogeneity, we should consider the term "heterogeneity" itself. Cells within a given population can be said to exhibit heterogeneity once a certain minimum (but generally unspecified) level of variation in one or more of their characteristics has been demonstrated. Thus, and this can't be emphasized strongly enough, heterogeneity is a purely descriptive term. A cell type may exhibit heterogeneity with respect to size, ultrastructure, mediator content, response to drugs, and/or other characteristics, taken alone or in combination. Yet individual examples of such phenotypic heterogeneity may reflect the operation of different underlying mechanisms.

Discussions of mast cell heterogeneity also frequently include two additional terms: "differentiation" and "maturation." Differentiation may be defined as "specialization; the acquisition or the possession of character or function different from that of the original type" (250). By contrast, "maturation" can be defined as "the process of achieving full development or growth" (250). Thus, most or all processes of cellular differentiation can be included within the broader process of maturation, but certain maturational events (*e.g.*, the storage of increasing amounts of histamine by maturing mast cells), may not properly be considered examples of differentiation. To avoid potential confusion, and to acknowledge that in many cases it is not yet clear which of the terms is more appropriate, the entire process by which mature mast cells develop from their precursors will be designated herein as "maturation/differentiation."

EVIDENCE FOR HETEROGENEITY OF MAST CELL PHENOTYPIC CHARACTERISTICS *IN VIVO*

Mast Cell Heterogeneity in Rats and Mice. Although mast cell heterogeneity has only recently attracted widespread interest, the initial observations that mast cells in different anatomical locations exhibit readily discernible differences in morphology are nearly 100 years old. Maximow is usually credited with the first observation that certain mast cells in the rat intestinal mucosa were "atypical" in their histochemical staining characteristics, that differed from those of mast cells observed in other anatomical sites (172). However, Hardy and Wesbrook published in 1895 what may be the first evidence of morphologic differences among mast cells ("basophile cells") observed in different anatomical locations in the rat (112).

Beginning in the 1960s, Enerbäck (65, 66) greatly extended the early observations of mast cell heteroge-

TABLE 3. MORPHOLOGIC FEATURES OF MATURE BASOPHILS AND MAST CELLS IN HUMANS

Characteristic	Basophils	Mast Cells
Size	5–7 μm	6–12 μm
Surface	Irregular, short, thick processes	Numerous, relatively uniformly distributed, elongated thin processes
Nucleus	Segmented	Non-segmented (usually round-to-oval in electron micrographs)
Nuclear chromatin condensation	Marked	Moderate
Cytoplasmic granules	Fewer and larger than in mast cells; contain predominantly electron-dense particulate material with occasional membranous whorls	Smaller, more numerous and generally more variable in appearance than in basophils; contain scroll-like structures, particles and crystals, alone or in combination
Aggregates of cytoplasmic glycogen	Present	Absent
Cytoplasmic lipid bodies	Rare	Common (but not present in all cells)
Granule-granule fusion during "anaphylactic" degranulation	Rare (granule membranes usually fuse individually with plasma membrane)	Common

Reproduced with permission, from (84).

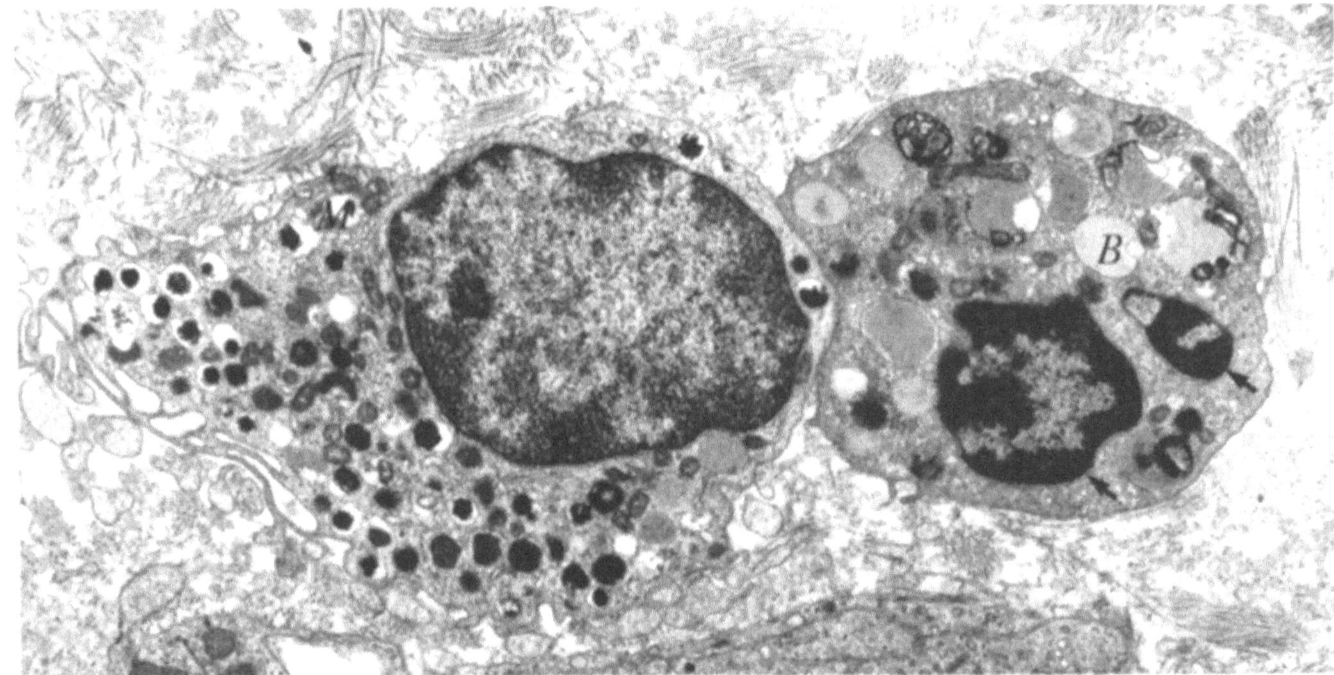

FIG. 1. A basophil (*B*) adjacent to a mast cell (*M*) in the ileal submucosa of a patient with Crohn's disease. The basophil exhibits a bilobed nucleus (*solid arrows*) whose chromatin is strikingly condensed beneath the nuclear membrane. The basophil surface is relatively smooth with a few blunt processes. The mast cell nucleus is larger, and its chromatin less condensed than that of the basophil. The mast cell's granules are smaller, more numerous, and more variable in shape and content than those of the basophil. The mast cell surface has numerous elongated, thin folds. Reproduced with permission from Dvorak *et al.* (57). ×8,700.

neity and defined in detail the conditions of fixation and histochemical staining which discriminated between the "atypical" or "mucosal" mast cells (MMC) observed in the intestinal lamina propria and the "connective-tissue-type" mast cells (CTMC) of the skin, peritoneal cavity, and other sites in the rat. Enerbäck and others also showed that in addition to differing in morphologic and histochemical characteristics, rat and mouse MMC and CTMC appear to differ in many other aspects of natural history, biochemistry, function and roles in inflammation and immunity (reviewed in 3, 12, 15, 65, 66, 135, 173, 182, 228, 260). One of the most striking of these differences, discussed in greater detail below, is that populations of MMC expand remarkably during T cell-dependent immune responses to certain intestinal parasites (173, 228). By contrast, CTMC exhibit little or no "T cell dependence," and occur in athymic nude mice or rats in numbers similar to those present in normal animals (3, 173, 228).

The terms "mucosal" and "connective tissue-type" mast cell (*i.e.*, MMC and CTMC) are the designations for mast cell "subtypes" most frequently encountered in the literature. As pointed out by Enerbäck (66) and others, these terms are least confusing when used to refer to the mature mast cell phenotype typical of a particular anatomical site, *e.g.*, the rat or mouse small intestinal mucosa (for MMC); the rat or mouse peritoneal cavity or skin (for "serosal" or CTMC). Nevertheless, one occasionally finds the term "MMC" used to refer to populations of mast cells which share characteristics of true MMC, but which are derived from non-mucosal sites (*e.g.*, certain growth factor-dependent mast cells gener-

ated *in vitro*). To distinguish such cells from MMC observed *in situ* in the gut, and to indicate that they may not be identical to true MMC, these cells will be designated herein as "MMC-like."

Finally, it should be emphasized that not all rat and mouse mast cells observed *in situ* can readily be categorized as classical MMC or CTMC. Aldenborg and Enerbäck (4) showed that while most dermal mast cells in the rat express a typical CTMC phenotype, some subepidermal mast cells have dye-binding properties and other features intermediate between those of MMC and CTMC (4). These investigators found no evidence indicating that these subepidermal mast cells can develop into typical CTMC. But even if such a transformation were to be demonstrated, the findings illustrate that phenotypically distinct "subpopulations" of mast cells can exist in different regions of the same anatomical site in adult animals.

Mast Cell Heterogeneity in Man. Human mast cells also exhibit variation in multiple aspects of their phenotype, including morphologic characteristics such as size (216) and cytoplasmic granule ultrastructure (49, 70, 131, 143), histochemical properties (11, 67, 229, 255), quantity of stored histamine (216), content of granule-associated neutral proteases (39, 126, 232, 238), sensitivity to stimulation by various secretogogues (13, 35, 36, 158), and susceptibility to various drugs (35, 36, 162). The potential clinical significance of mast cell heterogeneity in man is stimulating great efforts to define the spectrum of phenotypic characteristics exhibited by different populations of human mast cells. But data demonstrating phenotypic heterogeneity in human mast cells (and in mast cells of other species) must be examined very critically. When histochemical, immunochemical, or morphologic approaches are used to define heterogeneity, comparisons of results of different studies are simplest when the different groups of investigators have employed identical methods. Similarly, when functional criteria (*e.g.*, responsiveness to different secretogogues) are used, the data are most useful if the different populations of mast cells being evaluated have been isolated and tested using exactly the same techniques (of mechanical tissue dispersion, enzymatic digestion, etc.), since details of isolation methods may influence the properties of the cells being examined.

At the present time, these criteria have been met too infrequently to attempt a comprehensive summary of the phenotypic characteristics of different populations of human mast cells. Nor is it possible to define human human mast cell subpopulations that are analogous in all respects to murine MMC and CTMC. Perhaps the most attractive currently available potential "marker" for human mast cell "subpopulations" is cytoplasmic granule protease content. Proteases are a quantitatively important component of mast cell granules (157, 182, 238, 274, 281). In addition, the substrate specificity and solubility characteristics of these proteases can be used to fashion hypotheses about the special biologic functions of different populations of mast cells *in vivo* (182, 238, 274). Indeed, while most mast cell-associated mediators can be produced by other cell types (78, 90, 117, 179, 239), the granule-associated neutral proteases may represent constituents restricted to the mast cell. They thus may provide important insights into the unique functions of this cell.

Like rats (161, 182, 271–274) and mice (182), humans have mast cell subpopulations which differ in neutral protease content. Some human mast cells contain measurable levels of both tryptase and chymase (39, 126, 238), whereas other human mast cells contain tryptase but no detectable chymase (<0.04 pg/cell) (126, 238). These mast cells were initially designated TC or T mast cells to denote their predominant granule-associated neutral protease content (126, 238). However, this review will use the newer designations MC^{TC} and MC^{T}, as recommended in the consensus statement of a recent conference on mast cell heterogeneity (14). It is not yet clear whether MC^{T}, which contain substantially less tryptase than MC^{TC}, entirely lack chymase or have small amounts that are undetectable with current techniques (238). Nevertheless, it is possible to classify human mast cells in multiple anatomical sites on the basis of their predominant protease content as MC^{T} or MC^{TC} (39, 238). Such studies indicate that most anatomical sites contain a mixture of these mast cells (238). Thus, while MC^{T} predominate in lung and small intestinal mucosa and MC^{TC} predominate in skin and small intestinal submucosa, all of these sites contain representatives of both mast cell subtypes (238). As a result, human mast cells cannot be classified as MC^{T} or MC^{TC} based on tissue location alone (238).

Transmission electron microscopic studies of human mast cells established that their cytoplasmic granules can exhibit a variety of substructural patterns, referred to as scrolls, particles, and crystals (49, 52, 143). Granules of the scroll pattern are shown in Figures 2 and 3, granules with a crystalline substructural pattern are shown in Figure 4, and a mast cell containing granules with a particulate substructure is shown in Figure 1. Recent immunoelectron microscopic analysis (39, 238) indicates that MC^{T} have tryptase-containing cytoplasmic granules with the scroll-like configurations. By contrast, MC^{TC} lack scroll-containing granules but characteristically have tryptase- and chymase-positive granules with the crystalline or "grating/lattice" substructure (40, 41). The exact frequency with which mast cells with features of both MC^{T} and MC^{TC} occur, and the implications of this finding for the relationship between these subtypes, remain to be determined (238). However, occasional human mast cells contain cytoplasmic granules of scroll, particle, and crystal type, and some individual granules exhibit mixtures of these substructural patterns (49).

Numbers of intestinal mucosal and submucosal MC^{T}, but not MC^{TC}, are reduced in patients with either congenital combined immunodeficiency diseases or the acquired immunodeficiency syndrome, consistent with a T cell-dependent requirement for generation and/or maintenance of normal populations of MC^{T} (125). In this respect, MC^{T} seem similar to rat or mouse MMC, and MC^{TC} resemble murine CTMC. However, not all of the properties of MC^{T} and MC^{TC} may be predictable based on the properties of rat MMC and CTMC. In the rat, there appears to be a good correlation between mast cell protease phenotype, the ability to release histamine in response to stimulation with basic compounds such as compound 48/80 or substance P, and susceptibility for inhibition of activation by disodium cromoglycate (DSCG, reviewed in 204, 249). Thus rat peritoneal or skin mast cells (CTMC) contain the protease RMCP I,

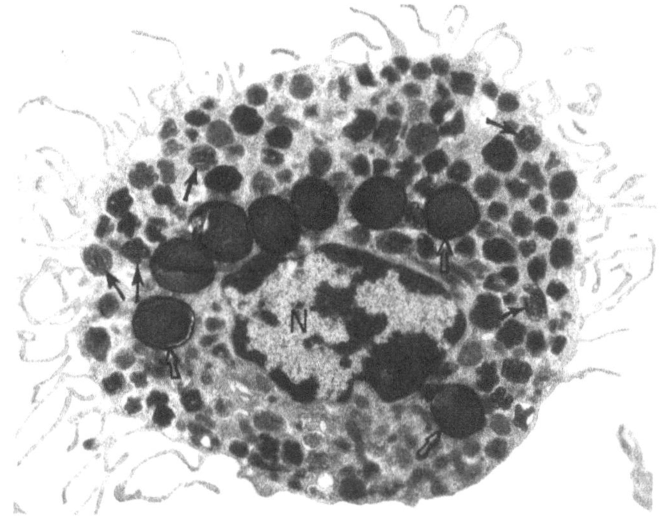

FIG. 2. Mast cell purified from human lung. The cell contains many cytoplasmic granules with scroll-like substructural elements (*solid arrows*) and eight large nonmembrane-bound lipid bodies (*open arrows*). The plasma membrane has prominent folds. N, nucleus. Reproduced with permission from Galli *et al.* (86) ×6,900.

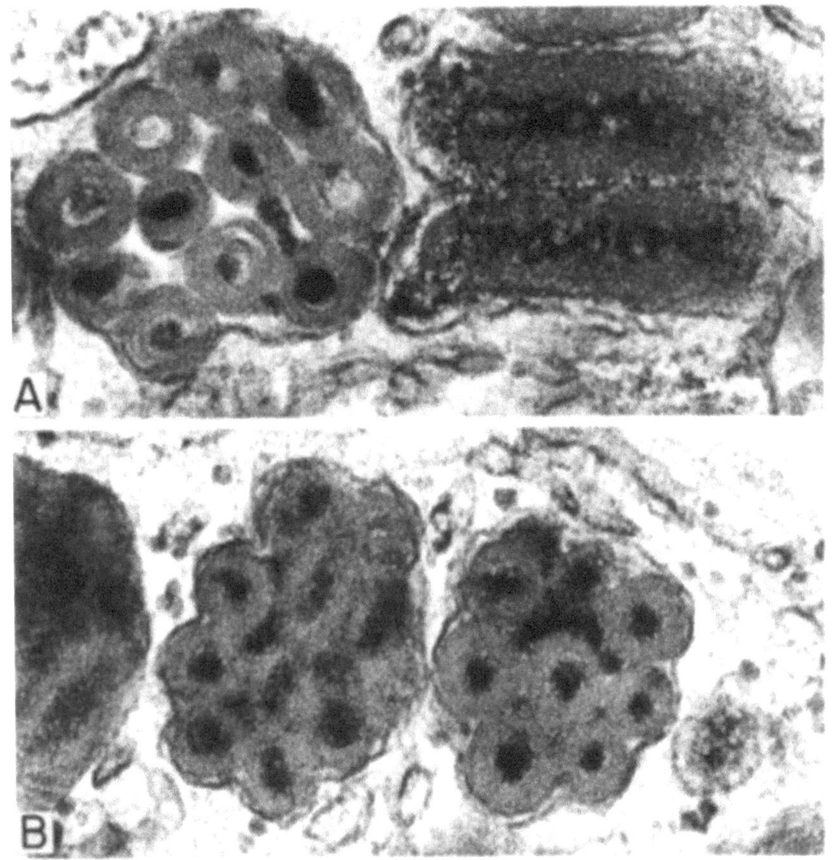

FIG. 3. Higher magnification view of scroll-containing cytoplasmic granules in purified human lung mast cells. The scrolls are shown both in cross-section (*A* and *B*) and in longitudinal section (*A*). Electron-dense material is present within and focally between the scrolls, whose lamellae exhibit a periodic cross-banding. *A* and *B*, Osmium tetroxide potassium ferrocyanide technique. Reproduced with permission from Dvorak (49). Figure 3*A*, ×100,000; *B*, ×90,000.

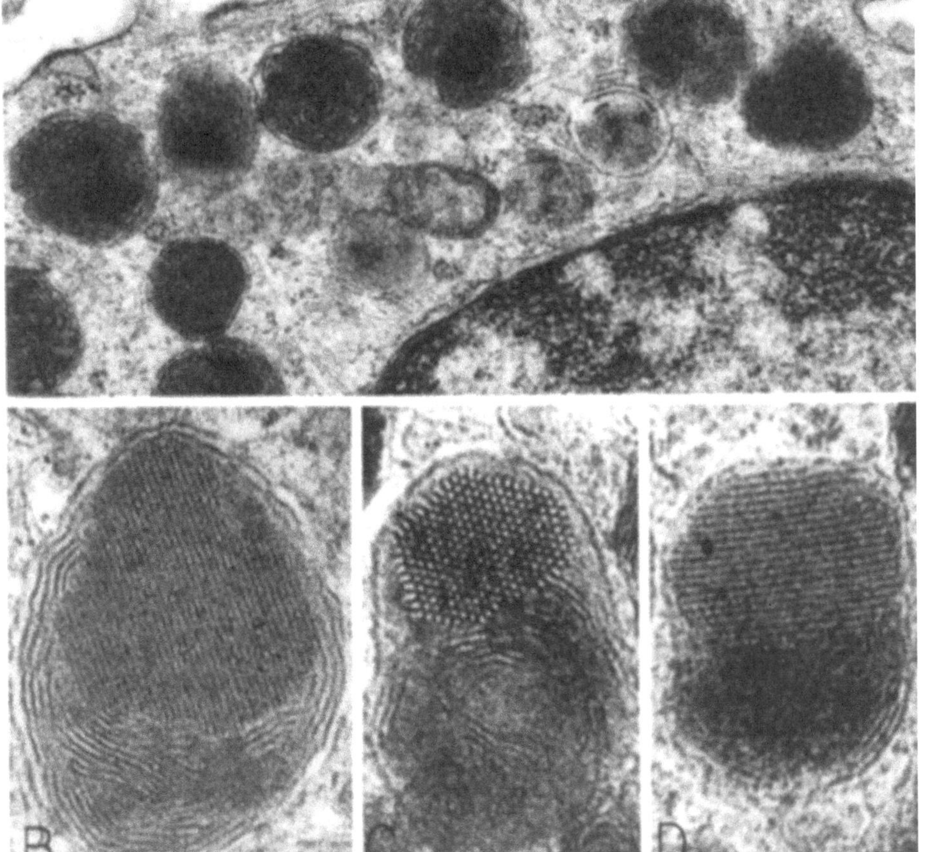

FIG. 4. Human skin mast cell granules with crystalline substructural patterns (*A-D*). When cut in cross-section, these exhibit a hexagonal pattern (*C*). (*A*. × 41,500; *B*. × 86,200; *C,D*. × 104,000). Reproduced with permission from Dvorak (49).

are sensitive to stimulation by compound 48/80 or substance P, and are susceptible to inhibition by DSCG; rat intestinal MMC contain predominantly RMCP II, are relatively insensitive to stimulation with compound 48/80 or substance P, and are not inhibited by DSCG. By contrast, Church *et al.* (35) reported that partially purified preparations of human skin mast cells (>85% MC^{TC}) were very sensitive to stimulation by substance P and other basic secretogogues, but not to inhibition by disodium cromoglycate, whereas mast cells isolated from lung (<10% MC^{TC}) and from colon mucosa or muscle (60% MC^{TC}) were insensitive to substance P stimulation but sensitive to inhibition of histamine release by disodium cromoglycate.

Conclusions. Studies such as those just outlined indicate that while human mast cell populations certainly exhibit heterogeneity, it may not be possible to identify one or two key phenotypic characteristics that can accurately predict many others. On the contrary, identification of the full spectrum of phenotypic characteristics of mast cells in different organs or anatomical sites probably will require analysis of multiple features of each mast cell population. Such detailed analysis of the individual characteristics of particular mast cell populations may represent a critical element in efforts to elucidate the roles of mast cells in health and disease. The potential value of this approach is illustrated by studies of the complex interactions between cutaneous mast cells and neuropeptides.

Human cutaneous mast cells (31, 35, 36, 104, 116, 158), like rat CTMC (249), are very sensitive to activation by substance P. Human cutaneous mast cells also express optimal mediator release at 30° C, a temperature likely to be representative of the conditions of activation of skin mast cells *in vivo* (158). And while substance P can produce multiple effects *in vivo* besides those mediated by mast cells, studies in mast cell-deficient and mast cell-reconstituted mice indicate that virtually all of the acute augmentation in local vascular permeability (275), tissue swelling (275), and infiltration of granulocytes (170, 275) induced by intradermal injection of substance P is mast cell dependent. Taken together, these findings suggest that mast cell activation significantly contributes to augmentation of cutaneous vascular permeability induced by the release of endogenous substance P.

Several lines of evidence now indicate that mast cell products also might down-regulate certain vascular changes induced by release of neuropeptides. *In vitro* studies showed that the rat CTMC protease RMCP I can effectively hydrolyze a variety of polypeptides, including neurotensin (161). Although RMCP I does not effectively degrade substance P (161), proteases isolated from dog mastocytoma cells can hydrolyze this peptide (32). And hydrolysis of polypeptides by RMCP I is particularly resistant to inhibition by rat serum or α_1-antitrypsin when the protease remains associated with the mast cell granules, as it would under physiologic conditions *in vivo* (161). *In vivo* studies indicate that degranulated rat cutaneous mast cells may be able to degrade the potent vasodilator calcitonin gene-related peptide (CGRP) (22), which can occur together with substance P in the same nerves (92, 167). Moreover, the duration of vasodilation which follows injection of CGRP into rat or human skin is markedly diminished when substance P is injected at the same time, suggesting that substance P-induced mast cell degranulation can result in attenuation of CGRP-induced vasodilatation (22).

This example by no means exhausts the potentially important interactions between neuropeptides, mast cells, and the nervous system, a subject of intense current interest (16, 100, 249). Indeed, certain populations of mast cells may themselves be able to generate molecules similar to neuropeptides (100). Nor do I wish to imply that all aspects of "neurogenic inflammation" are mast cell-dependent, as this is very unlikely (153). However, the available evidence does illustrate how the particular phenotypic characteristics of cutaneous mast cells may permit them to participate in both the augmentation and the subsequent down-regulation of certain manifestations of neuropeptide-induced inflammation. Further analysis of the physiologic and/or pathological consequences of interactions among neuropeptides, mast cells, and the nervous system in the skin and other organs will continue to require careful consideration of multiple specific phenotypic characteristics of the mast cell populations thought to participate in these processes. The same general point applies to the analysis of any other potential role for the mast cell in health and disease.

ALTERNATIVE MECHANISMS WHICH MIGHT ACCOUNT FOR MAST CELL HETEROGENEITY

Distinct Mast Cell Lineages. Mast cell phenotypic variation theoretically might reflect the following mechanisms, acting alone or in combination: (a) the existence of distinct mast cell lineages; (b) the process of cellular maturation/differentiation; (c) the functional status of the cell; and (d) the acquisition of molecules derived from other cell types (77).

Of these four possible mechanisms, evidence reviewed below indicates that the last three actually occur. By contrast, it is not yet clear whether distinct mast cell lineages exist. While definitions of cell "lineage" may vary, the term is used here in the sense in which it is applied to populations of granulocytes or lymphocytes. Two important sets of observations support the conclusion that neutrophils, eosinophils and basophils represent three distinct lineages of granulocytes (212). First, the three types of granulocyte exhibit clear qualitative and/or quantitative differences in multiple characteristics, including morphology, biochemistry and function. Second, the commitment of these cells to their own particular phenotype appears to be irrevocable, reflecting a stereotyped and, under physiological conditions, apparently irreversible alteration in the pattern of gene expression during their maturation/differentiation from a common precursor. Lymphocytes also can express apparently irrevocable commitment to distinct lineages of maturation/differentiation (202). But in contrast to the differentiation of the three granulocyte lineages, which may be readily monitored using morphological approaches, conventional morphology is considerably less useful in assessing the process of lymphocyte differentiation.

By analogy to the natural history of granulocytes, proof of the existence of distinct mast cell lineages should include not only demonstration of predictable differences in *phenotype* among the putative subsets, but also evidence of *irrevocable commitment* to the expression of such differences. On the other hand, consideration of the natural history of lymphocyte differentiation makes a different, but equally important, point: cells which *appear* quite similar by morphology can exhibit striking differences in gene expression and function. Thus, the existence of distinct mast cell lineages cannot be *excluded* simply because the population of mast cells studied appears homogeneous with respect to those particular phenotypic characteristics (whether of morphology, biochemistry, or function) which happen to have been analyzed.

Given the enormous number of distinct molecules comprising any particular cell, how many irreversible differences must there be in the phenotype of two different cells for them to be assigned to distinct lineages? While no single answer to this question is likely to satisfy all investigators, one important consideration might be the biologic significance of the molecules involved. Let's postulate: (a) that a single cell in the mouse mast cell lineage can generate two distinct types of progeny, one of which can synthesize only histamine and the other only serotonin (or, alternatively, the two cells can synthesize only one of two possible types of neutral protease); (b) that these patterns of mediator synthesis were shown to be irreversible under various conditions *in vivo* and *in vitro*; and (c) that when these two types of mast cell were induced to proliferate they continued to adhere to their own particular pattern of mediator production (*i.e.*, histamine$^+$, serotonin$^-$; histamine$^-$, serotonin$^+$). This evidence might convince many investigators to concede that the two types of mast cells represented distinct lineages, even if they were found to be identical by all other criteria tested. But what if proliferation of either "type" of mast cell produced mature progeny of both histamine$^+$ serotonin$^-$ and histamine$^-$, serotonin$^+$ type? The latter occurrence would provide important information about the relationship of proliferation to patterns of gene expression in the mast cell, but would also cast into serious doubt the conclusion that histamine$^+$, serotonin and histamine$^-$, serotonin$^+$ mast cells represented distinct "lineages."

In summary, the notion that at least some of the mast cell populations expressing different patterns of phenotypic characteristics, like the three types of mammalian granulocytes, represent distinct lineages has heuristic value and is consistent with some of the available data. On the other hand, it is not yet clear that phenotypically distinct "subsets" of mast cells are irrevocably committed to the expression of particular unique patterns of phenotypic characteristics.

Cellular Maturation/Differentiation. Another mechanism which may account for at least some of the phenotypic diversity observed in mast cell populations *in vivo* is the process of cell maturation/differentiation occurring within a single lineage. Circulating monocytes and tissue or peritoneal exudate macrophages exhibit many quantitative and qualitative differences in phenotype,

yet the latter populations clearly are derived from the former (243). B cells exhibit what is arguably an even more complex natural history, which includes striking alterations in their mitotic potential, morphology, and gene expression (38). For example, the immunoglobulin "isotype switch" represents a critical and characteristic feature of B cell maturation/differentiation. But if the underlying mechanisms accounting for this "change of phenotype" were not appreciated, it might be tempting to speculate that B cells synthesizing IgM must represent a "lineage" distinct from those synthesizing IgG.

Others already have pointed out certain similarities between the natural history of monocytes/macrophages and mast cells: both are derived from the bone marrow, and both circulate as forms which differ morphologically from the corresponding mature populations in the tissues (150, 284). In addition, like murine mast cells, the derivatives of circulating monocytes may express distinct phenotypes in different anatomical locations (*e.g.* alveolar macrophages, Kupffer cells, etc.) (243). While the extent to which these distinct derivatives of circulating monocytes are irrevocably committed to their particular pattern of phenotypic expression remains to be determined, at least some of the properties of monocytes/macrophages may be strikingly (and perhaps irrevocably) altered in response to microenvironmental factors (243). For example, under certain circumstances tissue macrophages may transform into "epithelioid" cells, or form different varieties of multinucleated giant cells (243). As discussed in detail below, murine mast cells also exhibit striking phenotypic changes during their maturation/differentiation.

Changes Associated with Functional Activation. Profound alterations in mast cell ultrastructure accompany the stimulus-induced release of the cells' stored and newly generated mediators (49, 51, 86, 154, 156, 227). While rapid, "anaphylactic" patterns of mast cell degranulation have been the most intensively studied, Dvorak and Dvorak proposed that basophils and mast cells may also be able to release granule-associated mediators in a slower, more gradual "piecemeal" fashion (reviewed in 61, 86). Both "anaphylactic" and "piecemeal" patterns of mast cell degranulation can alter the staining characteristics of the cell, probably because of changes in the physicochemical properties of granule-associated proteoglycans and other granule constituents. Furthermore, mast cells stimulated to undergo degranulation can synthesize a new complement of cytoplasmic granules, and these newly synthesized granules may differ in size, morphometric characteristics and appearance (and perhaps in mediator content) from those in mature, unstimulated cells (reviewed in 49, 59, 86, 110, 111, 154 and I. Hammel and D. Lagunoff, personal communication).

Indeed, morphological evidence indicates that mast cells in the process of replenishing their cytoplasmic granules after undergoing degranulation can exhibit many features of cellular "immaturity" including changes in nuclear chromatin condensation, as well as the appearance in the cytoplasm of the machinery of protein synthesis (49, 59, 154). However, the full extent of the similarities and differences between morphologically "immature" mast cells which have never previously achieved full cellular maturation ("authentically" immature mast cells) and the morphologically "immature" mast cells which are synthesizing a new complement of granules after having reached maturity and undergone degranulation (herein designated "born again" immature mast cells) remains to be determined. For example, it is not yet clear whether truly immature mast cells and "born again" immature mast cells have a similar potential for proliferation.

Acquisition of Molecules Derived from Other Cell Types. Although discussions of mast cell heterogeneity generally focus on factors that might influence patterns of *mast cell* gene expression, it has been recognized for some time that mast cells can take up a variety of exogenous or endogenous substances from their immediate environment and store them in their cytoplasmic granules (reviewed in 200). This process clearly represents a potential mechanism of mast cell phenotypic heterogeneity. For example, there has been some controversy about whether basophils or mast cells contain peroxidase activity (reviewed in 52, 53, 76). Michel *et al.* (181) recently reported that the acquisition of cytochemically detectable peroxidase activity in the nuclear envelope and endoplasmic reticulum of growth factor-dependent, bone marrow-derived mouse mast cells generated *in vitro* was associated with the dexamethasone-induced maturation of these cells.

These findings suggest that one source of variation in the peroxidase activity of mast cell populations may be the extent of the cells' maturation/differentiation. However, Dvorak *et al.* (52, 53) reported another possible explanation for variable expression of peroxidase activity by basophils and mast cells. Freshly isolated guinea pig peripheral blood basophils (53), cloned mouse mast cells maintained *in vitro* (53), and human basophils generated *in vitro* (52) lacked cytochemically detectable peroxidase activity in Golgi structures and rough endoplasmic reticulum, a finding that suggested that the cells were not synthesizing significant amounts of the enzyme. But all three cell types were able to take up exogenous eosinophil peroxidase within endocytotic vesicles that fused with the cytoplasmic granules (52, 53).

Apart from representing a mechanism that can alter aspects of mast cell phenotype, the ability of mast cells to take up molecules such as eosinophil peroxidase may constitute an important part of the cells' functional repertoire. Mast cell uptake of eosinophil peroxidase and other exogenous or endogenous compounds (a) may limit the biologic effects of these substances by withdrawing them from the microenvironment into which they had been initially liberated (whether or not uptake results in denaturation of the compound); and (b) may place expression of the biologic activity of these compounds (or the derivatives of these compounds as they exist within mast cell granules) under the regulation of signals which stimulate mast cell activation, rather than those governing the behavior of the cells or other sources of the original compounds. Evidence for the last possibility has been reported by Henderson *et al.* (115) who showed that mast cell granule-dependent killing of schistosomula

of *Schistosoma mansoni in vitro* was potentiated when the mast cell granules were permitted to bind EPO to their surface before their use in assays of cytotoxicity.

"MICROENVIRONMENTAL" REGULATION OF MAST CELL DEVELOPMENT AND PHENOTYPE

Introduction. The notion that mast cell phenotype can be importantly regulated by the cell's "microenvironment" has been the subject of much recent discussion and interest. Like "heterogeneity" itself, "microenvironment" is a descriptive term that may mean different things to different investigators. It will be used here in its broadest sense, to mean simply "the immediate vicinity of the cell." There are many possible sources of variation in microenvironmental factors which might have an effect on mast cell phenotype, and each of these potentially might influence mast cell phenotype by any of a variety of mechanisms.

As indicated in Table 4, such sources of variation in microenvironmental factors may be classified as constitutive or acquired. The mucosa and muscularis propria of certain regions of the rat or mouse gastrointestinal tract represent examples of constitutively distinct microenvironments, since MMC ordinarily predominate in the former, whereas CTMC normally occur in the latter (65, 66). However, inflammatory, immunologic or disease processes might induce transient changes in anatomical microenvironments which affect the mast cell populations residing in such areas. For example, the site of an intense T cell-dependent inflammatory response may have levels of lymphocyte-derived and other cytokines influencing mast cell proliferation or maturation/differentiation which are quite different than the "baseline" levels of these products expressed at the same anatomical location under normal circumstances. And certain microenvironments, such as sites of inflammation containing large numbers of eosinophils, may have high concentrations of molecules which can be internalized by mast cells. Alternatively, a particular microenvironment might be rich in substances (*e.g.*, IgE and specific antigen) which alter mast cell phenotype as a consequence of inducing mast cell degranulation. Finally, it is important to recognize that the mast cell itself, through the production of cytokines such as IL-3, GM-CSF, and/or IL-4 (26, 28, 210, 270, and see below) or by other potential mechanisms outlined in the Table, might participate in the regulation of its own numbers and phenotype, especially during immunological or disease processes.

Cytokine-Dependent Regulation of Mast Cell Proliferation and Maturation/Differentiation. A large number of histologic studies, some of them quite old, demonstrated that the size of different mast cell populations can increase significantly during a wide variety of immunologic or pathologic processes (65, 86, 179, 241). The development of techniques to grow mast cell populations *in vitro* provided a new approach for identifying and characterizing the actual cell-cell interactions and molecules which might regulate such proliferation. The seminal studies in this area were conducted by Ginsburg and his associates, who showed that mast cell populations developed in tissue culture systems incorporating lymphoid cells and

TABLE 4. MECHANISMS BY WHICH MICROENVIRONMENTAL FACTORS MIGHT REGULATE ASPECTS OF MOUSE MAST CELL PHENOTYPE AND REPRESENTATIVE SOURCES OF VARIATION IN SUCH FACTORS[a]

Mechanisms which may regulate mast cell phenotype	Examples/comments	Mechanisms which may regulate mast cell phenotype	Examples/comments
1. Factors promoting branching within the mast cell lineage	It is not yet certain whether "branching," *i.e.*, irrevocable commitment to more than one pattern of gene expression, occurs within the mast cell lineage	2. Acquired variation (in systemic and/or local levels of factors) in association with immune responses, disease processes, hormonal fluctuations, aging, etc.	Expansion of numbers of MMC in mice during T cell-dependent responses to intestinal parasites, probably reflecting, at least in part, increased production of IL-3 and IL-4; increased numbers of mast cells during a wide variety of pathological processes in man and experimental animals
2. Factors influencing differentiation/maturation (within a single or, if they occur, multiple pathway(s))	IL-3, IL-4, products of fibroblasts and possibly other cells present in the tissues		
3. Factors modulating aspects of function—*e.g.*, stimuli of secretory activity	IgE and specific antigen; many other "mast cell secretogogues," including C3a, C5a, and certain neuropeptides	3. "Mast cell-dependent"	Production by mast cells of cytokines influencing mast cell proliferation or phenotype, such as IL-3, IL-4, and GM-CSF; changes in microenvironmental levels of factors present in the plasma, or derived from leukocytes, as a consequence of mast cell-dependent changes in local vascular permeability or leukocyte infiltration; or mast cell-dependent changes in the properties of other cells resident in the tissues (*e.g.*, fibroblasts, endothelial, mesothelial or epithelial cells) which might be able to influence mast cell phenotype
4. Factors influencing local concentrations of exogenous substances not derived from mast cells but which are taken up and stored in mast cell granules	Agents which recruit and/or activate eosinophils		
Sources of variation in expression/levels of factors[b] influencing mast cell phenotype[c]			
1. Constitutive, based on anatomical site	Such variation probably accounts for differences in the phenotype of MMC and CTMC (or "serosal") mast cells in rats and mice, and for the special characteristics of cutaneous mast cells in man and other species		

[a] While some factors, such as IL-3, may influence both mast cell numbers and phenotype, others theoretically might influence only one aspect of mast cell biology, such as maturation/differentiation.

[b] "Factors" refers to signals presented on the surface of other cells, as soluble secreted products, or in association with other constituents of the microenvironment, such as proteoglycans, or other environmental conditions that affect mast cell phenotype. Variation in such factors may be qualitative and/or quantitative.

[c] Each source of variation theoretically might influence mast cell phenotype through any combination of the four mechanisms listed above.

embryonic fibroblasts derived from mice, and that mast cell growth in these systems was enhanced by products of antigen or mitogen-activated T cells (43, 95–99). Ishizaka *et al.* reported similar findings in the rat (128, 130).

As important as these studies were in defining approaches for the *in vitro* growth of mast cells, several fundamental questions about mast cell biology remained unresolved. One of these was the observation that T cell-dependent immune responses to certain intestinal nematodes in mice and rats were associated with striking (>100-fold) amplifications of numbers of intestinal MMC (reviewed in 66, 86, 135, 173, 228). Burnet and others pointed out that such "T cell-dependent" mast cell proliferation might reflect either the derivation of mast cells from T cells or the influence of a T cell-derived factor(s) on mast cell proliferation (29). Currently available evidence clearly favors the latter possibility. Several groups reported that cells with features of mast cells could be generated *in vitro* from normal mouse hematopoietic cells maintained in the presence of defined cell

supernatants including those derived from T cells (188, 192, 214, 236, 261). Moreover, both T cells that produced factor(s) required for mast cell proliferation *in vitro* (Ly1$^+$2$^-$ "inducer" T cells) and mast cells that proliferated in response to such factors could be cloned and characterized in detail (189). Taken together with similar evidence derived from uncloned cells (189, 214, 236, 261), this work provided a clear explanation for "T cell-dependent" mast cell proliferation.

Because suspension cultures of normal mouse bone marrow cells maintained for several weeks in T cell-conditioned medium consisted almost entirely of cells committed to the mast cell lineage, we (88, 189) and Moore and his associates (261, 279, 280) tentatively named the responsible activity in these supernatants "mast cell growth factor." However, it soon became clear that the major properties of "mast cell growth factor" (and other factors which have been designated in the literature as multipotential colony-stimulating factor (Multi-CSF, ref. 177), persisting cell-stimulating factor, panspecific hematopoietin, hemopoietic cell growth factor and burst-promoting activity), are expressed by interleukin-3 (IL-3) (reviewed in 74, 123, 177, 220, 276). IL-3, a glycoprotein first defined by its ability to induce expression of the enzyme 20-α-hydroxysteroid dehydrogenase in cultures of splenocytes derived from athymic (nu/nu) mice, can be produced *in vitro* by "helper" T cells and certain tumor cells of "myelomonocytic" origin (reviewed in 123, 124). IL-3 promotes the proliferation/maturation of multiple hematopoietic lineages in short-term cultures of normal mouse bone marrow cells (123, 220), but after a few weeks *in vitro* these cultures consist almost entirely of mast cells.

When recombinant IL-3 is given to mice *in vivo* (144, 178), it induces proliferation of multiple hematopoietic lineages, including certain populations of mast cells similar to MMC (178). And administration of IL-3 to athymic nude mice confers on these animals the ability to exhibit MMC proliferation in response to infection with the parasite *Strongyloides ratti* (1) or even in the absence of parasite infection (2). These findings strongly suggest that IL-3 is a critical signal for the expansion of the MMC population observed in the intestinal mucosa of mice during parasitic infections.

While the effects of T cell products on mast cells have been discussed primarily with reference to proliferation of mouse or rat MMC, modest proliferation of *cutaneous* mast cells has been observed in association with T-cell-dependent reactions in human skin (55). Although the factors that regulate human skin mast cell proliferation *in vivo* remain to be defined, *in vitro* evidence suggests that mouse CTMC proliferation might reflect the combined influence of IL-3 and IL-4 (107, 193). IL-4 (also designated B cell stimulation factor 1) has many effects on B cells, including a critical role in the production of IgE class antibodies (68, 69, 119, 203). In the mouse, IL-4 also augments production of IgG$_1$ antibodies (69, 203), the other immunoglobulin isotype that can sensitize mast cells in this species. Although it has little or no ability to stimulate mast cell proliferation *in vitro* when tested in the absence of other factors, IL-4 augments the IL-3-dependent proliferation of "MMC-like" mouse mast cells generated *in vitro* (159) and also appears to favor the *in vitro* growth and/or maturation of mouse mast cells with properties of CTMC (107, 193). In the mouse, the same inducer T cells can produce both IL-3 and IL-4 upon appropriate activation (21, 87). Such cells, therefore, can importantly regulate both the remarkable elevations in levels of IgE, and the changes in mast cell numbers and phenotype, that accompany adaptive or pathologic immune responses with components of immediate hypersensitivity.

Discussions of cytokines that promote mouse mass cell proliferation or maturation/differentiation traditionally focus on IL-3 and IL-4, but additional cytokines with regulatory effects on mast cells await full characterization. Some of these may be previously unknown molecules derived from spleen cells (121, 185) or fibroblast products distinct from IL-3 or IL-4 (see next section); others may be molecules already identified on the basis of other activities. Nerve growth factor (NGF) represents such a candidate. Administration of exogenous NGF to neonatal rats causes increased levels of mast cells in multiple tissues (5, 16, 249), but the molecule is apparently without effect on mast cell numbers in adult mammals (5, 249). Whether endogenous NGF has an important role in mast cell development, and, if so, the circumstances under which such effects are observed, remain to be defined.

Although considerable effort has been devoted to characterization of agents which promote mast cell proliferation, it may also be important to search for molecules that limit mast cell division (or maturation/differentiation). Infections with the parasite *Nematospiroides dubius* are *not* associated with MMC proliferation in mice, perhaps because of the production of cytokines (? interferonγ, ref. 120) with effects on mast cell proliferation or differentiation (217, 218). Other agents which limit mast cell development may be derived from the mast cell itself. Kanakura *et al.* have provided evidence that a mast cell-dependent mechanism limits the invasion of mast cell precursors into the peritoneal cavity of mice and inhibits the differentiation of these cells into morphologically identifiable mast cells (138). Aldenborg and Enerbäck have suggested a similar mechanism as one of the factors contributing to the slower growth rate of peritoneal mast cell mass in athymic as opposed to the corresponding euthymic rats (3). Granulocyte-macrophage colony-stimulating factor (GM-CSF) can suppress the growth of IL-3-dependent mast cells *in vitro* (23). Notably, some appropriately stimulated IL-3-dependent mast cells can themselves produce GM-CSF (28, 270), IL-3 (28, 210) and, possibly, interferon-γ (28). Thus, some mast cells may be able to release factors with both positive and negative effects on their own proliferation.

The valuable information about mast cell biology obtained using murine tissue culture systems has spurred efforts to employ similar approaches with human material. This work is difficult to summarize briefly at this time, since the different investigators working in this area have used different sources of hematopoietic cells and growth factors, and, importantly, different criteria to characterize and name their cells. Nevertheless, it is clear that cells containing histamine and expressing IgE receptors can be generated *in vitro* from precursors present in human bone marrow or peripheral or umbilical cord blood "mononuclear cell" sources and grown in the presence of a variety of "growth factor" preparations which are distinct from IL-2 (47, 53, 94, 129, 131, 197, 215, 231, 240, 258, 259).

However, the cells generated in suspension cultures that have been characterized in the most detail according to ultrastructural, biochemical and functional criteria have been identified as basophils, not mast cells (47, 53, 129, 131, 231). Furthermore, another granulocyte, the eosinophil, represents a major "contaminating" cell type in these cultures (47, 53, 129, 131, 231). Although some investigators have tentatively identified the histamine-containing cells they have derived from normal human hematopoietic cells in suspension culture as mast cells, the extent of the similarities between such cells and human mast cell populations isolated from tissue sources remains to be determined. Horton and O'Brien have reported the *in vitro* growth of cells with multiple characteristics of mast cells from the bone marrow of a patient with mastocytoma (118), and Butterfield *et al.*

have established a long-term cell line with many features of mast cells (but not detectable IgE receptors) from a patient with mast cell leukemia (30). But it is not yet clear whether similar approaches will lead to the establishment of mast cell lines from normal human bone marrow or peripheral blood cells. Thus, it now appears that suspension culture approaches that routinely result in the generation of mast cells in mice and rats usually result in the generation of basophils in humans. While the reasons for this important species difference are not clear, many findings indicate that T cell products can influence basophil production in a variety of mammalian species (reviewed in 79, 86). Based on these observations, the growth of basophils from human hematopoietic cells maintained with T cell-associated products perhaps should come as no surprise.

On the other hand, recent reports indicate that at least limited growth of human mast cells *in vitro* is possible. Cells with morphologic, histochemical and immunohistochemical characteristics of mast cells developed in "interphase" cultures of human bone marrow cells layered over agar in the presence of human rIL-3 (145) and in semisolid agar cultures of human bone marrow or cord blood cells (278). The latter candidate mast cells exhibited reactivity with a monoclonal antibody reported to be specific for human mast cells (174), but did not react with a monoclonal antibody reactive with human basophils (20). Another approach that appears very promising is to use complex tissue culture systems incorporating both hematopoietic and non-hematopoietic cell types. Thus, Furitsu *et al.* (75) have identified cells with multiple phenotypic characteristics of mast cells in long-term cultures of human cord blood cells and mouse 3T3 fibroblasts.

Use of Mast Cells Generated In Vitro to Demonstrate Unidirectional Changes in Mast Cell Phenotype. The most extensive studies of the ability of microenvironmental factors to induce unidirectional change in mast cell phenotype have been performed with growth factor-dependent mouse mast cells generated *in vitro*. It was apparent from the beginning that the features of such mast cells were not identical to those of mature peritoneal mast cells, the most well-characterized mouse mast cell population available for comparison (77, 88, 248, 253). These two populations expressed differences in ultrastructure (58, 88, 189, 261), content of histamine (189, 192, 214, 236, 248, 261) and serotonin (265), type of sulfated glycosaminoglycans (88, 216, 248), number of "high affinity" receptors for IgE (88), and responsiveness to secretogogues (248) (Table 5). On the other hand, growth factor-dependent mouse mast cells shared some features with the MMC which proliferate in the intestinal lamina propria of rats and mice during certain T cell-dependent responses to intestinal parasites (77, 88, 248, 252) (Table 5).

Unfortunately, mouse MMC had not been purified (as is still the case), and little was known about their mediator content. Consequently, there could be little direct comparison of the properties of cultured mouse mast cells with the MMC of the same species. Techniques for purifying rat MMC had been described (12), however, as well as methods for growing rat mast cells *in vitro* either

TABLE 5. PHENOTYPIC CHARACTERISTICS OF MAST CELL POPULATIONS IN THE MOUSE

Characteristic	"Connective tissue" or "serosal" (peritoneal) mast cells	"Mucosal" mast cells[a]	Growth factor-dependent cultured mast cells[b]
Cytoplasmic granule ultrastructure	Uniformly electron-dense	Variably electron-dense	Variably electron-dense
"T cell dependence"[c]	No	Yes	Yes
Major granule-associated proteoglycan	Heparin (biochemical analysis)	Chondroitin sulfates (by histochemistry)	Chondroitin sulfates
Staining with berberine sulfate[d]	Yes	No	No
Histamine content	High	Low (by histochemistry)	Low
Serotonin content	Variable	Low (by histochemistry)	High[e]
Surface expression of globopentaosylceramide	High	Not determined	Low
High affinity surface receptors for IgE	Yes	(Yes)	Yes[f]
Sensitivity to stimulation with compound 48/80	High	Low	Low
Staining with alcian blue	Yes	Yes	Yes
Staining with safranin	Yes	No	No

Modified, by permission, from (84).

[a] "Mucosal" mast cells have not been purified from mouse tissues. Therefore, information about biochemical content, IgE receptors, etc. is based on histochemical or immunological characterization, or analysis of homogenates of tissues containing these cells.

[b] Under usual conditions of culture of bone marrow cells or other sources of hematopoietic cells with IL-3/Multi-CSF-containing media. Under certain circumstances *in vivo* or *in vitro*, these populations can acquire many of the phenotypic characteristics of "connective tissue-type" or "serosal" mast cells (see text).

[c] Nude mice have CTMC populations but do not develop proliferation of MMC during parasite infections. However, T cell products may influence the proliferation or maturation/differentiation of CTMC under certain circumstances *in vitro* or *in vivo* (see text). Products derived from T cells (IL-3) can maintain proliferating populations of bone marrow-derived mouse mast cells *in vitro*. It is not yet clear whether cells other than T cells (including mast cells, refs. 28, 210, 270) can represent a biologically significant source of IL-3 (or IL-4) *in vivo*.

[d] Berberine sulfate is a cationic fluorescent dye that binds to heparin-containing cytoplasmic granules of mast cells (64). The specificity of staining should be confirmed by demonstrating that treatment with heparinase abolishes reactivity (64, 196).

[e] The high serotonin content of these cells may, in part, reflect uptake of serotonin from the tissue culture medium (265).

[f] Growth factor-dependent cultured mast cells express ~50% fewer Fc,R/cell than do freshly isolated peritoneal mast cells, but these two populations bind IgE with a similar equilibrium constant (88).

in the absence (128, 129) or presence (46) of T cells activated by specific antigen. Moreover, rat MMC and CTMC can be distinguished on the basis of their predominant cytoplasmic granule-associated chymotryptic protease (272, 273). Haig *et al.* (105, 106) showed that rat mast cells, generated *in vitro* in medium conditioned by antigen-activated T cells, expressed a number of properties shared by rat MMC, including synthesis of the same chymotryptic protease (RMCP II). Broide *et al.* (24, 25) demonstrated additional similarities between rat bone marrow-derived mast cells and rat MMC. These studies complemented and extended those performed with mouse cells in calling attention to certain remarkable parallels between the phenotype of murine growth factor-dependent mast cells and MMC.

But other findings indicated that it might be premature to conclude that growth factor-dependent cultured mast cells were irrevocably committed to expression of a MMC phenotype. Thus, murine mast cell populations in the skin and peritoneal cavity, sites classically containing CTMC, were themselves known to be heterogeneous with respect to morphology, proliferative ability, histochemistry and density (37, 211). Moreover, certain morphologic and histochemical features of these "immature" connective tissue or peritoneal mast cells resembled those of MMC (reviewed in 88, 280). We therefore suggested that the ultrastructure and mediator content of cultured, growth factor-dependent mouse mast cells may have reflected their immaturity or the influence of their culture conditions, rather than their derivation from a distinct mast cell subpopulation (such as MMCs) (88).

We speculated further that the phenotypic differences among mast cell populations *in vivo* may also be regulated by microenvironmental factors affecting morphology, mediator content or maturation (88).

To evaluate whether growth factor-dependent cultured mast cells could be induced to mature in suspension culture *in vitro*, we exposed the cells to sodium butyrate (88), an agent that increased the development of cytoplasmic granules and storage of granule-associated mediators in mouse mastocytoma cells (186). Exposure to butyrate did induce partial maturation of clonal mast cells, as judged both by ultrastructure (Fig. 5) and by increased storage of the granule-associated mediators histamine and ^{35}S-labeled chondroitin sulfates (88). These changes were accompanied by a marked diminution of the cells' proliferative ability (88). DuBuske *et al.* (48) confirmed the effect of butyrate on cultured mast cell histamine content, and also showed that butyrate-treated mast cells stored increased quantities of cytoplasmic granule-associated serine neutral proteases. But butyrate treatment did not induce full maturation (compare the cell in Fig. 5B to the mature peritoneal mast cell in Fig. 6) nor did it induce the cells to synthesize detectable quantities of ^{35}S-labeled heparin glycosaminoglycans (88).

Pitton *et al.* (209) recently demonstrated that treatment of growth factor-dependent, bone marrow-derived cultured mast cells (BMCMC) with dexamethasone (DM) induced changes similar to those observed with sodium butyrate, including reduced proliferation, increased histamine content, and morphological evidence

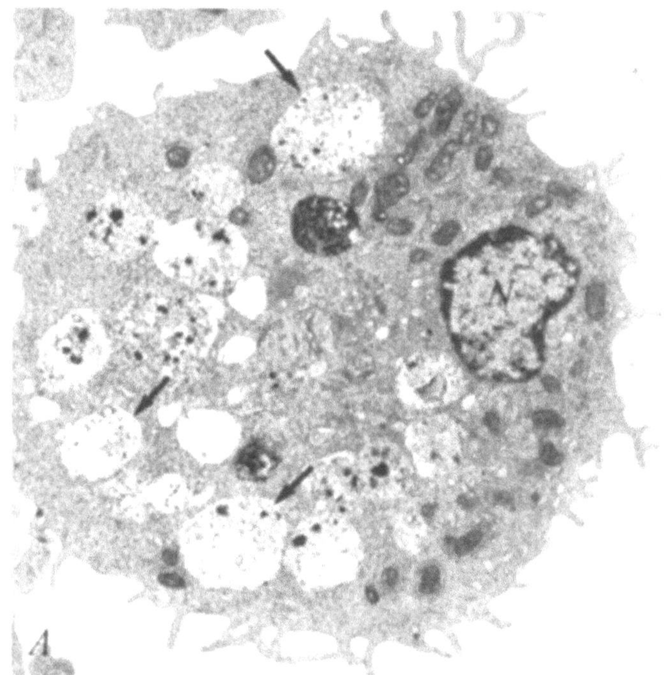
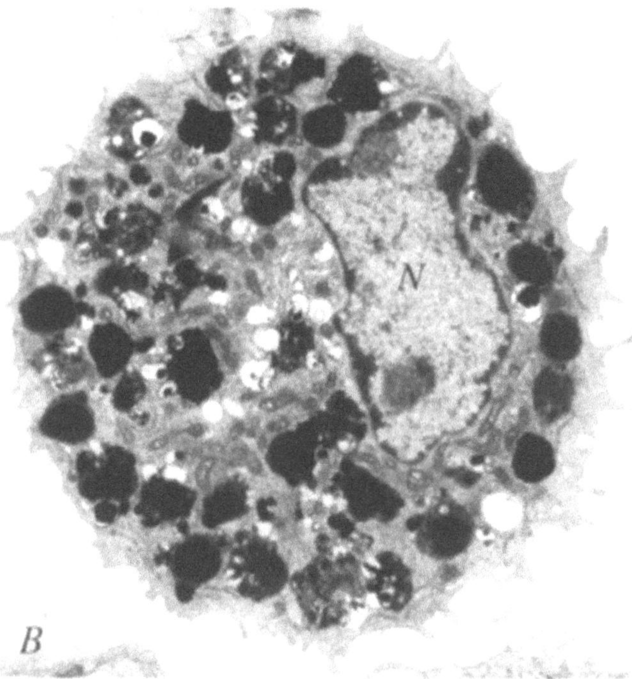
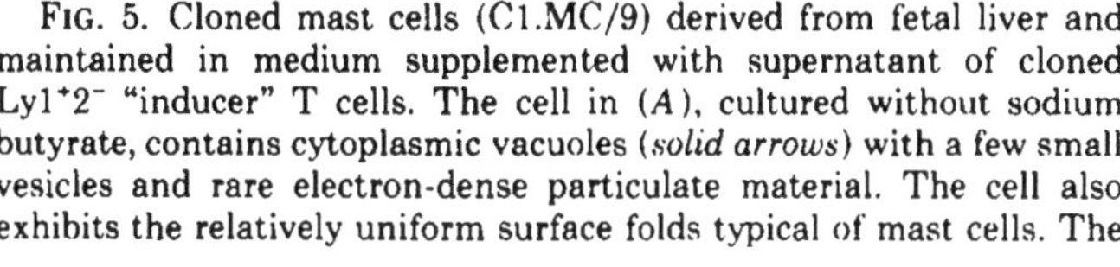

FIG. 5. Cloned mast cells (C1.MC/9) derived from fetal liver and maintained in medium supplemented with supernatant of cloned Ly1⁺2⁻ "inducer" T cells. The cell in (A), cultured without sodium butyrate, contains cytoplasmic vacuoles (*solid arrows*) with a few small vesicles and rare electron-dense particulate material. The cell also exhibits the relatively uniform surface folds typical of mast cells. The cell in (B) was cultured for 4 days in the same medium as the cell in (A), except that the medium also contained 1 mM sodium butyrate. The cytoplasmic granules appear more "mature" than in (A), with abundant electron-dense granule content. N, nucleus. Reproduced with permission from Galli *et al.* (88). Figure 5A, ×6,300; B, ×6,100.

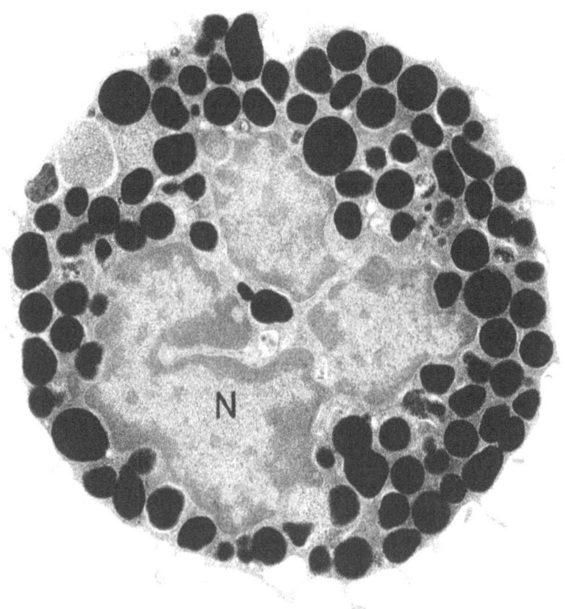

FIG. 6. Mature peritoneal mast cell from an adult C57BL/6J mouse. The short, narrow surface processes appear similar to those of the cultured mast cells in Figure 5. But the cytoplasmic granules of this cell are more homogeneously electron-dense than those in the butyrate-treated cell shown in Figure 5B. N, nucleus. Reproduced with permission from Dvorak *et al.* (58). ×5,400.

of maturation/differentiation. DM treatment also augmented by tenfold the mast cells' ability to generate PGD_2 upon stimulation with IgE and specific antigen, but decreased both $Fc_\epsilon RI$ expression and antigen-induced release of histamine, paf-acether, LTB_4 and LTC_4 (209). While the proteoglycans of the DM-treated mast cells were not analyzed, many of the cells became positive for staining with safranin (a feature of CTMC).

The apparent lack of heparin synthesis by growth factor-dependent mouse mast cells was regarded as a particularly important finding. Histochemical evidence suggested that rat MMC contained little or no heparin (260), whereas heparin had been detected in both rat (19, 155, 233, 282) and mouse (19, 88, 216) peritoneal mast cells. The initial inability to detect heparin in IL-3-dependent mouse mast cells (88, 216, 248), and the recognition that the cells' chondroitin sulfate proteoglycans included a species with 30-50% of its chondroitin sulfate disaccharides consisting of glucuronic acid → *N*-acetylglucosamine-4,6-disulfate (chondroitin sulfate E) (216), raised the possibility that mast cell subsets might be identified by detailed biochemical characterization of their sulfated glycosaminoglycans (252, 253).

However, it was known that at least some mastocytoma cells synthesized both heparin and chondroitin sulfates (226). Moreover, exposure of such mastocytoma cells (226), or isolated rat peritoneal mast cells (251), to the exogenous glycosaminoglycan acceptor β-D-xyloside greatly increased synthesis of chondroitin sulfates rather than heparin. Subsequent studies of BMCMC generated *in vitro* indicated that these populations did in fact synthesize small amounts of ^{35}S-heparin proteoglycan

(199, 242), which was stored as a complex with granule-associated proteases (242). Thus, the difference in heparin content of BMCMC and classical "serosal" mast cells isolated from the peritoneal cavity was, after all, quantitative rather than qualitative. Nevertheless, until 1985, it was not clear whether any conditions would permit "MMC-like" BMCMC to acquire multiple features of CTMC.

To address this issue, Nakano *et al.* (196) adopted a combined *in vitro* and *in vivo* approach: analysis of the phenotype of the mast cells which develop in genetically mast cell-deficient $WBB6F_1$-W/W^v mice after systemic or local injection of genetically compatible mast cell populations generated *in vitro*. This strategy was based on a straightforward assumption: since the $WBB6F_1$-W/W^v mouse provides an environment suitable for the development, from pluripotent bone marrow-derived precursors, of both CTMC (148) and MMC (42), it should also be able to reveal potential for phenotypic change in more differentiated cells in the mast cell lineage, such as BMCMC.

In the first stuides (196), mast cell phenotype was assessed according to light and electron microscopic criteria, histamine content, staining with alcian blue and safranin, and staining with berberine sulfate, a cationic fluorescent dye that binds to phosphate- and/or sulfate-containing polyanions including DNA and heparin (64). The binding to DNA and heparin are distinguishable according to the subcellular localization and characteristics of the fluorescence, and, importantly, the sensitivity of the staining to treatment with heparinase (64, 196). BMCMC whose phenotype resembled that of MMC gave rise to two phenotypically distinct populations of mast cells in $WBB6F_1$-W/W^v recipients (196). In anatomical sites that in $WBB6F_1$-+/+ mice ordinarily contain berberine sulfate-positive (heparin-rich) CTMC (dermis, peritoneal cavity, muscularis propria of the stomach), the adoptively-transferred mast cells were berberine sulfate-positive and expressed other phenotypic characteristics of typical CTMC, including ultrastructural features (Fig. 7). But in anatomical sites populated in $WBB6F_1$-+/+ mice by berberine sulfate-negative MMC (e.g., the gastric musoca), the adoptively-transferred mast cells in $WBB6F_1$-W/W^v recipients were also berberine sulfate-negative. These initial observations showing that BMCMC can undergo the change "MMC-like" → "CTMC-like" were later confirmed by biochemical characterization of the proteoglycans of the mast cells before and after transfer into W/W^v mice, and by demonstrating that the transferred mast cell population gradually acquired increased surface expression of globopentaosylceramide (199), another feature resembling that of native mouse peritoneal mast cells (140–142). The change "MMC-like" → "CTMC-like" may also occur *in vivo* in pulmonary mast cell populations during infections with *Nippostrongylus brasiliensis*, a classical stimulus for the proliferation of MMC in the gut (6).

Nakano *et al.* (196) also reported that findings similar to those observed after injection of BMCMC were obtained when partially purified, berberine sulfate-positive mast cells derived from the peritoneal cavities of

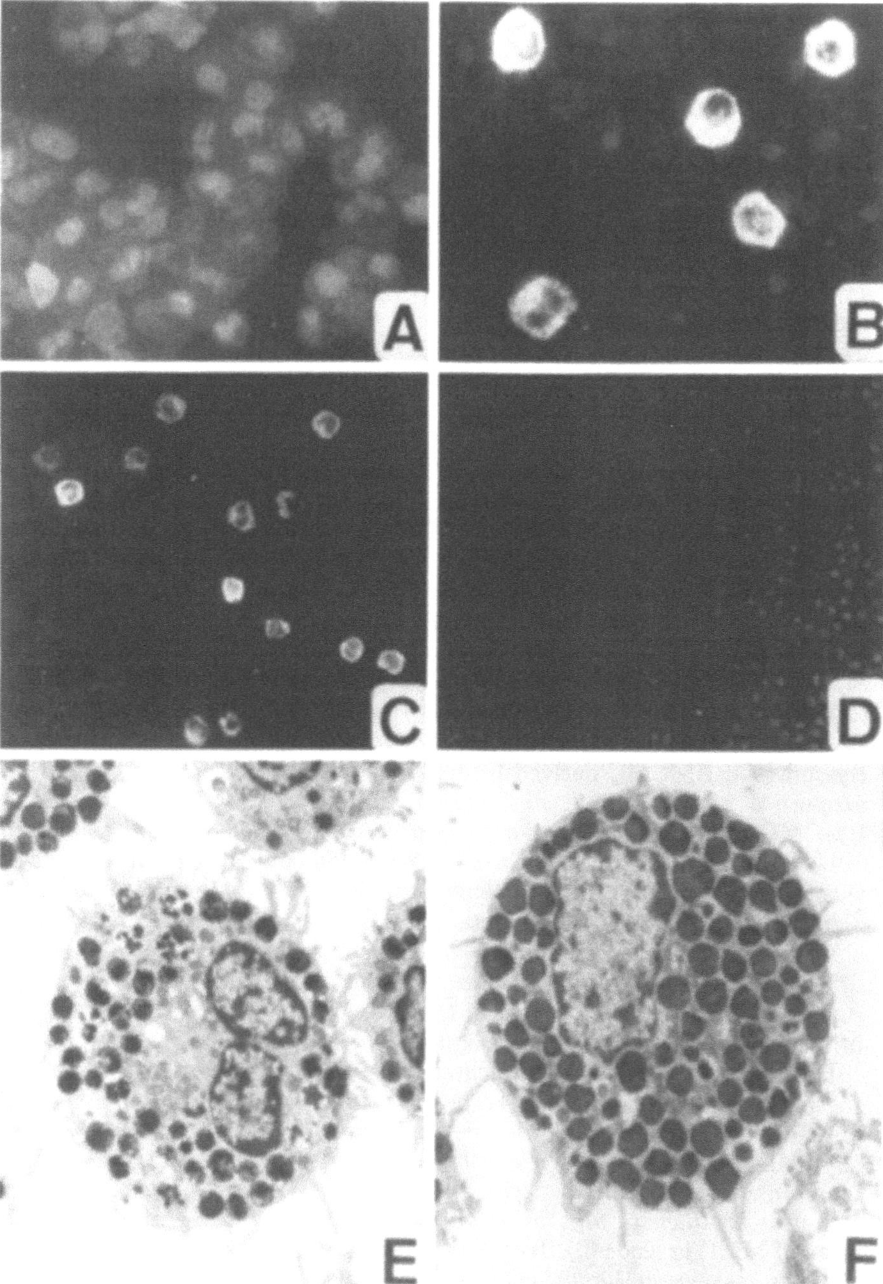

FIG. 7. *A* to *D*, Cytocentrifuge preparations stained with berberine sulfate. *A*, Cultured mast cells 4 weeks after initiation of culture; only nuclei showed faint fluorescence. *B*, Peritoneal cells recovered from a WBB6F$_1$-*W/W^v* mouse 10 weeks after the intraperitoneal injection of 10^6 cultured mast cells of WBB6F$_1$-+/+ mouse origin. The cytoplasm of the mast cells exhibited intense fluorescence. *C*, A specimen made from the same cell suspension shown in *B*, but treated with chondroitinase ABC before staining. Bright cytoplasmic fluorescence of mast cells was retained. *D*, A specimen made from the same cell suspension shown in *B* and *C*, but treated with heparinase before staining. Heparinase treatment abolished staining of mast cells by berberine sulfate. *E*, The ultrastructure of a cultured mast cell 4 weeks after initiation of the culture. The cytoplasmic granules exhibited heterogeneous content. *F*, Ultrastructure of a mast cell recovered from the peritoneal cavity of a WBB6F$_1$-*W/W^v* mouse 10 weeks after intraperitoneal injection of cultured mast cells. The cytoplasmic granules appear uniformly electron dense. Reproduced with permission from Nakano *et al.* (196). Figure 7*A* and *B*, ×400; *C* and *D*, ×200; *E* and *F*, ×5,800.

WBB6F$_1$-+/+ mice (+/+ PMC) were injected into WBB6F$_1$-*W/W^v* mice, suggesting that mast cells with phenotypic features of CTMC might give rise to cells with characteristics of MMC (196). Kobayashi *et al.* (152) then showed that clonal mast cell populations derived *in vitro* from PMC could express features of MMC or CTMC *in vivo*, as appropriate for the anatomical microenvironment in which they resided. Sonoda *et al.* (247) demonstrated that single peritoneal mast cells, upon injection into the stomach of *W/W^v* mice, could give rise to progeny with the morphologic and histochemical features of either MMC or CTMC. These results established that at least some PMC, a classic example of a CTMC, can give rise to mast cells with phenotypic similarities to either CTMC or MMC.

In vitro approaches offer an attractive additional strategy for analyzing mast cell phenotypic change, since the environment in which these changes take place is simpler than that represented by an intact organism. In culture systems which also included both antigen-stimulated T cells and embryonic skin fibroblasts, Ginsburg and his associates recognized two morphologically distinct mouse mast cell populations, one of which resembled MMC or growth factor-dependent mass cells and one of which resembled CTMC (43, 97). When [^{35}S]sulfate was included in these cultures, both heparin (60-70%) and chondroitin sulfate (30 to 40%) proteoglycans were synthesized (17). Subsequently, similar results were obtained using X-irradiated embryonic fibroblast layers (43).

A culture system containing even fewer cell types which might potentially influence mast cell phenotype was developed by Levi-Schaffer et al. (163), who demonstrated that the viability and CTMC phenotype of purified rat peritoneal mast cells could be maintained for up to 30 days *in vitro* if the mast cells were co-cultured solely with the mouse 3T3 fibroblast cell line. Co-culture with 3T3 fibroblasts also induced IL3-dependent mouse mast cells to acquire several phenotypic characteristics of CTMC, including the ability to synthesize [^{35}S]heparin as the predominant [^{35}S]proteoglycan (165), and to alter their pattern of mediator production (166). Some of these findings were subsequently confirmed using cloned mast cell populations (45). Thus, co-culture of BMCMC on 3T3 fibroblasts resulted in the change: "MMC-like" → "CTMC-like."

While it appears that close association between the 3T3 cells and the BMCMC favor the induction of phenotypic change (reviewed in 149, 254), the nature of the actual factors involved await clarification. The 3T3 cells don't produce detectable IL-3 or IL-4 (72). However, recent work by Fujita, Kitamura and their associates indicate that 3T3 cells derived from 17 day embryos of Sl/Sl^d mice are defective in their ability to induce a transition from the G_1 to S phases of the cell cycle in BMCMC derived from the congenic +/+ mice (73, 149). By contrast, BMCMC derived from W/W^v mice, which express a more limited ability than congenic +/+ BMCMC to survive *in vitro* or *in vivo* (196, 257, 279), failed to enter the S phase of the cell cycle upon contact with NIH/3T3 fibroblasts (71). Taken together with the identification of *c-kit* as the product of the *W* locus, these observations raise the possibility that the critical mast cell maturation/differentiation factor expressed on the surface of 3T3 cells is a product of the *Sl* locus that can influence or interact with *c-kit* (33, 91).

However, recent evidence indicates that some cells in the mast cell lineage can also respond to soluble fibroblast-derived maturation/differentiation factors (133, 134). Mast cells can be grown *in vitro* from the mesenteric lymph nodes of rats infected with the nematode *Nippostrongylus brasiliensis*, a parasite which induces proliferation of MMC *in vivo* (46). Jarboe *et al.* recently reported that the mesenteric lymph nodes of mice infected with *N. brasiliensis* represent a rich source of "mast cell-committed progenitors" (MCCP), cells that lack cytoplasmic granules by light microscopy but that can acquire characteristics of either CTMC-like or MMC-like mast cells under appropriate circumstances *in vitro* (134). Thus, MCCP cultured in IL-3-containing medium generate berberine sulfate-negative mast cells, whereas MCCP cultured on 3T3 cells or mouse skin embryonic fibroblasts in the absence of IL-3 and IL-4 generate mast cells with granules that stain with berberine sulfate and exhibit a mixed pattern of staining with alcian blue and safranin (134). The ability of MMCP to undergo maturation/differentiation on 3T3 cells in the absence of additional sources of growth factors is reminiscent of previous observations made with BMCMC (71, 72, 149, 165, 166) or other hematopoietic cells (225). However, unlike BMCMC, MCCP can proliferate and acquire "CTMC-like" histochemical features in fibroblast conditioned medium (134). Moreover, cells with properties of MCCP are not detectable in the bone marrow of either normal or *N. brasiliensis*-infected mice (133).

Several lines of evidence indicate that the soluble, fibroblast-derived factor responsible for inducing maturation/differentiation of MCCP is distinct from IL-3 and IL-4 (134). And the effects of this factor could not be mimicked by a wide variety of other previously identified molecules including IL-1, IL-2, GM-CSF, G-CSF, M-CSF, IFNα/β, IFN-γ, nerve growth factor, epidermal growth factor, fibronectin, heparin, or several other glycosaminoglycans (134). Like the 3T3 cell-associated factor regulating maturation/differentiation of BMCMC, the agent influencing MCCP development may represent a product of the *Sl* locus that can interact with *c-kit*. Thus, even though the lymph nodes or bone marrow of W/W^v mice virtually lacked MCCP, W/W^v fibroblast-conditioned medium supported the proliferation and differentiation of mast cells from MCCP of congenic +/+ origin (133). By contrast, Sl/Sl^d mice could generate MCCP but Sl/Sl^d fibroblast-conditioned medium was markedly deficient in its ability to support the proliferation and differentiation of mast cells from MCCP (133).

Demonstration of Multiple, Bidirectional Changes in Mast Cell Phenotype. Both *in vivo* (196, 199) and *in vitro* (45, 165, 166) studies indicated that BMCMC with features of MMC could acquire multiple phenotypic characteristic of CTMC. And combined *in vitro* and *in vivo* studies indicated that the change CTMC → "MMC-like" also could occur (152, 196, 247). However, it was unclear to what extent such changes were reversible. Kanakura *et al.* (139) therefore devised combined *in vitro* and *in vivo* approaches, outlined in Figure 8, to evaluate whether clonal mast cell populations could exhibit reversible changes in "MMC-like" and "CTMC-like" phenotypic characteristics.

Peritoneal mast cells (PMC) were isolated in >99% purity from WBB6F$_1$-+/+ mice; 100% of the cells in these populations were reactive with the heparin-binding dye berberine sulfate and the cells incorporated [^{35}S] sulfate predominantly (~88% of total [^{35}S]proteoglycans) into heparin. When the purified PMC were placed in methylcellulose culture with medium containing IL-3 and IL-4, ~25% of the PMC formed clonal colonies containing both berberine sulfate-positive and berberine-sulfate negative cells, as in previous studies (152). When the latter colonies were transferred to suspension cultures containing IL-3 and IL-4, they generated populations of variable proliferative ability, all of which contained cells that were entirely berberine sulfate-negative, a characteristic similar to that of MMC. These cells incorporated [^{35}S]sulfate predominantly into chondroitin sulfate proteoglycans, of which ~64% were chondroitin 4-sulfate and ~35% were chondroitin sulfate E, a result similar to that obtained with BMCMC generated under similar conditions of suspension culture (199). Together with the results of ultrastructural studies and measurements of histamine content, these findings indicated that the derivation of suspension cultures of clonal mast cell populations from individual PMC in IL-3- and IL4-

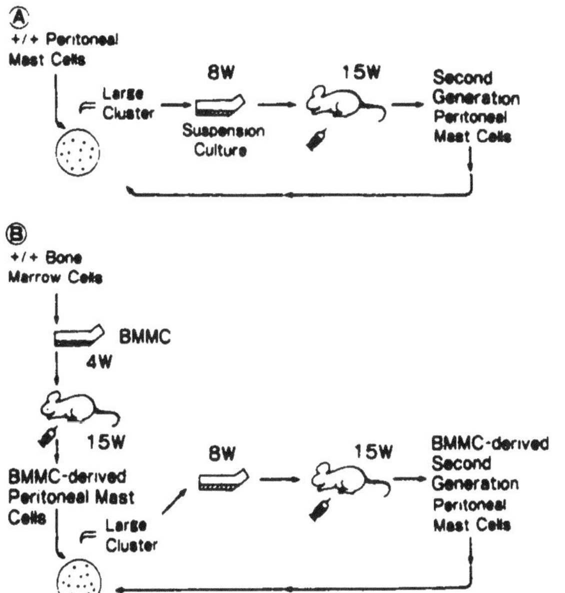

FIG. 8. Diagrammatic representation of experimental protocols for evaluating the potential of clonal mast cell populations to express reversible alterations of phenotypic characteristics. *A*, Peritoneal mast cells are purified (>99% purity) from WBB6F$_1$-+/+ mice and seeded into methycellulose. Individual large colonies are picked up 2 weeks later and placed in suspension culture, expanded *in vitro* for 8 weeks, and then injected intraperitoneally into genetically mast cell-deficient WBB6F$_1$-W/W^v mice, each W/W^v recipient receiving cells derived from a single clonal population of suspension culture-expanded mast cells. Fifteen weeks later, "second generation peritoneal mast cells" are recovered from the peritoneal cavities of the W/W^v mice and placed into methylcellulose culture. *B*, W/W^v mice receive an intraperitoneal injection of mast cells derived in suspension culture from WBB6F$_1$-+/+ bone marrow cells (*BMMC*). Fifteen weeks later, "BMMC-derived peritoneal mast cells" are recovered from the peritoneal cavities of the W/W^v mice and used to begin the same sequence of manipulations shown in *A*. Reproduced with permission from Kanakura *et al.* (139).

containing medium was associated with the phenotypic change: CTMC → "MMC-like." These findings also represented the first evidence to indicate that the pattern of [^{35}S]proteoglycan synthesis in a clonal population of non-neoplastic mast cells can change from predominantly heparin to predominantly chondroitin sulfate(s).

Morphological and histochemical criteria then were used to show that certain of these phenotypic changes were reversible. As indicated in Figure 8*A*, the berberine sulfate-negative clonal populations of WBB6F$_1$-+/+ PMC-derived mast cells were injected intraperitoneally into mast cell-deficient WBB6F$_1$-W/W^v mice. After 15 weeks *in vivo* in W/W^v mice, the +/+ mast cells resembled PMC morphologically and were entirely berberine sulfate-positive, like native PMC (i.e., CTMC → "MMC-like" → "CTMC-like"). And when the latter "second generation PMC" were returned to methylcellulose and then suspension cultures, the clonal populations contained mast cells that were negative for reactivity with berberine sulfate (*i.e.*, CTMC → "MMC-like" → "CTMC-like" → "MMC-like"). A similar pattern of phenotypic change was demonstrated when clonal mast cell populations were established from PMC derived originally from +/+ BMCMC (Figure 8*B*).

These findings provided direct evidence that clonal mast cell populations can exhibit multiple and reversible changes in phenotype. However, the number of times such clonal mast cell populations can undergo cycles of proliferation and phenotypic change may be limited. Assessment of the proliferative potential of various mast cell populations *in vitro* indicated that the sequential alterations of mast cell phenotype as the cells were passed through different environments (*in vitro* or *in vivo*) were associated with a progressive diminution in the cells' proliferative ability.

It is important to emphasize that the numbers of mast cells available for study at many steps of the schemes shown in Figure 8 are quite limited, making difficult the extensive biochemical and functional characterization which would be required to determine the extent of the similarities between classic BMCMC and the "MMC-like" progeny of PMC. And in the absence of techniques to purify and extensively analyze actual mouse MMC, it will not be clear to what extent either classical BMCMC or "MMC-like" derivatives of PMC resemble true MMC. It may be of particular interest to characterize the protease content of these cells, since recent data suggest that native mouse MMC and BMCMC populations can express considerable qualitative and quantitative heterogeneity in this aspect of phenotype (182). But whatever the results of such studies, the findings of Kanakura *et al.* showed unequivocally that clonal mast cell populations derived from single PMC are not irrevocably committed to expression of the mature CTMC phenotype, and that having "lost" certain of these characteristics, the same clonal population can later regain them.

Conclusions. Studies of mouse mast cells illustrate the remarkable facility of mast cell populations to respond to changes in the environment (either *in vitro* or *in vivo*) by significant alterations in multiple aspects of their phenotype, including morphology, mediator content, sensitivity to stimuli of activation, and proliferative potential. The notion that such changes are regulated by "microenvironmental signals" is useful in focusing the search for such signals in the immediate vicinity of the responding mast cell population (or in products of the mast cell itself). However, as pointed out in Table 4, such microenvironmental signals might regulate mast cell phenotype by any of a number of different mechanisms.

It should be emphasized that while all of the currently available data derived from mouse studies can be explained without reference to irreversible branching within the mast cell lineage, the existence of this mechanism has by no means been ruled out. We showed that ~75% of purified PMC failed to generate even small colonies when placed in methylcellulose culture with IL-3 and IL-4 (139). Did these PMC fail to receive an adequate signal for proliferation under the conditions tested, or were they a terminally differentiated subpopulation capable neither of proliferation nor of expression of "MMC-like" features? The data don't permit discrimination between these (or other) possibilities. Similarly, these are insufficient data to decide to what extent phenotypic plasticity can be expressed by single mast cells, as opposed to clonal populations of mast cells.

AN *IN VIVO* MODEL FOR EVALUATING THE ROLES OF MAST CELLS OF DISTINCT PHENOTYPE IN HEALTH AND DISEASE

One of the important reasons to elucidate the regulation of mast cell heterogeneity is the belief that mast cells of distinct phenotypes may have different roles in human health and disease. However, opportunities actually to test hypotheses about mast cell function in human subjects *in vivo* are obviously quite limited. It is true that human mast cells have been the subject of a wide variety of morphologic, biochemical, pharmacologic and functional studies. But, for reasons discussed in detail elsewhere, even in aggregate such approaches cannot establish with certainty that mast cells express a particular function in the complex setting of an intact organism (78, 90, 267). However, there is an approach for testing hypotheses about mast cell function under conditions where the presence or absence of mast cells, and the phenotypic characteristics of the mast cell populations participating in the response, can be controlled experimentally (Table 6). This method consists of investigating potential mast cell functions in mast cell-deficient and congenic normal (+/+) mice, and in W/W^v mice selectively reconstituted with congenic +/+ mast cells (78, 83, 90, 267).

We have used this general approach to confirm the long-held belief that mast cells are essential for the augmented vascular permeability and other aspects of inflammation occurring at sites of IgE-dependent immediate hypersensitivity reactions, whether these are elicited by CTMC in the skin (268) or by MMC in the stomach (266). Using the same approach, Matsuda *et al.* have provided evidence that cutaneous mast cell degranulation, which may be IgE-dependent, importantly contributes to immune resistance to the feeding of larval *Haemaphysalis longicornis* ticks (171). Mast cells also appear to contribute importantly to the pulmonary and cardiovascular effects, and death, associated with certain systemic IgE-dependent reactions (169, 170). By contrast, we and others have not detected a contribution of mast cells in T cell-dependent contact sensitivity responses (reviewed in 82, 175, 176, 267).

Experiments in mast cell-reconstituted mice have also identified significant mast cell-dependent augmentation of the vascular permeability changes, tissue swelling, and leukocyte infiltration associated with the acute inflammatory responses induced by epicutaneous application of phorbol 12-myristate 13-acetate (PMA, ref. 269) or intradermal administration of substance P (170, 275), and have demonstrated mast cell-dependent effects on the kinetics (but not the magnitude) of the neutrophil infiltration which occurs after intraperitoneal injection of thioglycollate (213). Mast cells may also significantly augment the area of acute gastric injury induced by oral ethanol (89), although this finding has not yet been confirmed using W/W^v mice which have undergone local reconstitution of gastric mast cell populations.

Taken together, these studies indicate that CTMC and MMC are essential for the expression of certain IgE-dependent immediate hypersensitivity responses, and

TABLE 6. GENERAL SCHEME FOR INVESTIGATING MOUSE MAST CELL FUNCTION *IN VIVO*[a]

1. Search for quantitative differences in the expression of biologic responses in genetically mast cell-deficient WBB6F$_1$-W/W^v (W/W^v) and WCB6F$_1$-Sl/Sl^d (Sl/Sl^d) mice and the congenic normal (+/+) mice.

   Note: The *lack* of a difference between the W/W^v and Sl/Sl^d mice and the congenic +/+ mice strongly suggests that mast cells are not *essential* for the response. However, the demonstration of a difference in the response of W/W^v and Sl/Sl^d mice and congenic normal (+/+) mice does not *prove* that this difference is mast cell-dependent.

2. Compare the responses in W/W^v mice and W/W^v mice which have received bone marrow transplantation from congenic +/+ mice.

   Note: Intravenous injection of +/+ bone marrow cells repairs the mast cell deficiency of W/W^v mice but also cures the mutants' anemia and theoretically might result in additional bone marrow cell-dependent effects unrelated to correction of the mast cell deficiency.

3. Analyze the response in W/W^v mice *selectively* reconstituted with mast cells.

   Note: A useful approach is to test the expression of the response in paired anatomical sites in the same mice, with only one site of each pair selectively reconstituted with mast cells (by injection of cultured mast cells). By testing the mice at different intervals after selective reconstitution with cultured mast cells, one can evaluate whether the cells' function varies as their phenotype gradually changes from that expressed by the cultured cells to that which is more appropriate for mast cells at the same anatomical sites in normal mice.

4. Define the mechanism(s) by which mast cells contribute to the response.

[a] Studies should include appropriate analysis of the tissues in which the response is taking place, to assess the numbers, phenotypic characteristics, and anatomical distribution of mast cells potentially participating in the responses in normal or mast cell-reconstituted mice (the characteristics of mast cell populations may change during the course of the response, references 6 and 90), and to search for evidence of mast cell degranulation. Such studies are also important to determine whether the biological responses under investigation might be associated with the development of endogenous mast cell populations in mast cell-deficient mice (85, 101).

can also significantly augment the expression of certain inflammatory responses of nonimmunologic origin.

The majority of studies using the approach shown in Table 6 have been conducted by eliciting responses 10 weeks or more after transfer of +/+ mast cell populations into W/W^v recipients, when the adoptively transferred mast cell populations have acquired phenotypic characteristics similar to those of the native mast cell populations present at the same sites in normal mice (196). However, the function of culture-derived mast cell populations can also be evaluated shortly after their transfer into W/W^v recipients (213, 268), when the phenotype of the adoptively transferred cells still resembles that of BMCMC. Alternatively, one could attempt to alter the phenotype of the adoptively transferred +/+ mast cell population before eliciting the biological response under investigation. While the general approach outlined above thus is quite versatile, the interpretation of results obtained in such studies must be guided by several important considerations, as indicated in Table 6 and discussed in detail elsewhere (83, 90, 168, 267).

CONCLUSIONS AND DIRECTIONS FOR FUTURE STUDY

Understanding the regulation of mast cell development and the biological significance of mast cell phenotypic heterogeneity now represent central goals of mast cell research. While the first observations of mast cell heterogeneity were published nearly 100 years ago, shortly after the discovery of this cell type, widespread interest in this phenomenon is a very recent development. Indeed, despite Enerbäck's careful documentation of distinctions between "mucosal" and "connective tissue-type" mast cells in the rat (65, 66), and clear descriptions of phenotypic variation in rat mast cells observed in single anatomical sites (37, 211), serious students of the mast cell could ask each other, not so long ago, whether one was a "believer" in the concept of mast cell heterogeneity, particularly with respect to human cells.

No one who has critically evaluated the evidence can now doubt the existence of significant variation in phenotypic characteristics of mast cell populations observed in different anatomical sites, and even within single anatomical sites, in man as well as in experimental animals. Moreover, it is now clear that phenotypic variation in mast cell populations can reflect the operation of several processes, acting alone or in combination. These include the process of cellular maturation/differentiation, consequences of the functional activation of the cells, and the acquisition and storage by mast cells of products derived from other cell types.

Because variation in mast cell phenotype includes at least quantitative (and perhaps qualitative) differences in the mediators produced by these cells, as well as in their pattern of sensitivity to stimuli of activation or therapeutic agents, it is reasonable to consider that mast cells of different phenotype may have different roles in health and disease. This assumption clearly complicates the task of developing a comprehensive understanding of mast cell biology. Even more complexity has been introduced by recent findings establishing that the phenotypic characteristics of different mouse mast cell populations are not fixed, but can vary predictably as the cells experience different microenvironmental conditions *in vitro* or *in vivo*. While most studies have focused on unidirectional phenotypic change, e.g., "MMC-like" → "CTMC-like" (45, 165, 166, 196, 199, 209) or CTMC → "MMC-like" (152, 196, 247), recent evidence using cloned mast cell populations indicates that at least some of these changes are reversible (139). The fact that many of the experiments documenting mast cell phenotypic changes have been performed *in vivo* is especially important, since such studies demonstrate that all of the signals necessary to regulate these phenotypic alterations are operative in intact animals.

In vitro experiments have begun to define the types of cell-cell interactions that may regulate mast cell phenotype *in vivo*. These studies are likely to permit the identification and detailed molecular characterization of a panel of candidate factors that might be responsible for microenvironmental regulation of mast cell phenotype. Some of these factors may function in soluble form, whereas others may function on the surface of the cells that produce them (or on other cells), or when presented in association with other molecules in the interstitium. Such factors theoretically might regulate mast cell phenotype in several ways, through effects on the proliferation, maturation/differentiation, or function of cells in the mast cell lineage, by favoring different patterns of irreversible change in some of the properties of the cell (*i.e.*, favoring "branching" within the mast cell lineage), or through effects regulating the type and local concentrations of products of other cells which are taken up and stored by mast cells.

While *in vivo* and *in vitro* studies of mast cell development and heterogeneity have already provided important new information, they have also called attention to significant gaps in our understanding of mast cell biology. In part, these reflect the limitations of some of the methods currently available for addressing these issues. For example, *in vivo* and *in vitro* studies of mast cell phenotypic change primarily have analyzed populations of mast cells, not individual cells. Thus, while we know that clonal populations of mast cells derived from a single peritoneal mast cell can express multiple bidirectional phenotypic alterations (139), we do not yet know whether such changes can be expressed by a single cell independently of proliferation.

Technical considerations also influence efforts to identify and purify the factors regulating mast cell phenotype. Generally, soluble factors derived from cell populations that can be grown in large numbers *in vitro* can be more readily studied than those not released in soluble form or that are produced by cells difficult to isolate and propagate in tissue culture. One example of this sort of problem can be cited. Several lines of evidence indicate that interactions between mast cells and "fibroblasts" (*e.g.*, embryonal fibroblasts (17, 43, 95–99, 133, 134) or 3T3 fibroblasts (45, 71–73, 133, 134, 163–166)), if not essential for the induction or maintenance of mast cell maturation/differentiation at least greatly favor this process. This observation may have considerable biologic relevance, since, in many tissues, CTMC develop in close proximity to fibroblasts. Moreover, mast cells appear to be able to influence multiple phenotypic characteristics of fibroblasts, including their movement (98), functional activity (256), and proliferation (44) *in vitro*.

But there is one anatomical site within which maturation of mast cells of the "connective tissue" or "serosal" type takes place, *i.e.*, the peritoneal cavity (138, 139, 196, 211), where the opportunity for direct contact between immature mast cells and fibroblasts would appear to be quite limited. How then is serosal mast cell maturation regulated *in vivo*? Are mesothelial cells (or other nonfibroblasts resident in the peritoneal cavity) producing a factor(s) identical to that produced by 3T3 cells, does a fibroblast-derived factor diffuse into and function within the peritoneal cavity, or is peritoneal mast cell maturation regulated by signals distinct from those produced by 3T3 cells?

Other examples could be given, but the point would be the same. The biologic significance of factors identified by *in vitro* studies as capable of regulating mast cell maturation/differentiation, or the expression of various phenotypic characteristics of fully mature mast cells, eventually will have to be established by providing evidence that such factors actually function *in vivo*. And it will not be enough to demonstrate that infusion of large amounts of purified factor *in vivo* induces a particular effect on mast cell populations. While this represents a useful first step, it will then be necessary to show that endogenous levels of factor sufficient to produce the particular effect can be achieved under appropriate circumstances *in vivo*. The issues that should be addressed in evaluating the biologic significance of factors identified as candidates for regulating mast cell proliferation and/or phenotype *in vivo* are outlined in Table 7. Similar considerations also apply to the characterization of the factors that might mediate mast cell-dependent effects on other cells or structures in the microenvironment of the mast cell.

One mechanism by which immunologic or disease processes might alter mast cell numbers or phenotype is by influencing the local concentrations of the same factors which regulate mast cell numbers or phenotype under normal circumstances, *e.g.*, by increasing a factor's production or expression or by decreasing its metabolism or degradation. Another possibility is that some of the factors influencing mast cell populations during immunologic or pathologic processes are entirely distinct from those of physiologic importance. In either case, the mast cell itself represents a likely candidate as an important regulator of microenvironmental signals which affect mast cells. Not only can mast cell products augment local vascular permeability (thus influencing microenvironmental levels of regulatory molecules which might be present in the circulation), but mast cells might also recruit or activate other cells able to produce and/or degrade molecules with effects on mast cell populations. And these represent just a few of the potential mechanisms by which mast cells might influence their own phenotypic characteristics. For example, certain mast cells may themselves produce cytokines promoting mast cell proliferation or maturation/differentiation (26, 28, 210, 270); under other circumstances, mast cells may help to limit the further expansion of their own numbers

(3, 138). Mast cell-derived cytokines also may influence multiple other cell types and biologic processes (26, 28, 202, 210, 270, 277).

In summary, it is clear that extensive variation in multiple important aspects of mast cell phenotype occurs in both man and experimental animals. Some of the mechanisms regulating mast cell phenotype are beginning to be defined, but many important issues await resolution. These questions include: (a) whether mast cells of different phenotype are in a single cell lineage or represent products of irreversible branch points of mast cell differentiation; (b) whether elucidation of the patterns and mechanisms of mast cell phenotypic variation will result in a comprehensive understanding of the actual roles of particular mast cell populations in health and disease, and (c) whether such understanding will lead to the design of more effective strategies for the management of allergic diseases and other disorders influenced by the mast cell.

Acknowledgments: I thank Dr. Ann M. Dvorak for providing electron micrographs and she and many other colleagues for helpful discussions and suggestions.

REFERENCES

1. Abe T, Nawa Y: Worm expulsion and mucosal mast cell response induced by repetitive IL-3 administration in *Strongyloides ratti*-infected nude mice. Immunology 63:181, 1988
2. Abe T, Ochiai H, Mimamishima Y, Nawa Y: Induction of intestinal mastocytosis in nude mice by repeated injection of interleukin-3. Int Arch Allergy Appl Immunol 86:356, 1988
3. Aldenborg F, Enerbäck L: Thymus dependence of connective tissue mast cells: A quantitative cytofluorometric study of the growth of peritoneal mast cells in normal and athymic rats. Int Arch Allergy Appl Immunol 78:277, 1985
4. Aldenborg F, Enerbäck L: Histochemical heterogeneity of dermal mast cells in athymic and normal rats. Histochemical J 20:19, 1988
5. Aloe J, Levi-Montalcini R: Mast cell increase in tissues in neonatal rats injected with the nerve growth factor. Brain Res 133:358, 1977
6. Arizono N, Koreto O, Nakao S, Iwai Y, Kushima R, Takeoka O: Phenotypic changes in mast cells proliferating in the rat lung following infection with *Nippostrongylus brasiliensis*. Virchows Arch B 54:1, 1987
7. Barrett KE, Metcalfe DD: Mast cell heterogeneity: evidence and implications. J Clin Immunol 4:253, 1984
8. Barsumian EL, McGivney A, Basciano L, Siraganian R: Establishment of four mouse mastocytoma cell lines. Cell Immunol 90:131, 1985
9. Bascom R, Wachs M, Naclerio RM, Pipkorn U, Galli SJ, Lichtenstein LM: Basophil influx occurs after nasal antigen challenge: effects of topical corticosteroid pretreatment. J Allergy Clin Immunol 81:580, 1988
10. Befus AD, Bienenstock MD, Denburg JA (editors): Mast Cell Differentiation and Heterogeneity. New York, Raven Press, 1986
11. Befus AD, Goodacre R, Dyck N, Bienenstock J: Mast cell heterogeneity in man. I. Histologic studies of the intestine. Int Arch Allergy Appl Immunol 76:232, 1985
12. Befus AD, Pearce FL, Gauldie J, Horsewood P, Bienenstock J: Mucosal mast cells. I. Isolation and functional characteristics of rat intestinal mast cells. J Immunol 128:2474, 1982
13. Benyon RC, Lowman MA, Church MK: Human skin mast cells: their dispersion, purification, and secretory characterization. J Immunol 138:861, 1987
14. Bienenstock J, Austen KF, Galli SJ: Nomenclature of mast cells and basophils. In Mast Cell and Basophil Differentiation and Function in Health and Disease, edited by Galli SJ, Austen KF, p 329. New York, Raven Press, 1989

TABLE 7. ISSUES TO BE CONSIDERED IN EVALUATING THE BIOLOGIC SIGNIFICANCE OF PUTATIVE FACTORS[a] REGULATING MAST CELL PROLIFERATION OR MATURATION/DIFFERENTIATION, OR OTHER ASPECTS OF MAST CELL PHENOTYPE

1. Is there evidence that the factor is produced *in vivo* in sufficient quantities, and in the appropriate microenvironments, to orchestrate in the intact animal the effects on mast cell populations which have been observed when the factor is tested *in vitro*?
2. If the factor has been originally isolated from a particular cell type *in vitro*, to what extent is it produced by the corresponding cell types *in vivo*?
3. Which cell types, in addition to those defined in 2, are capable of producing the factor *in vivo*, either in normal tissues or at sites of immunologic or pathologic responses?
4. Are constant levels of the factor expressed constitutively? How is expression (and metabolism/degradation) of the factor regulated?

[a] "Factors" are defined as in footnote [a] of Table 4.

15. Bienenstock J, Befus AD, Denburg JA: Mast cell heterogeneity: basic questions and clinical implications. In Mast Cell Differentiation and Heterogeneity, edited by Befus AD, Bienenstock J, Denburg JA, p 391. New York, Raven Press, 1986

16. Bienenstock J, Blennerhassett M, Kakuta Y, MacQueen G, Marshall J, Perdue M, Siegel S, Tsuda T, Denburg J, Stead R: Evidence for central and peripheral nervous system interaction with mast cells. In Mast Cell and Basophil Differentiation and Function in Health and Disease, edited by Galli SJ, Austen KF, p 275. New York, Raven Press, 1989

17. Bland EC, Ginsburg H, Silbert JE, Metcalfe DD: Mouse heparin proteoglycan: synthesis by mast cell fibroblast monolayers during lymphocyte-dependent mast cell proliferation. J Biol Chem 257:8661, 1982

18. Blank U, Ra C, Miller L, White K, Metzger H, Kinet J-P: Complete structure and expression in transfected cells of high affinity IgE receptor. Nature (London) 337:187, 1989

19. Bloom G, Ringertz NR: Acid polysaccharides of peritoneal mast cells of the rat and mouse. Ark Kemi 16:51, 1960

20. Bodger MP, Mounsey GL, Nelson J, Fitzgerald PH: A monoclonal antibody reacting with human basophils. Blood 69:1414, 1987

21. Bottomly K: A functional dichotomy in CD4$^+$ T lymphocytes. Immunol Today 9:268, 1988

22. Brain SD, Williams TJ: Substance P regulates the vasodilator activity of calcitonin gene-related peptide. Nature (London) 335:73, 1988

23. Bressler RB, Thompson HL, Keffer JM, Metcalfe DD: Inhibition of the growth of IL-3-dependent mast cells from murine bone marrow by recombinant granulocyte-macrophage colony-stimulating factor. J Immunol 143:135, 1989

24. Broide DH, Metcalfe DD, Wasserman SI: Functional and biochemical characterization of rat bone marrow-derived mast cells. J Immunol 141:4298, 1988

25. Broide D, Barrett K, Wasserman SI: Characterization and functional analysis of rat mucosal mast cells. In Mast Cell and Basophil Differentiation and Function in Health and Disease, edited by Galli SJ, Austen KF, p 195. New York, Raven Press, 1989

26. Brown MA, Pierce JH, Watson CJ, Falco J, Ihle JN, Paul WE: B cell stimulatory factor-1/interleukin-4 mRNA is expressed by normal and transformed mast cells. Cell 50:809, 1987

27. Brown SJ, Galli SJ, Gleich GJ, Askenase PW: Ablation of immunity to *Amblyomma americanum* by anti-basophil serum: cooperation between basophils and eosinophils in expression of immunity to ectoparasites (ticks) in guinea pigs. J Immunol 129:790, 1982

28. Burd PR, Rogers HW, Gordon JR, Martin CA, Jayaraman S, Wilson SD, Dvorak AM, Galli SJ, Dorf ME: IL-3-dependent and -independent mast cells stimulated with IgE and antigen express multiple cytokines. J Exp Med 143:135, 1989

29. Burnet FM: The probable relationship of some or all mast cells to the T-cell system. Cell Immunol 30:358, 1977

30. Butterfield JH, Weiler D, Dewald G, Gleich GJ: Establishment of an immature mast cell line from a patient with mast cell leukemia. Leuk Res 12:345, 1988

30. Casale TB, Bowman S, Kaliner M: Induction of human cutaneous mast cell degranulation by opiates and endogenous opioid peptides: evidence for opiate and nonopiate receptor participation. J Allergy Clin Immunol 73:775, 1984

32. Caughey GH, Leidig F, Viro NF, Nadel JA: Substance P and vasoactive intestinal peptide degradation by mast cell tryptase and chymase. J Pharmacol Exp Ther 244:133, 1988

33. Chabot B, Stephenson DA, Chapman VM, Besmer P, Bernstein A: The proto-oncogene *c-kit* encoding a transmembrane tyrosine kinase receptor maps to the mouse *W* locus. Nature 335:88, 1988

34. Chi E, Lagunoff D: Abnormal mast cell granules in the beige (Chediak-Higashi syndrome) mouse. J Histochem Cytochem 23:117, 1975

35. Church MK, Benyon RC, Rees PH, Lowman MA, Campbell AM, Robinson C, Holgate ST: Functional heterogeneity of human mast cells. In Mast Cell and Basophil Differentiation and Function in Health and Disease, edited by Galli SJ, Austen KF, p 161. New York, Raven Press, 1989

36. Cohan VL, Massey WA, Gittlen SD, Charlesworth EN, Warner JA, Kagey-Sobotka A, Lichtenstein LM: The heterogeneity of human histamine containing cells. In Mast Cell and Basophil Differentiation and Function in Health and Disease, edited by Galli SJ, Austen KF, p 149. New York, Raven Press, 1989

37. Combs JW, Lagunoff D, Benditt EP: Differentiation and proliferation of embryonic mast cells of the rat. J Cell Biol 25:577, 1965

38. Cooper MD, Kearney J, Scher I: B Lymphocytes. In Fundamental Immunology, edited by Paul WE, p 43. New York, Raven Press, 1984

39. Craig SS, DeBlois G, Schwartz LB: Mast cells in human keloid, small intestine, and lung by an immunoperoxidase technique using a murine monoclonal antibody. Am J Pathol 124:427, 1986

40. Craig SS, Schechter NM, Schwartz LB: Ultrastructural analysis of human T and TC mast cells identified by immunoelectron microscopy. Lab Invest 58:682, 1988

41. Craig SS, Schechter NM, Schwartz LB: Ultrastructural analysis of maturing human T and TC mast cells in situ. Lab Invest 60:147, 1989

42. Crowle PK, Reed ND: Bone marrow origin of mucosal mast cells. Int Arch Allergy Appl Immunol 73:242, 1984

43. Davidson S, Kinarty A, Coleman R, Reshef A, Ginsburg H: Fibroblasts are required for mast cell granule synthesis. In Mast Cell Differentiation and Heterogeneity, edited by Befus AD, Bienenstock J, Denburg JA, p 155. New York, Raven Press, 1986

44. Dayton ET, Caulfield JP, Hein A, Austen KF, Stevens RL: Regulation of the growth rate of mouse fibroblasts by IL-3-activated mouse bone marrow-derived mast cells. J Immunol 142:4307, 1989

45. Dayton ET, Pharr P, Ogawa M, Serafin WE, Austen KF, Levi-Schaffer F, Stevens RL: 3T3 fibroblasts induce cloned interleukin 3-dependent mouse mast cells to resemble connective tissue mast cells in granular consistency. Proc Natl Acad Sci USA 85:569, 1988

46. Denburg JA, Befus AD, Bienenstock J: Growth and differentiation in vitro of mast cells from mesenteric lymph nodes of *Nippostrongylus brasiliensis* infected rats. Immunology 41:195, 1980

47. Denburg JA, Tanno Y, Bienenstock J: Growth and differentiation of human basophils, eosinophils, and mast cells. In Mast Cell Differentiation and Heterogeneity, edited by Befus AD, Bienenstock J, Denburg JA, p 71. New York, Raven Press, 1986

48. DuBuske L, Austen KF, Czop J, Stevens RL: Granule-associated serine neutral proteases of the mouse bone marrow-derived mast cell that degrade fibronectin: their increase after sodium butyrate treatment of the cells. J Immunol 133:1535, 1984

49. Dvorak AM: Human mast cells. Advances in Anatomy Embryology and Cell Biology, Vol 114, edited by Beck F, Hild W, Kriz W, Ortmann R, Pauly JE, Schiebler TH. Springer-Verlag, 1989

50. Dvorak AM, Dvorak HF, Galli SJ: Ultrastructural criteria for identification of mast cells and basophils in humans, guinea pigs, and mice. Am Rev Respir Dis 128:S49, 1983

51. Dvorak AM, Galli SJ, Schulman ES, Lichtenstein LM, Dvorak HF: Basophil and mast cell degranulation: ultrastructural analysis of mechanisms of mediator release. Fed Proc 42:2510, 1983

52. Dvorak AM, Hammel I, Schulman ES, Peters SP, MacGlashan DW Jr, Schleimer RP, Newball HH, Pyne K, Dvorak HF, Lichtenstein LM, Galli SJ: Differences in the behavior of cytoplasmic granules and lipid bodies during human lung mast cell degranulation. J Cell Biol 99:1678, 1984

53. Dvorak AM, Ishizaka T, Galli SJ: Ultrastructure of human basophils developing in vitro. Evidence for the acquisition of peroxidase by basophils, and for different effects of human and murine growth factors on human basophil and eosinophil maturation. Lab Invest 53:57, 1985

54. Dvorak AM, Klebanoff SJ, Henderson WR, Monahan RA, Pyne K, Galli SJ: Vesicular uptake of eosinophil peroxidase by guinea pig basophils and by cloned mouse mast cells and granule-containing lymphoid cells. Am J Pathol 118:425, 1985

55. Dvorak AM, Mihm MC Jr, Dvorak HF: Morphology of delayed-type hypersensitivity reactions in man. II. Ultrastructural alterations affecting the microvasculature and the tissue mast cells. Lab Invest 34:179, 1976.

56. Dvorak AM, Mihm MC Jr, Osage JE, Kwan TH, Austen KF, Wintroub BU: Bullous pemphigoid, an ultrastructural study of the inflammatory response: eosinophil, basophil and mast cell granule changes in multiple biopsies from one patient. J Invest Dermatol 78:91, 1982

57. Dvorak AM, Monahan RA, Osage JE, Dickersin GR: Crohn's

disease: transmission electron microscopic studies. II. Immunologic inflammatory response. Alterations of mast cells, basophils, eosinophils, and the microvasculature. Hum Pathol 11:606, 1980

58. Dvorak AM, Nabel G, Pyne K, Cantor H, Dvorak HF, Galli SJ: Ultrastructural identification of the mouse basophil. Blood 59:1279, 1982

59. Dvorak AM, Schleimer RP, Lichtenstein LM: Human mast cells synthesize new granules during recovery from degranulation. *In vitro* studies with mast cells purified from human lungs. Blood 71:76, 1988

60. Dvorak AM, Schulman ES, Peters SP, MacGlashan DW Jr, Newball HH, Schleimer RP, Lichtenstein LM: Immunoglobulin E-mediated degranulation of isolated human lung mast cells. Lab Invest 53:45, 1985

61. Dvorak HF, Dvorak AM: Basophilic leukocytes: structure, function, and role in disease. In Clinics in Haematology, Granulocyte and Monocyte Abnormalities, Vol 4, edited by Lichtman MA, p 651. London, WB Saunders Co, Ltd, 1975

62. Ehrlich P: Beiträge zur Theorie und Praxis der histologischen Färbung. Leipzig; 1878 Thesis

63. Ehrlich P: Über die spezifischen Granulationen des Blutes. Arch Anat Physiol Abt 571–577, 1879

64. Enerbäck L: Berberine sulfate binding to mast cell polyanions: a cytofluorometric method for the quantitation of heparin. Histochemistry 42:301, 1974

65. Enerbäck L: The gut mucosal mast cell. Monogr Allergy 17:222, 1981

66. Enerbäck L: Mast cell heterogeneity: the evolution of the concept of a specific mucosal mast cell. In Mast Cell Differentiation and Heterogeneity, edited by Befus AD, Bienenstock J, Denburg JA, p 1. New York, Raven Press, 1986

67. Enerbäck L, Pipkorn U, Aldenborg F, Wingren U: Mast cell heterogeneity in man: properties and function of human mucosal mast cells. In Mast Cell and Basophil Differentiation and Function in Health and Disease, edited by Galli SJ, Austen KF, p 27. New York, Raven Press, 1989

68. Finkelman FD, Katona IM, Urban Jr JF, Holmes J, Ohara J, Tung AS, Sample JvG, Paul WE: IL-4 is required to generate and sustain *in vivo* IgE responses. J Immunol 141:2335, 1988

69. Finkelman FD, Ohara J, Goroff DK, Smith J, Villacreses N, Mond JJ, Paul WE: Production of BSF-1 during an *in vivo*, T-dependent immune response. J Immunol 137:2878, 1986

70. Fox CC, Dvorak AM, Peters SP, Kagey-Sobotka A, Lichtenstein LM: Isolation and characterization of human intestinal mucosal mast cells. J Immunol 135:483, 1985

71. Fujita J, Nakayama H, Onoue H, Ebi Y, Kanakura Y, Kuriu A, Kitamura Y: Failure of *W/W^v* mouse derived cultured mast cells to enter S phase upon contact with NIH/3T3 fibroblasts. Blood 72:463, 1988

72. Fujita J, Nakayama H, Onoue H, Kanakura Y, Nakano T, Asai H, Takeda S, Honjo T, Kitamura Y: Fibroblast-dependent growth of mouse mast cells *in vitro*: duplication of mast cell depletion in mutant mice of *W/W^v* genotype. J Cell Physiol 134:78, 1988

73. Fujita J, Onoue H, Ebi Y, Nakayama H, Kanakura Y: *In vitro* duplication and *in vivo* cure of mast cell deficiency of *Sl/Sl^d* mutant mice by cloned 3T3 fibroblasts. Proc Natl Acad Sci USA 86:2888, 1989

74. Fung MC, Hapel AJ, Ymer S, Cohen DR, Johnson RM, Campbell HD, Yung IG: Molecular cloning of cDNA for murine interleukin-3. Nature (London) 307:233, 1984

75. Furitsu T, Saito H, Dvorak AM, Schwartz LB, Irani AA, Burdick JF, Ishizaka K, Ishizaka T: Development of human mast cells *in vitro*. Proc Natl Acad Sci USA, in press 1989

76. Gabriel LC, Escribano LM, Marie J-P, Zittoun R, Navarro JL: Peroxidase activity in circulating mast cells in blast crisis of chronic granulocytic leukemia. Am J Clin Pathol 86:212, 1986

77. Galli SJ: Mast cell heterogeneity: can variation in mast cell phenotype be explained without postulating the existence of distinct mast cell lineages? In Mast Cell Differentiation and Heterogeneity, edited by Befus AD, Bienenstock J, Denburg JA, p 167. New York, Raven Press, 1986

78. Galli SJ: New approaches for the analysis of mast cell maturation, heterogeneity, and function. Fed Proc 46:1906, 1987

79. Galli SJ, Askenase PW: Cutaneous basophil hypersensitivity. In The Reticuloendothelial System: A Comprehensive Treatise, Vol IX, edited by Abramoff P, Phillips SM, Escobar MR, p 321. New York, Plenum, 1986

80. Galli SJ, Austen KF (editors): Mast Cell and Basophil Differentiation and Function in Health and Disease. New York, Raven Press, 1989

81. Galli SJ, Goetzl EJ: Eosinophils, basophils, and mast cells. In Blood: Principles and Practice of Hematology, edited by Handin RI, Lux SE, Stossel TP. Philadelphia, JB Lippincott Company, in press 1990

82. Galli SJ, Hammel I: Unequivocal delayed hypersensitivity in mast cell-deficient and beige mice. Science 226:710, 1984

83. Galli SJ, Kitamura Y: Animal model of human disease. Genetically mast cell-deficient *W/W^v* and *Sl/Sl^d* mice: their value for the analysis of the roles of mast cells in biological responses *in vivo*. Am J Pathol 127:191, 1987

84. Galli SJ, Lichtenstein LM: Biology of mast cells and basophils. In Allergy. Principles and Practice, Ed 3, edited by Middleton Jr E, Reed CE, Ellis EF, Adkinson Jr NF, Yunginger JW, p 106. St. Louis, The CV Mosby Company, 1988

85. Galli SJ, Arizono N, Murakami T, Dvorak AM, Fox JG: Development of large numbers of mast cells at sites of chronic idiopathic dermatitis in genetically mast cell-deficient WBB6F₁-*W/W^v* mice. Blood 69:1661, 1987

86. Galli SJ, Dvorak AM, Dvorak HF: Basophils and mast cells: Morphologic insights into their biology, secretory patterns and function. Prog Allergy 34:1, 1984

87. Galli SJ, Dvorak AM, Dvorak HF: Morphology, biochemistry, and function of basophils and mast cells. In Hematology, 4th edition, edited by Williams WJ, Beutler E, Erslev AJ, Lichtman MA. New York, McGraw Hill, p 840, 1990

88. Galli SJ, Dvorak AM, Marcum JA, Ishizaka T, Nabel G, Der Simonian H, Pyne K, Goldin JM, Rosenberg RD, Cantor H, Dvorak HF: Mast cell clones: a model for the analysis of cellular maturation. J Cell Biol 95:435, 1982

89. Galli SJ, Wershil BK, Bose R, Walker PA, Szabo S: Ethanol-induced acute gastric injury in mast cell-deficient and congenic normal mice: evidence that mast cells can augment the area of damage. Am J Pathol 128:131, 1987

90. Galli SJ, Wershil BK, Yano H, Arizono N, Gordon JR, Murakami T: Analysis of the roles of phenotypically distinct mast cell populations in non-immunological responses. In Mast Cell and Basophil Differentiation and Function in Health and Disease, edited by Galli SJ, Austen KF, p 255. New York, Raven Press, 1989

91. Geissler EN, Ryan MA, Housman DE: The dominant-white spotting (*W*) locus of the mouse encodes the *c-kit* proto-oncogene. Cell 55:185, 1988

92. Gibbins IL, Furness JB, Costa M, MacIntyre I, Hillyard CJ, Girgis S: Co-localization of calcitonin gene-related peptide-like immunoreactivity with substance P in cutaneous, vascular and visceral sensory neurons of guinea pigs. Neurosci Lett 57:125, 1985

93. Gilbert HS, Ornstein L: Basophil counting with a new staining method using alcian blue. Blood 46:279, 1975

94. Gilead L, Rahamim E, Ziv I, Or R, Razin E: Cultured human bone marrow-derived mast cells, their similarities to cultured murine E-mast cells. Immunology 63:669, 1988

95. Ginsburg H: The *in vitro* differentiation and culture of normal mast cells from mouse thymus. Ann NY Acad Sci 103:20, 1963

96. Ginsburg H, Lagunoff D: The *in vitro* differentiation of mast cells. Cultures of cells from immunized mouse lymph nodes and thoracic duct lymph on fibroblast monolayers. J Cell Biol 35:685, 1967

97. Ginsburg H, Ben-Shahar D, Ben-David E: Mast cell growth on fibroblast monolayers. Two cell entities. Immunology 45:371, 1982

98. Ginsburg H, Nir I, Hammel I, Eren R, Weissman B-A, Naot Y: Differentiation and activity of mast cells following immunization in cultures of lymph node cells. Immunology 35:485, 1978

99. Ginsburg H, Olson EC, Huff TF, Okudaira H, Ishizaka T: Enhancement of mast cell differentiation *in vitro* by T cell factor(s). Int Arch Allergy Appl Immunol 66:447, 1981

100. Goetzl EJ, Finch RJ, Peterson KE, Turck CW, Sneedharan SP: Mast cell and basophil mediation of lymphocytic functions. In Mast Cell and Basophil Differentiation and Function in Health and Disease, edited by Galli SJ, Austen KF, p 247. New York, Raven Press, 1989

101. Gordon JR, Galli SJ: PMA induces mast cell (MC) development

in genetically mast cell-deficient WBB6F$_1$-W/W^v mice (abstr). FASEB J 2:A1233, 1988

102. Gordon JR, Galli SJ: Mast cells as a source of preformed and immunologically inducible TNA-α/cachectin FASEB J, in press 1990

103. Green MC: Mutant genes and linkages. In Biology of the Laboratory Mouse, Ed 2, edited by Green EL, p 87. New York, McGraw-Hill, 1966

104. Hägermark O, Hökfelt T, Pernow B: Flare and itch induced by substance P in human skin. J Invest Dermatol 71:233, 1978

105. Haig DM, McKee, TA, Jarrett EEE, Woodbury R, Miller HRP: Generation of mucosal mast cells is stimulated *in vitro* by factors derived from T cells of helminth infected rats. Nature (London) 300:188, 1982

106. Haig DM, McMenamin C, Jarrett EEE: Mast cell development in the rat. In Mast Cell Differentiation and Heterogeneity, edited by Befus AD, Bienenstock J, Denburg JA, p 55. New York, Raven Press, 1986

107. Hamaguchi Y, Kanakura Y, Fujita J, Takeda S, Nakano T, Tarui S, Honjo T, Kitamura Y: Interleukin 4 as an essential factor for *in vitro* clonal growth of murine connective tissue-type mast cells. J Exp Med 165:268, 1987

108. Hammel I, Dvorak AM, Galli SJ: Defective cytoplasmic granule formation. I. Abnormalities affecting tissue mast cells and pancreatic acinar cells of beige mice. Lab Invest 56:321, 1987

109. Hammel I, Dvorak AM, Peters SP, Schulman ES, Dvorak HF, Lichtenstein LM, Galli SJ: Differences in the volume distributions of human lung mast cell granules and lipid bodies: evidence that the size of these organelles is regulated by distinct mechanisms. J Cell Biol 100:1488, 1985

110. Hammel I, Lagunoff D, Bauza M, Chi E: Periodic, multimodal distribution of granule volumes in mast cells. Cell Tissue Res 228:51, 1983

111. Hammel I, Lagunoff D, Krüger P-G: Studies on the growth of mast cells in rats. Changes in granule size between one and six months. Lab Invest 59:549, 1988

112. Hardy WB, Westbrook FF: The wandering cells of the alimentary canal. J Physiol 18:490, 1895

113. Harper ST, Wells E, Mann J, Eady RP: The pharmacology of the Macaque bronchial lavage mast cell. In Mast Cell and Basophil Differentiation and Function in Health and Disease, edited by Galli SJ, Austen KF, p 171. New York, Raven Press, 1989

114. Hasthorpe S: A hemopoietic cell line dependent upon a factor in pokeweed mitogen-stimulated spleen cell conditioning medium. J Cell Physiol 105:379, 1980

115. Henderson WR, Chi EY, Jong EC, Klebanoff SJ: Mast cell-mediated toxicity to schistosomula of *Schistosoma mansoni*: potentiation by exogenous peroxidase. J Immunol 137:2695, 1986

116. Hermens JM, Ebertz JM, Hanafin JM, Hirshman CA: Comparison of histamine release in human skin mast cells induced by morphine, fentanyl and oxomorphine. Anesthesiology 62:124, 1985

117. Holgate ST, Robinson C, Church MK: Mediators of immediate hypersensitivity. In Allergy. Principles and Practice. Third Edition, edited by Middleton Jr E, Reed CE, Ellis EF, Adkinson Jr NF, Yunginger JW, p 135. St. Louis, The CV Mosby Company, 1988

118. Horton MA, O'Brien HAW: Characterization of human mast cells in long-term culture. Blood 62:1251, 1983

119. Howard M, Farrar J, Hilfiker M, Johnson B, Takatsu K, Hamaoka T, Paul WE: Identification of a T cell-derived B cell growth factor distinct from interleukin 2. J Exp Med 155:194, 1982

120. Huff TF, Justus DE: Mast cell differentiation in cultures of T cell-depleted mesenteric lymph node cells from *Nippostrongylus brasiliensis*-infected mice. Int Arch Allergy Appl Immunol 85:137, 1988

121. Hültner L, Moeller J, Schmitt E, Jäger G, Reisbach G, Ring J, Dörmer P: Thiol-sensitive mast cell lines derived from mouse bone marrow respond to a mast cell growth-enhancing activity different from both IL-3 and IL-4. J Immunol 142:3440, 1989

122. Hurtado I, Urbina C: Ultrastructure of the mouse blood basophil. J Submicrosc Cytol 15:1041, 1983

123. Ihle JN, Keller J, Oroszlan S, Henderson LE, Copeland RD, Fitch F, Prystowsky MB, Goldwasser E, Schrader JW, Palaszynski E, Dy M, Lebel B: Biological properties of homogeneous interleukin 3. I. Demonstration of WEHI-3 growth-factor activity, mast cell growth-factor activity, P cell-stimulating factor activity and histamine-producing factor activity. J Immunol 131:282, 1983

124. Ihle JN, Rebar L, Keller J, Lee JC, Hapel A: Interleukin 3: possible roles in the regulation of lymphocyte differentiation and growth. Immunol Rev 63:101, 1981

125. Irani AA, Craig SS, DeBlois G, Elson CO, Schechter NM, Schwartz LB: Deficiency of the tryptase-positive, chymase-negative mast cell type in gastrointestinal mucosa of patients with defective T lymphocyte function. J Immunol 138:4381, 1987

126. Irani AA, Schechter NM, Craig SS, DeBlois G, Schwartz LB: Two human mast cell subsets with distinct neutral protease compositions. Proc Natl Acad Sci USA 83:4464, 1986

127. Ishizaka T: Mechanisms of IgE-mediated hypersensitivity. In Allergy. Principles and Practice, Ed 3, edited by Middleton Jr E, Reed CE, Ellis EF, Adkinson Jr NF, Yunginger JW, p 71. St. Louis, The CV Mosby Company, 1988

128. Ishizaka T, Adachi T, Chang TH, Ishizaka K: Development of mast cells *in vitro*. II. Biologic function of cultured mast cells. J Immunol 118:211, 1977

129. Ishizaka T, Dvorak AM, Conrad DH, Niebyl JR, Marquette JP, Ishizaka K: Morphological and immunological characterization of human basophils developed in cultures of cord blood mononuclear cells. J Immunol 134:532, 1985

130. Ishizaka T, Okudaira H, Mauser LE, Ishizaka K: Development of rat mast cells *in vitro*. I. Differentiation of mast cells from thymus cells. J Immunol 116:747, 1976

131. Ishizaka T, Saito H, Furitsu T, Dvorak AM: Growth of human basophils and mast cells *in vitro*. In Mast Cell and Basophil Differentiation and Function in Health and Disease, edited by Galli SJ, Austen KF, p 39. New York, Raven Press, 1989

132. Jacoby W, Cammarata PV, Findlay S, Pincus SH: Anaphylaxis in mast cell-deficient mice. J Invest Dermatol 83:302, 1984

133. Jarboe DL, Huff TF: The mast cell-committed progenitor. III. W/W mice do not make mast cell-committed progenitors and Sl/Sl^d fibroblasts do not support development of normal mast cell-committed progenitors. J Immunol 142:2418, 1989

134. Jarboe DL, Marshall JS, Randolph TR, Kukolja A, Huff TF: The mast cell-committed progenitor. I. Description of a cell capable of IL-3-independent proliferation and differentiation without contact with fibroblasts. J Immunol 142:2405, 1989

135. Jarrett EEE, Haig DM: Mucosal mast cells *in vivo* and *in vitro*. Immunol Today 5:115, 1984

136. Juhlin L: Basophil leukocyte differential in blood and bone marrow. Acta Haematol 29:89, 1963

137. Juhlin L, Michaëlsson G: A new syndrome characterized by absence of eosinophils and basophils. Lancet 1:1233, 1977

138. Kanakura Y, Kuriu A, Waki N, Nakano T, Asai H, Yonezawa T, Kitamura Y: Changes in numbers and types of mast cell colony-forming cells in the peritoneal cavity of mice after injection of distilled water: evidence that mast cells suppress differentiation of bone marrow-derived precursors. Blood 61:573, 1988

139. Kanakura Y, Thompson H, Nakano T, Yamamura T, Asai H, Kitamura Y, Metcalfe DD, Galli SJ: Multiple bidirectional alterations of phenotype and changes in proliferative potential during the *in vitro* and *in vivo* passage of clonal mast cell populations derived from mouse peritoneal mast cells. Blood 72:877, 1988

140. Katz HR, Austen KF: Mast cell glycosphingolipids. In Mast Cell and Basophil Differentiation and Function in Health and Disease, edited by Galli SJ, Austen KF, p 107. New York, Raven Press, 1989

141. Katz HR, Dayton ET, Levi-Schaffer F, Benson AC, Austen KF, Stevens RL: Coculture of mouse IL-3-dependent mast cells with 3T3 fibroblasts stimulates synthesis of globopentaosylceramide (Forssman glycolipid) by fibroblasts and surface expression on both populations. J Immunol 140:3090, 1988

142. Katz HR, LeBlanc PA, Russell SW: Two classes of mouse mast cells delineated by monoclonal antibodies. Proc Natl Acad Sci USA 80:5916-5918, 1983

143. Kawanami O, Ferrans VJ, Fulmer JD, Crystal RG: Ultrastructure of pulmonary mast cells in patients with fibrotic lung disorders. Lab Invest 40:717, 1979

144. Kindler V, Thorens B, de Kossodo S, Allet B, Eliason JF, Thatcher D, Farber N, Vassalli P: Stimulation of hematopoiesis *in vivo* by recombinant bacterial murine interleukin 3. Proc Natl

Acad Sci USA 83:1001, 1986

145. Kirshenbaum AS, Goff JP, Dreskin SC, Irani A-M, Schwartz LB, Metcalfe DD: IL 3-dependent growth of basophil-like cells and mast-like cells from human bone marrow. J Immunol 142:2424, 1989

146. Kitamura Y: Heterogeneity of mast cells and phenotypic changes between subpopulations. Ann Rev Immunol, in press 1989

147. Kitamura Y, Go S: Decreased production of mast cells in *Sl/Sl^d* anemic mice. Blood 53:492, 1979

148. Kitamura Y, Go S, Hatanaka S: Decrease of mast cells in *W/W^v* mice and their increase by bone marrow transplantation. Blood 52:447, 1978

149. Kitamura Y, Nakayama H, Fujita J: Mechanism of mast cell deficiency in mutant mice of *W/W^v* and *Sl/Sl^d* genotype. In Mast Cell and Basophil Differentiation and Function in Health and Disease, edited by Galli SJ, Austen KF, p 15. New York, Raven Press, 1989

150. Kitamura Y, Sonoda T, Yokoyama M: Differentiation of tissue mast cells. In Hematopoietic Stem Cells, Alfred Benzon Symposium 18, edited by Killman SA, Cronkite EP, Muller-Berat CN, p 350. Copenhagen, Munksgaard, 1984

151. Kitamura Y, Yokoyama M, Matsuda H, Ohno T, Mori KJ: Spleen colony-forming cell as common precursor for tissue mast cells and granulocytes. Nature (London) 291:159, 1981

152. Kobayashi T, Nakano T, Nakahata T, Asai H, Yagi Y, Tsuji K, Komiyama A, Akabane T, Kojima S, Kitamura Y: Formation of mast cell colonies in methylcellulose by mouse peritoneal cells and differentiation of these cloned cells in both the skin and the gastric mucosa of *W/W^v* mice: evidence that a common precursor can give rise to both "connective tissue-type" and "mucosal" mast cells. J Immunol 136:1378, 1986

153. Kowalski ML, Kaliner MA: Neurogenic inflammation, vascular permeability, and mast cells. J Immunol 140:3905, 1988

154. Krüger PG, Lagunoff D: Mast cell restoration. A study of the rat peritoneal mast cells after depletion with polymyxin B. Int Arch Allergy Appl Immunol 65:278, 1981

155. Lagunoff D: Structural aspects of histamine binding: the mast cell granule. In Mechanisms of Release of Biogenic Amines, edited by von Euler US, Rosell S, Uvnäs B, p 79. Oxford, Pergamon Press, 1966

156. Lagunoff D: Contributions of electron microscopy to the study of mast cells. J Invest Dermatol 58:296, 1972

157. Lagunoff D, Benditt EP: Proteolytic enzymes of mast cells. Ann NY Acad Sci 103:185, 1963

158. Lawrence ID, Warner JA, Cohan VL, Hubbard WC, Kagey-Sobotka A, Lichtenstein LM: Purification and characterization of human skin mast cells: evidence for human mast cell heterogeneity. J Immunol 139:3062, 1987

159. Lee F, Yokota T, Otsuka T, Meyerson P, Villaret D, Coffman R, Mosmann T, Rennick D, Roehm N, Smith C, Zlotnick A, Arai K-I: Isolation and characterization of a mouse interleukin cDNA clone that expresses B cell stimulatory factor 1 activities and T-cell- and mast cell-stimulating activities. Proc Natl Acad Sci USA 83:2061, 1986

160. Lemanske Jr RF, Kaliner MA: Late-phase allergic reactions. In Allergy. Principles and Practice, edited by Middleton Jr E, Reed CE, Ellis EF, Adkinson Jr NF, Yunginger JW, p 224. St. Louis, The CV Mosby Company, 1988

161. Le Trong H, Neurath H, Woodbury RG: Substrate specificity of the chymotrypsin-like protease in secretory granules isolated from rat mast cells. Proc Natl Acad Sci USA 84:364-367, 1987

162. Leung KBP, Fling KC, Brostoff J, Hudspith BN, Johnson NMcI, Lau HYA, Liu WL, Pearce FL: Effects of sodium cromoglycate and nedocromil sodium on histamine secretion from human lung mast cells. Thorax 43:756, 1988

163. Levi-Schaffer F, Austen KF, Caulfield JP, Hein A, Bloes WF, Stevens RL: Fibroblasts maintain the phenotype and viability of the rat heparin-containing mast cells *in vitro*. J Immunol 135:3454, 1985

164. Levi-Schaffer F, Austen KF, Caulfield JP, Hein A, Gravallese PM, Stevens RL: Co-culture of human lung-derived mast cells with mouse 3T3 fibroblasts: morphology and IgE mediated release of histamine, prostaglandin D2, and leukotrienes. J Immunol 139:494, 1987

165. Levi-Shaffer F, Austen KF, Gravallese PM, Stevens RL: Cocul-ture of interleukin 3-dependent mouse mast cells with fibroblasts results in a phenotypic change of the mast cells. Proc Natl Acad Sci USA 83:6485, 1986

166. Levi-Schaffer F, Dayton ET, Austen KF, Hein A, Caulfield JP, Gravallese PM, Liu FT, Stevens RL: Mouse bone marrow-derived mast cells cocultured with fibroblasts: morphology and stimulation-induced release of histamine, leukotriene B$_4$, leukotriene C$_4$, and prostaglandin D$_2$. J Immunol 139:3431, 1987

167. Lundberg JM, Franco-Cereceda A, Hua X, Hökfeit T, Fischer JA: Co-existence of substance P and calcitonin gene-related peptide-like immunoreactivities in sensory nerves in relation to cardiovascular and bronchoconstrictor effects of capsaicin. Eur J Pharmacol 108:315, 1985

168. Martin TR, Galli SJ, Katona IM, Drazen JM: The role of mast cells in anaphylaxis. Evidence for the importance of mast cells in the cardiopulmonary alterations and death induced by anti-IgE in mice. J Clin Invest 83:1375, 1989

169. Martin TR, Drazen JM, Galli SJ: Active anaphylaxis is associated with tachycardia in normal but not mast cell (MC)-deficient mice (abstr). FASEB J 3:A790, 1989

170. Matsuda H, Kawakita K, Kiso Y, Nakano T, Kitamura Y: Substance P induces granulocyte infiltration through degranulation of mast cells. J Immunol 142:927, 1989

171. Matsuda H, Nakano T, Kiso Y, Kitamura Y: Normalization of anti-tick response of mast cell-deficient *W/W^v* mice by intracutaneous injection of cultured mast cells. J Parasitol 73:155, 1987

172. Maximow A: Über die Zellformen des lockeren Bindegewebes. Arch mikrosk Anat Entw Mech 67:680, 1905

173. Mayrhofer G, Fisher R: Mast cells in severely T-cell depleted rats and the response to infestation with *Nippostrongylus brasiliensis*. Immunology 37:145, 1979

174. Mayrhofer G, Gadd SJ, Spargo LDJ, Ashman LK: Specificity of a mouse monoclonal antibody raised against acute myeloid leukaemia cells for mast cells in human mucosal and connective tissues. Immunol Cell Biol 65(pt 3):241, 1987

175. Mekori YA, Chang JCC, Wershil BK, Galli SJ: Studies of the role of mast cells in contact sensitivity responses: passive transfer of the reaction into mast cell-deficient mice locally reconstituted with cultured mast cells; effect of reserpine on transfer of the reaction with DNP-specific cloned T cells. Cell Immunol 109:39, 1987

176. Mekori YA, Weitzman GL, Galli SJ: Reevaluation of reserpine-induced suppression of contact sensitivity. Evidence that reserpine interferes with T lymphocyte function independently of an effect on mast cells. J Exp Med 162:1935, 1985

177. Metcalf D: The molecular biology and functions of the granulocyte-macrophage colony stimulating factors. Blood 67:257, 1986

178. Metcalf D, Begley CG, Johnson NA, Nicola NA, Lopez AF, Williamson DJ: Effects of purified bacterially synthesized murine Multi-CSF (IL-3) on hematopoiesis in normal adult mice. Blood 68:46, 1986

179. Metcalfe DD, Kaliner M, Donlon MA: The mast cell. CRC Crit Rev Immunol 2:23, 1981

180. Metzger H, Alcaraz G, Hohman R, Kinet JP, Pribluda V, Quarto R: The receptor with high affinity for immunoglobulin E. Ann Rev Immunol 4:419, 1986

181. Michel L, Pitton C, Prost C, Masse J-M, Mencia-Huerta J-M, Burtin C, Maclouf J, Breton-Gorius J, Benveniste J, Dubertret L: Prostaglandin D$_2$ generation in mouse bone marrow-derived mast cells exposed to dexamethasone is associated with endogenous peroxidase activity. Lab Invest 59:613, 1988

182. Miller HRP, Huntley JF, Newlands GFJ, Mackellar A, Irvine J, Haig DM, MacDonald A, Lammas AD, Wakelin D, Woodbury RG: Mast cell granule proteases in mouse and rat: a guide to mast cell heterogeneity and activation in the gastrointestinal tract. In Mast Cell and Basophil Differentiation and Function in Health and Disease, edited by Galli SJ, Austen KF, p 81. New York, Raven Press, 1989

183. Miller L, Blank U, Metzger H, Kinet J-P: Expression of high-affinity binding of human immunoglobulin E by transfected cells. Science 244:334, 1989

184. Mitchell EB, Platts-Mills TAE, Pereira RS, Malkovska V, Webster AD: Basophil and eosinophil deficiency in a patient with hypogammaglobulinemia associated with thymoma. In Primary Immunodeficiency Diseases - Birth Defects Original Article Se-

ries, Vol 19, No 3, edited by Wedgwood RJ, Rosen FS, Paul NW, p 331. March of Dimes Birth Defects Foundation, New York, Alan R. Liss, Inc, 1983

185. Moeller J, Hültner L, Schmitt E, Dörmer P: Partial purification of a mast cell growth-enhancing activity and its separation from IL-3 and IL-4. J Immunol 142:3447, 1989

186. Mori Y, Akedo Y, Tanigaki K, Tanaka KM, Okada M, Nakamura N: Effect of sodium butyrate on the production of serotonin, histamine, and glycosaminoglycans by cultured murine mastocytoma cells. Exp Cell Res 127:465, 1980

187. Mosmann TR, Cherwinski H, Bond MW, Giedlin MA, Coffman RL: Two types of murine helper T cell clone. I. Definition according to profiles of lymphokine activities and secreted proteins. J Immunol 136:2348, 1986

188. Murakami I, Ogawa M, Amo H, Ota K: Studies on kinetics of human leukocytes in $vivo$ with ^{3}H-thymidine autoradiography. II. Eosinophils and basophils. Acta Haematol Jpn 32:384, 1969

189. Nabel G, Galli SJ, Dvorak AM, Dvorak HF, Cantor H: Inducer T lymphocytes synthesize a factor that stimulates proliferation of cloned mast cells. Nature (London) 291:332, 1981

190. Naclerio RM, Meier HL, Kagey-Sobotka A, Norman PS, Lichtenstein LM: Mediator release after nasal airway challenge with allergen. Am Rev Respir Dis 128:597, 1983

191. Naclerio RM, Proud D, Togias AG, Adkinson Jr NF, Meyers DA, Kagey-Sobotka A, Plaut M, Norman PS, Lichtenstein LM: Inflammatory mediators in late antigen-induced rhinitis. N Engl J Med 313:65, 1985

192. Nagao K, Yokoro K, Aaronson SA: Continuous lines of basophil/mast cells derived from normal mouse bone marrow. Science 212:333, 1981

193. Nakahata T, Kobayashi T, Ishiguro A, Tsuji K, Naganuma K, Ando O, Yagi Y, Tadokoro K, Akabane T: Extensive proliferation of mature connective tissue type mast cells in $vitro$. Nature (London) 324:65, 1986

194. Nakahata T, Spicer SS, Cantey JR, Ogawa M: Clonal origin of murine mast cell colonies in methylcellulose culture. Blood 60:352, 1981

195. Nakano T, Kanakura Y, Nakahata T, Matsuda H, Kitamura Y: Genetically mast cell-deficient W/W^v mice as a tool for studies of differentiation and function of mast cells. Fed Proc 46:1920, 1987

196. Nakano T, Sonoda T, Hayashi C, Yamatodani A, Kanayama Y, Yamamura T, Asai H, Yonezawa Y, Kitamura Y, Galli SJ: Fate of bone marrow-derived cultured mast cells after intracutaneous intraperitoneal and intravenous transfer into genetically mast cell-deficient W/W^v mice. Evidence that cultured mast cells can give rise to both connective tissue-type and mucosal mast cells. J Exp Med 162:1025, 1985

197. Ogawa M, Nakahata T, Leary AG, Sterk AR, Ishizaka K, Ishizaka T: Suspension culture of human mast cells/basophils from umbilical cord blood mononuclear cells. Proc Natl Acad Sci USA 80:4494, 1983

198. Osgood EE: Culture of human marrow: length of life of the neutrophils, eosinophils and basophils of normal blood as determined by comparative cultures of blood and sternal marrow from healthy persons. J Am Med Assoc 109:933, 1937

199. Otsu K, Nakano T, Kanakura Y, Asai H, Katz HR, Austen KF, Stevens RL, Galli SJ, Kitamura Y: Phenotypic changes of bone marrow-derived mast cells after intraperitoneal transfer into W/W^v mice that are genetically deficient in mast cells. J Exp Med 165:615, 1987

200. Padawer J: The mast cell and immediate hypersensitivity. In Immediate Hypersensitivity, Vol 7, edited by Bach MD, p 301. New York, Marcel Dekker, 1979

201. Parwaresch MR: The Human Blood Basophil, New York, Springer-Verlag, 1976

202. Paul WE: The immune system: an introduction. In Fundamental Immunology, edited by Paul WE, p 3. New York, Raven Press, 1984

203. Paul WE, Ohara J: B-cell stimulatory factor-1/interleukin 4. Ann Rev Immunol 5:429, 1987

204. Pearce FL: Functional differences between mast cells from various locations. In Mast Cell Differentiation and Heterogeneity, edited by Befus AD, Bienenstock J, Denburg JA, p 215. New York, Raven Press, 1986

205. Pearce FL, Ali H, Barrett KE, Befus AD, Bienenstock J, Brostoff

J, Ennis M, Flint KC, Hudspith B, Johnson NM, Leung KBP, Peachell PT: Functional characteristics of mucosal and connective tissue mast cells of man, the rat and other animals. Int Arch Allergy Appl Immunol 77:274, 1985

206. Pharr PN, Ogawa M: A stochastic model for mast cell/basophil differentiation from pluripotent hemopoietic stem cells. In Mast Cell Differentiation and Heterogeneity, edited by Befus AD, Bienenstock J, Denburg JA, p 63. New York, Raven Press, 1986

207. Pharr PN, Suda T, Bergmann KL, Avila LA, Ogawa M: Analysis of pure and mixed mast cell colonies. J Cell Physiol 120:1, 1984

208. Pierce JH, Di Fiore PP, Aaronson SA, Potter M, Pumphrey J, Scott A, Ihle JN: Neoplastic transformation of mast cells by Abelson-MuLV: abrogation of IL-3 dependence by a nonautocrine mechanism. Cell 41:685, 1985

209. Pitton C, Michel L, Salem P, Benhamou M, Mencia-Huerta J-M, Maclouf J, Prost C, Burtin C, Dubertret L, Benveniste J: Biochemical and morphological modifications in dexamethasone-treated mouse bone marrow-derived mast cells. J Immunol 141:2437, 1988

210. Plaut M, Pierce JH, Watson CJ, Hanley-Hyde J, Nordan RP, Paul WE: Mast cell lines produce lymphokines in response to cross-linkage of Fc,RI or to calcium ionophores. Nature (London) 339:64, 1989

211. Pretlow TG, Cassady IM: Separation of mast cells in successive stages of differentiation using programmed gradient sedimentation. Am J Pathol 61:323, 1970

212. Quesenberry PJ: The concept of the hemopoietic stem cell. In Hematology, 3rd Edition, edited by Williams WJ, Beutler E, Erslev AJ, Lichtman MA, p 129. New York, McGraw-Hill, 1983

213. Qureshi R, Jakschik BA: The role of mast cells in thioglycollate-induced inflammation. J Immunol 141:2090, 1988

214. Razin E, Cordon-Cardo C, Good RA: Growth of a pure population of mouse mast cells in $vitro$ with conditioned medium derived from concanavalin A-stimulated splenocytes. Proc Natl Acad Sci USA 28:2559, 1981

215. Razin E, Rifkind AB, Cordon-Cardo C, Good RA: Selective growth of a population of human basophil cells in $vitro$. Proc Natl Acad Sci USA 78:5793, 1981

216. Razin E, Stevens RL, Akiyama F, Schmidt K, Austen KF: Culture from mouse bone marrow of a subclass of mast cells possessing a distinct chondroitin sulfate proteoglycan with glycosaminoglycans rich in N-acetylgalactosamine-4, 6-disulfate. J Biol Chem 257:7229, 1982

217. Reed ND: Function and regulation of mast cells in parasite infections. In Mast Cell and Basophil Differentiation and Function in Health and Disease, edited by Galli SJ, Austen KF, p 205. New York, Raven Press, 1989

218. Reed ND, Dehlawi MS, Wakelin D: Medium conditioned by spleen cells of $Nematospiroides$ $dubius$-infected mice does not support development of cultured mast cells. Int Arch Allergy Appl Immunol 85:113, 1988

219. Rein A, Keller J, Schultz AM, Holmes KL, Medicus R, Ihle JN: Infection of immune mast cells by Harvey sarcoma virus: immortalization without loss of requirement for interleukin-3. Mol Cell Biol 5:2257, 1985

220. Rennick D, Lee FD, Yokota T, Arai K-I, Cantor H, Nabel G: A cloned MCGF cDNA encodes a multilineage hematopoietic growth-factor: multiple activities of interleukin 3. J Immunol 134:910, 1985

221. Reshef A, MacGlashan DW: Immunogold probe for the light-microscopic phenotyping of human mast cells and basophils. J Immunol Methods 99:213, 1987

222. Reynolds DS, Serafin WE, Faller DV, Wall DA, Abbas AK, Dvorak AM, Austen KF, Stevens RL: Immortalization of murine connective tissue-type mast cells at multiple stages of their differentiation by coculture of splenocytes with fibroblasts that produce Kirsten Sarcoma virus. J Biol Chem 263:12783, 1988

223. Riley JF: The riddle of the mast cells - a tribute to Paul Ehrlich. Lancet i:841, 1954

224. Rimmer EF, Turberville C, Horton MA: Cell membrane glycoproteins of human mast cells: a biochemical comparison with basophils. Exp Hematol 14:809, 1986

225. Roberts RA, Spooncer E, Parkinson EK, Lord BI, Allen TD, Dexter TM: Metabolically inactive 3T3 cells can substitute for marrow stromal cells to promote the proliferation and develop-

ment of multipotent haematopoietic stem cells. J Cell Physiol 132:203, 1987

226. Robinson HC, Lindahl U: Effect of cyclohexamide, β-D-xylosides and β-D-galactosides on heparin biosynthesis in mouse mastocytoma. Biochem J 194:575, 1981

227. Röhlich R, Anderson P, Uvnäs B: Electron microscopic observations on compound 48/80-induced degranulation in rat mast cells. Evidence for sequential exocytosis of storage granules. J Cell Biol 51:465, 1971

228. Ruitenberg RJ, Elgersma A: Absence of intestinal mast cell responses in congenitally athymic mice during *Trichinella spiralis* infection. Nature (London) 264:258, 1976

229. Ruitenberg EJ, Gustowska L, Elgersma A, Ruitenberg HM: Effects of fixation on the light microscopical visualization of mast cells in the mucosa and connective tissue of the human duodenum. Int Arch Allergy Appl Immunol 67:233, 1982

230. Russell ES: Hereditary anemias of the mouse: a review for geneticists. Adv Genet 20:357, 1979

231. Saito H, Hatake K, Dvorak AM, Leiferman KM, Donnenberg AD, Arai N, Ishizaka K, Ishizaka T: Selective differentiation and proliferation of hematopoietic cells induced by recombinant human interleukins. Proc Natl Acad Sci USA 85:2288, 1988

232. Schechter NM, Franki JE, Geesin JC, Lazarus GS: Human skin chymotryptic proteinase. I. Isolation and relation to cathepsin G and rat mast cell protease. J Biol Chem 258:2973, 1983

233. Schiller S, Dorfman A: The isolation of heparin from mast cells of the normal rat. Biochim Biophys Acta 31:276, 1959

234. Schleimer RP, MacGlashan Jr DW, Gillespie E, Lichtenstein LM: Inhibition of basophil histamine release by antiinflammatory steroids. II. Studies on the mechanism of action. J Immunol 129:1632, 1982

235. Schleimer RP, Schulman ES, MacGlashan Jr DW, Peters SP, Hayes EC, Adams 3rd GK, Lichtenstein LM, Adkinson Jr NF: Effects of dexamethasone on mediator release from human lung fragments and purified human lung mast cells. J Clin Invest 71:1830, 1983

236. Schrader JW: The *in vitro* production and cloning of the P cell, a bone marrow-derived null cell that expresses H-2 and Ia-antigens, has mast cell-like granules, and is regulated by a factor released by activated T cells. J Immunol 126:452, 1981

237. Schulman ES, Kagey-Sobotka A, MacGlashan DW Jr, Franklin-Adkinson N Jr, Peters SP, Schleimer RP, Lichtenstein LM: Heterogeneity of human mast cells. J Immunol 131:1936, 1983

238. Schwartz LB: Heterogeneity of mast cells in humans. In Mast Cell and Basophil Differentiation and Function in Health and Disease, edited by Galli SJ, Austen KF, p 93. New York, Raven Press, 1989

239. Schwartz LB, Austen KF: Structure and function of the chemical mediators of mast cells. Prog Allergy 34:271, 1984

240. Seldin DC, Caulfield CP, Hein A, Osathanondh R, Nabel G, Schlossman SF, Stevens RL, Austen KF: Biochemical and phenotypic characterization of human basophilic cells derived from dispersed fetal liver with murine T cell factors. J Immunol 136:2222, 1986

241. Selye H: The Mast Cells, Washington, D.C., Butterworths, 1965

242. Serafin WE, Katz HR, Austen KF, Stevens RL: Complexes of heparin proteoglycans, chondroitin sulfate E proteoglycans, and (^{3}H)-diisopropyl fluorophosphate-binding proteins are exocytosed from activated mouse bone marrow-derived mast cells. J Biol Chem 261:15017, 1986

243. Shevach EM: Macrophages and other accessory cells. In Fundamental Immunology, edited by Paul WE, p. 71. New York, Raven Press, 1984

244. Shimizu A, Tepler I, Benfey PN, Berenstein EH, Siraganian RP, Leder P: Human and rat mast cell high-affinity immunoglobulin E receptors: characterization of putative α-chain gene products. Proc Natl Acad Sci USA 85:1907, 1988

245. Shohet SB, Blum SF: Coincident basophilic chronic myelogenous leukemia and pulmonary tuberculosis. Cancer 22:173, 1968

246. Slifman NR, Adolphson CR, Gleich GJ: Eosinophils: biochemical and cellular aspects. In Allergy. Principles and Practice, edited by Middleton Jr E, Reed CE, Ellis EF, Adkinson Jr NF, Yunginger JW, p 179. St. Louis, The CV Mosby Company, 1988

247. Sonoda S, Sonoda T, Nakano T, Kanayama Y, Kanakura Y, Asai H, Yonezawa T, Kitamura Y: Development of mucosal mast cells after injection of a single connective tissue-type mast cell in the stomach mucosa of genetically mast cell-deficient W/W^v mice. J Immunol 137:1319, 1986

248. Sredni B, Friedman MM, Bland CE, Metcalfe DD: Ultrastructural, biochemical and functional characteristics of histamine-containing cells cloned from mouse bone marrow: tentative identification as mucosal mast cells. J Immunol 131:915, 1983

249. Stead RH, Perdue MH, Blennerhassett MG, Kakuta Y, Sestini P, Bienenstock J: The innervation of mast cells. In The Neuroendocrine-Immune Network, edited by Freier S. Boca Raton, Florida, CRC Press (in press)

250. Stedman's Medical Dictionary: Ed 23, Baltimore, Williams and Wilkins Company, 1976

251. Stevens RL, Austen KF: Effect of p-nitrophenyl-β-D-xyloside on proteoglycan and glycosaminoglycan biosynthesis in rat serosal mast cells. J Biol Chem 257:253, 1982

252. Stevens RL, Katz JR, Seldin DS, Austen KF: Biochemical characteristics distinguish subclasses of mammalian mast cells. In Mast Cell Differentiation and Heterogeneity, edited by Befus AD, Bienenstock J, Denburg JA, p 183. New York, Raven Press, 1986

253. Stevens RL, Rothenberg ME, Levi-Schaffer F, Austen KF: Ontogeny of *in vitro*-differentiated mouse mast cells. Fed Proc 46:1915, 1987

254. Stevens RL, Serafin WE, Reynolds DS, Dayton ET, Gravallese PM, Austen KF: Development and characterization of in vitro-differentiated transformed and non-transformed mouse connective tissue-like mast cells, and the regulation of fibroblasts by these mast cells. In Mast Cell and Basophil Differentiation and Function in Health and Disease, edited by Galli SJ, Austen KF, p 1. New York, Raven Press, 1989

255. Strobel S, Miller HRP, Ferguson A: Human intestinal mucosal mast cells: evaluation of fixation and staining techniques. J Clin Pathol 34:851, 1981

256. Subba Rao PV, Friedman MM, Atkins FM, Metcalfe DD: Phagocytosis of mast cell granules by cultured fibroblasts. J Immunol 130:341, 1983

257. Suda T, Suda J, Spicer SS, Ogawa M: Proliferation and differentiation in culture of mast cell progenitors derived from mast-cell deficient mice of genotype W/W^v. J Cell Physiol 122:187, 1985

258. Tadokoro K, Stadler BM, de Weck AL: Factor-dependent *in vitro* growth of human normal bone-marrow-derived basophil-like cells. J Exp Med 158:857, 1983

259. Tadokoro K, Stadler GM, de Weck AL: Further biochemical characterization of human basophil-like cell-promoting activity and its distinction from human interleukin-3-like activity. Int Arch Allergy Appl Immunol 86:162, 1988

260. Tas J, Bernsden RG: Does heparin occur in mucosal mast cells of the rat small intestine? J Histochem Cytochem 25:1058, 1977

261. Tertian G, Yung YP, Guy-Grand D, Moore MAS: Long term *in vitro* culture of murine mast cells. I. Description of a growth-factor dependent culture technique. J Immunol 127:788, 1981

262. Tracey R, Smith H: An inherited anomaly of human eosinophils and basophils. Blood Cells 4:291, 1978

263. Urbina C, Ortiz C, Hurtado I: A new look at basophils in mice. Int Arch Allergy Appl Immunol 66:158, 1981

264. Vanderhoek JY, Tare NS, Bailey JM, Goldstein AL, Pluznik DH: New role for 15-hydroxyeicosatetraenoic acid. Activator of leukotriene biosynthesis in PT-18 mast/basophil cells. J Biol Chem 257:12191, 1982

265. Weitzman G, Galli SJ, Dvorak AM, Hammel I: Cloned mouse mast cells and normal mouse peritoneal mast cells. Determination of serotonin content, and ability to synthesize serotonin *in vitro*. Int Arch Allergy Appl Immunol 77:189, 1985

266. Wershil BK, Galli SJ: ^{125}I-fibrin deposition in IgE-dependent gastric reactions in the mouse: the role of mast cells (MCs) (abstr). FASEB J 3:A789, 1989

267. Wershil BK, Mekori YA, Galli SJ: The contribution of mast cells to immunological responses with IgE- and/or T cell-mediated components. In Mast Cell and Basophil Differentiation and Function in Health and Disease, edited by Galli SJ, Austen KF, p 229. New York, Raven Press, 1989

268. Wershil BK, Mekori YA, Murakami T, Galli SJ: ^{125}I-Fibrin deposition in IgE-dependent immediate hypersensitivity reactions in mouse skin. Demonstration of the role of mast cells using genetically mast cell-deficient mice locally reconstituted with cultured

mast cells. J Immunol 139:2605, 1987

269. Wershil BK, Murakami T, Galli SJ: Mast cell-dependent amplification of an immunologically nonspecific inflammatory response. Mast cells are required for the full expression of cutaneous acute inflammation induced by phorbol 12-myristate 13-acetate. J Immunol 140:2356, 1988

270. Wodnar-Filipowicz A, Heusser CH, Moroni C: Production of the haemopoietic growth factors GM-CSF and interleukin-3 by mast cells in response to IgE receptor-mediated activation. Nature (London) 339;150, 1989

271. Woodbury RG, Neurath H: Structure, specificity, and localization of the serine proteases of connective tissue. FEBS Lett 114:189, 1980

272. Woodbury RG, Everitt M, Katanuma N, Lagunoff D, Neurath H: A major serine protease in skeletal muscle. Evidence for its mast cell origin. Proc Natl Acad Sci USA 75:5311, 1978

273. Woodbury RG, Gruzenski GM, Lagunoff D: Immunofluorescent localization of a serine protease in rat small intestine. Proc Natl Acad Sci USA 75:2785, 1978

274. Woodbury RG, Le Trong H, Cole K, Neurath H, Miller HRP: Rat mast cell proteases. In Mast Cell and Basophil Differentiation and Function in Health and Disease, edited by Galli SJ, Austen KF, p 71. New York, Raven Press, 1989

275. Yano H, Wershil BK, Arizono N, Galli SJ: Substance P-induced augmentation of cutaneous vascular permeability and granulocyte infiltration in mice is mast cell dependent. J Clin Invest 84:1276, 1989

276. Yokota T, Lee F, Rennick D, Hall C, Arai N, Mosmann T, Nabel G, Cantor H, Arai K: Isolation and characterization of a mouse cDNA clone that expresses mast-cell growth-factor activity in monkey cells. Proc Natl Acad Sci USA 81:1070, 1984

277. Young J D-E, Liu CC, Butler G, Cohn ZA, Galli SJ: Identification, purification and characterization of a mast cell-associated cytolytic factor related to tumor necrosis factor. Proc Natl Acad Sci USA 84:9175, 1987

278. Yuen E, Brown RD, van der Lubbe L, Rickard KA, Kronenberg H: Identification and characterization of human hemopoietic mast cell colonies. Exp Hematol 16:896, 1988

279. Yung Y-P, Moore MAS: Long-term *in vitro* culture of murine mast cells. III. Discrimination of mast cell growth-factor and granulocyte CSF. J Immunol 129:1256, 1982

280. Yung Y-P, Moore MAS: Mast cell growth-factor. Lymphokine Res 2:127, 1983

281. Yurt RW, Austen KF: Preparative purification of rat mast cell chymase. Characterization and interaction with granule components. J Exp Med 146:1405; 1977

282. Yurt RW, Leid RW, Austen KF, Silbert JE: Native heparin from rat peritoneal mast cells. J Biol Chem 252:518, 1977

283. Zucker-Franklin D: Electron microscopic study of human basophils. Blood 29:878, 1967

283. Zucker-Franklin D, Grusky G, Hirayama N, Schnipper E: The presence of mast cell precursors in rat peripheral blood. Blood 58:544, 1981

Section II

INFLAMMATION AND IMMUNITY

From: *Pathology Reviews • 1990* Edited by: E. Rubin and I. Damjanov Copyright © 1990 The Humana Press Inc., Clifton, NJ

Biology of Disease

HLA Class II Polymorphism: Implications for Genetic Susceptibility to Autoimmune Disease

PETER K. GREGERSEN

Division of Molecular Medicine, Department of Medicine, North Shore University Hospital, Cornell University Medical College, Manhasset, New York

Human leukocyte antigen (HLA) class II molecules, encoded within the human major histocompatibility complex, play a central role in the immune response by presenting peptide antigens to helper (T4+) lymphocytes. One striking feature is their extraordinary variability between individuals in the population. These molecules, which are expressed on the surface of antigen presenting cells such as monocytes, B cells, and dendritic cells, are the products of the immune response genes originally discovered in the mouse and guinea pig (52). It is now apparent that allelic polymorphisms of class II genes are directly involved in regulating patterns of immune responsiveness in mammalian organisms (6, 74). This realization has provoked a major effort to define the nature and extent of class II polymorphism in the human population. Now almost completed, this endeavor has provided considerable insight into the complexity of the class II gene family and has stimulated new ap-

proaches to understanding the relationship between HLA polymorphism and autoimmune disease.

After reviewing the basic structural features of class II molecules and the genes encoding them, this article will focus on the patterns of polymorphism observed in the two most thoroughly studied isotypic groups of class II alleles, namely those encoded within the DR and DQ subregions of the HLA class II gene cluster. For each subregion, a specific autoimmune disease will be discussed to illustrate how detailed knowledge of sequence polymorphism has enhanced our understanding of HLA and disease associations. The accumulating data have focused attention on the DR subregion in the case of rheumatoid arthritis (RA), whereas DQ polymorphisms appear to be primarily involved in conferring risk for insulin dependent diabetes mellitus (IDDM). For these and other HLA associated autoimmune diseases, it appears increasingly likely that specific polymorphisms of the class II molecules are directly involved in disease pathogenesis. Therefore, their identification is essential for an overall understanding of the cause of these illnesses.

Address reprint requests to: Peter Gregersen, Division of Molecular Medicine, North Shore University Hospital, Cornell University Medical College, Manhasset, New York 11030.

STRUCTURES AND FUNCTION OF HLA MOLECULES

STRUCTURAL FEATURES OF HLA MOLECULES

Human leukocyte antigens are membrane glycoproteins that can be divided into two major types designated class I and class II (45). Both are heterodimers with structural features that are schematically diagrammed in Figure 1. HLA class I molecules consist of a transmembrane 45-kDa α chain associated noncovalently with $\beta2$ microglobulin. Class I molecules function in antigen presentation to T8+ lymphocytes and are primarily involved in cell-mediated cytotoxicity. HLA class II molecules are composed of a pair of noncovalently associated α and β chains (43). The α chain is ~32 kDa and the β chain 28 kDa. This difference in molecular weight is in large part due to the number of N-linked sugars present on each chain: two on the α chain and only one on the β chain. Both chains of the class II heterodimer are inserted into the cell membrane by means of a hydrophobic transmembrane segment and contain a short intracytoplasmic segment ranging from 8 to 15 residues.

HLA molecules are members of the immunoglobulin (Ig) gene family (94) and, as such, share a domain structure similar to immunoglobulin. Both α and β chains of HLA class II molecules contain two external domains that are ~90–95 amino acids long. The membrane proximal, or second, domains (designated $\alpha2$ and $\beta2$ in Fig. 1) are homologous to Ig constant region domains and include an internal disulfide loop similar to that found in Ig. Like Ig constant regions, the second domains of class II chains show little variability between alleles. In contrast the N-terminal, or first, domain is the major site of variation between the different class II alleles. Only the β chains contain an internal disulfide loop in the first domain. It should be apparent from Figure 1 that class I and class II molecules are highly similar in structure, the main difference between them being that the membrane distal domains are encoded by one protein (the α chain) in the case of class I but by separate α and β chains in the case of class II. As discussed below, this overall homology between class I and class II molecules allows a prediction of class II conformation to be derived from the recent x-ray crystallographic analysis of the structure of an HLA class I molecule.

CLASS II MOLECULES BIND ANTIGENIC PEPTIDE FRAGMENTS: BJORKMAN STRUCTURE

A major advance in understanding HLA molecules has come from the x-ray crystallographic analysis of the class I molecule HLA-A2 by Bjorkman and colleagues (9). This has clearly shown that the $\alpha1$ and $\alpha2$ domains form a cleft that may bind peptide fragments. Indeed, evidence of such bound fragments was seen in the cleft of the crystallized HLA-A2 molecule (9). The three-dimensional structure of class II molecules has not yet been directly determined. However, on the basis of predicted homologies with class I as well as alignment of disulfide loops, a tentative model for class II structure has been proposed (16).

Figure 2 shows the probable general features of the class II peptide binding cleft, as adapted from the Bjorkman class I structure. The first (N-terminal) domains of the α and β chains of class II are treated as homologous to the $\alpha1$ and $\alpha2$ domains of class I, respectively. Figure 2 shows the binding cleft as viewed from above. The floor of the cleft is composed of four β strands, two from each class II chain. The sides of the cleft are formed by two largely uninterrupted stretches of α helix. The cleft is therefore in the shape of a groove measuring ~10 Å across and 25 Å long (9). This would accommodate a linear peptide of approximately eight amino acids. However, if the bound peptide were to assume an α helical conformation, peptides as long as 20 residues could be accommodated within the binding cleft. Direct binding of antigenic peptides in this size range has been demonstrated for class II molecules (4, 17, 32).

One striking finding to emerge from the class I structural analysis was that polymorphic residues tended to reside either on the β sheets on the floor of the cleft or along the α helices (10). These polymorphisms can often be related to effects on immune responsiveness (10). As will be discussed, polymorphisms among class II β chains also appear to lie in analogous regions of the molecule and likewise may influence immune recognition events.

T CELLS RECOGNIZE "PROCESSED" FRAGMENTS OF FOREIGN ANTIGEN BOUND TO HLA MOLECULES

The direct demonstration of an antigen binding cleft on HLA molecules has lent strong support to models of T cell recognition in which a single T cell receptor binding site confers specificity for both the antigen and the HLA molecule to which it is bound (27). This is consistent with longstanding observations that T cells simultaneously recognize antigen and self major histocompatibility complex (MHC) molecules; under normal circumstances antigen T cells fail to respond to antigen when it is presented by non-self MHC molecules (75, 97). Furthermore, the size of the antigen binding cleft on HLA molecules is consistent with the requirement for "processing" of antigens into smaller peptide fragments before they can be presented to T cells (91); many

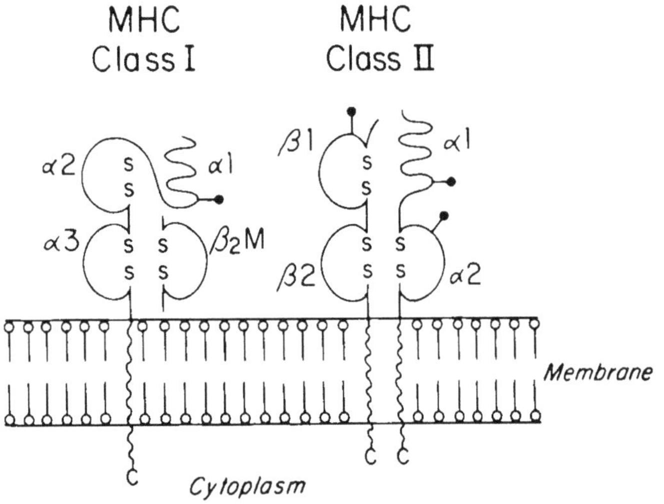

FIG. 1. Comparison of structural features of HLA class I and class II molecules.

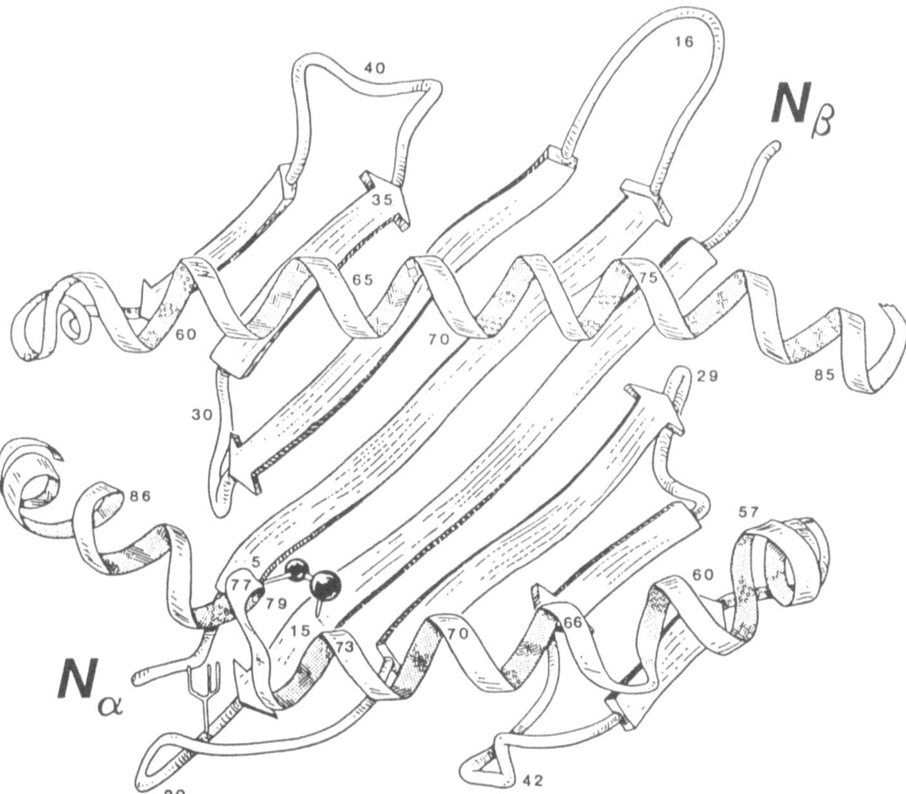

FIG. 2. General structural model of the antigen binding cleft on an HLA class II molecule [adapted from Bjorkman *et al.* (9)]. Numbers indicate amino acid positions on α and β chains. N, N terminus.

antigens would be far too large to fit into the HLA binding cleft in their native configuration. Such antigen processing events are conducted by antigen presenting cells such as monocytes and macrophages (91). These requirements for T cell recognition (outlined schematically in Fig. 3) contrast to the ability of the immunoglobulin receptor on B cells to recognize soluble antigens in their native (unprocessed) configuration in the absence of MHC molecules. The underlying reason for this strategic difference in T cell *versus* B cell recognition remains a mystery.

In general, class II molecules can bind many different peptides and therefore can present various antigens to T cells. However, the way in which a given antigenic peptide is bound may vary between different class II alleles. Some peptide antigens may not bind at all to a given class II allele, and this may explain a lack of an immune response to that peptide in some instances (32). In the final analysis, T cells probably recognize specific conformational determinants formed by a particular antigen/MHC combination (27, 91). It is apparent that the influence of specific HLA polymorphisms on this antigen/MHC conformation may be quite complex. Some HLA polymorphisms may predominantly affect T cell recognition by interacting directly with the T cell receptor molecule; others by affecting antigen binding (66). It seems likely that some amino acid substitutions in the MHC molecule may also have more complicated effects on the overall tertiary structure of the antigen/MHC combination. The detailed geometry of these interactions is not known. The elucidation of the basic HLA structure as an antigen binding cleft is a major first step toward this goal.

GENETIC ORGANIZATION OF MHC

The human MHC is located on the short arm of chromosome 6 and occupies ~3,000,000 base pairs of DNA (89). As shown in Figure 4, it encodes the two major classes of membrane HLA molecules, as well as many other genes including complement components C2 and C4, factor B, 21 hydroxylase genes, and the genes for tumor necrosis factor α and β (89). Located centromerically is the HLA-D, or class II region. As indicated in Figure 4, over the last 5 years the application of recombinant DNA techniques to the study of this region has revealed the presence of many class II genes distributed over ~1,000,000 base pairs of the MHC (34, 90).

HLA CLASS II GENES ARE LOCATED IN THREE MAJOR SUBREGIONS

The class II region is divided into three major subregions designated DR, DQ, and DP (90). Each subregion contains at least one pair of functional α and β chain genes. In most cases, the DR subregion encodes two functional β chains, both of which may pair with the α chain encoded by the single DRα gene. Many nonfunctional pseudogenes are also present in the DR and DP subregions. The DQ subregion contains a set of genes designated DXα and DXβ (59) that are not pseudogenes (40) but have not been found to be expressed. In addition, the DZα (90) and DOβ (76, 88) genes are located between the DQ and DP subregions; however, they do not appear to form a functional heterodimeric pair. The class II region is unusual in that both chains of the various heterodimeric class II molecules are encoded in the same

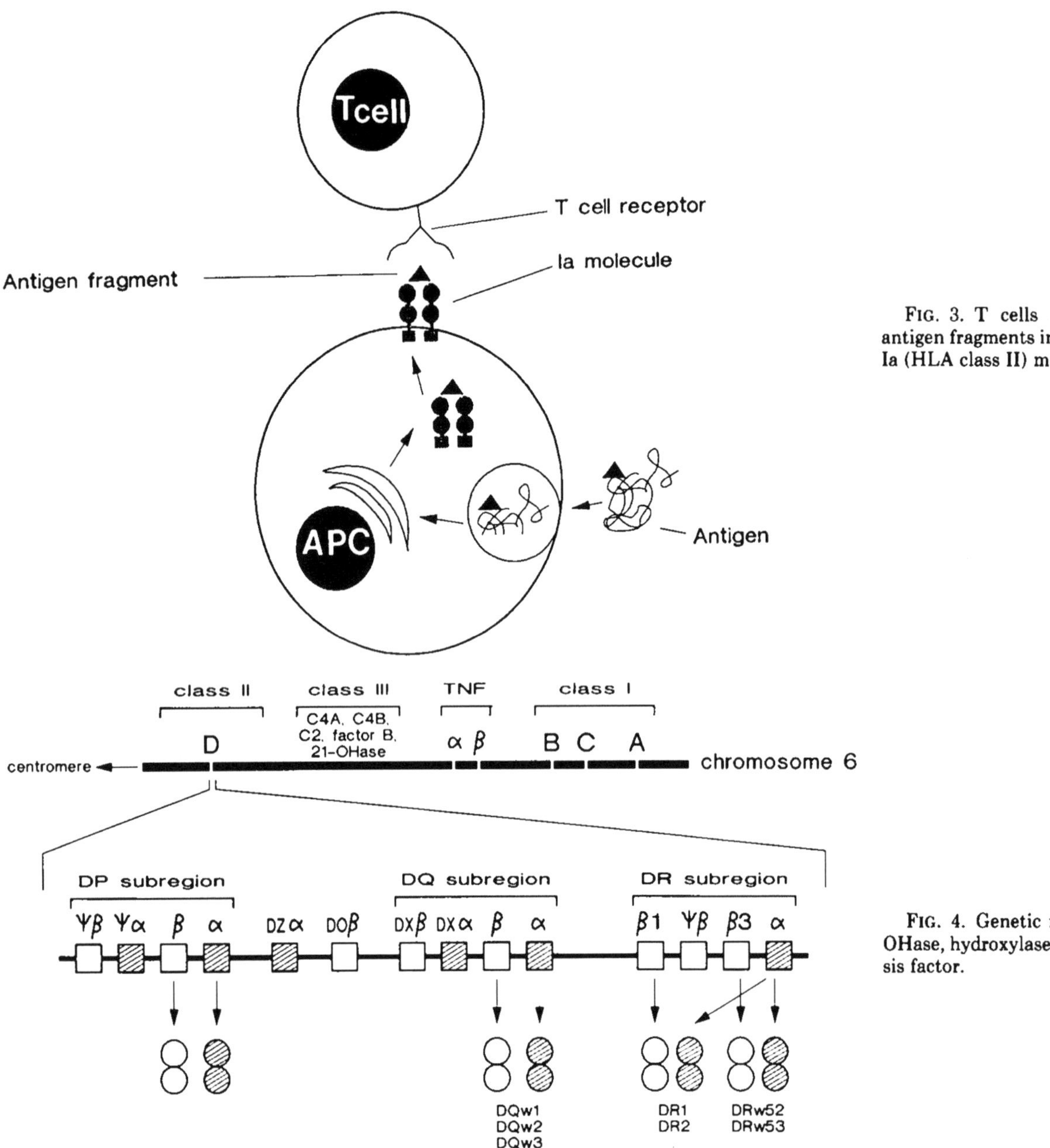

FIG. 3. T cells recognize processed antigen fragments in association with an Ia (HLA class II) molecule.

FIG. 4. Genetic map of HLA region. OHase, hydroxylase; TNF, tumor necrosis factor.

genetic region. This contrasts to other heterodimeric molecules such as immunoglobulin, T cell receptor, hemoglobin, or even HLA class I, where each chain is encoded on different chromosomes. The functional significance, if any, of the localization of both α and β chain genes to the same genetic region is unknown.

The subregion localization of a given class II α or β chain implies both structural and functional correlations. For example, β chain genes within the DR subregion are more closely related to each other in sequence than they are to β chain genes within the DQ subregion. A comparison of nucleotide sequences of DRβ1 and DRβ3 coding regions shows them to be over 90% similar (21), whereas DRβ1 and DQβ chains have ~70% nucleotide sequence similarity (33). Therefore, assignment of a given β (or α) chain allele to a subregion can be made on the basis of its nucleotide sequence alone. These features correlate with the generally restricted ability of β chains to form α/β heterodimers only with α chains encoded within the same subregion. Thus, DRβ chains form heterodimers with DRα chains, and DQβ chains form heterodimers only with DQα chains. Exceptions have been reported. For example, interisotypic heterodimers of DRα and DQβ have been detected in human B cell lines (49). However, the physiological relevance of this phenomenon *in vivo* has not yet been demonstrated.

RELATIONSHIP OF CLASS II GENES TO SEROLOGICALLY DEFINED HLA CLASS II ALLELES: CONCEPT OF HAPLOTYPE

Classical serologic analysis of class II polymorphism has defined three major allelic series: DR1–14, DRw52 and DRw53, and DQw1-DQw4 (11). As indicated in

Figure 4, the DR series is encoded by the DRβ1 locus and the DRw52 and DRw53 alleles by the DRβ3 locus. The DRα chain is identical (with minor exceptions) in all individuals and thus does not contribute to the allelic variability of DR molecules (90). The DQ series of alleles is encoded by the DQ α and β chain genes. Although both DQα and DQβ chains vary in sequence, it appears that the β chain is primarily responsible for the serologic typing, at least in the case of DQw2, 3, and 4.

Serological typing methods have established the existence of characteristic patterns of linkage disequilibrium in the population. Thus, particular alleles are commonly found together on the same chromosome, forming what is referred to as a haplotype. A summary of the patterns of linkage disequilibrium found commonly in caucasian populations is shown in Figure 5. As indicated in Figure 5, DR4, -7, and -9 haplotypes are always associated with the DRw53 specificity (encoded by the DRβ3 locus). Likewise, DR3, -5, and -6 haplotypes are always associated with the DRw52 specificity. These patterns of linkage disequilibrium reflect the evolutionary relationships among these various haplotypes. Thus, an analysis of DRβ chain sequences (29) as well as restriction fragment length polymorphisms (13) have established that DRw52 and DRw53 are serologic markers of distinct haplotype family groups. It appears likely that DR1, -2, and -10 also form a third haplotype family group, although the molecular organization of these haplotypes has not been as well characterized (13, 28).

As shown in Figure 5, serologically defined alleles encoded within the DR subregion are also in linkage disequilibrium with DQ subregion alleles. For example, in the caucasian population, DR4 is almost always associated with DQw3; likewise DR3 is almost always associated with DQw2. These patterns of linkage disequilibrium between DR and DQ are a stable characteristic of class II haplotypes within the caucasian population. However, these DR/DQ associations may differ in noncaucasian populations such as American blacks (37) or Asians (62).

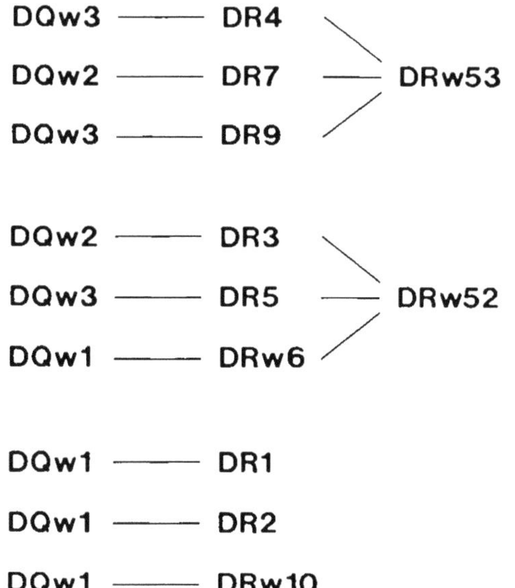

FIG. 5. Patterns of linkage disequilibrium found commonly on HLA class II haplotypes in caucasian populations.

The gene organization within each subregion that is shown in Figure 4 is generalized. In fact, there is considerable variation between different haplotypes, particularly in the DR subregion. For example, DR1 and DRw10 haplotypes appear to contain just two DRβ genes (13), only one of which is expressed. In contrast, most other haplotypes contain at least three DRβ genes and generally two of these are expressed. In addition, fragments of additional DRβ genes may be scattered in the DR subregion (79). These haplotype differences in DR subregion organization probably arose through a complex series of genetic events including gene duplication, deletions, and insertions. Extrapolating from the murine MHC, many of these events may have preceded speciation of *Homo sapiens* and thus are hard to reconstruct (51). Only two haplotypes, DR3 (64) and DR4 (3), have been studied in detail with respect to the number and organization of their DRβ genes. In some cases, this variability in gene organization between different haplotypes has led to confusion about allelic relationships. For example, it is debated whether the DRw52 and DRw53 serologic specificities reflect allelic variants at a single locus (the DRβ3 locus shown in Fig. 2) or whether they are encoded by different genes (26). A detailed map of the DR subregion has not been worked out for most haplotypes. Although serologic typing remains the standard method for detecting HLA polymorphism, it is now clear that serologic methods do not distinguish many common allelic variants. Therefore, the standard DR and DQ allelic series greatly underestimate the number of alleles present in the population. This additional complexity has been defined by the DNA sequence analysis of many DR and DQ alleles over the last several years.

POLYMORPHISM WITHIN DR SUBREGION

SEQUENCE VARIATION OF DRβ CHAINS: THREE REGIONS OF DIVERSITY

Allelic polymorphism in the DR subregion is found only in the β chain genes. The DRα chains are invariant in structure except for minor variations in the cytoplasmic portion of the molecule (90). The sequence analysis of DRβ chains encoded by most common haplotypes found in caucasian populations has now been completed (5, 18, 25, 28, 30, 33, 42, 59, 79, 84, 96). This has shown that most of the allelic variability is localized to the first or N-terminal domain of the DRβ chain. Furthermore, this polymorphism tends to be restricted to three major diversity regions. Figure 6 is a variability plot calculated from the reported DRβ chain sequences. This shows the first diversity region tightly clustered around residues 9–13, the second diversity region extending from residues 25–38, and a broader third diversity region extending from residues 57–86 but centered around position 70. Note that the most polymorphic residues in the first and second diversity regions tend to have a periodicity of every other residue. This correlates with the β sheet conformation in these regions predicted from the Bjorkman class I structure (9, 16) (Fig. 2). In contrast, the third diversity region tends to have a periodicity of approximately every third residue for the most polymorphic positions. This is consistent with the α

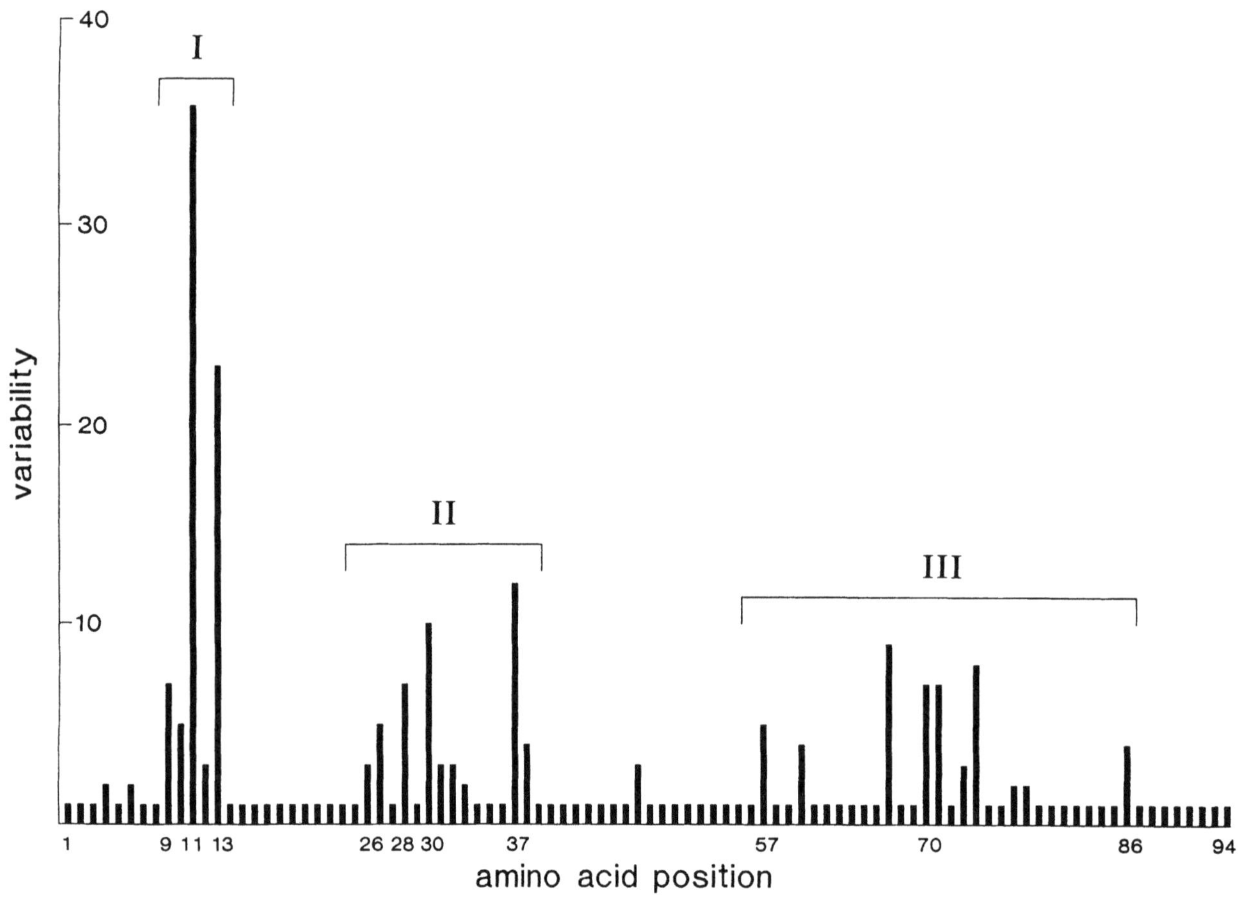

FIG. 6. Plot of variability at each amino acid position of first (variable) domain of DRβ chains. *Brackets*, three principal regions of diversity. Variability values are calculated by the following formula:

no. of different amino acids found at position/(no. of times most frequent amino acid occurs/total no. of different alleles)

helical conformation (~3.6 residues/turn for an idealized α helical peptide) predicted for the region between positions 57 and 86.

Therefore, as predicted from the Bjorkman class I structure, the third diversity region of DRβ is distinct in that its polymorphic residues appear to be located on the edge of the peptide binding cleft. These residues may face toward the cleft or upward away from the cleft, depending on their position on the α helix (10, 16). In contrast, polymorphisms in the first and second diversity regions probably lie at the base of the cleft, pointing up into the cleft from the β sheets (10, 16).

Sequence Variation of DRβ Chains: Sharing of Third Diversity Region Sequences by Multiple Alleles—Gene Conversion

One characteristic feature of DRβ polymorphisms is the patchwork pattern of variation between alleles; *i.e.*, extended segments of sequence are shared between different DRβ alleles. A representative collection of DRβ alleles is shown in Figure 7 to illustrate these sequence relationships. Some sequence sharing probably reflects the common evolutionary origin of some alleles. For example, DR3, -5, and -6 β chains share an identical first diversity region sequence, EYSTS. As mentioned above, DR3, -5, and -6 haplotypes belong to a closely related family of haplotypes that carry the serologic specificity DRw52 and have probably diverged from a common

ancestral haplotype. DR8 haplotypes also belong to this DRw52 family of haplotypes.

However, the most dramatic examples of these patchwork patterns of variation are found in the third diversity region. Here, identical sequences are shared between DRβ alleles from different haplotype family groups. For example, the DR1, DR4 Dw14, and the DR6c (AMALA) alleles all have identical third diversity region sequences. Likewise, DR6a, DR5(JVM), and the DR4, Dw10 chains have extended regions of sequence identity in the third diversity region. Other examples may be found by simple inspection of the sequences in Figure 7.

It has been proposed that this pattern of sequence sharing among different alleles is the result of gene conversion events that occurred during the evolution of class II haplotypes (25, 96). Gene conversion involves the unidirectional transfer of a segment of DNA from one gene (a donor gene) to another homologous recipient gene and has been described in many different gene families (7, 35). The net result of gene conversion is to produce multiple changes in the recipient gene in a single mutational event. This must occur during gametogenesis for the changes to be transmitted into the population. A schematic representation of a hypothetical gene conversion event is outlined in Figure 8. As shown Figure 8, the modern DR6a and DR6c alleles differ by 10 nucleotides. By invoking a gene conversion mechanism with a DR1 allele acting as the "donor" gene, it is apparent that the

```
                  10                  20                  30                  40                  50
DR1           G D T R P R F L W Q   L K F E C H F F N G   T E R V R L L E R C   I Y N Q E E S V R F   D S D V G E Y R A V
DR2 Dw2       - - - - - - - - Q -   D - Y - - - - - - -   - - - - - F - H - D   - - - - - - D L - -   - - - - - - - - - -
DR3           - - - - - - - E Y   S T S - - - - - - -   - - - - - Y - D - Y   F H - - - - N - - -   - - - - - - F - - -
DR4 Dw4       - - - - - - - E -   V - H - - - - - - -   - - - - - F - D - Y   F - H - - - Y - - -   - - - - - - - - - -
DR4 Dw10      - - - - - - - E -   V - H - - - - - - -   - - - - - F - D - Y   F - H - - - Y - - -   - - - - - - - - - -
DR4 Dw14      - - - - - - - E -   V - H - - - - - - -   - - - - - F - D - Y   F - H - - - Y - - -   - - - - - - - - - -
DR5 Dw5       - - - - - - - E Y   S T S - - - - - - -   - - - - - F - D - Y   F - - - - - Y - - -   - - - - - - F - - -
DR5 JVM       - - - - - - - E Y   S T S - - - - - - -   - - - - - F - D - Y - F - - - - - Y - - -   - - - - - - F - - -
DRw6a         - - - - - - - E Y   S T S - - - - - - -   - - - - - F - D - Y   F H - - - - N - - -   - - - - - - F - - -
DRw6b         - - - - - - - E Y   S T S - - - - - - -   - - - - - F - D - Y   F H - - - - F - - -   - - - - - - - - - -
DRw6c(AMALA)  - - - - - - - E Y   S T S - - - - - - -   - - - - - F - - - Y   F H - - - - N - - -   - - - - - - - - - -
DR7           - - - Q - - - - -   G - Y K - - - - - -   - - - - Q F - - - L   F - - - - - F - - -   - - - - - - - - - -
DRw8          - - - - - - - E Y   S T G - - Y - - - -   - - - - - F - D - Y   F - - - - - Y - - -   - - - - - - - - - -
DRw9          - - - Q - - - K -   D - - - - - - - - -   - - - - - Y - H - G   - - - - - - N - - -   - - - - - - - - - -
DRw10         - - - - - - - E E   V - - - - - - - - -   - - - - - - - - - R   V H - - - - Y A - Y   - - - - - - - - - -
DRw52a        - - - - - - - E L   R - S - - - - - - -   - - - - - Y - D - Y   F H - - - - F L - -   - - - - - - - - - -
DRw52b        - - - - - - - E L   - - S - - - - - - -   - - - - - F - - - H   F H - - - - Y A - -   - - - - - - - - - -
DRw53         - - - Q - - - E -   A - C - - - - L - -   - - - - W N - I - Y   - - - - - - Y A - Y   N - - L - - - Q - -


                  60                  70                  80                  90
DR1           T E L G R P D A E Y   W N S Q K D L L E Q   R R A A V D T Y C R   H N Y G V G E S F T   V Q R R
DR2 Dw2       - - - - - - - - - -   - - - - - - F - - D   - - - - - - - - - -   - - - - - - - - - -   - - - -
DR3           - - - - - - - - - -   - - - - - - - - - -   K - G R - - N - - -   - - - - - V - - - -   - - - -
DR4 Dw4       - - - - - - - - - -   - - - - - - - - - -   K - - - - - - - - -   - - - - - - - - - -   - - - -
DR4 Dw10      - - - - - - - - - -   - - - - - - I - - D   E - - - - - - - - -   - - - - - V - - - -   - - - -
DR4 Dw14      - - - - - - - - - -   - - - - - - - - - -   - - - - - - - - - -   - - - - - V - - - -   - - - -
DR5 Dw5       - - - - - - - E - -   - - - - - - F - - D   - - - - - - - - - -   - - - - - - - - - -   - - - -
DR5 JVM       - - - - - - - E - -   - - - - - - I - - D   E - - - - - - - - -   - - - - - V - - - -   - - - -
DRw6a         - - - - - - - E - -   - - - - - - I - - D   E - - - - - - - - -   - - - - - V - - - -   - - - -
DRw6b         - - - - - - A - - H   - - - - - - - - - R   - - - E - - - - - -   - - - - - V - - - -   - - - -
DRw6c(AMALA)  - - - - - - - - - -   - - - - - - - - - -   - - - - - - - - - -   - - - - - - - - - -   - - - -
DR7           - - - - - - V - - S   - - - - - - I - - D   - - G Q - - - V - -   - - - - - - - - - -   - - - -
DRw8          - - - - - - S - - -   - - - - - - F - - D   - - - L - - - - - -   - - - - - - - - - -
DRw9          - - - - - - V - - S   - - - - - - F - - R   - - - E - - - V - -   - - - - - - - - - -   - - - -
DRw10         - - - - - - - - - -   - - - - - - - - - R   - - - - - - - - - -   - - - - - - - - - -   - - - -
DRw52a        - - - - - - V - - S   - - - - - - - - - -   K - G R - - N - - -   - - - - - - - - - -   - - - -
DRw52b        R - - - - - - - - -   - - - - - - - - - -   K - G Q - - N - - -   - - - - - V - - - -   - - - -
DRw53         - - - - - - - - - -   - - - - - - - - - R   - - - E - - - - - -   Y - - - - V - - - -   - - - -
```

FIG. 7. Comparison of amino acid sequences of DRβ chains (first domain only).

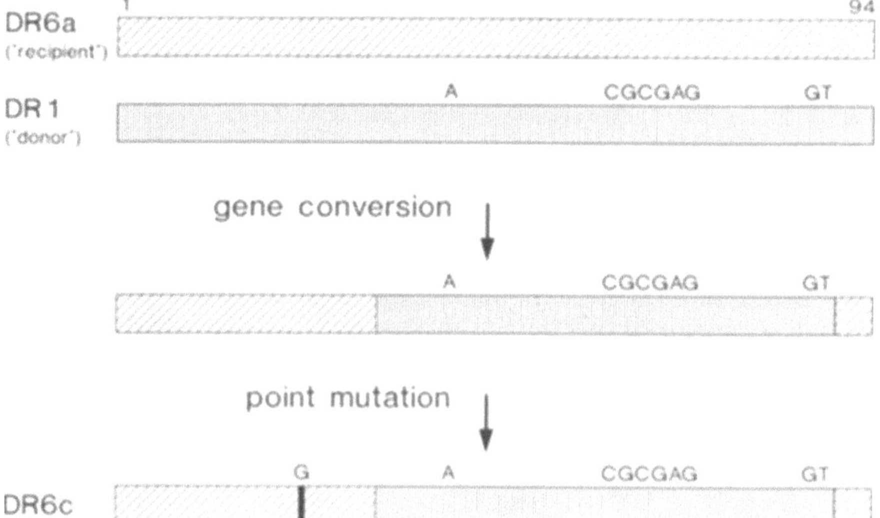

FIG. 8. Generation of DRβ allelic diversity by gene conversion and point mutation.

DR6c allele may have diverged from DR6a by virtue of only two mutational events, a gene conversion event plus a single point mutation. Of course these nucleotide differences may have been produced by 10 independent point mutations. However, gene conversion offers a more parsimonious explanation for the presence of stretches of shared sequence between otherwise dissimilar alleles. Furthermore, these shared sequences often include silent mutations, making it more difficult to argue that selection alone has acted to preserve identical sequences in various different genes.

H-2^{bm12} Mouse: Third Diversity Region Polymorphisms Influence Immune Responsiveness

The role of gene conversion events in generating class II diversity is further supported by examples of this phenomenon in the mouse. The H-2^{bm12} mutant is an inbred strain of mouse that arose spontaneously from the wild-type parental strain, H-2^b (53). The bm12 mouse differs by three nucleotides and three amino acid differences at one class II locus, I-Aβ (the murine homologue of DQβ). These sequence differences are located around position 70 of the I-Aβ chain and appear to have been donated in a gene conversion event by an adjacent class II gene on the same haplotype, I-Eβ (53). These sequence relationships are outlined schematically in Figure 9.

In addition to providing a classical example of gene conversion in the class II region, the bm12 mutant is also an instructive mutant from a functional standpoint. As indicated in Figure 9, the bm12 mutant differs from the wild type H-2^b mouse in its immune response patterns (36). The three amino acid differences in the I-Aβ chain result in reciprocal patterns of responsiveness to sheep and beef insulin, antigens that differ themselves by only one amino acid. Furthermore, the bm12 mutant is relatively resistant to a model autoimmune disease, experimentally induced myasthenia gravis (20). These data indicate that small numbers of amino acid changes in a circumscribed region of the class II molecule can profoundly influence its function and may affect susceptibility to autoimmune disease. One caveat has recently arisen in regard to the latter point, namely that bm12 mice also appear to express lower levels of I-A molecules (65), possibly explaining their decreased susceptibility to myasthenia gravis. Nevertheless, the bm12 mutant remains an instructive example of how class II polymorphisms generated by gene conversion events may produce differences in immune response patterns in the intact organism.

The example of the bm12 mutant indicates that amino acid substitutions in the region around position 70 (structurally analogous to the third diversity region of DRβ)

may have important functional consequences for immune responsiveness. Inasmuch as this region constitutes an α helical rim of the peptide binding cleft, polymorphisms in this portion of the class II molecule might reasonably be expected to interact directly with the T cell receptor molecule as well as influence antigenic peptide binding. One of the first indications in humans that third diversity region polymorphisms might affect T cell recognition came from a study of the molecular basis for alloreactive T cell responses to the various subtypes of HLA-DR4.

Third Diversity Region DRβ Polymorphisms Influence T Cell Responsiveness: MLC Subtypes of HLA-DR4

Even before the availability of sequence data on class II genes it was apparent that classical serological typing methods could not detect many of the allelic polymorphisms present in the population. For example, haplotypes that encoded the serologic determinant HLA-DR4 could be shown to be heterogeneous by means of the mixed lymphocyte culture (MLC) assay (63). Thus, serologically identical DR4 individuals in the population could occasionally be shown to cross-stimulate in an MLC, indicating that they were in fact not identical in class II phenotype. In this manner, many MLC subtypes of DR4 were defined that have been designated Dw4, Dw10, Dw13, Dw14, and Dw15 (39). Table 1 summarizes the serological features and predominant ethnic distribution of these various DR4 subtypes.

The molecular bases for these MLC typing differences, as well as others in the DR4 family, have now been defined (18, 30) (see Table 2). At the time it was somewhat surprising to discover that the sequence differences between these MLC subtypes were all localized to the third diversity region of the DRβ molecule. Furthermore, some MLC subtypes of DR4 differed by only one amino acid. For example, Dw13 and Dw14 differ by an Ala to Glu change at position 74. Other alleles, such as Dw10, have many distinctive amino acid substitutions. The Dw10 allele has two negatively charged residues, Asp and Glu at positions 70 and 71, compared with positively charged or neutral residues at these positions in the other DR4 subtypes. These data indicated that third diversity

TABLE 1. Major MLC Subtypes of DR4

MLC subtype designation	Serologic type	Predominant ethnic origin
Dw4	DR4, DRw53, DQw3	Caucasian
Dw10	DR4, DRw53, DQw3	Caucasian/Jewish
Dw13	DR4, DRw53, DQw3	Caucasian
Dw14	DR4, DRw53, DQw3	Caucasian
Dw15	DR4, DRw53, DQw4	Japanese

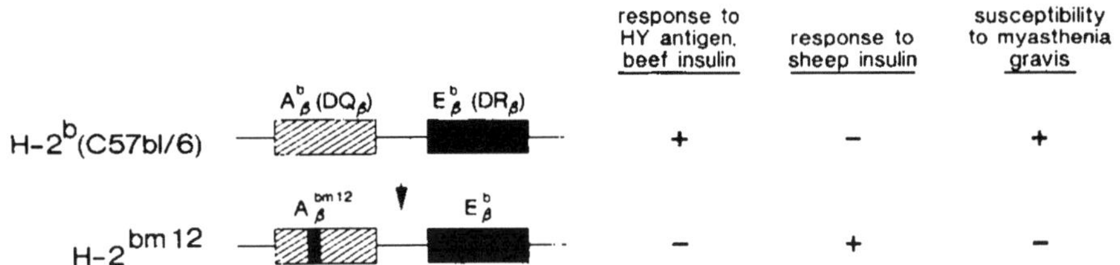

Fig. 9. Summary of sequence relationships and immune response differences between H-2^b and H-2^{bm12} mice. Aβ chain of H-2^{bm12} mouse differs from wild type H-2 Aβ chain by three amino acids that were derived from adjacent E locus in a gene conversion event (see text.

region differences at even a single position in the α helical region of DRβ can profoundly influence T cell responsiveness.

SIMILAR THIRD DIVERSITY REGION POLYMORPHISMS MAY BE FUNCTIONALLY EQUIVALENT EVEN WHEN PRESENT ON DIFFERENT DRβ ALLELES

As discussed above, identical third diversity region sequences may be shared by many otherwise different DRβ chains, possibly as the result of recurrent gene conversion events. An important question then becomes whether this sharing of third diversity region sequence results in functional equivalence of these DRβ chains with respect to T cell recognition or indeed for peptide binding. Studies by Weyand and colleages (93) have shown that alloreactive T cell clones specific for the Dw14 subtype of DR4 may also be stimulated by DR1 haplotypes (24). By referring to the DRβ sequences listed in Figure 6, it can be seen that DR1 and DR4, Dw14 share almost identical third diversity region sequences, indicating that this region may explain the functional similarity of these two alleles.

T cell reactivity patterns that cross react between DR1 and DR4 haplotypes have been termed "MC1-like" after a serologic specificity designated MC1. The MC1 specificity was originally described using alloantisera by Duquesnoy *et al.* (22) and, interestingly, was strongly associated with risk for rheumatoid arthritis (see below). Recently a DRw6 haplotype that stimulates MC1-like T cell clones (77) has been sequenced (83) and is shown in Figure 7 as the DR6c allele found in cell line AMALA. The DR6c allele also shares complete sequence identity with DR1 in the third diversity region, probably as a result of a gene conversion event similar to that outlined in Figure 8. These data strongly support the hypothesis that third diversity region sequences retain a degree of functional equivalence even when they are present in otherwise quite different DRβ chains.

THIRD DIVERSITY REGION POLYMORPHISMS IN DRβ CHAIN MAY CONFER RISK FOR RHEUMATOID ARTHRITIS

A reconsideration of the previously defined HLA associations with RA in light of the patterns of DRβ polymorphism outlined above indicates that third diversity region sequences may be of central importance in conferring disease risk. The association of RA with both DR4 and Dw4 was first defined by Stastny in the mid-1970s (80, 81). Subsequently, the association with DR4 has been confirmed in numerous different ethnic groups including North American and Northern European caucasian, Japanese, Hispanic, and North American black populations (85). A prominent exception to this is the Israeli Jewish population in which no association with DR4 is seen (72). The probable explanation of this relates to the prevalence of the various MLC subtypes of DR4 in these populations. In particular, the Dw10 subtype is present in high frequency in the Israeli population (2). This finding indicated that the Dw10 allele may not confer risk for RA. Note that the Dw10 sequence is conspicuously different from the other DR4 subtypes in the third diversity region, having two negatively charged residues at positions 70 and 71 (Table 1). In contrast, studies by Nepom and colleagues have demonstrated a positive association with the Dw4 and Dw14 subtypes in both the juvenile (56) and adult (57) rheumatoid populations. Likewise, the Dw15 subtype, found predominantly in Japanese populations, is also positively associated with RA (58). The Dw4, Dw14, and Dw15 alleles have similar sequences surrounding position 70 (Table 1 and Fig. 7).

HLA-DR1 has also been associated with RA; indeed DR1 is the predominant risk conferring haplotype in some populations, such as Asian Indians (95). Weaker associations with DR1 have been described in populations where DR4 is the predominant RA-associated haplotype (48). It should now be apparent that the likely explanation for this is the fact that DR1 and RA-associated DR4 alleles such as Dw14 have third diversity region sequence similarity. The clear implication from these relationships is that susceptibility to RA is in fact due to a group of similar third diversity region sequences that share certain conformational and functional attributes (31). These disease associated sequences may be found on many different DRβ chain alleles.

These considerations raise the question whether the DR6c (AMALA) allele may also confer risk for RA. This allele is identical to DR1 in the third hypervariable region (Figs. 7 and 8) but appears to be rare in white caucasian populations. It is however, found commonly in some Venezuelan Indian populations (47) as well as in North American Indians of the Pacific Northwest (G. Nepom, personal communication). The role of DR6c in predisposing to RA in these populations is an interesting avenue for further study. A related question concerns the distinct subtypes of DR1 that exist in the population. Variant DR1 alleles have been identified in patients with RA (54) as well as in normal individuals (38). It has not been established whether either of these DR1 subtypes is preferentially associated with RA. It is therefore likely that further study of class II sequences in rheumatoid populations will reveal additional insights into the specific polymorphisms that may predispose to this disease.

POLYMORPHISM WITHIN DQ SUBREGION

Unlike the DR subregion, polymorphism in the DQ subregion is found in both the DQα and DQβ chain

TABLE 2. SUMMARY OF AMINO ACID DIFFERENCES IN FIRST DOMAIN OF DRβ1 CHAINS FROM DIFFERENT DR4 SUBTYPES

	Amino acid position							
	57	 67	.. 69	70	71	.. 74	......	86
Dw4	Asp	.... Leu	. Glu	Gln	Lys	.. Ala	.....	Gly
Dw10	–	.... Ile	. –	Asp	Glu	.. –	.....	Val
Dw13	–	.... –	. –	–	Arg	.. Glu	.....	Val
Dw14	–	.... –	. –	–	Arg	.. –	.....	Val
Dw15	Ser	.... –	. –	–	Arg	.. –	.....	–

DRβ1 molecules are identical except at positions shown. Dashes signify identity with the Dw4 allele. See Figure 6 for complete first domain sequence.

genes. Furthermore, only a single α and β chain pair is expressed in all haplotypes, as indicated in Figure 4. In general, the degree of variation of DQα and DQβ chains is less than that seen in DRβ chains, both in terms of the number of different alleles as well as the degree of variability at particular polymorphic residues. Nevertheless, these loci are highly polymorphic, and the overall polymorphism of DQ molecules is further enhanced by the various possible combinations of α and β chains.

DQα CHAIN POLYMORPHISM: THREE MAJOR GROUPS OF RELATED ALLELES

A representative collection of DQα alleles is shown in Figure 10. It is apparent by simple inspection that the degree of variability of DQα chains is considerably less than the variability found in the DRβ chains just discussed. The DQα chains are shown in three general groupings reflecting the sequence similarity within each group. These groups most probably reflect the evolutionary relationships of the various haplotypes on which they are found. For example, two of these DQα groups follow the DRw52 and DRw53 haplotype family groupings discussed above. These relationships again reflect the strong linkage disequilibrium seen between alleles of the DR and DQ subregions. A third group of DQα chain alleles is found on haplotypes that bear the DQw1 specificity. These include DR1 and DR2 haplotypes that may form a third broad family analogous to the DRw52 and DRw53 families. Note, however, that DRw6, DQw1 haplotypes, which are members of the DRw52 haplotype family, nevertheless carry DQα chain alleles that belong to this third group. This indicates that the DRw6, DQw1 haplotypes, a common group of haplotypes in caucasian populations (see Fig. 5), may have arisen by recombination between the DRβ and DQα loci (28).

DQβ POLYMORPHISM: A PATCHWORK PATTERN OF SEQUENCE RELATIONSHIPS

Figure 11 displays the amino acid sequences of most reported DQβ alleles. They are divided into four groups according to the serological specificities with which they are associated. Note that the number of alleles within each group is quite variable. Only one sequence has been found for DQw2 (14). Three variants of the DQw3 DQβ chain have been reported: DQ3.1, DQ3.2, and DQ3.3 (46, 78, 87). They differ by one to four amino acids. Two minor variants of the DQw4 DQβ chain have also been reported (30, 37). For each of these groups, DQw2, DQw3, and DQw4, it appears that the DQβ chains are primarily responsible for the serological specificities with which

they are associated. In contrast, many quite distinct DQβ chains are found on haplotypes that encode the DQw1 serological specificity (87). This has led to the suggestion that the DQw1 specificity may be encoded by the DQα chain on these haplotypes (87). The DQw1 associated DQα chain is nearly identical in all haplotypes, as shown in Figure 10. Nevertheless, common amino acid substitutions found on DQw1 associated DQβ chains (for example between positions 84–90) may also contribute to the serological characteristics of DQw1 haplotypes.

The overall variability of DQβ chains is less than that found in DRβ chains. The most variable positions are at 57 and 71, each of which may have one of four possible amino acids, with a calculated variability index of about 7. In contrast, the most polymorphic positions of DRβ exhibit considerably greater variability. For example, position 11 of DRβ may have any of nine amino acid substitutions with a calculated variability index of 36 at this position (Fig. 6). Nevertheless, DQ and DRβ chains share many common features. First, segments of variable region sequence may be shared by several serologically unrelated alleles, lending a patchwork quality to the pattern of DQβ sequence variation. This can be observed by simple inspection of the sequences in Figure 11. As in DRβ, this may also reflect gene conversion events during the course of the evolution of these alleles. Secondly, the general distribution of diversity regions in DQβ also corresponds to the floor (β pleated sheets) and the α helical rim of the class II peptide binding cleft (Fig. 2). Note that position 57 appears to be located at the end of the α helix. As will be discussed, this position is not only one of the most variable in the DQβ chain but may play a special role in conferring risk for insulin dependent diabetes mellitus.

DQ α/β COMBINATORIAL DIVERSITY

Since both the α and β chains of the DQ molecule may vary, it is clear that additional diversity may be produced by the mixing of α and β chain alleles. For example, DR3,DQw2 and DR7,DQw2 haplotypes express an identical DQβ chain that appears to be responsible for the DQw2 serologic specificity (Fig. 11). Nevertheless, these two haplotypes express very different DQα chains (Fig. 10) that the DQw2 specific typing sera fail to distinguish. Likewise, DQ molecules on DR4,DQw3 and DR5,DQw3 haplotypes may differ in both the DQα chain as well as the DQβ chain (DR5 haplotypes express the DQ3.1 allele, whereas DR4 haplotypes may express either the DQ3.1 or the DQ3.2 chain (44).

A corollary to the principle of combinatorial diversity is the possibility of forming "hybrid" DQ molecules

	20	30	40	50	60	70	80
DR4,DQw3	YGVNLYQSYG	PSGQYSHEFD	GDEEFYVDLE	RKETVWQLPL	FRRFRRFDPQ	FALTNIAVLK	HNLNIVIKRS
DR7,DQw2	----------	--- FT--	----------	-- K---	-H-L -----	---	---- -L----
DR9,DQw3	- --------	----------	---- ---- -	----------	-- -----	----------	------
DR3,DQw2	- ---------	--- -T--	--Q--- --G	--- --C--V	L-Q -- -	----------	----SL-----
DR5,DQw3	----------	--- -T --	---Q --G	------C -V	L-Q- -----	----------	SL----
DR1,DQw1	C----- F--	---- T----	- -------	---A-RW E	SK-GG----	G--R-M--A-	-M---Y
DR2,DQw1	C- ---F--	-----T-- --	---Q --- -	-- -A-RW-F	-SK-GG- ---	G-- R-M--A-	--- M---Y
DRw6,DQw1	C------ F--	-----T----	----------	----A-RW-E	-SK- GG---	G--R-M A	-----M- Y

FIG. 10. Comparison of amino acid sequences of first (variable) domain (positions 20–86) of DQα chains. DQα alleles can generally be divided into three broad groups on the basis of sequence similarity. Upper two groups follow the DRw53 and DRw52 family groupings of the DR subregion genes. Lower group of DQα alleles are found on haplotypes that type as DQw1.

```
                    10          20          30          40          50
DQw1.1    R D S P E D F V Y Q  F K G L C Y F T N G  T E R V R G V T R H  I Y N R E E Y V R F  D S D V G V Y R A V
DQw1.2    - - - - - - - F -    - - - M - - - - - -  - - - - - L - - - Y  - - - - - - - - A -  - - - - - - - - - -
DQw1.12   - - P - - - - L -    - - A M - - - - - -  - - - - - Y - - - Y  - - - - - - - D - -  - - - - - - - - - -
DQw1.AZH  - - - - - - - - -    - - - - - - - - - -  - - - - - - - - - -  - - - - - - - - - -  - - - - - - - - - -
DQw1.9                                              - - - - - - - - - -  - - - - - - - - - -  - - - - - - - - - -
DQw1.18                                             - - - L - - - - - -  - - - - - - - A - -  - - - - - - - - - -
DQw1.19   - - - - - - - - - -  - - - M - - - - - -  - - - - - L - - - -  - - - - - - - A - -  - - - - - - - - - -

DQw2      - - - E - - - - - -  - - - M - - - - - -  - - - - - L - S - S  - - - - - - I - - -  - - - - - E F - - -

DQw3.1    - - - - - - - - - -  - - A M - - - - - -  - - - - - Y - - - Y  - - - - - - - A - -  - - - - E - - - - -
DQw3.2    - - - - - - - - - -  - - - M - - - - - -  - - - - - L - - - Y  - - - - - - - A - -  - - - - - - - - - -
DQw3.3    - - - - - - - - - -  - - - M - - - - - -  - - - - - L - - - Y  - - - - - - - A - -  - - - - - - - - - -

DQw4.1    - - - - - - - F -    - - - M - - - - - -  - - L - - - - - Y    - - - - - - - A - -  - - - - - - - - - -
DQw4.2    - - - - - - - F -    - - - M - - - - - -  - - - - - - - - Y    - - - - - - - A - -  - - - - - - - - - -


                    60          70          80          90
DQw1.1    T P Q G R P V A E Y  W N S Q K E V L E G  A R A S V D R V C R  H N Y E V A Y R G I  L Q R R
DQw1.2    - - - - - D - - -    - - - - - - - - - -  T - - E L - T - - -  - - - - - - F - - -  - - - -
DQw1.12   - - - - - D - - -    - - - - - D I - - R  T - - E L - T - - -  - - - - - - F - - -  - - - -
DQw1.AZH  - - - - - S - - -    - - - - - - - - - -  - - - - - - - - - -  - - - - - - - - - -
DQw1.9    - - - - - D - - -    - - - - - - - - - -  - - - - - - - -
DQw1.18   - - - - - D - - -    - - - - - - - - - -  T - - E L - T -
DQw1.19   - - - - - - - - -    - - - - - - - - - R  T - - E L - T - - -  - - - - - - G - - -  - - - -

DQw2      - L L - L - A - - -  - - - - - D I - - R  K - - A - - - - -    - - - Q L E L - T T  - - - -

DQw3.1    - - L - P - D - - -  - - - - - - - - - R  T - - E L - T - - -  - - - Q L E L - T T  - - - -
DQw3.2    - - L - P - A - - -  - - - - - - - - - R  T - - E L - T - - -  - - - Q L E L - T T  - - - -
DQw3.3    - - L - P - D - - -  - - - - - - - - - R  T - - E L - T - - -  - - - Q L E L - T T  - - - -

DQw4.1    - - L - - L D - - -  - - - - - D I - - E  D - - - - - T - - -  - - - Q L E L - T T  - - - -
DQw4.2    - - L - - L D - - -  - - - - - D I - - E  D - - - - - T - - -  - - - Q L E L - T T  - - - -
```

FIG. 11. Comparison of amino acid sequences of DQβ chains (first domain).

through trans association of DQα and DQβ chains encoded on different haplotypes (19). This situation is outlined schematically in Figure 12. In this example, a heterozygous individual carries two haplotypes: DR4,DQw3 from the father and DR3,DQw2 from the mother. As a result, four distinct DQ α/β heterodimers may be present at the cell surface. The DQα chain from each haplotype may pair with the DQβ chain from the same haplotype (cis pairing) as well as with that encoded on the opposite haplotype (trans pairing). Evidence for such trans associated "hybrid" DQ molecules has in fact been obtained in DR3/DR4 heterozygous individuals (55). In theory this mechanism effectively doubles the diversity of DQ molecules in a heterozygous individual. It also yields a heterozygous class II phenotype distinct from either parent. It has not been established that all the possible DQ α/β combinations can indeed be formed. Experiments with transfected α and β chains from the I-A subregion (the murine homologue of DQ) have indicated that some restriction of pairing may occur in the mouse (15). Analogous experiments using transfected DQα and DQβ chain pairs should establish whether any restrictions on DQ α/β chain pairing exist in humans.

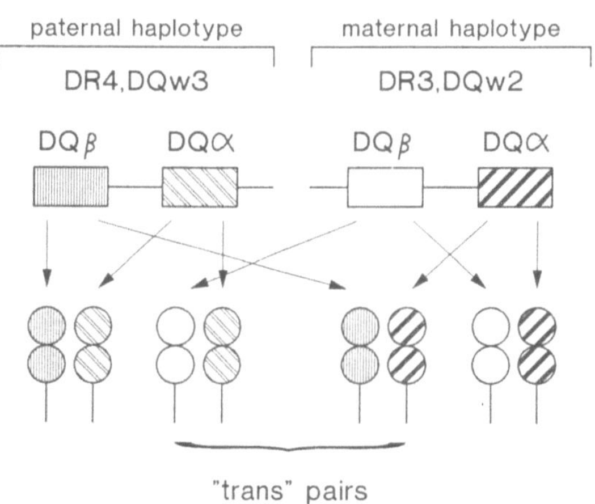

FIG. 12. DQ combinatorial complexity in a heterozygous individual: formation of trans associated DQ α/β pairs.

SUSCEPTIBILITY TO INSULIN DEPENDENT DIABETES MELLITUS: INFLUENCE OF ASP^{57} ON DQβ CHAIN

The definition at the sequence level of the range of allelic diversity in the DQ subregion has already increased understanding of the HLA class II associations with IDDM. IDDM is a heritable disorder thought to have an autoimmune pathogenesis, perhaps induced by viral infection (67). Like rheumatoid arthritis, IDDM has been associated with several different DR specificities, most notably DR3 and DR4 (8). Moreover, DR3/DR4 heterozygotes are at especially high risk for developing the disease (69). Intriguingly, DR2 is strongly *negatively* associated with the disease (69). A unique feature of IDDM that distinguishes it from most other autoimmune diseases, including RA, is the fact that its pattern of inheritance appears to be recessive (69). Attention was focused on the DQ subregion when it was reported that DQβ RFLPS could distinguish between DR4 haplotypes associated with risk for IDDM from those that are not (13, 73). This distinction is now known to be correlated with the two DQβ alleles found commonly on DR4 haplotypes: DQ3.2 (associated) and DQ3.1 (not associated). These two alleles differ by only four amino acids (Fig. 10), one of which is at position 57.

Todd *et al.* (87) have recently analyzed DQβ sequence diversity in a population of IDDM patients. These investigators confirmed the positive association with the DQ3.2 allele on DR4 haplotypes. However, they also noted that non-DR4 haplotypes associated with IDDM share a common feature with the DQ3.2 allele: the absence of aspartic acid at residue 57 of the DQβ chain. This correlation was particularly striking in the case of the DR2 haplotype designated AZH. As noted above, DR2 is generally negatively associated with IDDM; nevertheless, the AZH subtype of DR2 is positively associated with disease. The DQβ sequence found on the AZH haplotype contains serine at residue 57, in contrast to other DR2-associated DQ chains that have aspartic acid at this position (see Fig. 11). These correlations are further supported by the class II associations seen in strains of mice that spontaneously develop autoimmunity leading to diabetes. One such mouse strain, designated NOD (92), is homozygous for serine at position 57 of I-Aβ (the murine homologue of DQβ), whereas other reported I-Aβ alleles all have aspartic acid at this position (87). Homozygosity for this allele appears to be a requirement for development of disease in the NOD mouse (92).

The hypothesis that position 57 aspartic acid on the DQβ chain confers resistance to IDDM explains many observations. First, it is consistent with the apparent pattern of recessive inheritance for IDDM; one must lack aspartic acid on the DQβ chains of both haplotypes to be susceptible. Second, it explains the positive associations with some DR4, DR3, and DR1 haplotypes and the resistance conferred by most DR2 haplotypes, except for the AZH subtype of DR2. However, some features of the genetics of IDDM remain incompletely understood. For example, DR7 haplotypes that contain an identical DQβ chain as that found in DR3 haplotypes is not enriched in the diabetic population. One must therefore invoke other genes on DR7 haplotypes, perhaps the DQα allele, to explain this lack of association. In addition, some IDDM patients carry one DQβ allele with asp[57]. Therefore, other genes or environmental factors must be able to overcome this relative resistance. Finally, the very high risk for IDDM seen in DR3/DR4 heterozygotes is not fully explained by this hypothesis. Other heterozygote combinations are homozygous for the absence of aspartic acid at position 57 yet do not carry high risk for disease. Nevertheless, the correlations observed with this position 57 polymorphism has offered new insights and suggested further experiments to test the functional effects on antigen binding and T cell recognition of amino acid substitutions at this site. No doubt further refinements of the hypothesis will be forthcoming from these efforts.

SUMMARY AND CONCLUSIONS

Our understanding of HLA class II polymorphism has undergone a rapid evolution in the last few years. As in so many areas of modern biology, this progress has depended largely on the application of recombinant DNA techniques to the study of this gene family. In particular, the recent development of methods of gene amplification by means of the polymerase chain reaction (70) has allowed for the rapid assessment of polymorphism in the human population. In addition, the elucidation by x-ray crystallographic analysis of the three-dimensional structure of an HLA molecule (9) has been a major step. These areas of progress have now begun to converge to allow a more detailed approach to the problem of class II polymorphism and disease susceptibility. As discussed in this review, the data so far indicate that a few amino acid substitutions in class II molecules may exert a critical influence on susceptibility to autoimmune diseases such as RA and IDDM.

The mechanism by which these class II polymorphisms predispose to autoimmune disease is still unknown. It is tempting to speculate that differences in the binding affinity of HLA molecules for autoantigens might be involved; however, as yet no specific autoantigen has been identified for either RA or IDDM. Intriguingly, sequence similarities have been observed between some viral proteins and class II molecules, raising the possibility that these infectious agents might induce autoimmunity by "molecular mimicry." Examples include the human cytomegalovirus protein, IE2 (60, 86), as well as the Epstein Barr virus gp110 protein (68). Other possible mechanisms involve more complex immunoregulatory effects, such as the absence of suppressor functions that appear to be under the influence of the HLA genes (50, 71). To some extent, the persistent ignorance about the cause of autoimmunity reflects a general lack of knowledge concerning exactly how HLA polymorphisms exert immunoregulatory effects. For example, in addition to influencing antigen presentation, MHC molecules also affect the overall T cell repertoire during thymic selection (41). The relative importance of HLA class II polymorphism in exerting immunoregulatory effects by means of thymic selection of the T cell repertoire is unknown. For autoimmune diseases such as RA and IDDM, there is a need to identify a specific functional abnormality that is causing the disease before the etiological significance of the emerging associations with class II polymorphisms become clear.

Even in the absence of a precise etiologic mechanism, many therapeutic strategies are suggested by the existence of specific disease associated class II sequences. Among these is the use of monoclonal antibodies directed toward the disease associated class II alleles. Such monoclonal antibodies have been used successfully to prevent autoimmune disease in several animal models (1, 23, 82). Their mechanism of action is unclear, but may include specific blocking of antigen presentation, as well as more complex effects on the immune system (61). Alternatively, peptides might be designed to specifically interfere with the presentation of an autoantigen. These and other therapeutic approaches will undoubtedly be explored as the specific molecular interactions underlying autoimmunity are further defined.

REFERENCES

1. Adelman NE, Watling DL, McDevitt HO: Treatment of (NZB X NZW) F1 disease with anti Ia monoclonal antibodies. J Exp Med 158:1350, 1983
2. Amar A, Oksenberg J, Cohen N, Cohen I, Brautbar C: HLA-D locus in Israel. Characterization of 14 local HTC's and a population study. Tissue Antigens 20:198, 1982
3. Andersson G, Larhammar D, Widmark E, Servenius B, Peterson P, Rask L: Class II genes of the human major histocompatibility complex. Organization and evolutionary relationship of the DRβ genes. J Biol Chem 262:8748, 1987
4. Babbitt BP, Allen PM, Matsueda G, Haber E, Unanue ER: Binding of immunogenic peptides to Ia histocompatibility molecules. Nature 317:359, 1985
5. Bell JI, Denney D, Foster, Belt T, Todd JA, McDevitt HO: Allelic variation in the DR subregion of the human major histocompatibility complex. Proc Natl Acad Sci USA 84:6234, 1987
6. Benacerraf B: Role of MHC gene products in immune regulation. Science 212:1229, 1981
7. Bentley DL, Rabbits TH: Evolution of immunoglobulin V genes: Evidence indicating that recently duplicated V_k sequences have diverged by gene conversion. Cell 32:181, 1983
8. Betrams J and Baur MP: Disease reports: Insulin-dependent diabetes mellitus. In *Histocompatibility Testing, 1984*, edited by Albert ED, Baur MP, Mayr WR, pp 348–358. Berlin, Springer Verlag, 1984
9. Bjorkman PJ, Saper MA, Samraoui B, Bennett WS, Strominger JL, Wiley DC: Structure of the human class I histocompatibility antigen, HLA-A2. Nature 329:506, 1987
10. Bjorkman PJ, Saper MA, Samraoui B, Bennett WS, Strominger JL, Wiley DC: The foreign antigen binding site and T cell recognition regions of class I histocompatibility antigens. Nature 329:512, 1987
11. Bodmer WF: The HLA system, 1984. In Histocompatibility Testing 1984, edited by Albert ED, Baur MP, Mayr WR. Berlin, Springer Verlag, 1984
12. Böhme J, Andersson M, Andersson G, Möller E, Peterson P, Rask L: HLA-DR β genes vary in number between different DR specificities, whereas the number of DQ β genes is constant. J Immunol 135:2149, 1985
13. Böhme J, Carlson B, Wallin J, Moller E, Persson B, Peterson P, Rask L: Only one DQβ restriction fragment pattern of each DR specificity is associated with insulin dependent diabetes. J. Immunol. 137:941, 1986
14. Boss JM, Strominger JL: Cloning and sequence analysis of the human major histocompatibility complex gene DC-3β. Proc Natl Acad Sci USA 81:5199, 1984
15. Braunstein NS, Germain RN: Allele-specific control of Ia molecule surface expression and conformation: Implications for a general model of Ia structure-function relationships. Proc Natl Acad Sci USA 84:2921, 1987
16. Brown JH, Jardetzky T, Saper M, Samraoui B, Bjorkman PJ, Wiley DC: A hypothetical model of the foreign antigen binding site of class II histocompatibility molecules. Nature 332:845, 1988
17. Buus S, Sette A, Colon S, Miles C, Grey H: The relation between major histocompatibility complex restriction and the capacity of Ia to bind immunogenic peptides. Science 235:1353, 1987
18. Cairns JS, Curtsinger JM, Dahl CD, Freeman S, Alter BJ, Bach F: Sequence polymorphism of HLA-DRβ1 alleles relating to T cell recognized determinants. Nature 317:166, 1985
19. Charron D, Lotteau V, Tumel P: Hybrid HLA DC antigens provide molecular evidence for gene transcomplementation Nature 312:157, 1984
20. Christadoss P, Lindstrom JM, Melvold RW, Talal N: Mutation at I-A beta chain prevents experimental autoimmune myasthenia gravis. Immunogenetics 21:33, 1985
21. Curtsinger JM, Hilden JM, Cairns JS, Bach FH: Evolutionary and genetic implications of sequence variation in two nonallelic HLA-DR β chain cDNA sequences. Proc Natl Acad Sci USA 84:209, 1987
22. Duquesnoy RJ, Marrari M, Hackbarth S, Zeevi A: (1984) Serological and cellular definition of a new HLA-DR associated determinant, MC1, and its association with rheumatoid arthritis. Hum Immunol 10:165–176
23. Friedman A, Frankel G, Lorch Y, Steinman L: Monoclonal anti Ia antibody reverses chronic paralysis and demyelination in Theiler's virus infected mice: Critical importance of timing of treatment. J Virol 61:898, 1987
24. Gornzy J, Weyand CM, Fathman CG: Shared T cell recognition sites on human histocompatibility leukocyte antigen class II molecules of patients with seropositive rheumatoid arthritis. J Clin Invest 77:1042, 1986
25. Gorski J, Mach B: Polymorphism of human Ia antigens: Gene conversion between two DRβ loci results in a HLA-D/DR specificity. Nature 322:67, 1986
26. Gorski J, Rollini P, Mach B: Structural comparison of the genes of two HLA-DR supertypic groups: The loci encoding DRw52 and DRw53 are not truly allelic. Immunogenetics 25:397, 1987
27. Goverman J, Hunkapillar T, Hood L: A speculative view of the multicomponent nature of T cell antigen recognition. Cell 45:474, 1986
28. Gregersen PK, Kao H, Nunez-Roldan A, Hurley CK, Karr RW, Silver J: Recombination sites in the HLA class II region are haplotype dependent. J Immunol 141:1365, 1988
29. Gregersen PK, Moriuchi T, Karr RW, Obata F, Moriuchi J, Maccari J, Goldberg D, Winchester RJ, Silver J: Polymorphisms of HLA-DR β chains in DR4, -7, and -9 haplotypes: Implications for the mechanisms of allelic variation. Proc Natl Acad Sci USA 83:9149, 1986
30. Gregersen PK, Shen M, Song Q, Merryman P, Degar S, Seki T, Maccari J, Goldberg D, Murphy H, Schwenzer J, Wang CY, Winchester RJ, Nepom GT, Silver J: Molecular diversity of HLA-DR4 haplotypes. Proc Natl Acad Sci USA 83:2642, 1986
31. Gregersen PK, Silver J, Winchester RJ: The shared epitope hypothesis: an approach to understanding the molecular genetics of susceptibility to rheumatoid arthritis. Arthritis Rheum 30:1205, 1987
32. Guillet J-G, Lai M-Z, Briner T, Buus S, Sette A, Grey HM, Smith JA, Gefter ML: Immunological self, nonself discrimination. Science 235:865, 1987
33. Gustafsson K, Wiman K, Emmoth E, Larhammar D, Bohme J, Hyldig-Nielsen JJ, Ronne H, Peterson P, Rask L: Mutations and selection in the generation of class II histocompatibility antigen polymorphism. EMBO J 3:1655, 1984
34. Hardy DA, Bell JI, Long EO, Lindsten T, McDevitt HO: Mapping of the class II region of the human major histocompatibility complex by pulsed-field gel electrophoresis. Nature 323:453, 1986
35. Hill AVS, Nicholls RD, Thein SL, Higgs DR: Recombination within the human embryonic zeta-globin locus: A common zeta-zeta chromosome produced by gene conversion of the psuedo zeta gene. Cell 42:809, 1985
36. Hochman PS, Huber BT: A class II gene conversion event defines an antigen specific Ir gene epitope. J Exp Med 160:1925, 1984
37. Hurley CK, Gregersen PK, Steiner N, Bell J, Hartzman R, Nepom G, Silver J, Johnson AH: Polymorphism of the HLA-D region in American blacks. J Immunol 140:885, 1988
38. Hurley CK, Ziff BL, Silver J, Gregersen PK, Hartzman R, Johnson AH: Polymorphism of the HLA-DR1 haplotype in American blacks: Identification of a DR1 β chain determinant recognized in the mixed lymphocyte culture reaction. J Immunol 140:4019, 1988
39. Jaraquemada D, Reinsmoen NR, Ollier W, Okoye R, Bach FH,

Festenstein H: First level testing of HLA-DR4 associated new HLA-D specificities: Dw13(DB3), Dw14(LD40), Dw15(DYT) and DKT2. In Histocompatibility Testing 1984: Report on the Ninth International Histocompatibility Workshop and Conference, edited by Albert ED, Baur MP, Mayr WR. Heidelberg, Springer-Verlag, 1984

40. Jonsson A-K, Hyldig-Nielson J-J, Servenius B, Larhammar D, Andersson G, Jörgensen F, Peterson PA, Rask L: Class II genes of the human major histocompatibility complex. Comparisons of the DQ and DX α and β genes. J Biol Chem 262:8767, 1987

41. Kappler JW, Roehm N, Marrack P: T cell tolerance by clonal deletion in the thymus. Cell 49:273–280, 1987

42. Karr R, Gregersen PK, Obata F, Goldberg D, Maccari J, Alber C, Silver J: Analysis of DRβ and DQβ chain cDNA clones from a DR7 haplotype. J Immunol 137:2886, 1986

43. Kaufman JF, Auffray C, Korman AJ, Shackelford DA, Strominger JL: The class II molecules of the human and murine major histocompatibility complex. Cell 36:1, 1984

44. Kim SJ, Holbeck S, Nisperos B, Hansen JA, Maeda H, Nepom G: Identification of a polymorphic variant associated with HLA-DQw3 and characterized by specific restriction sites within the DQ β chain gene. Proc Natl Acad Sci USA 82:8139, 1985

45. Korman AJ, Boss JM, Spies T, Sorrentino R, Okada K, Strominger JL: Genetic complexity and expression of human class II histocompatibility antigens. Immunol Rev 85:45, 1985

46. Larhammar D, Hyldig-Nielsen JJ, Servenius B, Andersson G, Rask L, Peterson P: Exon-intron organization and complete nucleotide sequence of a human major histocompatibility antigen DCβ gene. Proc Natl Acad Sci USA 84:209, 1987

47. Layrisse Z, HD Heinen, and Simonney N: 1982 HLA-D typing with homozygous cells identified in an American indigenous isolate. II. Family studies and D/DR relationship. Tissue Antigens 20:86

48. LeGrande L, Lathrop GM, Marcelli-Barge A, Dryll A, Bardin T, Debeyre N, Poirier JC, Schmid M, Ryckewaert A, Dausset J: HLA-DR genotype risks in seropositive rheumatoid arthritis. Am J Hum Genet 36:690, 1984

49. Lotteau V, Teyton L, Burroughs D, Charron DJ: A novel HLA class II molecule (DR alpha-DQ beta) created by mismatched isotype pairing. Nature 329:339, 1987

50. Matsushita S, Muto M, Suemura M, Saito Y, Sasazuki T: HLA linked non-responsiveness to cryptomeria japonica pollen antigen. J Immunol 138:109, 1987

51. McConnell TJ, Talbot WS, McIndoe RA, Wakeland EK: The origin of MHC class II gene polymorphism within the genus *Mus*. Nature 332:651, 1988

52. McDevitt HO, Benacerraf B: Genetic control of specific immune responses. Adv Immunol 11:31, 1969

53. Mengle-Law L, Conner S, McDevitt HO, Fathman CG: Gene conversion between murine class II major histocompatibility complex loci: Functional and molecular evidence from the bm12 mutant. J Exp Med 160:1184, 1984

54. Merryman P, Gregersen PK, Lee S, Silver J, Nunez-Roldan A, Crapper R, Winchester RJ: Nucleotide sequence of a DRw10 β chain cDNA clone. J Immunol 140:2447, 1988

55. Nepom BS, Schwartz D, Palmer J, Nepom GT: Transcomplementation of HLA genes in IDDM. HLA DQα and β chains produce hybrid molecules in DR3/DR4 heterozygotes. Diabetes 36:114, 1987

56. Nepom BS, Nepom GT, Mickelson E, Schaller JG, Antonelli P, Hansen JA: Specific HLA-DR4-associated histocompatibility molecules characterize patients with seropositive juvenile rheumatoid arthritis. J Clin Inv 74:287, 1984

57. Nepom GT, Seyfried CE, Holbeck SL, Wilske KR, Nepom BS: Identification of HLA-Dw14 genes in DR4+ rheumatoid arthritis. Lancet 2:1002, 1987.

58. Ohta N, Nishimura YK, Tanimoto K, Horiuchi Y, Abe C, Shiokawa Y, Abe T, Katagiri M, Yoshiki T, Sasazuki T: Association between HLA and Japanese patients with rheumatoid arthritis. Hum Immunol 5:123, 1982

59. Okada K, Boss J, Prentice H, Spies T, Mengler R, Auffray C, Lillie J, Grossberger D, Strominger JL: Gene organization of DC and DX subregions of the human major histocompatibility complex. Proc Natl Acad Sci USA 82:3410, 1985

60. Oldstone MBA: Molecular mimicry and autoimmune disease. Cell 50:819, 1987

61. Perry L, Greene MI: Conversion of immunity to suppression by in vivo administration of Ia subregion specific antibodies. J Exp Med 156:480, 1982

62. Proceedings of the Third Asia-Oceania Histocompatibility Workshop and Conference, edited by Aizawa M. Sapporo, Hokkaido University Press, 1986

63. Reinsmoen NL, Bach F: Five HLA-D clusters associated with HLA-DR4. Hum Immunol 4:249, 1982

64. Rollini P, Mach B, Gorski J: Linkage map of three HLA-DRβ chain genes: Evidence for a recent duplication event. Proc Natl Acad Sci USA 82:3794, 1985

65. Ronchese F, Brown MA, Germain RN: Structure-function analysis of the Aβ^{bm12} mutation using site-directed mutagenesis and DNA-mediated gene transfer. J Immunol 139:629, 1987

66. Ronchese F, Schwartz RH, Germain RN: Functionally distinct sites on a class II major histocompatibility molecule. Nature 329:254, 1987

67. Rossini AA, Mordes JP, Like AA: Immunology of insulin dependent diabetes mellitus. Annu Rev Immunol 3:289, 1985

68. Roudier J, Rhodes GH, Petersen J, Vaughn J, Carson DJ: Two copies of the HLA Dw4,/Dw14/DR1 rheumatoid arthritis (RA) susceptibility determinant QKRAA/QRRAA are present on the Epstein-Barr virus (EBV) glycoprotein gp110 (abstr). FASEB J 2:A269, 1988

69. Rubinstein P, Rodriquez de Cordoba S: Insulin dependent diabetes mellitus: Immunogenic susceptibility, autoimmune components and environmental factors. Clin Aspects Autoimmun 2:18, 1988

70. Saiki RK, Bugawan TL, Horn GT, Mullis KP, Erlich HA: Genetic analysis of enzymatically amplified β globin and HLA-DQα genomic DNA with allele specific oligonucleotide probes. Nature 324:163, 1986

71. Sasazuki T, Nishimura Y, Muto M, Ohta N: HLA linked genes controlling immune response and disease susceptibility. Immunol Rev 70:51, 1983

72. Schiff B, Mizrachi Y, Orgad S, Gazit E: Association of HLA-Aw31 and HLA-DR1 with adult rheumatoid arthritis. Ann Rheumatic Dis 41:403, 1982

73. Schreuder G, Tilanus M, Bontrop RE, Bruining GJ, Giphart MJ, van Rood JJ, De Vries RRP: HLA-DQ polymorphism associated with resistance to type I diabetes detected with monoclonal antibodies, isoelectric point differences and restriction fragment length polymorphism. J Exp Med 164:938, 1986

74. Schwartz RH: Immune response (Ir) genes of the murine major histocompatibility complex. Adv Immunol 38:31, 1986

75. Schwartz RH: T lymphocyte recognition of antigen association with gene products of the major histocompatibility complex. *Ann Rev Immunol* 3:237, 1985

76. Servenius B, Rask L, Peterson PA: Class II genes of the human major histocompatibility complex. The DOβ gene is a divergent member of the class II β gene family. J Biol Chem 262:8759, 1987

77. Seyfried CE, Mickelson E, Hansen JA, Nepom GT: A specific nucleotide sequence defines a functional T cell recognition epitope shared by diverse HLA-DR specificities. Hum Immunol 21:289, 1988

78. Song QL, Gregersen PK, Karr RW, Silver J: Recombination between DQα and DQβ genes generates human histocompatibility leukocyte antigen class II haplotype diversity. J Immunol 139:2993, 1987

79. Speis T, Sorrentino R, Boss JM, Okada K, Strominger JL: Structural organization of the DR subregion of the human major histocompatibility complex. Proc Natl Acad Sci USA 82:5165, 1985

80. Stastny P: Association of the B-cell alloantigen DRw4 with rheumatoid arthritis. New Engl J Med 298:869, 1978

81. Stastny P: Mixed lymphocyte cultures in rheumatoid arthritis. J Clin Invest 57:1148, 1976

82. Subramaniam S, Topham DJ, Carroll L: Haplotype specific suppression of experimental allergic encephalomyelitis with anti Ia antibodies. J Immunol 139:1485, 1987

83. Takahasi PC, Kao HT, Tang JC, Gregersen PK, Silver J, Want CY: Molecular diversity of DRw6 haplotypes. In *Immunobiology of HLA: Immunogenetics and Histocompatibility*, Vol. 2, edited by Dupont B, Berlin, Springer Verlag, in press

84. Tieber VL, Abruzzini LF, Didier DK, Schwartz BD, Rotwein P: Complete characterization and sequence of an HLA class II β chain from the DR5 haplotype. J Biol Chem 261:2738, 1986

85. Tiwari JL, Terasaki PI: HLA and Disease Associations, pp 55–65.

Berlin, Springer Verlag, 1985
86. Todd JA, Acha-Orbea H, Bell JI, Chao N, Fronek Z, Jacob C, McDermott M, Sinha AA, Timmerman L, Steinman L, McDevitt HO: A molecular basis for MHC class II associated autoimmunity. Science 240:1003, 1988
87. Todd JA, Bell JI, McDevitt HO: HLA-DQβ gene contributes to susceptibility and resistance to insulin dependent diabetes mellitus. Nature 329:599, 1987
88. Tonelle C, DeMars R, Long EO: DOβ: A new β chain gene in HLA-D with a distinct regulation of expression. EMBO J 4:2839, 1985
89. Trowsdale J, Campbell RD: Physical map of the HLA region. Immunol Today 9:34, 1988
90. Trowsdale J, Young JAT, Kelly AP, Austin PJ, Carson S, Meunier H, So A, Erlich HA, Spielman RS, Bodmer J, Bodmer WF: Structure, sequence and polymorphism in the HLA-D region. Immunol Rev 85:5, 1985
91. Unanue ER, Allen PM: The basis for the immunoregulatory role of macrophages and other accessory cells. Science 236:551, 1987
92. Weyand CM, Goronzy J: Shared conformational T cell epitopes on DR-molecules of the HLA-DR1 and DR4 haplotypes associated with rheumatoid arthritis. Arth Rheum 30(Suppl):S25, 1987
93. Weyand CM, Goronzy J, Fathman CG: Human T cell clones used to define functional epitopes on HLA class II molecules. Proc Natl Acad Sci USA 83:762, 1986
93. Wicker LS, Miller BJ, Coker LZ, McNally SE, Scott S, Mullen Y, Appel MC: Genetic control of diabetes and insulinitis in the non-obese diabetic (NOD) mouse. J Exp Med 165:1639, 1987
94. Williams AF: A year in the life of the immunoglobulin superfamily. Immunol Today 8:298, 1987
95. Woodrow JC, Nichol FE, Zaphiropoulos G: DR antigens and rheumatoid arthritis: a study of two populations. Br Med J 283:1287, 1981
96. Wu S, Saunders TL, Bach FH: Polymorphism of human Ia antigens generated by reciprocal intergenic exchange between two DRβ loci. Nature 324:676, 1986
97. Zinkernagel RM, Doherty PC: MHC restricted cytotoxic T cells: Studies on the biological role of polymorphic major transplantation antigens determining T cell restricted specificity, function and responsiveness. Adv Immunol 27:51, 1979.

Biology of Disease

Interleukin 6: A Multifunctional Cytokine Regulating Immune Reactions and the Acute Phase Protein Response

JUNMING LE AND JAN VILČEK

Department of Microbiology and Kaplan Cancer Center, New York University Medical Center, New York, New York

INTRODUCTION

Cytokines are protein mediators of cell-to-cell communication important in a variety of physiologic and pathophysiologic processes. Only a decade ago information about cytokines was limited to the description of a multitude of ill-defined "factors" present in crude supernatants of cultures of mononuclear cells. Modern techniques of protein chemistry and molecular biology have led to the isolation and precise functional definition of many cytokines, including the interferons, colony-stimulating factors, and a heterogeneous group of agents termed interleukins. The name "interleukins" was originally conceived to designate proteins produced by lymphocytes or monocytes, affecting the growth and/or differentiation of lymphoid, monocytic or myeloid cells. With time it has become apparent that many interleukins are not produced exclusively by white blood cells, nor are their actions restricted to leukocytes. The terms "interleukin" or "lymphokine" are now being used for cytokines that can be produced by a variety of cell types and that can affect the functions of many nonhematopoietic cells.

Interleukin 6 (IL-6), to be reviewed in this article, is an example of a cytokine that acts as a messenger among cells both inside and outside the immune system. Originally described under a variety of different names, a group of scientists have recently recommended that the provisional names given this molecule by different investigators be replaced with the term "IL-6" (112).

Most cytokines are multifunctional. It is also apparent that certain biologic functions are shared by cytokines with distinct structural properties, and that many biologic actions *in vivo* are the result of synergistic or antagonistic actions involving two or more cytokines. These features are exemplified in the actions of IL-6 to be described in this review.

MULTIDISCIPLINARY ORIGINS OF IL-6 RESEARCH

IL-6 research, as it exists today, is the result of a convergence of several independent fields of investigation. In order to survey the properties and biologic activities of IL-6 it will be helpful to recall briefly the major developments that led to cloning of the IL-6 gene, the purification of the IL-6 protein and recognition of its major functions.

The earliest report of the cloning of IL-6 was by Weissenbach *et al.* (176); this accomplishment was the result of their efforts to clone human interferon (IFN)-β cDNA from cultured human fibroblasts. In order to induce IFN-β, Weissenbach *et al.* (176) treated fibroblasts with the double-stranded RNA, poly(I)·poly(C) in the presence of cycloheximide. (This induction procedure is widely employed for the stimulation of IFN-β synthesis in human fibroblasts.) The authors isolated two DNA clones complementary to a 1.3 kb mRNA inducible by poly(I)·poly(C) and cycloheximide. Weissenbach et al. (176) termed the protein coded by this mRNA "IFN-β_2" because, in their hands, injection of the 1.3 kb mRNA into *Xenopus laevis* oocytes yielded a protein with IFN-like antiviral activity and this antiviral activity was neutralized by antisera to IFN-β. However, the cloned "IFN-β_2" cDNA did not cross-hybridize with authentic IFN-β mRNA.

The same mRNA species was also found by Content et al. (25) in the course of their efforts to clone IFN-β from human fibroblasts. However, unlike Weissenbach et al. (176), these authors concluded that the 1.3 kb mRNA codes for a protein devoid of antiviral activity and unrelated to IFN-β. Unable to assign functional activity to this protein, they termed it provisionally "26-kDa protein." Content et al. (25) also showed that the 26-kDa protein was immunoprecipitated by antisera prepared against impure preparations of IFN-β, but not by an antiserum prepared against pure human IFN-β. They concluded that the apparent antigenic cross-reactivity reported by Weissenbach et al. (176) was more likely due to the presence of antibodies with two different specificities in antisera prepared against preparations of IFN-β contaminated with the 26-kDa protein.

An "IFN-β_2" mRNA was also described, but not cloned or sequenced, by Sehgal and Sagar (131). Their description was based on the observed presence of an IFN-like antiviral activity in the incubation medium of oocytes microinjected with a crude "14 S" mRNA fraction from induced fibroblasts. This mRNA was thought to be different from the smaller mRNA coding for classical IFN-β. The authors found that the antiviral action of the oocyte product injected with the "14 S" mRNA fraction was neutralized by antisera to IFN-β and hence, in agreement with Weissenbach et al. (176), they ascribed it to "IFN-β_2." Subsequently, Sehgal and his colleagues had postulated the existence of additional distinct IFN-β_3, -β_4 and -β_5 mRNAs and even had assigned structural genes for these "interferons" to various human chromosomes (126, 130). The "IFN-β_2" gene was assigned to chromosome 5, although subsequent studies by Sehgal et al. (133) that did not rely on antiviral activity showed that the structural gene for IL-6 is in fact on chromosome 7. In retrospect, it is likely that the antiviral activity found by these authors in the medium of oocytes injected with various crude mRNA fractions (126, 131) was not due to IL-6 but to contamination with authentic IFN-β mRNA or perhaps to some other unidentified material in the crude oocyte medium.

It is now widely believed that only one IFN-β protein exists in the human species, with its structural gene located on chromosome 9, along with all known IFN-α genes. (Interferon genes and proteins have been recently reviewed in references 32, 169, 177). Although in some cells IL-6 is co-induced with IFN-β upon certain treatments, IL-6 is not closely related to IFN-β structurally or functionally, as was first correctly pointed out by Content·et al. (25) and Haegeman et al. (43). In agreement with many other investigators, we believe that the assignment of antiviral activity to IL-6 was erroneous. Nevertheless, Weissenbach et al. (176) deserve enormous credit for the first reported cloning of IL-6.

Hirano et al. (50) described the cloning of a human B cell differentiation factor (BCDF) termed BSF2. This achievement was the culmination of a series of studies initiated by the demonstration of the presence of a characteristic late-acting BCDF activity in mitogen- or antigen-stimulated T cells. Cloning of BSF2 cDNA from a T cell line was preceded by the purification of the protein and determination of its partial amino acid sequence (49, 51). When the nucleotide and deduced amino acid sequences of the cloned BSF2 cDNA were compared with other known proteins, only human G-CSF showed a significant homology, with the position of four cysteine residues of BSF2 matching those of G-CSF (50). However, upon examination of the published BSF2 sequence, Billiau (12) noted that it was identical with the sequence of "IFN-β_2"/26 kDa protein which had been published only a few months earlier (43, 186).

Another totally unexpected discovery was the demonstration of molecular identity between "IFN-β_2"/26 kDa protein/BSF2 and a factor required for the survival and growth of murine B cell hybridomas or plasmacytomas (161). This discovery was preceded by the demonstration that a mouse T cell-derived factor, provisionally termed HP1, could sustain the growth of some murine B cell hybridomas and plasmacytomas (166). A similar growth-promoting activity, termed hybridoma/plasmacytoma growth factor (HPGF), was found in the supernatants of human fibroblasts stimulated with double-stranded RNA or IL-1 (159). HPGF from the MG-63 osteosarcoma cell line stimulated with IL-1 was purified to homogeneity and its NH_2-terminal amino acid sequence was determined (161). The sequence was identical with that of "IFN-β_2"/26 kDa protein and, as became apparent somewhat later, it also matched the sequence of BSF2.

Another line of studies led to the demonstration that IL-6 is a major regulator of the acute phase response. One of the characteristic reactions of the body to injury or infection is the increase in the release of liver-derived plasma proteins termed acute phase reactants (76). Regulation of the synthesis of acute phase proteins (which include C-reactive protein, serum amyloid A, fibrinogen and many others) is the function of monocyte-derived cytokines. The latter include IL-1, TNF and, most prominently, a protein termed hepatocyte-stimulating factor (HSF) (7, 8, 124). Gauldie et al. (40) observed that HSF activity from human monocytes was neutralized by antisera raised against IFN-β that also contained antibodies to "IFN-β_2". Conclusive evidence that HSF is identical with IL-6 derived from the demonstration that recombinant human BSF2/IL-6 (50) showed HSF activity similar to that seen with the purified natural protein (40). The identity of HSF and IL-6 was also confirmed by Andus et al. (4).

MOLECULAR CLONING AND EXPRESSION

In an effort to structurally define and genetically engineer the protein identified as "IFN-β_2", BSF-2, 26-kDa protein and HPGF, several groups have almost simultaneously reported the cloning of the cDNA for human IL-6 (17, 43, 50, 90, 186).

Hirano *et al.* (49) purified IL-6 (BSF-2) to homogeneity from the culture supernatant of the HTLV I-transformed T cell line, TCL-Na1 (140). The biological assay employed was based on the stimulation of IgM and IgG production by B lymphoblastoid SKW6-CL4 and CESS cells. Purified IL-6 (molecular weight 21 kDa) was digested with lysylendopeptidase to yield 9 fragments, and synthetic oligonucleotide probes were prepared based on the partial amino acid sequences of the NH_2-terminal and two other fragments. The cDNA for IL-6 was cloned by probing a cDNA library prepared from poly(A)$^+$RNA of the TCL-Na1 cell line with 11 groups of synthetic oligonucleotide mixtures (17 bases each) corresponding to these three fragments. A cDNA clone (pBSF2.38), specifically hybridizing with probes corresponding to all three fragments, was isolated from the cDNA library constructed in the pQ vector. The culture supernatant of COS7 cells transfected with pBSF2.38 DNA induced IgM production in SKW6-CL4 cells, indicating that pBSF2.38 contained the entire coding region of IL-6 (50).

The IL-6 cDNA contains a single large open reading frame, and the initiator ATG is followed by 211 codons before the termination triplet TAG. Sequence analysis of the NH_2-terminal region (51) indicated that the mature IL-6 containing 184 amino acids is processed by cleavage between the Ala(-1) and Pro(+1) residues from a precursor consisting of 212 amino acids. The first 28 amino acids (-28 to -1) form a strongly hydrophobic region, which appears to be a signal peptide required for IL-6 secretion. The calculated molecular weight of the entire mature IL-6 polypeptide is 20,781 daltons. Two potential N-glycosylation sites are present at amino acids 45 and 144. Northern blot analysis showed that IL-6 cDNA hybridized with a single species of 1.3 Kb mRNA in activated lymphocytes and TCL-Na1 cells (50). Recombinant IL-6 was also expressed in *E. coli* with the aid of a construct used for high-level expression of IL-2 (128). IL-6 was produced as a fusion protein with a part of IL-2, and the fusion protein was sequentially digested with kallikrein and amino-peptidase P to yield mature IL-6 (69).

Earlier, IL-6 ("IFN-β_2") cDNA was isolated by Weissenbach *et al.* (176). Full-length cDNA was formed by recombining through the *Xba*I site two cDNAs, which correspond to two overlapping segments of the 1.3 Kb "IFN-β_2" RNA isolated from FS11 fibroblasts stimulated with poly(I)·poly(C), cycloheximide and actinomycin D. This cDNA, fused to the SV40 early promoter, was transfected, amplified and expressed in CHO cells (186). "IFN-β_2" genomic clones were also isolated and expressed in hamster and mouse cells.

Independently, Haegeman *et al.* (43) isolated genomic clones coding for the 26-kDa protein from a total human DNA library, and cDNA clones were obtained from a library made with mRNA from human VGS fibroblasts induced by poly(I)·poly(C) and cycloheximide (33). Various vectors were used to express the isolated cDNA in *E. coli*, CHO cells and *Xenopus laevis* oocytes (115). Brakenhoff *et al.* (17) expressed cloned hybridoma growth factor (HGF) cDNA derived from human mono-cyte-poly(A)$^+$ RNA. Sequence analysis showed that HGF is identical with "IFN-β_2", 26-kDa protein, and BSF-2. It is interesting that the HGF activity produced in *E. coli* from a cDNA which encoded a recombinant product lacking the 28-amino acid signal peptide and the first 15 amino acids of the mature protein was found to be much higher than that produced from cDNAs containing the entire coding sequence. Deletion of the hydrophobic region may render the molecule less prone to aggregation. In a separate study, Jambou *et al.* (61) expressed a bioengineered, cysteine-free IL-6 protein, and found that removal of the cysteine residues did not affect the ability of IL-6 to induce B cell differentiation.

Comparison of the IL-6 protein sequence with other cytokines including human IL-1, IL-3, IL-4, IL-5, IFN-α, IFN-β, IFN-γ, G-CSF and GM-CSF, disclosed that only human G-CSF showed significant homology in a limited region with IL-6 (50). The positions of four cysteine residues in G-CSF and IL-6 molecules are precisely matched. In addition, a considerable similarity in genomic organization was observed between IL-6 and G-CSF. Both genes consist of five exons and four introns, and the sizes of the corresponding exons in the two genes are strikingly similar (183).

Revel (122) and May *et al.* (90) pointed out the presence of sequence homologies between limited regions of the IL-6 ("IFN-β_2") and IFN-β molecules. These authors speculated that the regions of homology may account for the claimed similarities in the actions of IL-6 and IFN-β. However, Haegeman *et al.* (43) -- while confirming the presence of limited sequence homologies between IL-6 and IFN-β as described by Revel (122) -- failed to find a statistically significant relationship between IL-6 and any IFN sequence available in the databases.

Genomic clones of IL-6 were isolated by Zilberstein *et al.* (186), Haegeman *et al.* (43) and Yasukawa *et al.* (183). S1 nuclease mapping and primer extension analyses revealed at least three transcription initiation sites, located approximately at nucleotide positions -63, -86 and -176 (relative to iniator ATG) (183). Several enhancer-like sequences, related to sequences found in the 5′ flanking regions of the IL-2 and IFN-β genes, were identified. Since it is already clear that the IL-6 gene can be activated by an unusually large variety of different signals, it is possible that different regulatory sequences control IL-6 gene expression (see below). Their identification is currently being pursued in several laboratories.

The structural gene for human IL-6 has been assigned to chromosome 7 by Southern blot analyses of DNA extracted from a panel of mouse/human somatic cell hybrids (133). *In situ* hybridization of IL-6 cDNA with human metaphase chromosomes localized this gene to 7p21 (16, 35).

Murine IL-6 was purified to homogeneity from a cloned helper T cell line and the macrophage cell line P388D1 (108, 165). A cDNA for murine IL-6 (interleukin-HP1) was recently isolated from a library prepared from mRNA derived from the murine helper T cell clone activated with a clonotypic antibody (167). The cDNA encodes a polypeptide consisting of 211 amino acids, with a signal peptide of 24 residues followed by 187 amino acid residues of the mature IL-6. There is a 42% homology between the amino acid sequences of human IL-6 and murine IL-6, and a 65% homology between their DNA sequences. The position of four cysteines in murine IL-6 also perfectly matches that in murine G-CSF. These results suggest that the genes coding for IL-6 and G-CSF may have evolved from a common ancestor gene (50). Chiu *et al.* (22) isolated functional murine IL-6 cDNA clones with identical characteristics from murine bone marrow stromal cell cDNA libraries. The genomic clone of mouse IL-6 has been isolated, and found to be similar to human IL-6 gene in overall structure and organization (152). The murine IL-6 gene has been localized to the proximal region of chromosome 5 (96).

REGULATION OF GENE EXPRESSION

Expression of IL-6 can be induced in various cell types including fibroblasts, monocytes/macrophages, T cells, B cells, endothelial cells, epidermal cells, synovial cells, keratinocytes and diverse tumor cells (13, 14, 54, 56, 62, 68, 134, 137, 145). Constituent cells of the endocrine system, such as endometrial stromal cells and folliculo-stellate cells of the anterior pituitary gland were also found capable of producing IL-6 (148, 168). Agents that enhance IL-6 gene expression in fibroblasts include cytokines (TNF, IL-1, IL-2, IL-3, colony-stimulating factors, IFN-β and platelet-derived growth factor) (26, 31, 63, 64, 72, 90, 125, 159, 186), lipopolysaccharide (LPS) (28, 44), bacteria (162), viruses (19, 136, 162), the double-stranded RNA poly(I)·poly(C) and/or cycloheximide (25, 73, 159, 176). TNF, IL-1, and LPS were also shown to stimulate IL-6 gene expression in monocytes/macrophages (91, 155), and endothelial cells (62, 145). In addition, treatment with IFN-γ and adherence induced IL-6 gene expression in monocytes (102). Induction of IL-6 gene expression in T cells can be triggered by concanavalin A (Con A), PHA and 12-0-tetradecanoyl phorbol 13-acetate (TPA) (50, 159, 165). However, production of IL-6 by PHA-stimulated T cells requires the presence of monocytes/macrophages or TPA (56).

In vivo studies showed that systemic administration of TNF, IL-1, or LPS resulted in a rapid induction of circulating IL-6 (18, 36, 60, 93). Treatment with high doses of IL-2 generated lower but consistent levels of circulating IL-6, presumably mediated by the synthesis of TNF (60, 93). IL-6 in the circulation is probably protected from the action of proteases by its binding to the carrier protein, α2-macroglobulin, which apparently does not affect the biologic activities of IL-6 (89). Whereas the cellular source of the circulating IL-6 remains to be elucidated, Tovey *et al.* (156) found that IL-6 as well as TNF and IL-1 genes were transcribed at high levels in the spleen, liver, kidney and peripheral blood leukocytes of normal individuals. Further studies are required to establish whether the constitutively produced IL-6 mRNA is actually translated *in vivo*.

Different mechanisms have been proposed for the regulation of IL-6 gene expression in human fibroblasts. Treatment of fibroblasts with synthetic diacylglycerols or the calcium ionophore A23187 resulted in a rapid increase in IL-6 mRNA levels due to increased transcription, indicating that both protein kinase C-activating and Ca^{++}-elevating agents can up-regulate IL-6 gene expression (135). In addition, various treatments that lead to an elevated cAMP accumulation also enhanced IL-6 gene expression in the apparent absence of protein kinase C activation (184). Treatment with TNF or IL-1, for instance, induced both IL-6 mRNA synthesis and a rapid increase in intracellular cAMP and cAMP-dependent protein kinase activity in fibroblasts without demonstrable protein kinase C activation. However, the cAMP-dependent pathway(s) appeared not to be the sole mechanism(s) mediating the activation of IL-6 gene by TNF and IL-1 (185). Moreover, TNF and IL-1 may enhance IL-6 gene transcription by somewhat different mechanisms, as cycloheximide inhibited the amplification of IL-6 gene transcription by IL-1α, but not by TNF, suggesting a requirement of newly-synthesized proteins for IL-1α-stimulated IL-6 transcription (175). Furthermore, it seems likely that pathways mediating IL-6 induction vary among different cell types.

To identify DNA sequences responsible for the activation of the IL-6 gene, Ray *et al.* (118) have linked various segments of the 5′ flanking region of the human IL-6 gene to the bacterial chloramphenicol acetyltransferase (CAT) gene. The constructs were transfected into HeLa cells and the ability of various stimuli to drive the IL-6 promoter was examined. The region between −225 and −113 in the IL-6 gene (relative to the major transcription start site) was found to contain the major elements responsible for the activation by TNF, IL-1, epidermal growth factor, serum, viruses, cAMP, 1,2-diacylglycerol and the calcium ionophore A23187. However, in similar studies carried out in our laboratory in human GM-637 cells transfected with various fragments of the 5′ flanking region of human IL-6 DNA, the major element controlling responsiveness to TNF and IL-1 (but not to forskolin) was located to a fragment of −110 to −50, containing a κB-like sequence (Y. Zhang and J. Vilček, manuscript in preparation). Gel shift and DNase I footprinting experiments revealed activation of a nuclear protein in TNF- or IL-1 treated human fibroblasts that binds to the κB-like sequence in the IL-6 gene.

Although only one structural gene for IL-6 has been clearly identified in man and mouse, there is evidence for size heterogeneity of the IL-6 protein product. For example, Content *et al.* (25) observed that human fibroblasts induced with poly(I)·poly(C) and cycloheximide secreted two forms of IL-6, with molecular masses of 22 and 27 kDa. When IL-6 mRNA was translated in an *in vitro* reticulocyte lysate supplemented with dog pancreas microsomes, a 19 and a 24 kDa form were identified by immunoprecipitation. May *et al.* (91) identified up to five molecular weight bands by sodium dodecyl sulfate-polyacrylamide gel electrophoresis (SDS-PAGE) analysis of IL-6 from human fibroblasts or monocytes, consisting of a 28-30 kDa triplet and 23-25 kDa doublet. Tunicamycin inhibited the appearance of the 28-30 kDa bands but not the 23-25 kDa bands, suggesting that at least some of the differences in molecular size are due to differential glycosylation. Whether the different molecular weight forms differ in specific activities or relative potencies in different types of assays has not been reported. The existence of multiple molecular weight forms is not unusual among glycoproteins and has been well-documented for some other cytokines, e.g., IFN-γ (67).

May *et al.* (92) obtained evidence indicating that the 28-30 kDa as well as the 23-25 kDa forms of IL-6 are phosphorylated. However, 28-30 kDa IL-6 from human monocytes appeared to be less extensively labeled with ^{32}P-orthophosphate than 28-30 kDa IL-6 from human fibroblasts. The authors suggested that phosphorylation may modulate IL-6 functions.

THE IL-6 RECEPTOR

Expression of specific IL-6 receptors (IL-6R) has been demonstrated in various cell types (reviewed in reference 54). The specificity of IL-6R was established by a number of observations. First, binding of radiolabeled IL-6 to CESS cells was competed for by recombinant or natural IL-6, but not by IL-1, IL-2, TNF, IFN-α_2, IFN-β, IFN-γ or G-CSF (29, 149). Second, IL-6 failed to bind to cell lines, such as K562 and Daudi, known to have binding sites for type I IFN (IFN-α and IFN-β). Moreover, cross-linking studies showed that the apparent molecular masses of IL-6R and type I IFN receptors are completely different (29). These observations clearly indicate that IL-6 and IFN-β act through distinct receptors, and make it very unlikely that IL-6 and IFN-β share an homology in the tertiary structure of their active sites, as was suggested by Zilberstein *et al.* (186).

Scatchard plot analyses showed that all EBV-transformed B cell lines tested expressed high affinity IL-6R (200-2700 per cell), with a Kd of 2 to 4 × 10^{-10} M. In contrast, none of the Burkitt's lymphoma lines examined expressed detectable IL-6R, and EBV failed to induce IL-6R on Burkitt's cells (149). Expression of the IL-6R was found on B cells activated with *Staphyloccocus aureus* Cowan I (100–600 sites/cell), but not on normal resting B cells. In contrast, normal resting T cells expressed the IL-6R (100 to 1000 sites/cell), whereas several T cell lines lacked detectable IL-6R. Cell lines expressing the IL-6R include the plasma cell lines ARH-77 and U266, the histiocytic line U937, the promyelocytic line HL60, the astrocytoma line U373, and the glioblastoma SK-MG-4 (149). The wide distribution of the IL-6R in the miscellaneous types of cells reflects the pleiotropic functions of this cytokine. Among the cell types studied so far, myeloma cells appear to express the highest number of IL-6R (over 10^4/cell), and both high-affinity (1.5 × 10^{-11} M) and low-affinity (1 × 10^{-9} M) receptors have been revealed. Three specific protein bands (145, 115 and 99 kD) were detected by SDS-PAGE analysis of [^{125}I]labeled IL-6 cross-linked to myeloma cells (70).

Yamasaki *et al.* (182) have isolated a cDNA encoding the human IL-6R utilizing a high-efficiency COS7 cell expression system with the CDM8 vector. A cDNA library was constructed from poly(A)$^+$ RNA of a human NK-like cell line, YT. The expressed receptors were detected with biotinated-recombinant IL-6 and fluorescein-conjugated avidin. The IL-6R consists of 468 amino acids, including a signal peptide of 19 residues, a presumed transmembrane domain of 28 residues, a cytoplasmic domain of 82 amino acids and a 339 amino acids-long extracellular portion. Most interesting is that sequence homologies were found between IL-6R and several members of the immunoglobulin superfamily. In this respect the IL-6R resembles the recently characterized receptor for IL-1 (144). Transfection of the IL-6R-negative human Jurkat T cell line with the cDNA for IL-6R resulted in a stable transfectant expressing both high-affinity (10^{-11} M) and low-affinity (10^{-9} M) binding sites, suggesting that both classes of IL-6R are coded for by the same cDNA (182). Recently, Taga *et al.* (149a) discovered an IL-6R-associated membrane protein (see note added in proof).

Not much information is available concerning the signal transduction mechanisms resulting from IL-6/IL-6R interaction. In a B lymphoblastoid cell line, in which IL-6 induced an increased transcription of mRNA for secretory-type heavy chains of Ig genes, treatment with IL-6 did not induce phosphoinositol metabolism, calcium ion mobilization, protein kinase C translocation, membrane depolarization, or protein phosphorylation (69). The possible involvement of tyrosine kinase activation in the signal transduction of IL-6 also seems unlikely in view of the recent finding that the intracytoplasmic portion of IL-6R lacks a tyrosine kinase domain (182).

BIOLOGIC ACTIVITIES

IL-6 is a pleiotropic cytokine exerting multiple biologic activities on different types of target cells (Table 1). IL-6 and IL-1 have overlapping activities, somewhat reminiscent of the earlier recognized interrelationship between TNF and IL-1 (78). Although in some cells IL-1 can induce IL-6, the similarity in the actions of IL-6 and IL-1 can not be fully explained by the ability of IL-1 to induce IL-6 production (103, 163). A synergism between IL-6 and IL-1 is often observed.

INDUCTION OF B CELL TERMINAL DIFFERENTIATION

The process of differentiation of antigen-stimulated B cells into antibody-forming plasma cells can be dissected into three stages, *i.e.*, activation, proliferation, and differentiation. Whereas IL-4 and IL-5 appear to be in-

TABLE 1. MAJOR BIOLOGIC ACTIVITIES OF IL-6

Action	References[a]
Induction of B cell differentiation	11, 49, 99
Stimulation of myeloma, hybridoma and plasmacytoma growth	65, 161, 166
Activation of T cells/thymocytes	85, 158
Induction of acute phase proteins	40
Stimulation of hemopoietic precursor cell growth and differentiation	181
Induction of myelomonocytic differentiation	23, 95, 138
Pyrogenic action	46
Induction of GM-CSF	125
Inhibition of TNF production	3
Induction of nerve cell differentiation	129
Inhibition of cell growth	21
Induction of ACTH synthesis[b]	179

[a] Only selected key references are included in this table, see text for other references.

[b] This action was observed with incompletely purified IL-6 and requires confirmation.

volved in the stages of activation and proliferation, IL-6 has been identified as a major inducer of B cell terminal differentiation (69). Because of this activity, IL-6 was originally also termed B cell differentiation factor (BCDF) (48, 109), or T cell-replacing factor (TRF) (98). Recombinant IL-6 at 1 and 10 ng/ml induced a 3- to 10-fold increase in IgM, IgG and IgA production in poke-weed mitogen (PWM)-stimulated mononuclear cells. To determine the target cells of IL-6 action, purified B cells were cultured with irradiated T cells and PWM prior to incubation with IL-6. That IL-6 induced a dose-dependent enhancement of IgG production in the activated B cells indicates a direct action of IL-6 on B cells. IL-6 showed no effect on the proliferation of PWM-activated B blasts, whereas IL-2 exerted a marked growth stimulation (99).

IL-6 appears to be one of the factors essential for Ig production in B cells, as addition of antibody specific for IL-6 inhibited over 90% of PWM-induced Ig production. The inhibition was evident even when the antibody was added 4 days after initiation in a total 8-day culture, indicating that IL-6 acts at the late stage of B cell differentiation (99). In contrast, neuroleukin, another essential factor for PWM-induced Ig production, was shown to function at the early stage of B cell differentiation (42). In a separate study, IL-6 was found to induce a high rate of IgA secretion by freshly isolated murine Peyer's patch B cells. IL-6 induced a sharp increase in numbers of IgA-secreting cells and failed to trigger B cell proliferation, indicating a role of IL-6 in promoting the terminal differentiation of Peyer's patch B cells into IgA-secreting plasma cells (11). IL-6 plays a similar role in the antigen specific antibody responses. Both primary and secondary antibody responses to sheep red blood cells were significantly enhanced by IL-6 *in vitro* and *in vivo* (151). It would be interesting to determine whether other cytokines, such as IL-1, can synergistically enhance the differentiation-inducing activity of IL-6, as suggested by Vink *et al.* (171).

Epstein-Barr virus (EBV)-transformed B lymphoblastoid cells can be induced to produce Ig by IL-6 (98, 99, 127, 153). Although these earlier studies suggested that IL-6 does not affect the growth of EBV-transformed B cell lines, Tosato *et al.* (155) recently observed a stimulatory effect of IL-6 on the growth of EBV-transformed B cells when the cells were cultured at low densities. However, this growth stimulatory action apparently can not be seen regularly with all preparations of recombinant IL-6 (G. Tosato, personal communication).

STIMULATION OF PLASMACYTOMA AND HYBRIDOMA GROWTH

It is well known that survival and growth of certain murine B cell hybridomas and plasmacytomas (the latter induced by injection of mineral oil into the peritoneal cavity) depends on soluble factor(s) secreted by macrophages (1, 10, 27, 101, 107, 146), T cells (142, 165, 166), endothelial cells (5), and fibroblasts (159, 174). The major active factor present in these conditioned media, originally designated hybridoma-plasmacytoma growth factor (HPGF) or interleukin-HP1, has been identified

as human or murine IL-6 (161, 167). To achieve a half-maximal growth, sensitive murine plasmacytoma cells required approximately 1 ng/ml (30 pM) of recombinant IL-6 (80, 166), which is about 100 to 200 times more than the amount required by murine B cell hybridomas (99, 115, 166). The high sensitivity of B cell hybridomas to IL-6 has been utilized to detect picogram levels of IL-6 (2, 88). Why B cell hybridomas are more sensitive to IL-6 than plasmacytomas or, in fact, any other target cells is not known. The difference might perhaps be due to the presence of IL-6R with a higher binding affinity on the hybridoma cells, which are formed by fusion of murine myeloma cells with B cells.

These studies suggest that IL-6 may play an essential role in the *in vivo* generation of plasmacytomas and myelomas. Indeed, it was found that freshly isolated human multiple myeloma cells constitutively produced autocrine IL-6 and expressed IL-6R (65). Moreover, exogenous IL-6 stimulated the *in vitro* proliferation of certain myeloma cells, and anti-IL-6 antibodies inhibited the growth of myeloma cells responsive to IL-6. IL-6-dependent human bone marrow-derived myeloma cell lines were also established (141). Adherent cells isolated from bone marrow were also found capable of producing IL-6 required for the growth of multiple myelomas (a paracrine regulation) (71). IL-1 too can stimulate the growth of human meyloma cells mostly through the induction of IL-6 (66). These results suggest that IL-6 functions as an important autocrine or paracrine growth factor for human myeloma cells.

INDUCTION OF ACUTE PHASE PROTEIN SYNTHESIS IN HEPATOCYTES

The acute phase response is a systemic reaction to tissue injury caused by infection or trauma, characterized by an increased synthesis of a series of hepatocyte-derived plasma proteins knows as acute phase reactants (including C-reactive protein, serum amyloid A, α_1-antitrypsin, fibrinogen, complement factors B and C3), and by reduced synthesis of albumin and transferrin (76). Several cytokines have been implicated in the induction of the acute phase response. In rat and human cell cultures of hepatic origin, IL-1 and TNF stimulated the generation of only a limited subset of the acute phase proteins, such as α_1-acid glycoprotein, complement C3, and factor B (7, 30, 40, 113, 116). Induction of a wide spectrum hepatic acute phase protein response can be achieved by a cytokine, originally termed hepatocyte-stimulating factor (HSF) and shown to be produced mainly by activated monocytes, macrophages, fibroblasts and some tumor cell lines (8, 40, 76, 178). Monocyte-derived HSF has been identified as IL-6, because antibodies specific for IL-6 were found to neutralize HSF activity (4, 40). However, another HSF, structurally different from IL-6, may be produced by human carcinoma cells (9).

E. coli-derived recombinant IL-6 induced the *in vitro* synthesis of all major acute phase proteins and also inhibited the production of albumin by hepatocytes. A maximal stimulation of α_2-macroglobulin synthesis by rat hepatocytes, or of fibrinogen synthesis by human hepatoma HepG2 cells was observed with 40 units/ml or 8 ng/ml of IL-6 (40). IL-6 acted as a potent inducer of some acute phase genes in human hepatoma Hep3B cells, exerting its effect at the level of transcription (97). Administration of recombinant IL-6 also induced a rapid acute phase response *in vivo* (117). Maximal increases in mRNA levels of several acute phase proteins in the liver were observed 4 hours after injection of IL-6 in the rat (41). Concomitant administration of glucocorticoids (*e.g.*, dexamethasone) can maximize the action of IL-6 in inducing the synthesis of acute phase proteins (87).

Although IL-6 emerges as a major regulator of the acute phase response, its potency varies depending on the experimental system involved. It is also apparent that in regulating acute phase protein synthesis IL-6 generally acts synergistically with IL-1 and TNF as well as glucocorticoids. Thus, the interaction among IL-1, TNF and IL-6 is at two levels: IL-1 and TNF promote IL-6 production and, in turn, all three cytokines cooperate in inducing the acute phase reactants. The details of regulation vary somewhat depending on the animal species, tissue and specific gene involved (reviewed in reference 137). Both IL-1 and IL-6 have also been reported to stimulate ACTH synthesis (179); the resulting generation of cortisol would then help to promote the acute phase response. On the other hand, cortisol would act to inhibit IL-1, TNF and IL-6 synthesis (84), eventually promoting the termination of both the inflammatory and acute phase responses.

STIMULATION OF HEMOPOIETIC PROGENITORS

The proliferation and development of hemopoietic progenitor cells is regulated by a number of cytokines including CSFs, IL-1, IL-3, IL-4 and IL-5. Recombinant human IL-6 was also found capable of supporting the proliferation of some mouse granulocyte/macrophage progenitors (181). In addition, IL-6 indirectly supported the formation of several types of multilineage hemopoietic colonies in cultures of mouse spleen cells, most likely through the induction of other cytokines in accessory cells present in the culture. IL-6 was found to stimulate myelopoiesis and erythropoiesis *in vivo*, as administration of IL-6 caused a mild myeloid hyperplasia and a striking erythroid hyperplasia in the bone marrow of rats (157). IL-6 also interacts with a variety of cytokines to regulate the growth of progenitor cells at different stages of lineage commitment and maturation. For example, IL-6 strongly synergized with M-CSF in stimulating macrophage colony formation from purified human bone marrow progenitor cells (15). IL-6 and IL-3 can act synergistically to support the proliferation of murine multipotential progenitors (75). The IL-3-dependent blast cell colony formation was enhanced by IL-6 via its ability to shorten the Go period of the quiescent progenitor cells (59). The same conclusion was drawn on the basis of a similar study with purified human bone marrow cells (82). In addition, bone marrow cultures prepared from mice treated 4 days earlier with 5-fluorouracil showed an enhanced GM colony formation when stimulated with IL-6 plus IL-4 or G-CSF. In bone marrow cultures from normal mice, IL-6 enhanced colony for-

mation by lineage-restricted megakaryocytic and erythroid progenitors in the presence of IL-3 and IL-4 plus erythropoietin, respectively (121). IL-6 was also found to stimulate early hemopoietic progenitors derived from patients with hairy cell leukemia. Formation of lymphomyeloid and erythroid colonies was markedly enhanced by IL-6 in hairy cell leukemia cells (123).

Recent studies showed that IL-6 is a potent inducer of terminal macrophage differentiation in a mouse myeloid leukemia cell line (M1) (95). Addition of IL-6 to M1 cell cultures resulted in an inhibition of proliferation, a decrease in *c-myc* mRNA accumulation and increases in FcγR, *c-fos* and *c-fms* mRNA expression (23). IL-6 also induced differentiation of human pre-monocytic U937 cells, which can be synergistically augmented by combined treatment with IL-1 (111). Along similar lines, Sachs *et al.* (125, 138) have recently shown that MGI-2, a protein that induces differentiation of myeloid leukemia cells to macrophages or granulocytes, is in fact IL-6.

ACTIVATION OF T CELLS AND THYMOCYTES

A series of studies have recently revealed that IL-6 can act as an important signal for T cell proliferation and differentiation. IL-6 is capable of inducing the differentiation of cytotoxic T lymphocyte (CTL) precursors activated by antigen and mitogen. In primary allogeneic mixed lymphocyte cultures, IL-6 caused an approximately 100-fold increase in the specific anti-H-2^d CTL response (158). IL-6 was also shown to induce the differentiation of Lyt-2$^+$ CTL from Con A-activated murine thymocytes in the presence of IL-2, and the cytotoxicity could be enhanced by murine IFN-γ. Serine esterase, a marker of cytotoxic granules in CTL, was induced only in the presence of IL-6, suggesting that IL-6 contributes to the CTL response at least partially by inducing proteins required for mediating target cell lysis (150). Similarly, IL-6 was found to augment CTL generation from human T cells or thymocytes stimulated with allogeneic cells in the presence of IL-2, and IL-6 apparently acts in the late phase of CTL generation (110).

It has been well documented that IL-6 stimulates the proliferation of both thymocytes and mature T cells depleted of macrophages in the presence of mitogen or antibodies specific for the T cell antigen receptors (39, 46, 58, 79, 85, 154, 158). To some extent, IL-6 can replace the function of monocytes/macrophages to serve as an accessory signal in support of T cell activation (6, 20). Several lines of evidence suggested that IL-2 and the IL-2 receptor (IL-2R) are involved in IL-6 action. First, purified murine T cells can be activated to produce low levels of IL-2 by IL-6 in the presence of Con A (39). Second, IL-6 enhanced the IL-2R expression in murine thymocytes co-stimulated with PHA (79). Enhancement of the IL-2R expression in a T cell line by IL-6 was also demonstrated (106). Third, monoclonal antibody specific for IL-2R (p55 chain) partially blocked IL-6-driven proliferation of T cells or thymocytes (39, 79, 85). However, the same antibodies failed to affect IL-6-stimulated proliferation under different experimental conditions (*e.g.*, low PHA concentration), suggesting the existence of an

IL-2-independent pathway (20, 58, 79, 154). The mechanism of the latter pathway remains to be established. It is interesting that IL-6 synergistically enhanced not only IL-1-stimulated T cell/thymocyte activation, but also IL-4 and TPA-driven thymocyte proliferation (34, 55, 58, 79).

Studies showed that IL-6 and IL-1 are functionally related cytokines in T cell activation. IL-1-stimulated thymocyte proliferation appears to be dependent on endogenous IL-6 production by a subpopulation of thymocytes with low buoyant density. IL-1 not only induces IL-6 production, but also renders thymocytes much more responsive to IL-6 (47). In primary MLC, presentation of alloantigen by non-activated B cells required the presence of both IL-1 and IL-6, suggesting that IL-1 and IL-6 play important roles in alloantigen-stimulated T cell activation (94).

Antiviral Activity?

As indicated earlier in this review, the first reported cloning of IL-6 cDNA by Weissenbach *et al.* (176) was accomplished in the course of the authors' efforts to clone IFN-β cDNA. These authors suggested that the newly isolated cDNA codes for a protein structurally and functionally related to IFN-β and proposed the name "IFN-β_2". Several years later Zilberstein *et al.* (186) reported the expression of the "IFN-β_2" cDNA in Chinese hamster ovary (CHO) cells by fusing the cDNA to the SV40 early promoter. In addition, two genomic clones of human "IFN-β_2" were isolated and expressed in mouse or hamster cells. When supernatants of the transfected cells were tested for antiviral activity in standard IFN assays they showed several hundred units/ml of antiviral activity. In general, the pattern of antiviral activity reported by Zilberstein *et al.* (186) resembled that of authentic human IFN-β. Antiviral activity of the preparations was neutralized by polyclonal or monoclonal antibodies to human IFN-β, although the same antibodies failed to immunoprecipitate the "IFN-β_2" protein. The authors speculated that neutralization of "IFN-β_2" by antibodies to IFN-β was possibly due to a resemblance of the active site in "IFN-β_2" to that of IFN-β. They did not explain, however, the lack of immunoprecipitation by the same antibodies. Antiviral activity of recombinant human IL-6 was also reported by Sehgal and May (132). The latter authors used a preparation of IL-6 expressed in *E. coli* as a fusion protein containing a 34-amino acid prokaryotic leader peptide. Although Sehgal and May (132) used an IL-6 preparation much more highly purified than the material employed by Zilberstein *et al.* (186), they too have not ruled out the contribution of some extraneous material to the observed antiviral action. For example, Helfgott *et al.* (44) reported that bacterial lipopolysaccharide can produce an antiviral state in human fibroblasts as well as induce IL-6 expression, and the possible contribution of LPS to the reported antiviral action of the IL-6 preparation used by Sehgal and May (132) has not been ruled out. In a recent study Chen *et al.* (21) indicate that the specific activity of an *E. coli*-derived human IL-6 in the antiviral assay is only 1.5 to 3 $\times$ 10^3 units/mg, i.e., about five orders of magnitude less than that of authentic IFN-β.

In contrast to the incomplete evidence for the antiviral activity of IL-6 reported by two groups of investigators, at least five laboratories have failed to show any antiviral action with a variety of IL-6 preparations. The first to point out a lack of detectable antiviral activity were Content *et al.* (25) who used a purified natural protein produced in human fibroblasts and the product of IL-6 mRNA translation in *Xenopus laevis* oocytes. A similar lack of antiviral activity was reported by other groups who had tested several natural and recombinant preparations of IL-6 (52, 115, 119, 160).

Our laboratory reported that TNF induces an antiviral action in human fibroblasts (72). In the same cells TNF also acted as an inducer of IL-6. In view of the claims of Weissenbach *et al.* (176) and Zilberstein *et al.* (186) that IL-6 shows IFN-β-like antiviral activity, Kohase *et al.* (72) initially suggested that IL-6 may act as a mediator of TNF's antiviral action. However, upon closer examination this interpretation became untenable (74). It is now apparent that the antiviral action of TNF in human fibroblasts is the result of a synergistic action of TNF with very small amounts of endogenously produced IFN-β (120, 170), and there is evidence against a role of IL-6 in this system (119). Studies similar to those with TNF have been done with IL-1, which also exerts an IFN-β-like antiviral effect on certain cells (160). In this case the authors have likewise considered the possibility that this antiviral effect might be mediated by the IL-6 induced by IL-1. However, careful studies done by the use of specific antibodies to IFN-β and to IL-6 led to the conclusion that IFN-β and not IL-6 was involved.

Other Biologic Activities

The list of actions associated with IL-6 is still growing. Like nerve growth factor, IL-6 induced differentiation of pheochromocytoma PC12 cells into neuronal cells (129). Furthermore, the neuropeptides substance P and K were found capable of inducing IL-6 production by monocytes (86). IL-6 also induced fever in rabbits with kinetics essentially identical with those observed with IL-1 (46).

In addition, IL-6 was found to inhibit the growth of a number of tumor cell lines, including breast carcinomas T-47 and MCF-7, histiocytic lymphoma U937, and T cell lymphoma Molt-4 (21). These data once again raise the interesting question whether in some cells IL-6 might act as an autocrine growth inhibitor, rather than growth stimulator. On the basis of indirect evidence (using polyclonal antibodies to IFN-β that also neutralized IL-6), Kohase *et al.* (72) suggested that IL-6 ("IFN-β_2") may act as a negative growth regulator in human diploid FS-4 fibroblasts. However, in subsequent experiments we found no significant effect of *E. coli*-derived recombinant human IL-6 on the proliferation of the same line of human fibroblasts (J. Le, V. J. Palombella, L. F. L. Reis, and J. Vilček, unpublished data). On the other hand, Chen *et al.* (21) found some inhibitory action of IL-6 on the growth of normal human skin fibroblasts, albeit only at high doses.

Aderka *et al.* (3) have observed an inhibitory action of IL-6 on LPS-induced synthesis of TNF. This inhibitory action was seen in cultured human peripheral blood monocytes, the myelomonocytic U937 cell line and in intact mice. The inhibition of TNF production by IL-6 is interesting because TNF is known to be a potent inducer of IL-6 (72). This finding raises the possibility that the generation of IL-6 in response to TNF serves as a negative regulatory mechanism controlling TNF production.

Earlier, TNF was found capable of increasing HLA-A,B (class I) antigen expression at both mRNA and protein levels in cultured endothelial cells and fibroblasts (24). Based on the observation that the stimulation of class I antigen expression by TNF could be inhibited by antibodies directed against IFN-β, May *et al.* (90) suggested that IL-6 functions as an intermediate of TNF action in these cells. However, some subsequent studies failed to demonstrate a significant stimulation of class I antigen expression by recombinant IL-6 preparations (83, 114, J. Le, unpublished data). Navarro *et al.* (102) reported that IL-6 slightly increased HLA class I, but had no effect on class II antigen expression in U937 cells.

ROLES IN DISEASES

Clinical studies suggest that IL-6 plays a role in the pathogenesis of systemic autoimmune diseases, in which the overproduction of IL-6 might lead to abnormal B cell differentiation and antibody production. Cardiac myxoma, a rare benign intraatrial heart tumor, is often associated with autoimmune symptoms, such as hypergammaglobulinemia and an elevated erythrocyte sedimentation rate (147). These symptoms often disappear upon surgical removal of the tumor. Cardiac myxoma cells, when cultured *in vitro*, produced substantial quantities of IL-6 (50, 51). Kishimoto and Hirano (69) reported on a patient in whom cervical cancer was associated with a Sjögren-like syndrome and high titers of serum autoantibodies. The patient's autoimmune symptoms disappeared 3 months after removal of the tumor, and the tumor cells in culture secreted large amounts of IL-6 (51). These authors also noted an abnormal production of IL-6 by the lymph nodes of patients with Castleman's disease, characterized by lymphadenopathy with massive infiltration of plasma cells, hypergammaglobulinemia, increased acute phase proteins and, in advanced stages, plasmacytomas (69).

High levels of IL-6 were detected in synovial fluids of patients with active rheumatoid arthritis, and the cells isolated from the synovial fluids expressed increased levels of IL-6 mRNA. Immunohistochemical analysis demonstrated that IL-6 was mainly produced by CD2$^+$ T cells and CD20$^+$ blastoid B cells (53). IL-6 was also present in synovial fluids of patients with inflammatory arthritis and traumatic arthritis, and there appears to be an association between the levels of IL-6 and disease activity (173).

Studies using highly sensitive IL-6-dependent hybridoma growth assays showed that IL-6 levels are elevated in patients who develop an acute phase response. In patients with severe burns, IL-6 levels in serum or plasma increased 2- to 100-fold within hours of injury, whereas C-reactive protein and α_1-antitrypsin rose relatively slowly. On the other hand, while the acute phase proteins

were still raised, IL-6 levels and the body temperature were already declining (104). In patients undergoing surgical operation, a rapid elevation of serum IL-6 after surgery was followed by increased levels of acute phase proteins (105, 139). High levels of IL-6 were also detected both in the serum and urine of renal transplant recipients after transplantation and during acute rejection episodes, possibly relating to the acute phase reaction (164).

Abnormal production of IL-6 may be associated with polyclonal B cell activation in viral infections. A feature common to viral infection of the brain is the intrathecal production of immunoglobulin by B cells infiltrating the brain tissue. IL-6 appears to play a role in this regard, as not only were high levels of IL-6 detected in cerebrospinal fluids of patients with acute viral infection of the central nervous system, but also viral infection *in vitro* (e.g., vesicular stomatitis virus) induced the secretion of IL-6 by microglial cells and astrocytes (37, 38). HIV also can induce IL-6 production (100). Mononuclear cells of healthy donors expressed increased levels of IL-6 mRNA and secreted IL-6 soon after exposure to live or inactivated HIV. The overproduction of IL-6 (mainly by monocytes) might contribute to the polyclonal B cell activation in AIDS patients.

IL-6 is possibly involved in the pathogenesis of acute bacterial infections. High levels of IL-6 were detected in the cerebrospinal fluid of patients with acute bacterial meningitis and in the serum of patients with various bacteriemias (45, 57). It was found that IL-6, IL-1 and TNF are released into the serum in patients with meningococcal septic shock, and that high levels of IL-6 and the presence of IL-1 are associated with a fatal outcome (172). IL-6 may also be involved in neoplasia. McIntosh *et al.* (93) observed that the sera of tumor-bearing mice contained detectable levels of IL-6 which rose linearly with increasing tumor burden. Although in this study circulating IL-6 was detected in mice bearing syngeneic sarcomas as well as melanomas or adenocarcinomas, further studies are required to elucidate the cellular source of endogenously produced IL-6, and to establish whether this phenomenon is common to all tumor-bearing hosts.

These results, together with the finding that IL-6 may act as an autocrine growth factor for multiple myeloma (65), suggest that specific inhibitors of IL-6, such as specific antibodies or recombinant soluble IL-6 receptor, may be potentially useful for the therapy of diseases in which some of the pathology may be caused by an overproduction of IL-6. A chimeric toxin composed of IL-6 attached to a portion of *Pseudomonas* exotoxin may be useful in the selective elimination of myeloma or other IL-6 receptor-bearing cells (143).

It is still too early to survey potential clinical applications of IL-6. In view of its ability to enhance immunoglobulin secretion, IL-6 may be useful in some forms of immunodeficiencies. It is conceivable that IL-6 may have adjuvant activity and that its administration (perhaps together with some other B cell differentiation agents) may enhance the immune responses to vaccines. Safe and effective adjuvants are needed especially for recombinant vaccines that may lack sufficient immunogenicity. It is also possible that the ability of IL-6 to stimulate the proliferation of hemopoietic progenitor cells could be beneficially exploited in some clinical situations, together with other hemopoietic growth factors.

CONCLUSIONS

The brief history of IL-6 research exemplifies the rapid progress in our understanding of the important roles played by cytokines in the regulation of immune responses, in inflammation and other vital processes. The enormous functional versatility of IL-6 (Table 1) no longer comes as a great surprise, since other cytokines, notably the interferons, IL-1 and TNF, were earlier shown to serve a multitude of biological functions (32, 78). It is also not unexpected that some of the actions of IL-6 complement and partially overlap the activities of other cytokines, e.g., IL-1 in the ability to activate T cells and to stimulate hepatocytes to produce acute phase proteins, or IL-3 in the stimulatory action on the growth of hemopoietic precursor cells.

IL-6 appears to be one of the most readily inducible cytokines, due mainly to two characteristics. One, an unusual variety of cell types can produce IL-6 and two, IL-6 production can be induced by an unusually large array of different stimuli. These features can explain why enhanced levels of IL-6 are being found in the serum and human body tissues in a large variety of infectious and autoimmune diseases (137). It is significant that in many cell types IL-6 is readily and directly inducible by invading bacteria or viruses, but the production of IL-6 is further amplified by other cytokines (especially IL-1 and TNF) also generated in response to infectious agents. Although the complete roles of IL-6 *in vivo* are not yet fully understood, it appears that during infection IL-6 serves a predominantly useful role. The major functions of IL-6 in the inflammatory process include an immunoenhancing action mediated by the activation of T and B lymphocytes, and the stimulation of the acute phase proteins, *i.e.*, a general anti-inflammatory response whose full significance is partly still a matter of conjecture (76). It seems that IL-6 shows less acute toxicity than some other cytokines produced during inflammation (*e.g.*, TNF or IL-1). The ability of IL-6 to inhibit TNF production (3) suggests that the generation of IL-6 (which is increased by TNF) may eventually lead to a decrease in the toxic effects due to TNF.

Despite the rapid recent progress, much more needs to be learned about the functions of IL-6.

Note Added in Proof: Brakenhoff *et al.* (17a) constructed recombinant IL-6 protein analogs with deletions at the *N*-terminal end. Removal of up to 28 amino acids failed to affect IL-6 activity in four different assays, but removal of amino acids 29 and 30 reduced all activities about 50-fold, suggesting that a single domain is responsible for most all of the biologic activities measured. Taga *et al.* (149a) provided new insights into the functioning of the IL-6 receptor by demonstrating the requirement for its association with a 130 kDa membrane glycoprotein (gp130). Binding with gp130 involves only the extracellular portion of the IL-6 receptor and the model proposed represents a completely novel form of receptor functioning and signal transduction. New evidence has been obtained for the role of IL-6 in the regulation of IgM, IgA (77a) and IgE (168a) synthesis. Other newly described activities of IL-6 include a stimulatory effect on the growth and differentiation of megakaryocytes (59a), and an activation of natural killer cells apparently mediated through an increase in IL-2 production (86a). Suematsu *et al.* (145a) generated transgenic mice overproducing human IL-6. Such mice displayed a massive plasmacytosis in the thymus, lymph nodes and spleen, and had infiltrates of plasma cells in the lungs, liver and kidneys; transgenic mice also showed a glomerulonephritis and an increase in megakaryocytes in the bone marrow. Grossman *et al.* (41a) showed that active psoriatic plaques from skin lesions of psoriasis patients contained a high concentration of immunoreactive Il-6; the authors suggested that IL-6 could both directly contribute to the epidermal hyperplasia and promote the function of local inflammatory cells.

Acknowledgments: We thank the numerous colleagues who sent us manuscripts before their publication and especially Drs. Alfons Billiau, Toshio Hirano, Jean Content, Jack Gauldie and Jacques Van Snick for the critical reading of this manuscript and for their comments. We also thank Mary Ann Singer and Ilene Toder for the preparation of the manuscript.

REFERENCES

1. Aarden LA, Lansdorp PM, DeGroot ER: A growth factor for B cell hybridomas produced by human monocytes. Lymphokines 10:175, 1985
2. Aarden LA, DeGroot ER, Schaap OL, Lansdorp PM: Production of hybridoma growth factor by human monocytes. Eur J Immunol 17:1411, 1987
3. Aderka D, Le J, Vilček J: Interleukin-6 inhibits lipopolysaccharide-induced tumor necrosis factor production in cultured human monocytes, U937 cells and in mice. J Immunol, in press 1989
4. Andus T, Geiger T, Hirano T, Northoff H, Ganter U, Bauer J, Kishimoto T, Heinrich PC: Recombinant human B cell stimulatory factor 2 (BSF-2/IFN-beta$_2$) regulates beta-fibrinogen and albumin mRNA levels in Fao-9 cells. FEBS Lett 221:18, 1987
5. Astaldi GCB, Janssen MC, Lansdorp P, Willems C, Zeijlemaker WP, Oosterhof F: Human endothelial culture supernatant (HECS): a growth factor for hybridomas. J Immunol 125:1411, 1980
6. Baroja ML, Ceuppens JL, Van Damme J, Billiau A: Cooperation between an anti-T cell (anti-CD28) monoclonal antibody and monocyte-produced IL-6 in the induction of T cell responsiveness to IL-2. J Immunol 141:1502, 1988
7. Baumann H, Onorato V, Gauldie J, Jahreis GP: Distinct sets of acute phase plasma proteins are stimulated by separate human hepatocyte-stimulating factors and monokines in rat hepatoma cells. J Biol Chem 262:9756, 1987
8. Baumann H, Richards C, Gauldie J: Interaction among hepatocyte-stimulating factors, interleukin 1, and glucocorticoids for regulation of acute phase plasma proteins in human hepatoma (Hep G2) cells. J Immunol 139:4122, 1987
9. Baumann H, Won K-A, Jahreis GP: Human hepatocyte-stimulating factor-III and interleukin-6 are structurally and immunologically distinct but regulate the production of the same acute phase plasma proteins. J Biol Chem 264:8046, 1989
10. Bazin R, Lemieux R: role of the macrophage-derived hybridoma growth factor in the *in vitro* and *in vivo* proliferation of newly formed B cell hybridomas. J Immunol 139:780, 1987
11. Beagley KW, Eldridge JH, Lee F, Kiyono H, Everson MP, Koopman WJ, Hirano T, Kishimoto T, McGhee JR: Interleukins and IgA synthesis. Human and murine interleukin 6 induce high rate IgA secretion in IgA-committed B cells. J Exp Med 169:2133, 1989
12. Billiau A: BSF-2 is not just a differentiation factor. Nature

(London) 324:415, 1986
13. Billiau A: Interferon-beta$_2$ as a promoter of growth and differentiation of B cells. Immunol Today 8:84, 1987
14. Biondi A, Rossi V, Bassan R, Barbui T, Bettoni S, Sironi M, Mantovani A, Rambaldi A: Constitutive expression of the interleukin-6 gene in chronic lymphocytic leukemia. Blood 73:1279, 1989
15. Bot FJ, Van Eijk L, Broeders L, Aarden LA, Löwenberg B: Interleukin-6 synergizes with M-CSF in the formation of macrophage colonies from purified human marrow progenitor cells. Blood 73:435, 1989
16. Bowcock AM, Kidd JR, Lathrop M, Daneshvar L, May LT, Ray A, Sehgal PB, Kidd KK, Cavalli-Sforza LL: The human "β_2 interferon/hepatocyte stimulating factor/interleukin-6" gene: DNA polymorphism studies and localization to chromosome 7p21. Genomics 3:8, 1988
17. Brakenhoff JPJ, DeGroot ER, Evers RF, Pannekoek H, Aarden LA: Molecular cloning and expression of hybridoma growth factor in *Escherichia coli*. J Immunol 139:4116, 1987
17a. Brakenhoff JPJ, Hart M, Aarden LA: Analysis of human IL-6 mutants expressed in *Escherichia coli*. Biologic activities are not affected by deletion of amino acids 1-28. J Immunol 143:1175, 1989
18. Brouckaert P, Spriggs DR, Demetri G, Kufe DW, Fiers W: Circulating interleukin 6 during a continuous infusion of tumor necrosis factor and interferon γ. J Exp Med 169:2257, 1989
19. Cayphas S, Van Damme J, Vink A, Simpson RJ, Billiau A, Van Snick J: Identification of an interleukin HP1-like plasmacytoma growth factor produced by L cells in response to viral infection. J Immunol 139:2965, 1987
20. Ceuppens JL, Baroja ML, Lorre K, Van Damme J, Billiau A: Human T cell activation with phytohemagglutinin. The function of IL-6 as an accessory signal. J Immunol 141:3868, 1988
21. Chen L, Mory Y, Zilberstein A, Revel M: Growth inhibition of human breast carcinoma and leukemia/lymphoma cell lines by recombinant interferon-beta$_2$. Proc Natl Acad Sci USA 85:8037, 1988
22. Chiu C-P, Moulds C, Coffman RL, Rennick D, Lee F: Multiple biological activities are expressed by a mouse interleukin 6 cDNA clone isolated from bone marrow stromal cells. Proc Natl Acad Sci USA 85:7099, 1988
23. Chiu C-P, Lee F: IL-6 is a differentiation factor for M1 and WEHI-3B myeloid leukemic cells. J Immunol 142:1909, 1989
24. Collins T, Lapierre LA, Fiers W, Strominger JL, Pober JS: Recombinant human tumor necrosis factor increases mRNA levels and surface expression of HLA-A,B antigens in vascular endothelial cells and dermal fibroblasts *in vitro*. Proc Natl Acad Sci USA 83:446, 1986
25. Content J, De Wit L, Pierard D, Derynck R, De Clercq E, Fiers W: Secretory proteins induced in human fibroblasts under conditions used for the production of interferon beta. Proc Natl Acad Sci USA 79:2768, 1982
26. Content J, De Wit L, Poupart P, Opdenakker G, Van Damme J, Billiau A: Induction of a 26-kDa-protein mRNA in human cells treated with an interleukin-1-related, leukocyte-derived factor. Eur J Biochem 152:253, 1985
27. Corbel C, Melchers F: The synergism of accessory cells and of soluble alpha-factors derived from them in the activation of B cells to proliferation. Immunol Rev 78:51, 1984
28. Coulie PG, Cayphas S, Vink A, Uyttenhove C, Van Snick J: Interleukin-HP1-related hybridoma and plasmacytoma growth factors induced by lipopolysaccharide *in vivo*. Eur J Immunol 17:1217, 1987
29. Coulie PG, Vanhecke A, Van Damme J, Cayphas S, Poupart P, De Wit L, Content J: High-affinity binding sites for human 26-kDa protein (interleukin 6, B cell stimulatory factor-2, human hybridoma plasmacytoma growth factor, interferon-beta$_2$), different from those of type I interferon (alpha, beta), on lymphoblastoid cells. Eur J Immunol 17:1435, 1987
30. Darlington GJ, Wilson DR, Lachman LB: Monocyte-conditioned medium, interleukin-1, and tumor necrosis factor stimulate the acute phase response in human hepatoma cells *in vitro*. J Cell Biol 103:787, 1986
31. Defilippi P, Poupart P, Tavernier J, Fiers W, Content J: Induction and regulation of mRNA encoding 26-kDa protein in human cell lines treated with recombinant human tumor necrosis factor. Proc Natl Acad Sci USA 84:4557, 1987
32. De Maeyer E, De Maeyer-Guignard J: Interferons and Other Regulatory Cytokines. New York, John Wiley and Sons, 1988
33. Derynck R, Content J, DeClercq E, Volckaert G, Tavernier J, Devos R, Fiers W: Isolation and structure of a human fibroblast interferon gene. Nature (London) 285:542, 1980
34. Elias J, Trinchieri G, Beck JM, Simon PL, Sehgal PB, May LT, Kern JA: A synergistic interaction of IL-6 and IL-1 mediates the thymocyte-stimulating activity produced by recombinant IL-1-stimulated fibroblasts. J Immunol 142:509, 1989
35. Ferguson-Smith AC, Chen Y-F, Newman MS, May LT, Sehgal PB, Ruddle FH: Regional localization of the beta$_2$-interferon/B-cell stimulatory factor 2/hepatocyte stimulating factor gene to human chromosome 7p15-p21 Genomics 2:203, 1988
36. Fong Y, Moldawer LL, Marano M, Wei H, Tatter SB, Clarick RH, Santhanam U, Sherris D, May LT, Sehgal PB, Lowry SF: Endotoxemia elicits increased circulating β_2-IFN/IL-6 in man. J Immunol 142:2321, 1989
37. Frei K, Leist TP, Meager A, Gallo P, Leppert D, Zinkernagel RM, Fontana A: Production of B cell stimulatory factor-2 and interferon gamma in the central nervous system during viral meningitis and encephalitis. Evaluation in a murine model infection and in patients. J Exp Med 168:449, 1988
38. Frei K, Malipiero UV, Leist TP, Zinkernagel RM, Schwab ME, Fontana A: On the cellular source and function of interleukin 6 produced in the central nervous system in viral diseases. Eur J Immunol 19:689, 1989
39. Garman RD, Jacobs KA, Clark SC, Raulet DH: B-cell-stimulatory factor 2 (beta$_2$ interferon) functions as a second signal for interleukin 2 production by mature murine T cells. Proc Natl Acad Sci USA 84:7629, 1987
40. Gauldie J, Richards C, Harnish D, Lansdorp P, Baumann H: Interferon beta$_2$/B-cell stimulatory factor type 2 shares identity with monocyte-derived hepatocyte-stimulating factor and regulates the major acute phase protein response in liver cells. Proc Natl Acad Sci USA 84:7251, 1987
41. Geiger T, Andus T, Klapproth J, Hirano T, Kishimoto T, Heinrich PC: Induction of rat acute-phase proteins by interleukin 6 *in vivo*. Eur J Immunol 18:717, 1988
41a. Grossman RM, Krueger J, Yourish D, Granelli-Piperno A, Murphy DP, May LT, Kupper TS, Sehgal PB, Gottlieb AB: Interleukin 6 is expressed in high levels in psoriatic skin and stimulates proliferation of cultured human keratinocytes. Proc Natl Acad Sci USA 86:6367, 1989
42. Gurney ME, Apatoff BR, Spear GT, Baumel MJ, Antel JP, Bania MB, Reder AT: Neuroleukin: a lymphokine product of lectin-stimulated T cells. Science 234:574, 1986
43. Haegeman G, Content J, Volckaert G, Derynck R, Tavernier J, Fiers W: Structural analysis of the sequence coding for an inducible 26-kDa protein in human fibroblasts. Eur J Biochem 159:625, 1986
44. Helfgott DC, May LT, Sthoeger Z, Tamm I, Sehgal PB: Bacterial lipopolysaccharide (endotoxin) enhances expression and secretion of beta$_2$ interferon by human fibroblasts. J Exp Med 166:1300, 1987
45. Helfgott DC, Tatter SB, Santhanam U, Clarick RH, Bhardwaj N, May LT, Sehgal PB: Multiple forms of IFN-β_2/IL-6 in serum and body fluids during acute bacterial infection. J Immunol 142:948, 1989
46. Helle M, Brakenhoff JPJ, DeGroot ER, Aarden LA: Interleukin 6 is involved in interleukin 1-induced activities. Eur J Immunol 18:957, 1988
47. Helle M, Boeije L, Aarden LA: IL-6 is an intermediate in IL-1-induced thymocyte proliferation. J Immunol 142:4335, 1989
48. Hirano T, Teranishi T, Lin B, Onoue K: Human helper T cell factor(s) IV Demonstration of a human late-acting B cell differentiation factor acting on *Staphylococcus aureus* Cowan I-stimulated B cells. J Immunol 133:798, 1984
49. Hirano T, Taga T, Nakano N, Yasukawa K, Kashiwamura S, Shimizu K, Nakajima K, Pyun KH, Kishimoto T: Purification to homogeneity and characterization of human B-cell differentiation factor (BCDF or BSFp-2). Proc Natl Acad Sci USA 82:5490, 1985
50. Hirano T, Yasukawa K, Harada H, Taga T, Watanabe Y, Matsuda T, Kashiwamura S, Nakajima K, Koyama K, Iwamatsu A, Tsun-

asawa S, Sakiyama F, Matsui H, Takahara Y, Taniguchi T, Kishimoto T: Complementary DNA for a novel human interleukin (BSF-2) that induces B lymphocytes to produce immunoglobulin. Nature (London) 324:73, 1986

51. Hirano T, Taga T, Yasukawa K, Nakajima K, Nakano N, Takatsuki F, Shimizu M, Murashima A, Tsunasawa S, Sakiyama F, Kishimoto T: Human B-cell differentiation factor defined by an anti-peptide antibody and its possible role in autoantibody production. Proc Natl Acad Sci USA 84:228, 1987

52. Hirano T, Matsuda T, Hosoi K, Okano A, Matsui H, Kishimoto T: Absence of antiviral activity in recombinant B cell stimulatory factor 2 (BSF-2). Immunol Lett 17:41, 1988

53. Hirano T, Matsuda T, Turner M, Miyasaka N, Buchan G, Tang B, Sato K, Shimizu M, Maini R, Feldmann M, Kishimoto T: Excessive production of interleukin 6/B cell stimulatory factor-2 in rheumatoid arthritis. Eur J Immunol 18:1797, 1988

54. Hirano T, Kishimoto T: Interleukin-6. In Handbook of Experimental Pharmacology, Peptide Growth Factors and Their Receptors, edited by Sporn MB, Roberts AB, Berlin, Springer-Verlag, in press 1990

55. Hodgkin PD, Bond MW, O'Garra A, Frank G, Lee F, Coffman RL, Zlotnik A, Howard M: Identification of IL-6 as a T cell-derived factor that enhances the proliferative response of thymocytes to IL-4 and phorbol myristate acetate. J Immunol 141:151, 1988

56. Horii Y, Muraguchi A, Suematsu S, Matsuda T, Yoshizaki K, Hirano T, Kishimoto T: Regulation of BSF-2/IL-6 production by human mononuclear cells. Macrophage-dependent synthesis of BSF-2/IL-6 by T cells. J Immunol 141:1529, 1988

57. Houssiau FA, Bukasa K, Sindic CJM, Van Damme J, Van Snick J: Elevated levels of the 26k human hybridoma growth factor (interleukin 6) in cerebrospinal fluid of patients with acute infection of the central nervous system. Clin Exp Immunol 71:320, 1988

58. Houssiau FA, Coulie PG, Olive D, Van Snick J: Synergistic activation of human T cells by interleukin 1 and interleukin 6. Eur J Immunol 18:653, 1988

59. Ikebuchi K, Wong GG, Clark SC, Ihle JN, Hirai Y, Ogawa M: Interleukin 6 enhancement of interleukin 3-dependent proliferation of multipotential hemopoietic progenitors. Proc Natl Acad Sci USA 84:9035, 1987

59a.Ishibashi T, Kimura H, Uchida T, Kariyone S, Friese P, Burstein SA: Human interleukin 6 is a direct promoter of maturation of megakaryocytes in vitro. Proc Natl Acad Sci USA 86:5953, 1989

60. Jablons DM, Mule JJ, McIntosh JK, Sehgal PB, May LT, Huang CM, Rosenberg SA, Lotze MT: IL-6/IFN-β_2 as a circulating hormone. Induction by cytokine administration in humans. J Immunol 142:1542, 1989

61. Jambou RC, Snouwaert JN, Bishop GA, Stebbins JR, Frelinger JA, Fowlkes DM: High-level expression of a bioengineered, cysteine-free hepatocyte-stimulating factor (interleukin 6)-like protein. Proc Natl Acad Sci USA 85:9426, 1988

62. Jirik FR, Podor TJ, Hirano T, Kishimoto T, Loskutoff DJ, Carson DA, Lotz M: Bacterial lipopolysaccharide and inflammatory mediators augment IL-6 secretion by human endothelial cells. J Immunol 142:144, 1989

63. Kasid A, Director EP, Rosenberg SA: Induction of endogenous cytokine-mRNA in circulating peripheral blood mononuclear cells by IL-2 administration to cancer patients. J Immunol 143:736, 1989

64. Katz Y, Strunk RC: IL-1 and tumor necrosis factor similarities and differences in stimulation of expression of alternative pathway of complement and IFN-β_2/IL-6 genes in human fibroblasts. J Immunol 142:3862, 1989

65. Kawano M, Hirano T, Matsuda T, Taga T, Horii Y, Iwato K, Asaoku H, Tang B, Tanabe O, Tanaka H, Kuramoto A, Kishimoto T: Autocrine generation and requirement of BSF-2/IL-6 for human multiple myelomas. Nature (London) 332:83, 1988

66. Kawano M, Tanaka H, Ishikawa H, Nobuyoshi M, Iwato K, Asaoku H, Tanabe O, Kuramoto A: Interleukin-1 accelerates autocrine growth of myeloma cells through interleukin-6 in human myeloma. Blood 73:2145, 1989

67. Kelker HC, Le J, Rubin BY, Yip YK, Nagler C, Vilček J: Three molecular weight forms of natural human interferon-gamma revealed by immunoprecipitation with monoclonal antibody. J Biol Chem 259:4301, 1984

68. Kirnbauer R, Köck A, Schwarz T, Urbanski A, Krutmann J, Borth W, Damm D, Shipley G, Ansel JC, Luger TA: IFN-β_2, B cell differentiation factor 2, or hybridoma growth factor (IL-6) is expressed and released by human epidermal cells and epidermoid carcinoma cell lines. J Immunol 142:1922, 1989

69. Kishimoto T, Hirano T: Molecular regulation of B lymphocyte response. Ann Rev Immunol 6:485, 1988

70. Kishimoto T, Taga T, Yamazaki K, Kawanishi K, Hirata Y, Yahata H, Hirano T: High and low affinity receptors for BSF-2/IL-6 and their organization (abstr 8912). FASEB J 2:A1830, 1988

71. Klein B, Zhang X-G, Jourdan M, Content J, Houssiau F, Aarden L, Piechaczyk M, Bataille R: Paracrine rather than autocrine regulation of myeloma-cell growth and differentiation by interleukin-6. Blood 73:517, 1989

72. Kohase M, Henriksen-DeStefano D, May LT, Vilček J, Sehgal PB: Induction of beta$_2$-interferon by tumor necrosis factor: a homeostatic mechanism in the control of cell proliferation. Cell 45:659, 1986

73. Kohase M, May LT, Tamm I, Vilček J, Sehgal PB: A cytokine network in human diploid fibroblasts: interactions of beta-interferons, tumor necrosis factor, platelet-derived growth factor, and interleukin-1. Mol Cell Biol 7:273, 1987

74. Kohase M, Zhang Y, Lin J-X, Yamazaki S, Sehgal PB, Vilček J: Interleukin-1 can inhibit interferon-beta synthesis and its antiviral action: comparison with tumor necrosis factor. J Interferon Res 8:559, 1988

75. Koike K, Nakahata T, Takagi M, Kobayashi T, Ishiguro A, Tsuji K, Naganuma K, Okano A, Akiyama Y, Akabane T: Synergism of BSF-2/interleukin 6 and interleukin 3 on development of multipotential hemopoietic progenitors in serum-free culture. J Exp Med 168:879, 1988

76. Koj A: Definition and classification of acute-phase proteins. In The Acute-Phase Response to Injury and Infection, edited by Gordon AH, Koj A, p 139, Amsterdam, Oxford, and New York, Elsevier, 1985

77. Koj A, Gauldie J, Sweeney GD, Regoeczi E, Sauder DN: A simple bioassay for monocyte-derived hepatocyte stimulating factor: increased synthesis of alpha 2-macroglobulin and reduced synthesis of albumin by cultured rat hepatocytes. J Immunol Methods 76:317, 1985

77a.Kunimoto DY, Nordan RP, Strober W: IL-6 is a potent cofactor of IL-1 in IgM synthesis and of IL-5 in IgA synthesis. J Immunol 143:2230, 1989

78. Le J, Vilček J: Tumor necrosis factor and interleukin 1: cytokines with multiple overlapping biological activities. Lab Invest 56:234, 1987

79. Le J, Fredrickson G, Reis LFL, Diamantstein T, Hirano T, Kishimoto T, Vilček J: Interleukin 2-dependent and interleukin 2-independent pathways of regulation of thymocyte function by interleukin 6. Proc Natl Acad Sci USA 85:8643, 1988

80. Le J, Reis LFL, Vilček J: Tumor necrosis factor and interleukin 1 can act as essential growth factors in a murine plasmacytoma line. Lymphokine Res 7:99, 1988

81. Le J, Fredrickson G, Pollack M, Vilček J: Activation of thymocytes and T cells by interleukin 6. Ann NY Acad Sci 557:444, 1989

82. Leary AG, Ikebuchi K, Hirai Y, Wong GG, Yang YC, Clark SC, Ogawa M: Synergism between interleukin-6 and interleukin-3 in supporting proliferation of human hematopoietic stem cells: comparison with interleukin-1 alpha. Blood 71:1759, 1988

83. Leeuwenberg JFM, Van Damme J, Jeunhomme GMAA, Buurman WA: Interferon-beta$_1$, an intermediate in the tumor necrosis factor alpha-induced increased MHC class I expression and an autocrine regulator of the constitutive MHC class I expression. J Exp Med 166:1180, 1987

84. Lew W, Oppenheim JJ, Matsushima K: Analysis of the suppression of IL-1α and IL-1β production in human peripheral blood mononuclear adherent cells by a glucocorticoid hormone. J Immunol 140:1895, 1988

85. Lotz M, Jirik F, Kabouridis P, Tsoukas C, Hirano T, Kishimoto T, Carson DA: B cell stimulating factor 2/interleukin 6 is a costimulant for human thymocytes and T lymphocytes. J Exp Med 167:1253, 1988

86. Lotz M, Vaughan JH, Carson DA: Effect of neuropeptides on

production of inflammatory cytokines by human monocytes. Science 241:1218, 1988

86a. Luger TA, Krutmann J, Kirnbauer R, Urbanski A, Schwarz T, Klappacher G, Köck A, Micksche M, Malejczyk J, Schauer E, May LT, Sehgal PB: IFN-β_2/IL-6 augments the activity of human natural killer cells. J Immunol 143:1206, 1989

87. Marinkovic S, Jahreis GP, Wong GG, Baumann H: IL-6 modulates the synthesis of a specific set of acute phase plasma proteins *in vivo*. J Immunol 142:808, 1989

88. Matsuda T, Hirano T, Kishimoto T: Establishment of an interleukin 6 (IL-6)/B cell stimulatory factor 2-dependent cell line and preparation of anti-IL-6 monoclonal antibodies. Eur J Immunol 18:951, 1988

89. Matsuda T, Hirano T, Nagasawa S, Kishimoto T: Identification of α2-macroglobulin as a carrier protein for IL-6. J Immunol 142:148, 1989

90. May LT, Helfgott DC, Sehgal PB: Anti-beta-interferon antibodies inhibit the increased expression of HLA-B7 mRNA in tumor necrosis factor-treated human fibroblasts: structural studies of the beta$_2$ interferon involved. Proc Natl Acad Sci USA 83:8957, 1986

91. May LT, Ghrayeb J, Santhanam U, Tatter SB, Sthoeger Z, Helfgott DC, Chiorazzi N, Grieninger G, Sehgal PB: Synthesis and secretion of multiple forms of beta$_2$-interferon/B-cell differentiation factor 2/hepatocyte stimulating factor by human fibroblasts and monocytes. J Biol Chem 263:7760, 1988

92. May LT, Santhanam U, Tatter SB, Bhardwaj N, Ghrayeb J, Sehgal PB: Phosphorylation of secreted forms of human beta$_2$-interferon/hepatocyte stimulating factor/interleukin-6. Biochem Biophys Res Commun 152:1144, 1988

93. McIntosh JK, Jablons DM, Mule JJ, Nordan RP, Rudikoff S, Lotze MT, Rosenberg SA: *In vivo* induction of IL-6 by administration of exogenous cytokines and detection of *de novo* serum levels of IL-6 in tumor-bearing mice. J Immunol 143:162, 1989

94. McKenzie D: Alloantigen presentation by B cells. Requirement for IL-1 and IL-6. J Immunol 141:2907, 1988

95. Miyaura C, Onozaki K, Akiyama Y, Taniyama T, Hirano T, Kishimoro T, Suda T: Recombinant human interleukin 6 (B-cell stimulatory factor 2) is a potent inducer of differentiation of mouse myeloid leukemia cells (M1). FEBS Lett 234:17, 1988

96. Mock BA, Nordan RP, Justice MJ, Kozak C, Jenkins NA, Copeland NG, Clark SC, Wong GG, Rudikoff S: The murine *IL-6* gene maps to the proximal region of chromosome 5. J Immunol 142:1372, 1989

97. Morrone G, Ciliberto G, Oliviero S, Arcone R, Dente L, Content J, Cortese R: Recombinant interleukin 6 regulates the transcriptional activation of a set of human acute phase genes. J Biol Chem 263:12554, 1988

98. Muraguchi A, Kishimoto T, Miki Y, Kuritani T, Kaieda T, Yoshizaki K, Yamamura Y: T cell-replacing factor (TRF)-induced IgG secretion in a human B blastoid cell line and demonstration of acceptors for TRF. J Immunol 127:412, 1981

99. Muraguchi A, Hirano T, Tang B, Matsuda T, Horii Y, Nakajima K, Kishimoto T: The essential role of B cell stimulatory factor 2 (BSF-2/IL-6) for the terminal differentiation of B cells. J Exp Med 167:332, 1988

100. Nakajima K, Martinez-Maza O, Hirano T, Breen EC, Nishanian PG, Salazar-Gonzalez JF, Fahey JL, Kishimoto T: Induction of IL-6 (B cell stimulatory factor-2/IFN-β_2) production by HIV. J Immunol 142:531, 1989

101. Namba Y, Hanaoka M: Immunocytology of cultured IgM-forming cells of mouse. I Requirement of phagocytic cell factor for the growth of IgM-forming tumor cells in tissue culture. J Immunol 109:1193, 1972

102. Navarro S, Debili N, Bernaudin J-F, Vainchenker W, Doly J: Regulation of the expression of IL-6 in human monocytes. J Immunol 142:4339, 1989

103. Neta R, Vogel SN, Sipe JD, Wong GG, Nordan RP: Comparison of *in vivo* effects of human recombinant IL-1 and human recombinant IL-6 in mice. Lymphokine Res 7:403, 1988

104. Nijsten MWN, DeGroot ER, Ten Duis HJ, Klasen HJ, Hack CE, Aarden LA: Serum levels of interleukin-6 and acute phase responses. Lancet ii:921, 1987

105. Nishimoto N, Yoshizaki K, Tagoh H, Monden M, Kishimoto S, Hirano T, Kishimoto T: Elevation of serum interleukin 6 prior to acute phase proteins on the inflammation by surgical operation. Clin Immunol Immunopathol 50:399, 1989

106. Noma T, Mizuta T, Rosen A, Hirano T, Kishimoto T, Honjo T: Enhancement of the interleukin 2 receptor expression on T cells by multiple B-lymphotropic lymphokines. Immunol Lett 15:249, 1987

107. Nordan RP, Potter M: A macrophage-derived factor required by plasmacytomas for survival and proliferation *in vitro*. Science 233:566, 1986

108. Nordan RP, Pumphrey JG, Rudikoff S: Purification and NH$_2$-terminal sequence of a plasmacytoma growth factor derived from the murine macrophage cell line P388D1. J Immunol 139:813, 1987

109. Okada M, Sakaguchi N, Yoshimura N, Hara H, Shimizu K, Yoshida N, Yoshizaki K, Kishimoto S, Yamamura Y, Kishimoto T: B cell growth factors and B cell differentiation factor from human T hybridomas. Two distinct kinds of B cell growth factor and their synergism in B cell proliferation. J Exp Med 157:583, 1983

110. Okada M, Kitahara M, Kishimoto S, Matsuda T, Hirano T, Kishimoto T: IL-6/BSF-2 functions as a killer helper factor in the *in vitro* induction of cytotoxic T cells. J Immunol 141:1543, 1988

111. Onozaki K, Akiyama Y, Okano A, Hirano T., Kishimoto T, Hashimoto T, Yoshizawa K, Taniyama T: Synergistic regulatory effects of interleukin 6 and interleukin 1 on the growth and differentiation of human and mouse myeloid leukemic cell lines. Cancer Res 49:3602, 1989

112. Paul WE, Laughlin CA, Johnston MI: Report of nomenclature discussion. Ann NY Acad Sci 557:579, 1989

113. Perlmutter DH, Dinarello CA, Punsal PI, Colten HR: Cachectin/tumor necrosis factor regulates hepatic acute-phase gene expression. J Clin Invest 78:1349, 1986

114. Pober JS: The multiple roles of tumor necrosis factor. Ann Inst Pasteur/Immunol 139:337, 1988

115. Poupart P, Vandenabeele P, Cayphas S, Van Snick J, Haegeman G, Kruys V, Fiers W, Content J: B cell growth modulating and differentiating activity of recombinant human 26-Kd protein (BSF-2, HuIFN-beta$_2$, HPFG). EMBO J 6:1219, 1987

116. Ramadori G, Sipe JD, Dinarello CA, Mizel SB, Colten HR: Pretranslational modulation of acute phase hepatic protein synthesis by murine recombinant interleukin 1 (IL-1) and purified human IL-1. J Exp Med 162:930, 1985

117. Ramadori G, Van Damme J, Rieder H, Meyer zum Büschenfelde K-H: Interleukin 6, the third mediator of acute-phase reaction, modulates hepatic protein synthesis in human and mouse. Comparison with interleukin 1β and tumor necrosis factor-α. Eur J Immunol 18:1259, 1988

118. Ray A, Tatter SB, May LT, Sehgal PB: Activation of the human "beta$_2$-interferon/hepatocyte-stimulating factor/interleukin 6" promoter by cytokines, viruses, and second messenger agonists. Proc Natl Acad Sci USA 85:6701, 1988

119. Reis LFL, Le J, Hirano T, Kishimoto T, Vilček J: Antiviral action of tumor necrosis factor in human fibroblasts is not mediated by B cell stimulatory factor 2/IFN-beta$_2$, and is inhibited by specific antibodies to IFN-beta. J Immunol 140:1566, 1988

120. Reis LFL, Lee TH, Vilček J: Tumor necrosis factor acts synergistically with autocrine interferon-β and increases interferon-β mRNA levels in human fibroblasts. J Biol Chem, 264:1635, 1989

121. Rennick D, Jackson J, Yang G, Wideman J, Lee F, Hudak S: Interleukin-6 interacts with interleukin-4 and other hematopoietic growth factors to selectively enhance the growth of megakaryocytic, erhthroid, myeloid, and multipotential progenitor cells. Blood 73:1828, 1989

122. Revel M: Genetic and functional diversity of interferons in man. In Interferon 1983, Vol 5, edited by Gresser I, p 205. London, Academic Press, 1983

123. Revel M, Zilberstein A, Ruggieri R, Chen L, Mory Y, Rubinstein M, Michalevicz R: Human interferon beta$_2$: a multifunctional cytokine. In Tumor Necrosis Factor/Cachectin and Related Cytokines, edited by Bonavida B, Gifford GE, Kirchner H, Old LJ, p 252. Karger, 1988

124. Ritchie DG, Fuller GM: Hepatocyte-stimulating factor: a monocyte-derived acute-phase regulatory protein. Ann NY Acad Sci 408:490, 1983

125. Sachs L, Lotem J, Shabo Y: The molecular regulators of macrophage and granulocyte development. Role of MGI-2/IL-6. Ann NY Acad Sci 557:417, 1989

126. Sagar AD, Sehgal PB, Slate DS, Ruddle FH: Multiple human beta interferon genes. J Exp Med 156:744, 1982

127. Saiki O, Ralph P: Clonal differences in response to T cell replacing factor (TRF) for IgM secretion and TRF receptors in a human B lymphoblast cell line. Eur J Immunol 13:31, 1983

128. Sato T, Matsui H, Shibahara S, Kobayashi T, Morinaga Y, Kashima N, Yamasaki S, Hamuro J, Taniguchi T: New approaches for the high-level expression of human interleukin-2 cDNA in *Escherichia coli*. J Biochem 101:525, 1987

129. Satoh T, Nakamura S, Taga T, Matsuda T, Hirano T, Kishimoto T, Kaziro Y: Induction of neuronal differentiation in PC12 cells by B-cell stimulatory factor 2/interleukin 6. Mol Cell Biol 8:3546, 1988

130. Sehgal PB: The interferon genes. Biochim Biophys Acta 695:17, 1982

131. Sehgal PB, Sagar AD: Heterogeneity of poly(I)poly(C)-induced human fibroblast interferon mRNA species. Nature (London) 288:95, 1980

132. Sehgal PB, May LT: Human interferon-beta$_2$. J Interferon Res 7:521, 1987

133. Sehgal PB, Zilberstein A, Ruggieri M-R, May LT, Ferguson-Smith A, Slate DL, Revel M, Ruddle FH: Human chromosome 7 carries the beta$_2$ interferon gene. Proc Natl Acad Sci USA 83:5219, 1986

134. Sehgal PB, May LT, Tamm I, Vilček J: Human beta$_2$ interferon and B-cell differentiation factor BSF-2 are identical. Science 235:731, 1987

135. Sehgal PB, Walther Z, Tamm I: Rapid enhancement of beta$_2$-interferon/B-cell differentiation factor BSF-2 gene expression in human fibroblasts by diacylglycerols and the calcium ionophore A23187. Proc Natl Acad Sci USA 84:3663, 1987

136. Sehgal PB, Helfgott DC, Santhanam U, Tatter SB, Clarick RH, Ghrayeb J, May LT: Regulation of the acute phase and immune responses in viral disease. Enhanced expression of the beta$_2$ - interferon/hepatocyte-stimulating factor/interleukin 6 gene in virus-infected human fibroblasts. J Exp Med 167:1951, 1988

137. Sehgal PB, Greininger G, Tosato G (Editors): Regulation of the Acute Phase and Immune Responses: Interleukin-6. Ann NY Acad Sci V. 557:1–583, 1989

138. Shabo Y, Lotem J, Rubinstein M, Revel M, Clark SC, Wolf SF, Kamen R, Sachs L: The myeloid blood cell differentiation-inducing protein MGI-2A is interleukin 6. Blood 72:2070, 1988

139. Shenkin A, Fraser WD, Series J, Winstanley FP, McCartney AC, Burns HJG, Van Damme J: The serum interleukin 6 response to elective surgery. Lymphokine Res 8:123, 1989

140. Shimizu K, Hirano T, Ishibashi K, Nakano N, Taga T, Sugamura K, Yamamura Y, Kishimoto T: Immortalization of BGDF (BCGF II)- and BCDF-producing T cells by human T cell leukemia virus (HTLV) and characterization of human BGDF (BCGF II). J Immunol 134:1728, 1985

141. Shimizu S, Yoshioka R, Hirose Y, Sugai S, Tachibana J, Konda S: Establishment of two interleukin 6 (B cell stimulatory factor 2/interferon β_2)-dependent human bone marrow-derived myeloma cell lines. J Exp Med 169:339, 1989

142. Shrestha K, Hiramoto RN, Ghanta VK: Regulation of MOPC 104E by T cells and growth factors induced by *C parvum* stimulation. Int J Cancer 33:845, 1984

143. Siegall CB, Chaudhary VK, FitzGerald DJ, Pastan I: Cytotoxic activity of an interleukin 6-*Pseudomonas* exotoxin fusion protein on human myeloma cells. Proc Natl Acad Sci USA 85:9738, 1988

144. Sims JE, March CJ, Cosman D, Widmer MB, MacDonald HR, McMahan CJ, Grubin CE, Wignall JM, Jackson JL, Call SM, Friend D, Alpert AR, Gillis S, Urdal DL, Dower SK; cDNA expression cloning of the IL-1 receptor, a member of the immunoglobulin superfamily. Science 241:585, 1988

145. Sironi M, Breviario F, Proserpio P, Biondi A, Vecchi A, Van Damme J, Dejana E, Mantovani A: IL-1 stimulates IL-6 production in endothelial cells. J Immunol 142:549, 1989

145a.Suematsu S, Matsuda T, Aozasa K, Akira S, Nakano N, Ohno S, Miyazaki J-I, Yamamura K-I, Hirano T, Kishimoto T: IgG1 plasmacytosis in interleukin 6 transgenic mice. Proc Natl Acad Sci USA 86:7547, 1989

146. Sugasawara RJ, Cahoon BE, Karu AE: The influence of murine macrophage-conditioned medium on cloning efficiency, antibody synthesis and growth rate of hybridomas. J Immunol Methods 79:263, 1985

147. Sutton MGJ, Mercier L, Giuliani E, Lie JT: Atrial myxomas. A review of clinical experience in 40 patients. Mayo Clin Proc 55:371, 1980

148. Tabibzadeh SS, Santhanam U, Sehgal PB, May LT: Cytokine-induced production of IFN-β/IL-6 by freshly explanted human endometrial stromal cells. Modulation by estradiol-17β. J Immunol 142:3134, 1989

149. Taga T, Kawanishi Y, Hardy RR, Hirano T, Kishimoto T: Receptors for B cell stimulatory factor 2. Quantitation, specificity, distribution, and regulation of their expression. J Exp Med 166:967, 1987

149a.Taga T, Hibi M, Hirata Y, Yamasaki K, Yasukawa K, Matsuda T, Hiaron T, Kishimoto T: Interleukin-6 triggers the association of its receptor with a possible signal transducer, gp130. Cell 58:573, 1989

150. Takai Y, Wong GG, Clark SC, Burakoff SJ, Herrmann SH: B cell stimulatory factor-2 is involved in the differentiation of cytotoxic T lymphocytes. J Immunol 140:508, 1988

151. Takatsuki F, Okano A, Suzuki C, Chieda R, Takahara Y, Hirano T, Kishimoto T, Hamuro J, Akiyama Y: Human recombinant IL-6/B cell stimulatory factor 2 augments murine antigen-specific antibody responses *in vitro* and *in vivo*. J Immunol 141:3072, 1988

152. Tanabe O, Akira S, Kamiya T, Wong GG, Hirano T, Kishimoto T: Genomic structure of the murine IL-6 gene. High degree conservation of potential regulatory sequences between mouse and human. J Immunol 141:3875, 1988

153. Teranishi T, Hirano T, Arima N, Onoue K: Human helper T cell factor(s) (ThF) II. Induction of IgG production in B lymphoblastoid cell lines and identification of T cell-replacing factor (TRF)-like factors. J Immunol 128:1903, 1982

154. Tosato G, Pike SE: Interferon-beta$_2$/interleukin 6 is a co-stimulant for human T lymphocytes. J Immunol 141:1556, 1988

155. Tosato G, Seamon KB, Goldman ND, Sehgal PB, May LT, Washington GC, Jones KD, Pike SE: Monocyte-derived human B-cell growth factor identified as interferon-beta$_2$ (BSF-2, IL-6). Science 239:502, 1988

156. Tovey MG, Content J, Gresser I, Gugenheim J, Blanchard B, Guymarho J, Poupart P, Gigou M, Shaw A, Fiers W: Genes for IFN-β_2 (IL-6), tumor necrosis factor, and IL-1 are expressed at high levels in the organs of normal individuals. J Immunol 141:3106, 1988

157. Ulich TR, del Castillo J, Guo K: *In vivo* hematologic effects of recombinant interleukin-6 on hematopoiesis and circulating numbers of RBCs and WBCs. Blood 73:108, 1989

158. Uyttenhove C, Coulie PG, Van Snick J: T cell growth and differentiation induced by interleukin-HP1/IL-6, the murine hybridoma/plasmacytoma growth factor. J Exp Med 167:1417, 1988

159. Van Damme J, Cayphas S, Opdenakker G, Billiau A, Van Snick J: Interleukin 1 and poly(rI)poly(rC) induce production of a hybridoma growth factor by human fibroblasts. Eur J Immunol 17:1, 1987

160. Van Damme J, De Ley M, Van Snick J, Dinarello CA, Billiau A: The role of interferon-beta$_1$ and the 26-kDa protein (interferon-beta$_2$) as mediators of the antiviral effect of interleukin 1 and tumor necrosis factor. J Immunol 139:1867, 1987

161. Van Damme J, Opdenakker G, Simpson RJ, Rubira MR, Cayphas S, Vink A, Billiau A, Van Snick J: Identification of the human 26-kD protein, interferon beta$_2$ (IFN-beta$_2$), as a B cell hybridoma/plasmacytoma growth factor induced by interleukin 1 and tumor necrosis factor. J Exp Med 165:914, 1987

162. Van Damme J, Schaafsma MR, Fibbe WE, Falkenburg JHF, Opdenakker G, Billiau A: Simultaneous production of interleukin 6, interferon-β and colony-stimulating activity by fibroblasts after viral and bacterial infection. Eur J Immunol 19:163, 1989

163. Van der Meer JWM, Helle M, Aarden L: Comparison of the effects of recombinant interleukin 6 and recombinant interleukin 1 on nonspecific resistance to infection. Eur J Immunol 19:413, 1989

164. Van Oers MHJ, Van der Heyden AAPAM, Aarden LA: Interleukin 6 (IL-6) in serum and urine of renal transplant recipients. Clin Exp Immunol 71:314, 1988

165. Van Snick J, Cayphas S, Vink A, Uyttenhove C, Coulie PG, Rubira MR, Simpson RJ: Purification and NH$_2$-terminal amino acid sequence of a T-cell-derived lymphokine with growth factor activity for B-cell hybridomas. Proc Natl Acad Sci USA 83:9679, 1986

166. Van Snick J, Vink A, Cayphas S, Uyttenhove C: Interleukin-HP1, a T cell-derived hybridoma growth factor that supports the *in vitro* growth of murine plasmacytomas. J Exp Med 165:641, 1987

167. Van Snick J, Cayphas S, Szikora J, Renauld J, Van Roost E, Boon T, Simpson RJ: cDNA cloning of murine interleukin-HP1: homology with human interleukin 6. Eur J Immunol 18:193, 1988

168. Vankelecom H, Carmeliet P, Van Damme J, Billiau A, Denef C: Production of interleukin-6 by folliculo-stellate cells of the anterior pituitary gland in a histiotypic cell aggregate culture system. Neuroendocrinology 49:102, 1989

168a. Vercelli D, Jabara HH, Arai K-I, Yokota T, Geha RS: Endogenous interleukin 6 plays an obligatory role in interleukin 4-dependent human IgE synthesis. Eur J Immunol 19:1419, 1989

169. Vilček J: Interferons. In Handbook of Experimental Pharmacology, Peptide Growth Factors and Their Receptors, edited by Sporn MB, Roberts AB, Berlin, Springer-Verlag, in press 1990

170. Vilček J, Palombella VJ, Zhang Y, Lin J-X, Feinman R, Reis LFL, Le J: Mechanisms and significance of the mitogenic and antiviral actions of TNF. Ann Inst Pasteur/Immunol 139:281, 1988

171. Vink A, Coulie PG, Wauters P, Nordan RP, Van Snick J: B cell growth and differentiation activity of interleukin-HP1 and related murine plasmacytoma growth factors. Synergy with interleukin 1. Eur J Immunol 18:607, 1988

172. Waage A, Brandtzaeg P, Halstensen A, Kierulf P, Espevik T: The complex pattern of cytokines in serum from patients with meningococcal septic shock. Association between interleukin 6, interleukin 1, and fatal outcome. J Exp Med 169:333, 1989

173. Waage A, Kaufmann C, Espevik T, Husby G: Interleukin-6 in synovial fluid from patients with arthritis. Clin Immunol Immunopathol 50:394, 1989

174. Walker KZ, Gibson J, Axiak SM, Prentice RL: Potentiation of hybridoma production by the use of mouse fibroblast conditioned media. J Immunol Methods 88:75, 1986.

175. Walther Z, May LT, Sehgal PB: Transcriptional regulation of the interferon-beta$_2$/B cell differentiation factor BSF-2/hepatocyte-stimulating factor gene in human fibroblasts by other cytokines. J Immunol 140:974, 1988

176. Weissenbach J, Chernajovsky Y, Zeevi M, Shulman L, Soreq H, Nir U, Wallach D, Perricaudet M, Tiollais P, Revel M: Two interferon mRNAs in human fibroblasts: *In vitro* translation and *Escherichia coli* cloning studies. Proc Natl Acad Sci USA 77:7152, 1980

177. Weissmann C, Weber H: The interferon genes. In Progr Nucl Acid Res Mol Biol, edited by Cohn WE, Moldave K, 33:251, Orlando, Academic Press, 1986

178. Woloski BMRNJ, Fuller GM: Identification and partial characterization of hepatocyte-stimulating factor from leukemia cell lines: comparison with interleukin 1. Proc Natl Acad Sci USA 82:1443, 1985

179. Woloski BMRNJ, Smith EM, Meyer WJ III, Fuller GM, Blalock JE: Corticotropin-releasing activity of monokines. Science 230:1035, 1985

180. Wong GG, Clark SC: Multiple actions of interleukin 6 within a cytokine network. Immunol Today 9:137, 1988

181. Wong GG, Witek-Giannotti JS, Temple PA, Kriz R, Ferenz C, Hewick RM, Clark SC, Ikebuchi K, Ogawa M: Stimulation of murine hemopoietic colony formation by human IL-6. J Immunol 140:3040, 1988

182. Yamasaki K, Taga T, Hirata Y, Yawata H, Kawanishi Y, Seed B, Taniguchi T, Hirano T, Kishimoto T: Cloning and expression of the human interleukin-6 (BSF-2/IFN-beta$_2$) receptor. Science 241:825, 1988

183. Yasukawa K, Hirano T, Watanabe Y, Muratani K, Matsuda T, Nakai S, Kishimoto T: Structure and expression of human B cell stimulatory factor-2 (BSF-2/IL-6) gene. EMBO J 6:2939, 1987

184. Zhang Y, Lin J-X, Vilček J: Synthesis of interleukin 6 (interferon-beta$_2$/B cell stimulatory factor 2) in human fibroblasts is triggered by an increase in intracellular cyclic AMP. J Biol Chem 263:6177, 1988

185. Zhang Y, Lin J-X, Yip YK, Vilček J: Enhancement of cAMP levels and of protein kinase activity by tumor necrosis factor and interleukin 1 in human fibroblasts: role in the induction of interleukin 6. Proc Natl Acad Sci USA 85:6802, 1988

186. Zilberstein A, Ruggieri R, Korn JH, Revel M: Structure and expression of cDNA and genes for human interferon-beta$_2$, a distinct species inducible by growth-stimulatory cytokines. EMBO J 5:2529, 1986

From: *Pathology Reviews • 1990* Edited by: E. Rubin and I. Damjanov Copyright © 1990 The Humana Press Inc., Clifton, NJ

Biology of Disease

IgA Nephropathy: Pathogenesis of the Most Common Form of Glomerulonephritis

STEVEN N. EMANCIPATOR, AND MICHAEL E. LAMM

Institute of Pathology, Case Western Reserve University, Cleveland, Ohio

Introduction
Definition and Clinical Features
Demographics and Genetics
Clinical Immunology of IgA Nephropathy
Therapy
The Mucosal Immune System and Properties of IgA
Clearance of IgA Immune Complexes
Pathogenesis of IgA Nephropathy
Pathophysiology
Role of Different Classes of Antibody
Nature of the Antigen in IgA Nephropathy
Antigen as a Factor in Nephritogenesis
Prospects for the Future
Conclusions

INTRODUCTION

IgA nephropathy (IgAN) is being recognized increasingly as a common form of glomerulonephritis with progressive potential (17, 29, 42). Our initial goal here is briefly to consider the definition, clinical features, and major clinical problems of IgAN, and the special characteristics of the secretory immune system, the major source of IgA in the body. Then follows a critical discussion of experimental and clinical observations which provide a conceptual framework for a scheme of pathogenesis based on distinctive features of immunity in mucous membranes and altered regulation of mucosal immune responses due to a defect in mucosal IgG/IgM tolerogenesis. We believe that, in the main, IgAN is an immune complex disease resulting from a poorly controlled mucosal immune response to environmental antigens to which the host is chronically subject. The deposited IgA is likely antibody to viral or dietary antigen. Evidence exists for other mechanisms, which we consider less likely.

The overall frequency of IgAN as determined by renal biopsy varies widely in different geographic regions, ranging from 5 to 10% in North America, the United Kingdom, and northern Europe, through 25 to 35% in southern Europe and Australia, to 50% or more in Asia (17, 42). Although not the only elements, biopsy policy

and health screening standards strongly influence this rate. Patients with low grade manifestations such as microhematuria and/or mild proteinuria are seldom biopsied in the United States, but frequently biopsied in Japan, particularly if the signs are persistent.

The important influence of urinalysis screening and biopsy policy is illustrated by the studies of Propper *et al.* (116) in Scotland and Woo *et al.* (171) in Singapore. In Aberdeen, where 26% of renal biopsies are from cases of IgAN, patients with persistent microhematuria are routinely biopsied (116); however, in another center in the United Kingdom, where the biopsy policy is less aggressive, only 4% of all glomerulonephritis is thought to be IgAN (143). Propper *et al.* (116) report that 37% of patients with asymptomatic microhematuria have IgAN diagnosed at renal biopsy; in another study from the United Kingdom, the figure was 54% (99). In Singapore, males, who are actively screened and biopsied in relation to military duty, represent 85% of the asymptomatic cases of IgAN diagnosed since females are only biopsied if overtly symptomatic (171). Japan has an aggressive urinalysis screening policy for all students, which may help explain the lower male:female ratio in Japanese IgAN patients compared to other countries (H. Sakai, personal communication).

The effect of biopsy policy on the prevalence of IgAN can be illustrated in the following way. In regions with a conservative biopsy policy and/or no active screening program, only symptomatic patients with obvious manifestations of renal disease, such as macrohematuria or heavy proteinuria, are biopsied. Hence, fewer patients with IgAN are actually diagnosed. The apparent incidence of IgAN will be inversely correlated with the frequency of severe signs among patients diagnosed as having the disease because the mild cases are being missed. On the other hand, in geographic areas with active urinalysis screening programs and a policy of performing renal biopsies for milder signs such as persistent microhematuria or low grade proteinuria, patients with these milder manifestations will be biopsied. In this case, more IgAN will be found (higher prevalence), but there will no longer be an inverse correlation with severity. Such shifts in correlation are observed in the world literature (Fig. 1).

In light of the size of the population of Asia and those parts of Europe where IgAN is the most prevalent form of glomerulonephritis and the likely underrecognition of IgAN in most of the United States, Canada, and the United Kingdom, IgAN is probably the most common form of glomerulonephritis in much of the world (17). Its incidence and progressive nature in many cases indicate that IgAN is an important disease.

DEFINITION AND CLINICAL FEATURES

IgA nephropathy was first described as an entity by Berger and Hinglais (8) based on immunohistologic criteria that included IgG as well as the more prominent

IgA deposits. Indeed, the first report seems prophetic 20 years later since IgAN is now more than ever a histopathologic diagnosis in which the predominant IgA deposits are at once the *sine qua non* and yet but a component of the disease. In addition to the striking deposits of IgA, which by definition must be the most prominent immunoglobulin (Ig), associated IgG and/or IgM are frequent, and C3 is nearly ubiquitous in symptomatic patients (Fig. 2) (42). The distribution of these deposits, while typically confined to the mesangium as originally described, is not a criterion, and some patients with capillary wall deposits, even when these are predominant, are considered to have IgAN. Most patients have mild to moderate mesangial proliferative glomerulonephritis associated with increased mesangial matrix and electrondense deposits demonstrable in the mesangium and paramesangium. However, patients with morphologically normal glomeruli, diffuse or focal endocapillary proliferative glomerulonephritis, crescentic and necrotizing lesions, and even occasional patients with membranous or membranoproliferative glomerulonephritis are included within the spectrum of IgAN when IgA is the predominaant glomerular Ig (Fig. 3) (42).

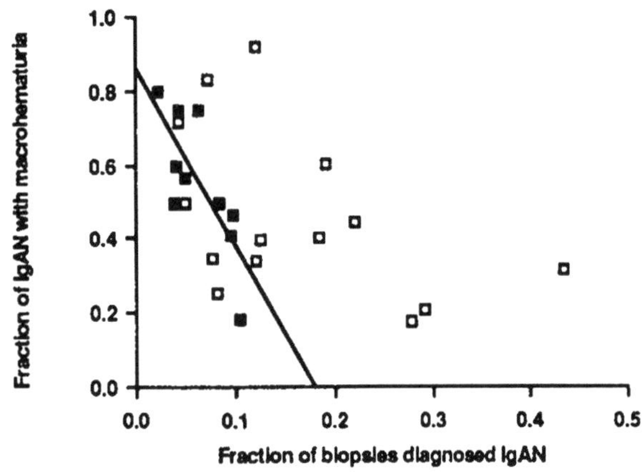

FIG. 1. Scattergrams depict the frequency at which patients with IgAN manifest macrohematuria *versus* the frequency at which IgAN is diagnosed among all renal biopsies. Included are data from 25 series of cases for which complete information was available (42). In studies from North America and the United Kingdom (■), biopsy policy is generally conservative, and where the frequency of diagnosis of IgAN is relatively low, the two frequencies are highly (inversely) correlated (solid line; $p < 0.01$). In contrast, in continental Europe, Australia, and Japan (□), where a more aggressive biopsy policy and more extensive urinalysis screening exist, there is no significant correlation. Since many patients with IgAN have only mild signs such as low grade proteinuria and/or microhematuria, IgAN patients are underrepresented in geographic areas with a conservative biopsy policy; diagnosis depends on severe manifestations such as macrohematuria and/or proteinuria. In countries with a more aggressive biopsy policy, even patients with only mild disease are biopsied, diagnosed, and included in the data. This increases the prevalence of IgAN, and at the same time removes the inverse correlation between macrohematuria (and also severe proteinuria, data not shown) and the rate of diagnosis of IgAN.

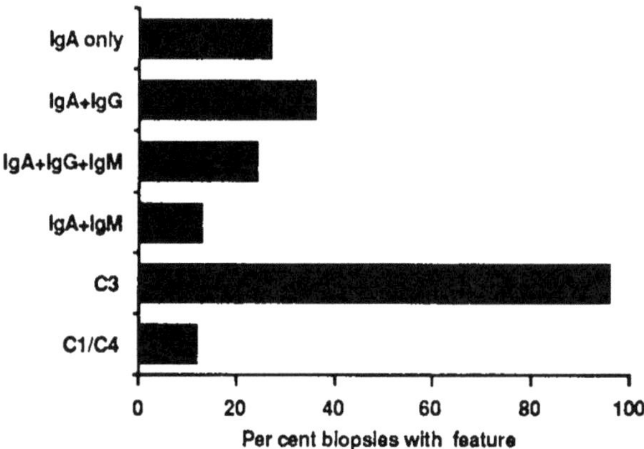

FIG. 2. The frequencies of immunohistochemical findings among 2,000 renal biopsies diagnosed as IgAN (42) are shown. Note that relatively few patients have IgA as the sole immunoglobulin and that virtually all have C3.

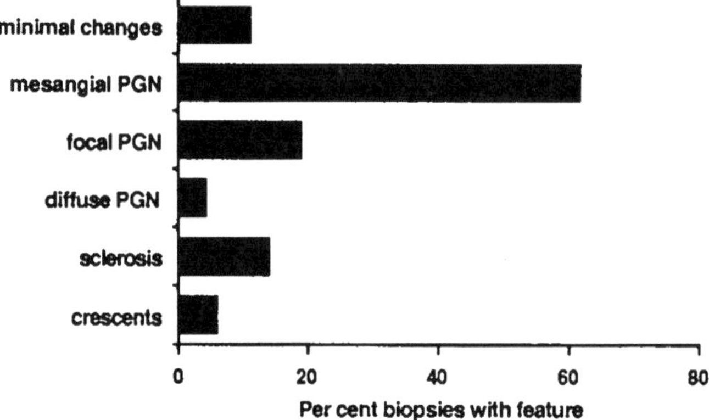

FIG. 3. The frequencies of histologic findings among 2,000 renal biopsies diagnosed as IgAN (42) are illustrated. Biopsies with more than 10% of glomeruli showing crescents or sclerosis are included in these categories. Vascular sclerosis and tubulointerstitial changes, increasingly recognized as important histologic features, are not included since only a few papers give details on these parameters. *PGN*, proliferative glomerulonephritis.

Clinical expression of glomerulopathy in patients with IgAN most consistently includes hematuria. Episodic macrohematuria and persistent microhematuria occur nearly equally; intermittent microhematuria is also common (Fig. 4). Proteinuria, azotemia, hypertension and nephrotic syndrome are all observed in patients with IgAN, with variable severity, in various combinations, and with or without hematuria. Each of these clinical features is the presenting sign or symptom in 5 to 10% of patients. Acute and chronic renal failure are also seen. Recurrent acute renal failure is frequently associated with episodic macrohematuria, often concomitant with viral syndromes (91). Chronic renal failure and progression to end stage kidney were once thought to be rare in IgAN, but are increasingly recognized as greater numbers of patients are being followed for longer periods (10, 17–20, 29, 30, 42, 85, 108, 110, 116, 117, 150, 164, 171, 173). Nearly one-third of patients with IgAN worldwide progress to hemodialysis or renal transplantation over a 20- or 30-year course. Some patients ultimately develop end stage kidney, whereas others enjoy longstanding good health, apparently without regard to the clinical signs and symptoms or histologic pattern of the glomerulonephritis. Association of disease exacerbation with viral syndromes in some patients but not others and the variable demographics further confound attempts to establish a cohesive definition and understanding of what constitutes IgAN (10, 42).

DEMOGRAPHICS AND GENETICS

The demographics of IgAN are interesting from several standpoints. Aside from the geographic differences already mentioned, there are suggestions of a genetic component to IgAN. Although there are no reports from Africa, it appears that the incidence of IgAN in blacks is much lower than the overall incidence of IgAN (76). Racial predilection, on the other hand, is evident in American Indians in new Mexico (144) and Utah (A. Haakenstad, personal communication).

There are also several series which describe familial clustering of patients with IgAN, particularly in geographically isolated or inbred regions (38, 39, 80, 82, 129, 151). Even in the largest of these series, however, the experience is not sufficient to identify a pattern of inheritance or suspect alleles, or to decide if a single or multiple genes underlie predisposition to IgAN (80). The gene cluster most heavily investigated, because of its general import in immune responses rather than by virtue of any genetic clues, is the major histocompatibility (HLA) complex. The DR, DQ and B loci of the HLA complex have been related to risk for IgAN and/or severity or progression of disease; however, critical statistical evaluations of larger series have contradicted the earlier inferences (10, 38, 42, 79, 80, 82, 129, 151, 173). In several cases the original authors themselves recanted their reported associations. The only unchallenged statistically significant associations between genetic loci and IgAN relate C3 and C4 phenotypes to relative risk (173) although there is no functional difference in C3 phenotypes. There is an association between IgAN and C4 null alleles in both the A and B loci. Disordered immunoregulation and a lupus-like syndrome occurs in such patients. Impaired immunoregulation could be related to a propensity for IgA response or failure of mucosal tolerance, but such relationships are speculative at present.

Study of restriction fragment length polymorphism of Ig heavy chain genes is a provocative approach that deserves continued emphasis (34, 79). The one result to date is the implication that heavy chain genes are involved in IgAN since patients are less frequently heterozygous for the switch regions of the IgM gene, with corresponding increases in both homozygous patterns. In addition, the frequency of homozygotes for the 7.4 kb allele of the switch region for IgA1 is greatly increased whereas the frequency of the 6.9 kb allele, homozygous or heterozygous, is markedly reduced in patients with IgAN compared to controls (27).

Among IgAN patients there is a predominance of males in most parts of the world, the major exception being Japan (42). IgAN patients also tend to be young, with most in the second or third decade of life at the time of initial diagnosis. Episodic macrohematuria with mild proteinuria and either transient acute renal failure or minimal insufficiency are most frequent in young males, and these patients infrequently progress to end stage kidney (29, 42).

CLINICAL IMMUNOLOGY OF IgA NEPHROPATHY

Serum IgA levels, particularly polymeric IgA, are significantly elevated in about half the patients with IgAN (36, 37, 42, 170). Increased spontaneous and/or pokeweed mitogen stimulated IgA synthesis has been described by some investigators and denied by others (6, 14, 37, 38, 42, 130, 135, 170). Likewise, T lymphocytes with Fc receptors for IgA and CD4$^+$ and CD8$^+$ subsets of these cells have been reported as increased, normal or decreased (6, 14, 38, 42, 48, 49, 130, 170). Although we later discuss a potential role for kidney-binding lectins or lectin-like compounds in the pathogenesis of IgAN, it is worth noting here that if the lectins were of appropriate

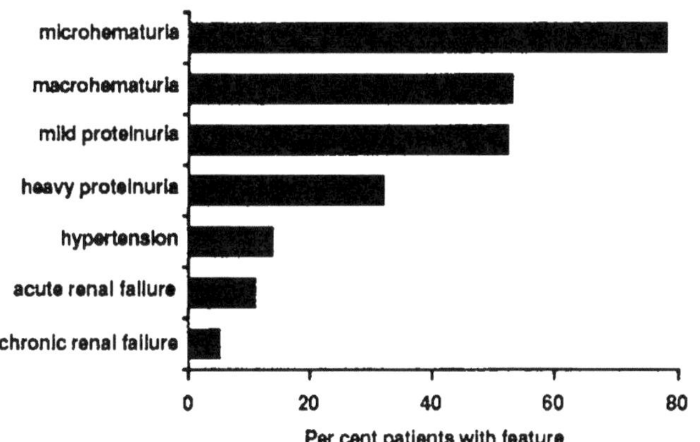

FIG. 4. The frequencies of clinical features at presentation of 2,000 patients with IgAN are depicted. Mild proteinuria is defined as excretion of less than 1 g/24 h, heavy proteinuria as greater than 1 g/24 h. Acute and chronic renal failure and microhematuria are as defined by the nephrologists initially evaluating the patients.

specificity, T cells could be stimulated as they course through the glomerulus since lectins can be T cell mitogens (37, 38, 130, 135, 170). Antilectin antibodies could deposit, and IgA positive B cells might even be selectively stimulated to secrete antilectin antibody. The pluripotential nature of lectins could therefore explain many of the diverse features of IgAN. Whereas lymphocyte function studies have primarily focused on IgA, some studies have also examined IgG and IgM production and regulation, again with varying results (37, 135). In some cases in which antithetical results were obtained, different methodologies were used, but this consideration cannot explain all conflicting findings (29, 30, 114, 118). Other variables, *e.g.*, phase of disease and clinical subgrouping of patients, have seldom been considered, yet these factors may be significant. For example, Egido *et al.* (38) observed a difference in the number of polymeric IgA-producing blood lymphocytes in IgAN patients during bouts of hematuria *versus* those without active hematuria.

In most studies of immunologic parameters, the scatter of data is large: coefficients of variation are frequently in excess of 50% and occasionally greater than 100%. The simple distinction of clinical phase of disease, remission *versus* exacerbation *versus* chronic renal failure, appreciably reduces variances (38, 135). Perhaps more critical than considering individual immunologic parameters to determine if there are immunologically distinct subgroups among patients with a common clinical status, the relative values of combinations of several immunologic parameters should be considered.

Application of a panel of uniformly performed immunologic assays could conceivably permit categorizations which are highly correlated with clinical presentation or course and which relate to a particular pathogenesis. For example, T cells with Fc receptors for IgA and IgA-binding suppressor factors are induced *in vitro* by IgA (64–67). Patients with high serum IgA and elevated levels of IgA suppressor cells might have a clinical status different from patients with similar serum IgA levels but normal or low IgA suppressors, and such patients would almost certainly differ in their immunologic status. High IgA without concomitant increases in IgA suppressors might signal a defect in suppressor function; immunomodulatory therapy might then be directed to enhancing IgA suppressors. On the other hand, if suppressors are already high in response to elevated serum IgA, an abnormally robust or autonomous B cell response could be the primary pathogenetic mechanism, and therapy would more logically be directed to down-regulating IgA B cells or IgA helper T cells.

THERAPY

As with glomerulonephritis in general, there is no specific therapy available. Supportive measures aimed at controlling hypertension and maintaining homeostasis during episodes of acute renal failure and at preserving renal function through dietary restriction are important therapeutic goals, although none of these interventions is specific or curative (19). A more tantalizing prospect is therapy to reduce glomerular IgA deposition. Diaminodiphenylsulfone and diphenylhydantoin reduce serum IgA, apparently by altering IgA synthesis. Although initial experience with these approaches has outwardly been disappointing, critical review suggests that modified regimens may in fact improve the longterm course of IgAN patients (19, and J. Egido and A. Woodroffe, personal communications). Another potentially worthwhile avenue is to use corticosteroids to treat patients with heavy proteinuria (85, 105, 171). This approach not only shows promise in initial studies but also accords with the observations of several centers that heavy proteinuria is a strong predictor of ultimate renal failure. Again, rational specific therapy can only develop after the pathogenesis and pathophysiology are elucidated.

THE MUCOSAL IMMUNE SYSTEM AND PROPERTIES OF IgA

The lymphoid cells and tissues structurally related to secretory mucosae are collectively considered as mucosal-associated lymphoid tissue, for which the gut associated lymphoid tissue is the archetype (87, 97, 114). Immune responses in the secretory immune system arise when lumenal antigen is imported into underlying lymphoid nodules, *e.g.*, the Peyer's patches, by specialized epithelial cells. Antigen is then "processed" by accessory cells and presented to helper T lymphocytes, apparently similarly to the same processes in the general systemic immune system. The helper cells subsequently augment clonal proliferation and differentiation of antigen-specific B and effector T lymphocytes in the lymphoid nodules. At this point, a number of differences apply to the secretory, as distinct from the systemic, immune system. The B cells in these mucosal sites are preferentially selected for or directed to IgA synthesis. They respond to antigenic stimulation by exiting the lymphoid nodules to enter the draining lymph nodes, where they further divide and differentiate. Mucosal T cells have been less extensively studied, but are believed to follow a similar path. Lymphoid progenitors are therefore initially close to the site where antigen enters the body. Stimulated cells migrate to the regional nodes for maturation, in contrast to the systemic immune system, where lymphocytes first encounter antigen in the draining lymph nodes. Subsequently, lymphocytes of mucosal origin leave the regional lymph nodes via efferent lymphatics, eventually reach the general blood circulation, and selectively settle in the lamina propria of mucous membranes, including sites that may be distant from their point of origin. In the lamina propria, the B cells complete their differentiation into IgA secreting plasma cells.

The widely distributed mucosal immune system is collectively immense, even greater in cell content than the systemic immune system. The mucosal immune system manifests other differences from the systemic immune system in terms of kinetics and regulation of immune responses. Unlike the systemic system, the entry of exogenous antigen appears to be an active process facilitated by specialized epithelial cells. Hence, the potential for developing an immune response is high, although immunologic memory is weak. In view of the extent and variety of mucosal exposure to foreign substances, immunoregulation becomes critical. Soluble antigen-specific T cell suppressor factors were first identified in mucosally derived T cells from orally immunized mice (16, 93), and both IgA specific and antigen specific regulatory cells and factors are well represented in mucosae. Although the humoral immune response to antigens entering via mucosal surfaces has initial IgM and IgG components, it rapidly shifts to an IgA predominant response under the influence of "switch" T cells that induce immature B cells to shift from IgM to the production of IgA (83, 94) and IgA specific helper T cells that promote secretion of IgA by B cells that previously switched (84). Active suppression of specific IgG and IgM responses also develops (16, 81, 93, 131). Recently, interleukin (IL)-5 has emerged as a factor which may preferentially elicit the differentiation and proliferation of IgA lymphocytes and promote IgA rather than IgG or IgM production by activated B cells (11, 22, 59). In this context, it may facilitate rearrangement of Ig heavy chain genes, similar to the effect IL-4 is thought to have on IgG1 expression (145). On the other hand, since the effects of IL-5 occur preferentially on B cells which express surface IgA, it may act in whole or in part by stimulating proliferation and/or differentiation of B cells already committed to IgA synthesis (59). The net effect of the various regulatory influences is a strong tendency for mucosal lymphoid tissue to generate IgA antibodies, with simultaneous attenuation of IgG and IgM responses. This latter phenomenon, termed "oral tolerance," may be important in protecting the host from hypersensitivity diseases that could be induced by environmental antigens entering the airways and intestines (46) even though such tolerance takes time to develop (16, 47, 93, 131). Reflecting their functional anatomy, the mucosae are necessarily more permeable to antigens than the skin and are therefore at higher potential risk for hypersensitivity injury, particularly before oral tolerance develops.

The secretory immune system is thus singularly well adapted to protect the host, not only by its concentration of elements of the afferent immune response close to the site of antigen entry, its large mass of cells carefully regulated and capable of wide dissemination and its potential for systemic tolerogenesis, but also because of the properties of its primary humoral product, IgA. The IgA synthesized at mucosal sites is predominantly dimeric, composed of two H_2L_2 Ig subunits (87, 97, 114). It therefore has four antigen-binding sites/molecule, improving its agglutinating ability. Locally synthesized dimeric IgA is also actively and selectively transported from the lamina propria across the epithelium into the lumen, which concentrates IgA antibody at the mucosal surface, outside the body proper and at sites where host defenses first encounter many pathogens (104). This scheme, which focuses immune defense mechanisms on pathogens early, is essentially preventive rather than reparative in nature. It also shifts immune defenses that are potentially noxious to the host toward the external environment. Moreover, IgA is distinctly less phlogistic than IgG or IgM, a property which seems to have been selected for in evolution (44, 87). For example, IgA immune complexes are not efficient activators of complement. Pfaffenbach, Lamm, and Gigli (113) and Johnson et al. (78) showed that murine IgA antibodies can promote assembly of an alternative pathway C3 convertase when immune complexes are incubated with fresh human, guinea pig, or rat serum, but maturation to an effective C5 convertase does not ensue. Rifai, Chen, and Imai (122) reported that model immune complexes prepared with IgA do not even consume C3 (122). In contrast, Hiemstra et al. concluded that human IgA generates functional alternative pathway C5 convertase and full assembly of membrane attack complexes (62); however, this group used highly chemically cross-linked high molecular weight IgA aggregates as model immune complexes, rather than complexes of IgA antibody and antigen. Waldo, Mestecky, and Kohaut (167) in turn found that human IgA cleaves C3 but not C5, consonant with the observations on murine IgA. This group also demonstrated that nascent C3b is more likely to hydrolyze its internal thiolester than to bind to IgA immune complexes. Admixture of progressive amounts of IgA with IgG in immune complexes diminished incorporation of C3 into the complex, and inhibited complement activation. Furthermore, complement components are either absent or at low concentration in mucosal secretions (120, 127, 174) and phagocytic cells tend not to exit in a major way into the lumens of normal mucosae (4, 9, 97, 160). IgA is thus a good agglutinin which is actively concentrated at sites of potential entry of pathogens into the body, and yet does not invoke effector mechanisms that are potentially noxious to the host and irrelevant in secretions.

CLEARANCE OF IgA IMMUNE COMPLEXES

An antigen which circumvents the immunologic barrier of lumenal IgA antibody and the mucus layer may gain access to the lamina propria, as can antigens shed from viruses that are replicating in mucosal epithelium. Here, there is also abundant IgA antibody available to bind the antigen. Resulting immune complexes must ultimately be eliminated. Transcellular transport of IgA and IgA immune complexes can occur in the liver since the hepatocytes of rodents (13, 88, 103, 112, 146) and the biliary epithelium of humans (33, 106) can actively transport dimeric IgA into bile via a secretory component-dependent mechanism. IgA immune complexes, like IgG complexes, are also subject to clearance by the mononuclear phagocyte system (123, 124). Monocytes and neutrophils bear IgA receptors although these appear more related to degranulation and antibody dependent cytotoxic responses than to phagocytosis (44, 61). Fixed phagocytes in the liver and spleen are important for removal of IgA immune complexes from the circulation (123, 124). Blockade of phagocytic function by colloidal carbon promotes glomerular deposition of IgA immune complexes (133). The extent to which such phagocytosis depends upon Fc receptors *versus* nonspecific phagocytosis of particulates is controversial. Consonant with the inefficient complement fixing ability of IgA immune complexes, enhanced binding of IgA immune complexes to phagocytes via immune adherence (complement) receptors does not appear to operate with IgA immune complexes, and is definitely less effective at promoting ingestion of IgA complexes than complexes containing IgG (44, 168).

PATHOGENESIS OF IgA NEPHROPATHY

Glomerulonephritis associated with deposits of Ig and complement is almost uniformly considered to be within the general category of immune complex disease. In the case of IgAN the original evidence in favor of an immune complex etiology, beyond the simple association of disease with Ig deposits, came from clinical studies. Initial presentation and exacerbations in IgAN frequently occur concurrently with or shortly after bouts of mucosal infection, and deposits can be present in other sites such as dermal blood vessels (35, 42, 161). Circulating immune complexes are frequent in patients with IgAN and often correlate with disease activity (24, 27, 32, 58, 75, 98, 132, 135, 155, 172). High molecular weight IgA from serum and renal eluates, presumably in the form of immune complexes, can be dissociated to predominantly dimeric IgA by acid pH (24, 42, 102). The aggregates often contain activated complement and can bind to phagocytes (24, 53, 54, 155, 167). These data collectively have been interpreted as evidence that the glomerular IgA is the antibody component of an immune complex resulting from an immune response to antigen derived from the pathogen that caused the preceding bout of infection. On the other hand, IgA rheumatoid factor (IgA anti-Fc of IgG), anti-IgA rheumatoid factors (IgG/IgM anti-Fc of IgA) and antibodies specific for the constant portion of the Fab fragment of IgA have also been demonstrated frequently and in high titer in the sera of patients with IgAN (see below) (27, 75, 141, 142). Aggregates formed in these last two instances would still be immune complexes, but the IgA would be acting as antigen rather than as antibody. Still another proposal envisions the macromolecular IgA to be aggregated by other than immunologically specific means.

Experimental models of IgAN in rodents have been useful for identifying potential pathogenetic mechanisms and predisposing factors for glomerular IgA deposits and for elucidating pathophysiologic mechanisms likely to be operative in nephritogenesis. Rifai *et al.* (125) originally demonstrated that IgA immune complexes injected into mice as preformed aggregates or formed within the circulation can lead to mesangial deposits of IgA, antigen and complement, microhematuria, and increased mesangial matrix. Beyond establishing that the salient features of IgAN could be elicited experimentally by IgA immune complexes, this study showed that polymeric rather than monomeric IgA is required and that the size of the immune lattice is important. Shortly thereafter, Isaacs *et al.* (72–74) emphasized the role of the size and charge of antigens, and, therefore, of the immune lattice in glomerular injury and its expression, in both active and passive systems. Only antigens 70 kilodaltons and greater in size were nephritogenic although antigens as small as 10 kilodaltons could elicit glomerular immune deposits. The demonstration that large immune complexes are more deleterious, though no more likely to deposit, agrees with the earlier emphasis of Rifai *et al.* (125) on polymeric IgA antibody, which would tend to form larger aggregates than would monomeric IgA.

Since IgA is the main Ig of the exocrine secretions, in our own experimental work we reasoned that mucosal antigenic stimulation should preferentially elicit an IgA immune response and under appropriate circumstances IgA immune complexes could form internally (41). Indeed, protracted oral immunization yields a highly selective IgA antibody response, and leads to glomerular mesangial deposits of antigen and specific IgA antibody. The antigens used range from 45 to 440 kilodaltons and the immune deposits appear to contain excess oligomeric IgA antibody, again suggesting that large aggregates tend to deposit. The same general experimental approach was later employed by Genin, Sabatier, and Berthoux (51) in two strains of congenic mice which differ markedly in their capacity to mount an IgA response; IgA responders developed glomerular deposits, whereas nonresponders did not. Both studies underscore the concept that the degree of IgA antibody synthesis and the concurrent availability of antigen, rather than some other feature of oral immunization, determine the development of mesangial IgA immune complex deposits.

Yet another animal model of IgAN develops spontaneously in the ddY strain of mice (71). Aged mice of this strain develop glomerular IgA deposits associated with glomerular C3 and proteinuria. These mice are congenitally infected with a retrovirus. Before the onset of clinically apparent IgA dominant nephritis, polyclonal IgA and IgG levels increase in serum. Mammary, ovarian and pulmonary carcinomas and malignant lymphomas arise in these mice; in particular, the mammary carcinomas become evident shortly after IgA increases and becomes dominant. The investigators proposed that the elevated IgA and IgG are antibodies to tumor antigens, particularly in mammary glands, or are specific for the retrovirus, which becomes more exposed at about the glomerulopathy begins. They further suggest that immune complexes of such antigens and antibodies underlie IgAN in these mice.

Aware of the prominence of IgA synthesis in the mucosal immune system and the association of viral syndromes with onset and exacerbation of clinical IgAN, we sought to induce IgAN in mice by immunization and challenge with Sendai virus, a parainfluenza virus that is a natural murine respiratory pathogen (77). In fact, mice immunized intranasally over 6 weeks and then subjected to systemic challenge with live virus developed IgA and IgG serum antibody and glomerular deposits containing IgA, IgG, C3 and Sendai virus antigen as well as microhematuria. Mice immunized but not challenged had less intense glomerular antigen and antibody and lacked C3 deposits and hematuria. Thus, exposure to a pathogen in an already mucosally immunized animal can result in glomerular immune deposits and nephritis. Hence, we propose that exacerbations of nephritis associated with flulike syndromes in humans could reflect episodes of mucosal infection in an immune host. In this context, it is well to recall that immunologic memory for IgA antibody responses is generally weak. Also, mucosal immune tolerance for IgG and IgM responses tends to be difficult to sustain. Episodic exposure to a given pathogen at wide intervals could thus introduce antigen into a mucous membrane, favoring combination with predominantly IgA but also IgG/IgM antibodies. Such conditions would be optimal for nephritogenesis.

Gormly *et al.* (52) and Melvin *et al.* (96) pursued yet another approach to the experimental study of the pathogenesis of IgAN. Aware that patients with hepatobiliary disease frequently have clinically inapparent deposits of glomerular IgA, these investigators used carbon tetrachloride and bile duct ligation, respectively, to induce hepatobiliary abnormalities in rats. Both groups concluded that elevated serum and mesangial IgA, associated with mild mesangial proliferation and matrix expansion and hematuria, followed impaired excretion of polymeric IgA from blood to bile, a route that is especially significant in the rat. These data, taken alone, are compatible with increased polymeric IgA depositing by itself in glomeruli, independent of immune complexes. We examined the effect of bile duct ligation on glomerular immune complex deposition in mice that had been orally immunized or injected with preformed, soluble immune complexes (43). In both instances the deposition of antigen, as well as IgA antibody, was enhanced in mice with ligated bile ducts. We therefore interpret the mesangial IgA observed in animals with ligated bile ducts but not deliberately immunized or given IgA immune complexes as antibody in immune complexes formed physiologically with a variety of environmental antigens, but inadequately cleared due to impaired bile flow. More recently, Sato, Idewa, and Koshikowa (133) focused on the role of the mononuclear phagocyte system in clearing circulating IgA immune complexes. Orally immunized mice given colloidal carbon to blockade the reticuloendothelial system developed mesangial lesions with predominantly IgA deposits, whereas orally immunized mice or mice given carbon alone did not (133).

Abramowsky *et al.* (1, 2, 32) demonstrated the effects of hepatobiliary disease on glomerular IgA deposits and circulating IgA immune complexes in patients with cystic fibrosis and biliary atresia. As expected, those patients in whom disease had progressed to cirrhosis had deposits of IgA, J chain and secretory component in glomeruli, and heightened levels of polymeric IgA and IgA immune complexes in serum. Age-matched controls or patients with less advanced stages of disease who had not developed cirrhosis lacked these changes. While the studies confirm the applicability of the bile duct ligation and hepatotoxin models of IgAN to humans and emphasize the role the liver can play in the clearance of IgA immune complexes, they do not shed light on the relative contributions of fixed hepatic mononuclear phagocytes *versus* secretory component-mediated transport.

PATHOPHYSIOLOGY

The nature of the molecular coupling of deposited immune complexes containing IgA antibody to altered glomerular function, like the coupling in glomerulonephritis in general, is a challenging problem. Experimental models and *in vitro* studies can, of course, illuminate the properties of immune complexes that are central to glomerular pathophysiology, and may reveal whether the complexes in IgAN have distinctive properties. Features of the nephritogenic complexes can potentially guide therapy. For example, if they share a single pathophysiologic sequence, therapy can perhaps be targeted to a particular mechanism. If different mechanisms are elucidated, correlations between clinical parameters and particular mechanisms must be sought and therapy perhaps tailored accordingly. Otherwise one is left with nonspecific regimens, which historically have been rather ineffective in glomerulonephritis.

Traditionally, considerations of the mechanisms of glomerular injury in IgAN have focused on the role of IgA and complement. More recently, attention has been directed to Ig classes other than IgA and to antigen in promoting hematuria and mesangial proliferation (45, 47, 69, 122). Deposition of C3, the third component of complement, is strongly implicated. Mice congenitally deficient in component C5 become hematuric if appropriately challenged with antigen, identically to congenic normocomplementemic mice. Both C5-deficient and C5 competent mice fail to develop hematuria associated with glomerular immune deposits if they are earlier depleted of complement with cobra venom factor (45, 47). Cobra venom factor depletes C3 and distal components by generating a homologue of the alternative pathway convertase (21). Whereas C4 can be consumed to a limited extent, cobra venom has little effect on C1, C2, B or D, the other complement components proximal to C3 in the classical and alternative pathways. The critical factor is therefore proximal to C5. C3 and perhaps C4 are thus candidates for agents of inflammation in IgAN.

The membrane attack complex of complement, C5b-9, has been recognized increasingly as an important mediator of glomerulonephritis in general (26). IgAN was among the first diseases recognized to have glomerular deposition of the membrane attack complex (119). However, in IgAN the regulatory S protein is invariably associated with C5b-9 (154). Since the S protein interferes with the biologic effects of C5b-9, inhibiting its insertion into cell membranes (115), it is questionable whether the membrane attack complex is physiologically relevant. Moreover, it is likely that S is bound in the circulation; if so, the C5b-9 deposited may be inert. It is possible, however, that S binds to C5b-9 *in situ* after glomerular deposition, in which case C5b-9 should be biologically active. Although it is definite from experimental studies in mice that C5 and therefore C5b-9 is not necessary for hematuria (45), the membrane attack complex may still augment hematuria and may be necessary for other aspects of altered glomerular performance and/or disease progression.

Although glomerular C3 seems to promote hematuria in mice, the mechanism is unknown. The role of C3 in other aspects of glomerular pathophysiology is also not known, nor can we be certain whether hematuria depends on C3 in human IgAN. Cultured rat mesangial cells and glomerular epithelial cells bear a receptor similar to CR1; binding of oligomeric activated C3 (C3b oligomers) to CR1 stimulates eicosanoid synthesis (57, 147). Although in our work we have focused on C3b interacting with CR1 on glomerular cells because this mechanism is established, the C3a split product could be important in IgAN. The effect of this anaphylatoxin on endogenous glomerular cells is unknown. Glomerular cells produce mediators such as eicosanoids, acylglycerylethers, ILs and free radicals in response to immune complexes, complement, and phagocytic stimuli (5, 57, 90, 134, 138,

140, 147, 169). The potential contribution of these mediators to glomerular injury in general has been studied in a number of laboratories, but these mediators have not yet been considered in IgAN.

The role of circulating leukocytes, stimulated with anaphylatoxins or not, has not been studied in IgAN. Although leukocytic infiltration of glomeruli is not present in experimental IgAN and is not typically a feature of patients with IgAN, small numbers of infiltrating leukocytes can be missed histologically, even with immunohistochemistry or histochemistry (139). Moreover, leukocyte products released in response to C3a, such as platelet-activating factor, platelet-derived growth factor, myeloperoxidase, proteases and IL-1, might act on the glomerulus from remote sites, without the need for glomerular leukocytic infiltration. Experimental IgAN induced in leukocyte-deficient animals would be informative, but such experiments are not feasible in the active models, which require several weeks for induction. There is clear involvement of T cells in some forms of glomerulonephritis, but their role in IgAN is uncertain, and the mechanisms of glomerular injury induced by T cells are unknown.

Noting the wide clinicopathologic spectrum encompassed by IgAN, some have questioned whether it should be considered a single disease entity. If a disease should reflect a single pathogenesis, elicit common signs and symptoms, and follow a defined course, IgAN may not fulfill the criteria (10). Such criteria, however, would seem to be unduly rigid. Within broader limits IgAN does constitute a disease, or at least a family of closely related diseases. Even if not a direct cause of altered glomerular function (see below), in our opinion the glomerular IgA or IgA containing immune complexes must be important pathogenetic factors in the altered renal function. The variability in clinical presentation and long-term course can be ascribed to qualitative and quantitative variations in the deposits and to the range of function of the target of this disease, the versatile glomerular mesangium (128, 162). Mesangial cells have smooth muscle-like properties, and may regulate intraglomerular hemodynamics via contraction or relaxation (134). Moreover, such cells produce a variety of vasoactive autacoids and are in close contact with the macula densa, and therefore can regulate afferent and efferent arteriolar tone to control total renal plasma flow. Mesangial cells bear Fc and complement receptors, produce IL-1, and are phagocytic (5, 90, 138, 140, 147). Furthermore, class II histocompatibility antigen expression by these cells is inducible. Mesangial cells are thus important in clearing intraglomerular immune deposits, and can potentially serve as antigen presenting cells. Since they produce reactive oxygen metabolites in response to immune complexes, or phagocytic stimuli and can release proteases, they may contribute to glomerular injury (50, 92, 140, 165). IgA immune deposits may modulate these functions in several ways: the intercalation of IgA among IgG antibodies in an immune aggregate, the altered ratio of Ig to complement, a change in lattice size, the relative proportion of Ig that is IgA, and perhaps the nature of the antigen (see below) could all dramatically influence the mesangial response, thereby widely varying the clinical expression of mesangial immune deposits. Finally, mesangiopathic lesions other than IgAN comprise a fascinating subset of glomerulonephritides which collectively incorporate many of the features of IgAN. Thus, when one considers the range of functions associated with mesangial cells, the spectrum of clinical manifestations and variable course of IgAN may well be more attributable to the site of immunopathologic injury than to varying pathogenesis or mechanisms. Although there may be more than one means whereby IgA deposits form, the proximate common pathogenesis relates to the deposition of glomerular deposits in which IgA is prominent, and the common response is altered glomerular ultrafiltration.

ROLE OF DIFFERENT CLASSES OF GLOMERULAR ANTIBODY

Complement appears central to nephritogenesis in IgAN. Since IgA by itself is an inefficient activator of complement (78, 113, 122), in our experimental studies of IgAN we have focused on the significance of complement-fixing codeposits of IgG and/or IgM (45, 47). While IgG *per se* is not nephritogenic in the sense that neither deposition of IgG immune complexes containing a non-complement fixing genetic variant of IgG (63) nor deposition of complexes containing normal IgG in complement depleted mice elicits nephritis, IgG complexes capable of fixing complement do promote hematuria in normocomplementemic mice. Complement fixation by IgG and IgM proceeds by both the classical and alternative pathways. To the extent that IgG and IgM codeposits are responsible for glomerular C3 in IgAN, classical pathway components like C1 and C4 should also be deposited, yet these are relatively infrequent in glomeruli of biopsies from IgAN patients. This may well relate to the sensitivity of immunofluorescence since C1 and C4 are detectable in renal eluates and in circulating immune complexes in IgAN (24, 135, 172). Certainly, the amplification of classical pathway complement activation via the alternative pathway favors conspicuous C3 deposits.

Prominent glomerular IgG or IgM associated with a strong IgA immune response may signal a defect in immunoregulation. Normally, persistent mucosal antigenic stimulation favors a vigorous IgA response, but suppresses IgG and IgM responses, *i.e.*, oral tolerance (16, 41, 81, 93, 131). Recently, we have used cyclophosphamide and estradiol to inhibit the usual suppression of IgG antibody in response to chronic oral immunization. In contrast to untreated mice, which had only IgA antibody in serum and glomeruli and no hematuria, mice treated with cyclophosphamide or estradiol to inhibit oral tolerance had a mixed IgA/IgG serum antibody response, IgA, IgG and C3 glomerular deposits, and microhematuria (L. Gesualdo, S. N. Emancipator, and M. E. Lamm unpublished observations). These studies are consistent with the suggestion that defective mucosal tolerance plays a role in the inflammatory component of IgAN.

Clinocopathologic observations also support the concept that codeposits of complement-fixing IgG and IgM are critical for nephritogenesis in IgAN. A sizable majority (85%) of patients with symptomatic IgAN have codeposits of IgG and/or IgM detectable by immunofluorescence, whereas few subjects with asymptomatic glomerular IgA have codeposits of IgG or IgM (42). Other reports indicate that patients with more severe or more frequent renal manifestations have IgG or IgM codeposits associated with a less favorable prognosis (50, 68, 148). Schena *et al.* (135) observed significant elevations in the numbers of IgG- and IgM-producing cells in peripheral blood of IgAN patients in exacerbation compared with those in remission. Immune complexes in IgAN are most frequently detected by the C1q binding assay, a technique which requires classical pathway complement activation. Since IgA does not activate complement via the classical pathway, other elements within the complex, such as admixed IgG and IgM, must be responsible. Other assays of immune complexes that are less sensitive to the large aggregates which activate the classical complement pathway all demonstrate immune complexes in patients with IgAN, but less well than the C1q-binding assay (24, 135, 172).

Since the correlation between serum immune complexes and disease activity is better with methods which depend on C1q, admixture of antibodies like IgG and IgM that can activate the classical pathway may have predictive value in patients with IgAN. This hypothesis fits with the increases in IgG and IgM production observed in IgAN patients in exacerbation compared with those in remission, with immunofluorescence studies of clinical biopsies, and with the aforementioned experimental results. In this context, a paradox therefore emerges with regard to the role IgA plays in the genesis of IgAN. If the IgA *per se* is not nephritogenic, what role does it play? Are the IgA deposits simply a bystander, or perhaps a necessary but not sufficient concomitant?

Miller and Nussenzweig (28, 101, 149) showed that insertion of complement into an immune lattice following complement activation can solubilize immune precipitates. Compared with IgG immune precipitates, complement-mediated solubilization of IgA immune complexes proceeds less efficiently and only via the alternative pathway (100, 126). Despite normal levels of individual complement components, the sera of IgAN patients are defective in solubilizing a standard IgG containing immune precipitate compared with both normal people and patients with other forms of glomerulonephritis (136, 137, 159). Rheumatoid factor can inhibit complement mediated solubilization by stabilizing the immune lattice; however, Schena *et al.* (136, 137) and Tomino *et al.* (159) reported that high molecular weight IgA in the sera of IgAN patients, presumably in immune complexes, is responsible for impaired complement-mediated dissociation of immune complexes independently of the presence of IgA rheumatoid factor. Since complement activation, at least to C3b generation, is required for complement-mediated solubilization, the inhibition of complement fixation via both classical and alternative pathways by oligomeric IgA which Waldo *et al.* (167) observed might account for the impaired solubilization of standard immune complexes.

The potential ramifications of polymeric IgA as an inhibitor of complement activation are striking. If IgA is incorporated into an immune lattice, the entire immune complex is less able to bind to erythrocyte immune adherence receptors, an important mechanism for clearing immune complexes from serum and preventing their deposition in tissues (60, 168). Clearance by mononuclear phagocytes would also be impaired by decreased binding to complement receptors. Thus, through its anticomplementary effects the IgA component of immune complexes may indirectly facilitate nephritis by inhibiting the normal mechanisms for handling immune complexes, consequently promoting their glomerular deposition.

Another potential way to promote glomerular deposits concerns interactions of IgA, which is much more highly glycolysated than IgG, with endogenous and exogenous lectins, *i.e.*, proteins with affinity for specific carbohydrate groups. It is increasingly apparent that fibronectin, a glycoprotein with carbohydrate binding specificity which is plentiful in the mesangial matrix, can bind IgA (A. Woodroffe, J. Mestecky and D. Schlondorff, independent personal communications and 98). The IgA component of immune complexes might thus serve to target complexes to the fibronectin rich glomerular mesangium. Once deposited, other components of the complex such as C3 could stimulate changes in glomerular function. Exogenous multivalent lectins might bridge glycosyl residues in the mesangium to IgA molecules, thereby targeting IgA immune complexes or IgA aggregates to the glomerulus. Saccharide antigens or lectin antigens complexed to IgA antibody could also bind to lectin-like molecules or glycosylated sites, respectively in the mesangium, with the same effect. Finally, deposited IgA could serve as a nidus upon which environmental or autologous lectin-like molecules could deposit. Moreover, many patients with IgAN have elevated titers of IgG antibodies specific for α-galactosyl residues, which are present on IgA (31). Such antibodies could be the anti-IgA rheumatoid factors described by others (75, 136, 141, 142) and may also further affect IgA-lectin-mesangial matrix interactions.

Collectively, the animal models demonstrate that the salient features of IgAN can be elicited experimentally by immune complexes that contain IgA antibody. Other mechanisms of pathogenesis whereby IgA is an autoantigen or is aggregated by other than immunologically specific means have not been experimentally established, but are nonetheless possible. In clinical IgAN, the deposited IgA could, for example, be an autoimmune antibody, i.e., a rheumatoid factor. The IgA could conceivably be an autoantigen in an immune complex or even represent nonspecific aggregation. Whatever their origin, the deposits of IgA do appear to be mechanistically related, though perhaps only indirectly, to the glomerular damage.

NATURE OF THE ANTIGEN IN IgA NEPHROPATHY

Cognizant of the temporal association between various viral-like, mucosally related illnesses and the onset or exacerbation of IgAN in many patients, several investigators have attempted to demonstrate viral antigens and/or antiviral antibodies in patients with IgAN (55, 107, 153, 156, 157, 172). Some patients, particularly in Japan, have antiviral antibodies that bind to virally infected cells in culture and to tonsillar cells and glomerular mesangium from other patients with IgAN, but not from patients with other forms of glomerulonephritis (153, 156, 157). Renal or tonsillar tissue from IgAN patients, as opposed to tissues from patients with other glomerulonephritides, can generate a cytopathic effect when added to cultured cells, again suggesting viral involvement (157). Gregory, Hammond, and Brewer (55) recently reported that 100% of 31 IgAN patients in Utah had glomerular deposits of cytomegalovirus antigens compared with only 4% of 55 patients with other glomerular diseases. However, the interpretation that the immune deposits represent immune complexes of cytomegalovirus antigen and anti-cytomegalovirus IgA antibody is not the only possibility. The authors, although favoring an immune complex etiology, proposed alternative explanations. One hundred percent of patients is certainly a striking result, particularly in light of studies from Japan, where cytomegalovirus antigen was not demonstrated; however, adenovirus and herpes simplex virus were found frequently (153, 156, 157). Nagy *et al.* (107) in Hungary observed that a high percentage of their IgAN patients had elevated anticytomegalovirus and/or antiherpes simplex virus serum antibody titers, but could not demonstrate viral antigens in the glomeruli. While dramatic demographic and geographic differences in etiology may well exist, other explanations should be kept in mind.

Significant numbers of patients in diverse geographic areas also have serum antibodies specific for dietary antigens, and immune complexes containing such antigens in their serum (15, 25, 95, 132, 163, 172). Moreover, there is provocative preliminary evidence that a gluten-free diet benefits some IgAN patients (25). In nearly all these studies, only a minority of patients had antibody specific for a particular antigen. The prevalence of the different antibodies is unknown, and their coexistence in individuals has not been established. Finally, in the renal eluates of some patients dietary antigens have been identified, and in others viral antigens (153, 156, 157, 172). Conceivably, therefore, some cases of IgAN may be due to immune complexes caused by dietary antigens, whereas others may be caused by infectious pathogens.

Anti-Ig levels have also been studied in IgAN. Once again, the results are intriguing but their significance unclear. IgA rheumatoid factor, anti-IgA rheumatoid factors, and most recently, antibody specific for the constant domain of the Fab region of IgA have all been described in IgAN patients at levels exceeding those in normals and/or patients with other forms of glomerulonephritis. generally, only a minority of IgAN patients exhibit such activities, but the levels correlate with disease activity in individual patients (27, 75, 136, 141, 142). Antibodies specific for the Fc region of IgA might be particularly effective at enhancing glomerular deposition of polymeric IgA, not only by generating immune complexes with IgA as antigen, but potentially also by blocking transepithelial transport of polymeric IgA or polymeric IgA-containing immune complexes by secretory component.

ANTIGEN AS A FACTOR IN NEPHRITOGENESIS

Antigen has also been recognized as a potential factor in glomerular injury. Related but distinct antigens which elicit the same degree of Ig deposits can be associated with marked differences in glomerular reactions. Imai *et al.* employed a passive serum sickness model in mice, using murine TEPC-15 antiphosphorylcholine monoclonal IgA antibody complexed with either the phosphorylcholine-containing pneumococcal C-polysaccharide or phosphorylcholine substituted complex polysaccharide (Ficoll®) (69). Although ensuing glomerular deposits of IgA and C3 were similar, differences in glomerular response were striking. Mice given complexes of polymeric IgA antibody and C-polysaccharide showed marked mesangial matrix expansion, mesangial hyperplasia and focal-segmental endocapillary proliferation, whereas mice given complexes prepared with phosphorylcholine-Ficoll had normal glomeruli (69). Parallel changes were observed in hematuria and in purpuric lesions of the ears (A. Rifai, personal communication).

Isaccs and Miller (72, 73) chronically immunized mice with dextrans of differing charge. All mice immunized with appropriately sized antigen developed comparable pronounced glomerular IgA deposits and similar antidextran serum titers. However, highly anionic antigen favored matrix expansion, while cationic antigen favored cellular proliferation. Neutral antigen was less noxious than either highly negative or highly positive antigen. The reasons for the different responses to antigens of different charge are unknown, but could provide clues to the nature of mesangial cellular responses to deposited immune aggregates. Perhaps, for example, cell receptors associated with proliferation are anionic, while those linked to synthesis of matrix are cationic.

At present these observations are more a warning that the particular antigen deposited in glomeruli can be an important factor than they are explanations of glomerular responses. Although little information regarding mechanisms is available, investigation of the influence of particular antigens on glomerular injury is warranted. As another example, consider the use of dinitrophenylated antigens in passive models of IgAN. It is now apparent that the hematuria and complement deposition observed in the initial report (125) were incited by the capacity of the dinitrophenyl group aggregated by antibody-induced cross-linking to activate complement, despite the fact that free, unaggregated antigen does not fix complement (86, 122).

PROSPECTS FOR THE FUTURE

Although the bulk of clinical and experimental evidence indicates that IgAN is a form of immune complex glomerulonephritis, the nature of the IgA as either antigen or antibody remains controversial. The possibility of deposition of nonimmunologically aggregated IgA as opposed to immune complexes containing IgA is still not excluded.

Recently a new method for isolating IgA immune complexes from serum by precipitation with polyethylene glycol was reported (70). This method is easily performed, reproducible, 70% efficient and allows quantification and analysis of immune complexes by a variety of techniques. Because several different tests can be applied to a single immune complex precipitate, standardized quantification of the immunochemical composition of immune complexes from large numbers of patients in multiple centers is practical. The amounts of various complement components and non-IgA Ig can be considered. Dissociation of immune complex precipitates may allow isolation or identification of antigens. The IgA subclass distribution of circulating complexes could be compared with the ratio of IgA1 and IgA2 in noncomplexed circulating IgA and in glomerular IgA. Finally, antiglobulin activity of the IgA in the complexes could be assessed. Correlation of these parameters with each other, with assessments of T cell immunity and with clinical presentation and course might prove to be a powerful approach to pathogenesis, prognosis, and perhaps therapy.

As with all glomerulonephritides, the cellular and molecular bases of the pathophysiologic changes in IgAN remain enigmatic, although clues are emerging. Prognostic ability is likewise advancing: severity of proteinuria, initial creatinine clearance, presence or absence of hypertension, and degree of tubulointerstitial change histologically appear collectively to enable retrospective distinction between patients with stable versus progressive renal disease in many centers (20, 29, 30, 85, 105, 108, 116, 164, 166, 171). These parameters are essentially the same as those found useful in membranous nephropathy (12). In addition, patients with IgAN behave similarly to patients with histologically comparable lesions but without predominance of IgA (111, 162). Hence, the special features of IgAN would seem to relate more to pathogenesis than to progression of the renal disease after the deposition of immune complexes. Effective treatment directed to the pathophysiology or progression of glomerulonephritis in general and IgAN in particular is not yet available and hinges upon a better understanding of the underlying mechanisms. To the extent that IgAN can be shown to have unique pathogenic elements, therapeutic strategies could be focused on these.

Many of the issues concerning IgAN converge on the special features of its pathogenesis as related to the preeminence of IgA in the deposits (6, 35, 68, 128). The mechanisms proposed for accumulation of IgA immune complexes reflect various features of immune function and dysfunction such as defective transport of polymeric Ig; primary B cell hyperresponsiveness; a defect in IgA-specific suppressor T cells, induction of oral tolerance, or humoral immunosuppressors in general; augmented helper function, perhaps specific for IgA; and development of an autoimmune state characterized by the production of anti-Igs. Careful and systematic grouping of patients according to immunologic parameters might help clarify the genesis of the immune complexes.

Parallel studies are required to determine to what extent the special characteristics of IgA, particularly its interaction with complement or its glycosyl moieties, are relevant to IgAN. As we gain insight into the network of immune receptors, effectors, mediators and cellular responses operative in glomerulonephritis in general, we must consider how the presence of IgA in immune deposits might influence the interplay. Such knowledge could guide therapeutic objectives.

Another aspect of IgAN which has received wide attention because it has etiologic and pathogenetic implications concerns a mucosal *versus* a bone marrow, *i.e.*, systemic, source of the mesangial IgA. The weight of evidence indicates that most of the deposited IgA belongs to the IgA1 subclass, even though there are technical reasons why the IgA2 subclass may be underrecognized immunohistochemically (3, 23, 24, 58, 89, 118, 152). The preponderance of the IgA also appears to be J chain-linked dimer, in keeping with experimental observations that monomeric IgA is not pathogenic, or at least much less pathogenic than dimeric IgA (3, 7, 24, 35, 36, 40, 89, 102, 158, 166). In humans, normal serum IgA is largely derived from marrow, 90% IgA1, and predominantly monomeric. In contrast, most IgA derived from mucosae is dimeric, containing J chain, and only abut half is IgA1 (56, 87, 97, 114). One would predict, therefore, that if plasma cells in marrow were the principal source of deposited IgA in IgAN, monomeric IgA1 lacking J chain would predominate in the deposits. In contrast, more nearly equal amounts of IgA1 and IgA2, both as J chain linked dimers, should be present if mucosa-derived plasmacytes are the source of the IgA. Neither of these extremes seems to apply, however. Rifai (121) has argued why this issue is unresolvable currently, and has offered a number of alternative interpretations and hypotheses compatible with all existing data.

CONCLUSIONS

Clinical and experimental observations strongly support the concept that IgAN is an immune complex glomerulonephritis. We believe the bulk of the glomerular IgA in most patients is mucosally derived antibody to infectious or environmental antigens, but acknowledge that alternative pathogenic routes may exist. Given the properties of the mucosal immune system, episodic exposure to pathogens capable of penetrating or replicating in mucosal linings emerges as a means of evoking IgAN in otherwise normal individuals, since IgA memory is weak and mucosal IgG and IgM tolerance decays over time. Environmental antigens to which mucosae are persistently exposed could elicit the same result were there also defective mucosal regulation of IgG and IgM. In either situation, defective clearance of immune complexes increases the likelihood of glomerular injury. Some of the avenues to IgAN are illustrated schematically in Figure 5.

The mucosae are under continuous barrage by an array of pathogens and environmental agents. Infections of mucosal sites require that host defenses, both immune and nonimmune, be overcome. If an infection develops in an immune host, whether through the pathogen being especially abundant or virulent or an insufficiency of mucosal antibody, a continuing immune response incorporating IgA, IgG, or IgM antibody could result in immune complexes with potential to deposit in glomeruli. It should be evident that individual exacerbations need not derive from reinfection with the same pathogen. Also, by focally damaging the mucosa, infection with one microorganism may predispose to superinfection with another, including a commensal to which the host is already immune. A mechanism whereby multiple episodes of infection with different pathogens elicit IgAN might explain the general difficulty in demonstrating the anti-

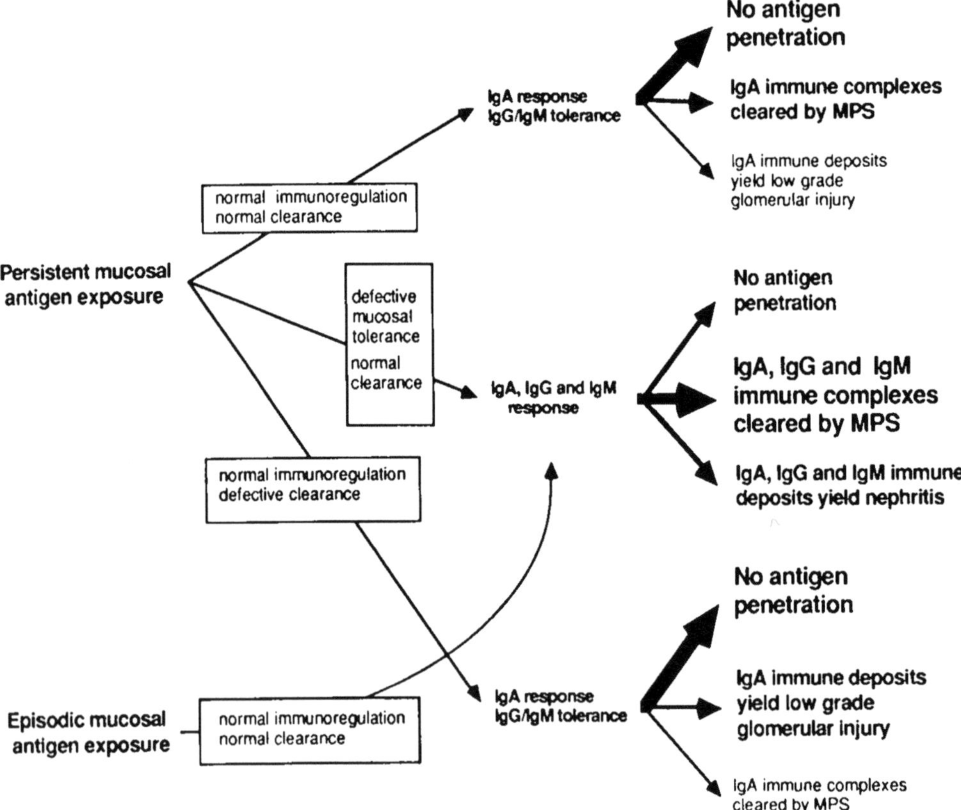

FIG. 5. Schematic diagram of some of the ways in which a host can respond to mucosal antigenic stimulation. The *heavy arrows* and *large type* represent those pathways and outcomes considered most likely, the *medium arrows* and *medium type* intermediate, and the *small arrows* and *small type* least likely. Note that combined defects in immunoregulation and clearance (not shown) would synergize to elicit more severe nephritis. In situations with episodic antigen exposure, either the same or different antigens could elicit individual bouts of nephritis; even in individuals with normal immunoregulation, the intrinsically weak memory of IgA responses and the interval usually required to establish mucosal tolerance with respect to IgG and IgM responses could promote nephritis. The responses in normal individuals with episodic antigen exposure could thus resemble the situation in which persistent antigen exposure occurs in individuals with defective mucosal tolerance. For simplicity, situations in which episodic antigen exposure occurs in hosts with abnormal immunoregulation or defective clearance are omitted. *MPS*, mononuclear phagocyte system.

gens of particular infectious agents in glomerular deposits. Similar arguments could apply to dietary antigens.

Improved comprehension of normal immune responses and immunoregulation of the mucosal and systemic immune systems, their interplay, and the effect of infections on the immune system will derive from basic studies. Systematic evaluation of the immune status of patients with IgAN, in both remission and exacerbation, should be capable of identifying features that can pinpoint immunopathogenesis. In parallel, understanding the biochemical and physiologic responses of glomeruli to immunologic stimuli in general and the effects of IgA on these responses is requisite for elucidating glomerular pathophysiology in IgAN. Progress towards rational therapy of IgAN is limited by our ability to develop sophisticated multidisciplinary investigations of the basic immunopathologic and pathophysiologic events. Large clinical studies guided by insights into basic immunology and pathophysiology will be the key to understanding the mechanisms of IgAN, its relationship to other glomerulonephritides, and to therapy. Needless to say, such studies will require a more aggressive policy of renal biopsy by nephrologists.

Acknowledgments: We are grateful to Sara Cechner for typing the manuscript and to Nancy J. Urankar for technical help, and to Randa B. Habib and Loreto Gesualdo for valuable discussion and review of the manuscript.

This work was supported by the John Lowey Research Grant from the Kidney Foundation of Ohio and National Institutes of Health Grants DK 38544 (S.N.E.), AI 26449 and HL 37117 (M.E.L.).

Address reprint requests to: Steven N. Emancipator, M.D., Institute of Pathology, Case Western Reserve University, 2085 Adelbert Road, Cleveland, OH 44106.

REFERENCES

1. Abramowsky CR, Christiansen, DM: Secretory immunoglobulin deposits in renal glomeruli of children with extrahepatic biliary atresia: studies in a human counterpart of experimental ligation of the bile ducts. Human Pathol 18:1126, 1987
2. Abranowsky CR, Dahms, B, Swinehart G: IgA-associated glomerular deposits in liver disease. Human Pathol 16:1243, 1985
3. Andre C, Berthoux FC, Andre F, Gillon J, Genin C, Sabatier JC: Prevalence of IgA2 deposits in IgA nephropathies: a clue to their pathogenesis. N Engl J Med 303:1343, 1980
4. Barbeau J, Bourget J, Deslauriers N: RFc alpha-bearing cells and IgA-mediated phagocytes in the mouse oral mucosa. Adv Exp Biol Med 216:563, 1987

5. Baud L, Hagege J, Sraer J, Rondeau E, Perez J, Ardaillou R: Reactive oxygen production by cultured rat glomerular mesangial cells during phagocytosis is associated with stimulation of lipoxygenase activity. J Exp Med 158:1836, 1983

6. Bene MC, Faure G: Mucosal immunity and IgA nephropathy. Semin Nephrol 7:297, 1987

7. Bene MC, Faure G, Duheille J: IgA nephropathy: characterization of the polymeric nature of mesangial deposits by *in vitro* binding of free secretory component. Clin Exp Immunol 47:527, 1982

8. Berger J, Hinglias N: Les depots intercapillaires d'IgA-IgG. J Urol Nephrol 74:694, 1968

9. Bernatowska E, Rejman E, Kus J, Madalinski K, Wooniewicz B: Subpopulations of lymphocytes and macrophages/monocytes in small intestine and blood of children with primary antibody immunodeficiency. Adv Exp Biol Med 216:1455, 1987

10. Beukhof JR, Kardaun O, Ockhuizen T, van der Hem GK: Kidney survival in IgA nephropathy: multiple regression analysis of genetically differing subpopulations; is IgA nephropathy a real disease entity? Semin Nephrol 7:367, 1987

11. Bond MW, Schrader B, Mosmann TR, Coffman RL: A mouse T cell product that preferentially enhances IgA production. II. Physiochemical characterization. J Immunol 139:3691, 1987

12. Braden G, Rastegar A, Hession J, Garb J, Siegel N, Fitzgibbons J, Kashgarian M: Predictors of progression to chronic renal failure (CRF) in idiopathic membranous glomerulonephritis (MG) (abstr). Kidney Int 33:183, 1988

13. Brown TA, Russell MW, Mestecky J: Hepatobiliary transport of IgA immune complexes: molecular and cellular aspects. J Immunol 128:2183, 1982

14. Cagnoli L, Zucchelli P: Lymphocyte dysfunctions and clinical outcome in primary IgA nephropathy. Semin Nephrol 7:318, 1987

15. Cairns SA, London A, Mallick NP: Circulating immune complexes following food: delayed clearance in idiopathic glomerulonephritis. J Clin Lab Immunol 6:121, 1981

16. Challacombe SJ, Tomasi TB: Systemic tolerance and secretory immunity after oral immunization. J Exp Med 152:1459, 1980

17. Clarkson AR: Preface. In IgA Nephropathy, edited by Clarkson AR, p ix. Boston, Martinus Nijhoff Publishing, 1987

18. Clarkson AR, Seymour AE, Thompson AJ, Haynes WDG, Chan Y-L, Jackson B: IgA nephropathy: a syndrome of uniform morphology, diverse clinical features, and uncertain prognosis. Clin Nephrol 8:459–1977

19. Clarkson AR, Woodroffe AJ: Treatment tentatives in IgA nephropathy. Semin Nephrol 7:393, 1987

20. Clarkson AR, Woodroffe AJ, Aarons I: IgA nephropathy in patients followed up for at least ten years. Semin Nephrol 7:377, 1987

21. Cochrane CG, Muller-Eberhard HJ, Aikin BS: Depletion of plasma complement in vivo by a protein of cobra venom: its effect on various immunologic reactions. J Immunol 105:55, 1970

22. Coffman RL, Shrader B, Carty J, Mosmann TR, Bond MW: A mouse T cell product that preferentially enhances IgA production. I. Biologic characterization. J Immunol 139:3685, 1987

23. Conley ME, Cooper MD, Michael AF: Selective deposition of IgA$_1$ in IgA nephropathy, anaphylactoid purpura nephritis. amd systemic lupus erythematosus. J Clin Invest 66:1432, 1980

24. Coppo R, Basolo B, Piccoli G, Mazzucco G, Bulzoni MR, Roccatello D, De Marchi M, Carbonara AO, di Belgioioso GB: IgA$_1$ and IgA$_2$ immune complexes in primary IgA nephropathy and Henoch-Schonlein nephritis. Clin Exp Immunol 57:583, 1984

25. Coppo R, Basolo B, Rollino C, Roccatello D, Martin G, Amore A, Bogiorno G, Piccoli G: Mediterranean diet and primary IgA nephropathy. Clin Nephrol 26:72, 1986

26. Couser WG, Baker PJ, Adler S: Complement and the direct mediation of immune glomerular injury: a new perspective. Kidney Int 28:879, 1985

27. Czerkinsky C, Koopman WJ, Jackson S, Collins JE, Crago SS, Schrohenloher RE, Julian BA, Galla JH, Mestecky J: Circulating immune complexes and immunoglobulin A rheumatoid factor in patients with mesangial immunoglobulin A nephropathies. J Clin Invest 77:1931, 1986

28. Czop J, Nussenzweig V: Studies on the mechanism of solubilization of immune precipitates by serum. J Exp Med 143:615, 1976

29. D'Amico G: Natural history and prognosis. In IgA Nephropathy, edited by Clarkson AR, p 108. Boston, Martinus Nijhoff Publishing, 1987

30. D'Amico G, Colasanti G, di Belgioioso GB, Fellini G, Ragni A, Egidi F, Radaelli L, Fogazzi G, Ponticelli C, Minetti L: Long-term followup of IgA mesangial nephropathy: clinico-histological study in 374 patients. Semin Nephrol 7:355, 1987

31. Davin J-C, Malaise M, Foidart J, Mahieu P: Anti-α-galactosyl antibodies and immune complexes in children with Henoch-Schonlein purpura or IgA nephropathy. Kidney Int 31:1132, 1987

32. Davis CA, Abramowsky CR, Swinehart G: Circulating immune complexes and the nephropathy of cystic fibrosis. Human Pathol 15:244, 1984

33. Delacroix DL, Hodgson HJF, McPherson A, Dive C, Vaerman JP: Selective transport of polymeric immunoglobulin A in bile. J Clin Invest 70:230, 1982

34. Demaine AG, Rambausek M, Knight JF, Williams DG, Welsh KI, Ritz E: Relation of mesangial IgA glomerulonephritis to polymorphism of immunoglobulin heavy chain switch region. J Clin Invest 81:611, 1988

35. Dobrin RS, Knudson FE, Michael AF: The secretory immune system and renal disease. Clin Exp Immunol 21:318, 1975

36. Egido J: The role of polymeric IgA in the pathogenesis of IgA nephropathy. In IgA Nephropathy, edited by Clarkson AR, p 157. Boston, Martinus Nijhoff Publishing, 1987

37. Egido J, Blasco R, Sancho J, Lozano L, Sanchez-Crespo M, Hernando L: Increased rate of polymeric IgA synthesis by circulating lymphoid cells in IgA mesangial glomerulonephritis. Clin Exp Immunol 47:309, 1982

38. Egido J, Garcia-Hoyo R, Lozano L, Gonzalez-Cabrero J, de Nicolas R, Hernando L: Immunological studies in familial and sporadic IgA nephropathy. Semin Nephrol 7:311, 1987

39. Egido J, Julian BA, Wyatt RJ: Genetic factors in primary IgA nephropathy. Nephrol Dial Transplant 2:134, 1987

40. Egido J, Sancho J, Mampaso F, Lopez-Trascasa M, Sanchez-Crespo M, Blasco R, Hernando L: A possible common pathogenesis of the mesangial IgA glomerulonephritis in patients with Berger's disease and Schoenlein-Henoch syndrome. Proc Eur Dial Transplant Assoc 17:660, 1980

41. Emancipator SN, Gallo GR, Lamm ME: Experimental IgA nephropathy induced by oral immunization. J Exp Med 157:572, 1983

42. Emancipator SN, Gallo GR, Razaboni R, Lamm ME: Experimental cholestasis promotes the deposition of glomerular IgA Am J Pathol 113:19, 1983

44. Emancipator SN, Lamm ME: Pathways of tissue injury initiated by humoral immune mechanisms. Lab Invest 54:475, 1986

45. Emancipator SN, Lamm ME: The role of IgG, IgM and C3 in experimental murine IgA nephropathy. Semin Nephrol 7:286, 1987

46. Emancipator SN, Lamm ME: Oral tolerance as a protective mechanism against hypersensitivity disease. Monogr in Allergy, 24:244, 1987

47. Emancipator SN, Ovary Z, Lamm ME: The role of mesangial complement in the hematuria of experimental IgA nephropathy. Lab Invest 57:269, 1987

48. Endoh M, Sakai H, Suga T, Miura M, Tomino Y, Nomoto Y: Increase of peripheral blood B cells with Fc receptor for IgA in patients with IgA nephropathy. Scand J Immunol 17:437, 1983

49. Garcia-Hoyo R, Egido J, Lozano L, de Nicolas R, Hernando L: Disturbances of IgA immune regulation in lymphocytes from mucosae and peripheral blood in patients with IgA nephropathy. Semin Nephrol 7:301, 1987

50. Gartner HV, Vetter W, Bohle A: IgA nephritis-prognostic relevance of glomerular focal-segmental lesions. Proceedings of the IXth International Congress of Nephrology, I:281, 1984

51. Genin C, Sabatier JC, Berthoux FC: IgA mesangial deposits in C3H/HeJ mice after oral immunization. Proc Eur Dial Transpl Assoc-Eur Renal Assoc 21:703, 1985

52. Gormly AA, Smith PS, Seymour AF, Clarkson AR, Woodroffe, AJ: IgA glomerular deposits in experimental cirrhosis. Am J Pathol 104:50, 1981

53. Gorter A, Hiemstra PS, Klar-Mohamed N, van Es LA, Daha MR: Binding and degradation of soluble aggregates of IgA by rat peritoneal macrophages. Adv Exp Biol Med 216:1333, 1987

54. Gorter A, Hiemstra PS, Leijh PCJ, van Es LA, Daha MR: Stimulation of human polymorphonuclear leukocytes by serum IgA or secretory IgA. Adv Exp Biol Med 216:1325, 1987

55. Gregory MC, Hammond ME, Brewer ED: Renal deposition of cytomegalovirus antigen in immunoglobulin-A nephropathy. Lancet I:11, 1988

56. Grey HM, Abel CA, Yount WJ, Kunkel HG: A subclass of human γA globulins (γA2) which lacks the disulfide bonds linking heavy and light chains. J Exp Med 128:1223, 1968

57. Habib RB, Stork JE, Emancipator SN: Complement on immune complexes (IC) or zymosan (Z) stimulates prostaglandin (PG) E_2 synthesis by glomeruli and cultured glomerular epithelial cells (abstr). Fed Proc 46:1329, 1987

58. Hall RP, Stachura I, Cason J, Whiteside TL, Lawley TJ: IgA-containing circulating immune complexes in patients with IgA nephropathy. Am J Med 74:56, 1983

59. Harriman GR, Strober W: Interleukin 5, a mucosal lymphokine? J Immunol 139:3553, 1987

60. Hebert LA, Cosio FG: The erythrocyte-immune complex-glomerulonephritis connection in man. Kidney Int 31:877, 1987

61. Heremans JF: Immunoglobulin A. In The Antigens, Vol II, edited by Sela M, p 365. New York, Academic Press, 1974

62. Hiemstra PS, Gorter A, Stuurman ME, van Es LA, Daha MR: Activation of the alternative pathway of complement by human serum IgA. Eur J Immunol 17:321, 1987

63. Hirayama H, Hirano T, Kohler G, Kurata A, Okumura K, Ovary Z: Biological activities of anti-trinitrophenyl and anti-dinitrophenyl mouse monoclonal antibodies. Proc Natl Acad Sci USA 79:613, 1982

64. Hoover RG, Dieckgraefe BK, Lake J, Kemp JD, Lynch RG: Lymphocyte surface membrane immunoglobulin in myeloma. III. IgA plasmacytomas induce large numbers of circulating, adult-thymectomy-sensitive, Θ^+, Lyt-1⁻2⁺ lymphocytes with IgA-Fc receptors. J Immunol 129:2329, 1982

65. Hoover RG, Dieckgraefe BK, Lynch RG: T cells with Fc receptors for IgA: induction of Tα cells *in vivo* and *in vitro* by purified IgA. J Immunol 127;1560, 1981

66. Hoover RG, Lynch RG: Lymphocyte surface membrane immunoglobulin in myeloma. II. T cells with IgA-Fc receptors are markedly increased in mice with IgA plasmacytomas. J Immunol 125:1280, 1980

67. Hoover RG, Lynch RG: T cells with FC receptors in myeloma: suppression of growth and secretion of MOPC-315 by Tα cells. J Immunol 134:644, 1985

68. Hyman LR, Wagnild JP, Beirne GJ, Burkholder PM: Immunoglobulin A distribution in glomerular disease: analysis of immunofluorescence localization and pathogenic significance. Kidney Int 3:397, 1973

69. Imai H, Chen A, Endoh M, Rifai A: Influence of the antigen on experimental IgA nephropathy. Semin Nephrol 7:283, 1987

70. Imai H, Chen A, Wyatt RJ, Rifai A: Composition of IgA immune complexes precipitated with polyethylene glycol: a model for isolation and analysis of immune complexes. J Immunol Methods 103:239, 1987

71. Imai H, Nakamoto Y, Askaura K, Miki K, Yasuda T, Miura AB: Spontaneous glomerular IgA deposition in ddY mice: an animal model of IgA nephritis. Kidney Int 27:756, 1985

72. Isaacs K, Miller F: Role of antigen size and charge in immune complex glomerulonephritis. I. Active induction of disease with dextran and its derivatives. Lab Invest 47:198, 1982

73. Isaacs K, Miller F: Antigen size and charge in immune complex glomerulonephritis. II. Passive induction of immune deposits with dextran-anti-dextran immune complexes. Am J Pathol 111:298, 1983

74. Isaacs K, Miller F, Lane B: Experimental model for IgA nephropathy. Clin Immunol Immunopathol 20:419, 1981

75. Jackson S, Montgomery RI, Mestecky J, Julian BA, Galla JH, Czerkinsky C: Antibodies directed at Fab of IgA in the sera of normal individuals and IgA nephropathy patients. Adv Exp Biol Med 216:1537, 1987

76. Jennette JC, Wall SD, Wilkman S: Low incidence of IgA nephropathy in Blacks. Kidney Int 28:944, 1985

77. Jessen RH, Nedrud JG, Emancipator SN: A mouse model of IgA nephropathy induced by Sendai virus. Adv Exp Med Biol 216:1609, 1987

78. Johnson KJ, Ward PA, Kunkel RG, Wilson BS: Mediation of IgA induced lung injury in the rat: role of macrophages and reactive oxygen products. Lab Invest 54:499, 1986

79. Julian BA, Phillips III JA, Orlando PJ, Wyatt RJ, Butler MG: Analysis of immunoglobulin heavy chain restriction fragment length polymorphisms in IgA nephropathy. Semin Nephrol 7:306, 1987

80. Julian BA, Quiggins PA, Thompson JS, Woodford SY, Gleason K, Wyatt RJ: Familial IgA nephropathy: evidence of an inherited mechanism of disease. N Engl J Med 312:202, 1985

81. Kagnoff MF: Effects of antigen-feeding on intestinal and systemic immune responses. III. Antigen-specific serum-mediated suppression of humoral antibody responses after antigen feeding. Cell Immunol 40:186, 1978

82. Katz A, Karanicolas S, Falk JA: Family study in IgA nephritis: the possible role of HLA antigens. Transplantation 29:505, 1980

83. Kawanishi H, Saltzman L, Strober W: Mechanisms regulating IgA-class specific immunoglobulin production in murine gut-associated lymphoid tissues. 1. T cells derived from Peyer's patches which switch sIgM B cells to sIgA B cells *in vitro*. J Exp Med 157:433, 1983

84. Kiyono H, Cooper MD, Kearney JF, Mosteller LM, Michalek SM, Koopman WJ, McGhee JR: Isotype specificity of helper T cell clones: Peyer's patch Th cells preferentially collaborate with mature IgA B cells for IgA responses. J Exp Med 159:798, 1984

85. Kobayashi Y, Hiki Y, Fujii K, Kurokawa A, Tateno S: IgA nephropathy: heterogeneous clinical pictures and steroid therapy in progressive chases. Semin Nephrol 7:382, 1987

86. Konig W, Bitter-Suermann D, Dierich M, Limbert M, Schorlemmer HU, Hadding U: DNP-antigens activate the alternate pathway of the complement system. J Immunol 113:501, 1974

87. Lamm ME: Cellular aspects of immunoglobulin A. Adv Immunol 22:223, 1976

88. Lemaitre-Coelho I, Jackson GDF, Vaerman J-P: High levels of secretory IgA and free secretory component in the serum of rats with bile duct obstruction. J Exp Med 147:934, 1978

89. Lomax-Smith JD, Zabrowarny LA, Howarth GS, Seymour AE, Woodroffe AJ: The immunochemical characterization of mesangial IgA deposits. Am J Pathol 113:359, 1983

90. Lovett DH, Szamel M, Ryan JL, Sterzel RB, Gemsa D, Resch K: Interleukin 1 and the glomerular mesangium. I. Purification and characterization of a mesangial cell-derived auto-growth factor. J Immunol 136:3700, 1986

91. Lupo A, Rugiu C, Cagnoli L, Zucchelli P, Maschio G: Acute changes in renal function in IgA nephropathy. Semin Nephrol 7:359, 1987

92. Martin J, Lovett DH, Gemsa D, Sterzel RB, Davies M: Enhancement of glomerular mesangial cell neutral proteinase secretion by macrophages: role of interleukin 1. J Immunol 137:525, 1986

93. Mattingly JA, Kaplan JM, Janeway CA: Two distinct antigen-specific suppressor factors induced by the oral administration of antigen. J Exp Med 152:545, 1980

94. Mayer L: Switch T cell line, ST, induces an Ig class switch in surface isotype. Adv Exp Biol Med 216:39, 1987

95. McKenzie PE, Gormly AA, Clarkson AR, Seymour AE, Kwitko AO, Shearman DJC, Woodroffe AJ: Gut-derived antigens and immune complexes in IgA nephropathy. Aust N Z J Med 10:126, 1980

96. Melvin T, Burke B, Michael AF, Kim Y: Experimental IgA nephropathy in bile duct ligated rats. Clin Immunol Immunopathol 27:369, 1983

97. Mestecky J, McGhee JR: Immunoglobulin A (IgA): molecular and cellular interactions involved in IgA biosynthesis and immune response. Adv Immunol 40:153, 1987

98. Mestecky J, Tamana M, Czerkinsky C, Tarkowski, A, Matsuda S, Waldo FB, Moldoveanu Z, Julian BA, Galla JH, Russell MW, Jackson S: IgA-associated renal diseases: immunochemical studies of IgA1 proteins, circulating immune complexes, and cellular interactions. Semin Nephrol 7:332, 1987

99. Michael J, Jones NF, Davies DR, Tighe JR: Recurrent haematuria: role of renal biopsy and investigative morbidity. Br Med J 1:686, 1976

100. Miller GW: Solubilization of IgA immune precipitates by complement. J Immunol 127:1374, 1976

101. Miller GW, Nussenzweig V: A new complement function: solubilization of antigen-antibody aggregates. Proc Natl Acad Sci USA 72:418, 1975

102. Monteiro RC, Noel LH, Halbwachs-Mecarelli L, Berger J, Lesavre

P: Charge and size of mesangial IgA in IgA nephropathy. Kidney Int 28:666, 1985

103. Montgomery PC, Lemaitre-Coelho IM, Vaerman J-P: Molecular diversity of secretory IgA anti-DNP antibodies elicited in rat bile. J Immunol 125:518, 1980

104. Mostov KE, Kraehenbuhl JP, Blobel G: Receptor-mediated transcellular transport of immunoglobulin: synthesis of secretory component as multiple and larger transmembrane forms. Proc Natl Acad Sci USA 77:7257, 1980

105. Mustonen J, Pasternack A, henlin H: The course of the disease in patients with the nephrotic syndrome and IgA nephropathy. Semin Nephrol 7:374, 1987

106. Nagura H, Smith PD, Nakane PK, Brown WR: IgA in human bile and liver. J Immunol 126:587, 1981

107. Nagy J, Uj M, Szücs G, Trinn C, Burger T: Herpes virus antigens and antibodies in kidney biopsies and sera of IgA glomerulonephritic patients. Clin Nephrol 21:259, 1984

108. Neelakantappa K, Gallo GR, Baldwin DS: Proteinuria in IgA nephropathy. Semin Nephrol 7:344, 1987

109. Deleted in proof.

110. Noel LH, Droz D, Gascon M, Berger J: Primary IgA nephropathy: from the first described cases to the present. Semin Nephrol 7:351, 1987

111. Okada M, Okamura K, Ohmura N, Kitaoka T: Clinicopathological study of IgA nephropathy in comparison wtih mesangial proliferative glomerulonephritis without IgA deposits. Proceedings of the IXth International Congress of Nephrology, I:117, 1984

112. Peppard J, Orlans E, Payne AWR, Andrew E: The elimination of circulating complexes containing IgA by excretion in the bile. Immunol 42:83, 1981

113. Pfaffenbach G, Lamm ME, Gigli I: Activation of the guinea pig alternative complement pathway by mouse IgA immune complexes. J Exp Med 155:231, 1982

114. Phillips-Quagliata JM, Lamm ME: Circulation and differentiation of lymphocytes in gut associated lymphoid tissue and mammary gland. In Food Allergy and Intolerance, edited by Brostoff J, Challacombe SJ, p 54. London, Bailliere Tindall, 1987

115. Podack ER, Preissner KT, Muller-Eberhard HJ: Inhibition of C9 polymerization within the SC5b-9 complex by S-protein. Acta Pathol Microbiol Immunol Scand 284 (Suppl) 92:89, 1984

116. Propper DJ, Power DA, Simpson JG, Edward N, Catto GRD: The incidence, mode of presentation and prognosis of IgA nephropathy in northeast Scotland. Semin Nephrol 7:363, 1987

117. Rambausek M, Rauterberg E-W, Waldherr R, Demaine A, Krupp G, Ritz E: Evolution of IgA glomerulonephritis: relation to morphology, immunogenetics, and blood pressure. Semin Nephrol 7:370, 1987

118. Rambausek M, Seelig HP, Andrassy K, Waldherr R, Lenhard V, Ritz E: Clinical and serological features of mesangial IgA glomerulonephritis. Proc Eur Dial Transplat Assoc 19:663, 1982

119. Rauterberg EW, Gehrig T, Lieberknecht M: C5-9 neoantigen detection indicates a complete complement activation in various types of glomerulonephritis (abstr). Mol Immunol 19:1398, 1982

120. Reynolds HY, Thompson RE: Pulmonary host defenses. I. Analysis of protein and lipids in bronchial secretions and antibody responses after vaccination with *Pseudomonas aeruginosa*. J Immunol 111:358, 1973

121. Rifai A: Experimental models for IgA-associated nephritis. Kidney Int 31:1, 1987

122. Rifai A, Chen A, Imai H: Complement activation in experimental IgA nephropathy: an antigen-mediated process. Kidney Int 32:838, 1987

123. Rifai A, Mannik M: Clearance kinetics and fate of mouse IgA immune complexes prepared with monomeric or dimeric IgA. J Immunol 130:1826, 1983

124. Rifai A, Mannik, M: Clearance of circulating IgA immune complexes is mediated by a specific receptor on Kupffer cells in mice. J Exp Med 160:125, 1984

125. Rifai A, Small PA, Teague PO, Ayoub EM: Experimental IgA nephropathy. J Exp Med 150:1161, 1979

126. Rits M, Hiemstra PS, Van Es LA, Bazin M, Vaerman JP, Daha MR: Complement-mediated solubilization of rat IgA immune precipitates. Mol Immunol 24:1047, 1987

127. Robertson J, Caldwell JR, Castle JR, Waldman RH: Evidence for the presence of components of the alternative (properdin) pathway of complement activation in respiratory secretions. J Immunol 117:900, 1976

128. Roy LP, Fish AJ, Vernier RL, Michael AF: Recurrent macroscopic hematuria, focal nephritis, and mesangial deposition of immunoglobulin and complement. J Pediatr 82:767, 1973

129. Sabatier JC, Genin C, Assenat H, Colon S, Ducret F, Berthoux FC: Mesangial IgA glomerulonephritis in HLA-identical brothers. Clin Nephrol 11:35, 1979

130. Sakai H: Lymphocyte function in IgA nephropathy. In IgA Nephropathy, edited by Clarkson AR, p 176. Boston, Martinus Nijhoff Publishing, 1987

131. Saklayen MG, Pesce AJ, Pollak VE, Michael JG: Kinetics of oral tolerance: study of variables affecting tolerance induced by oral administration of antigen. Int Arch Allergy Appl Immunol 73:5, 1984

132. Sancho J, Egido J, Rivera F, Hernando L: Immune complexes in IgA nephropathy: presence of antibodies against diet antigens and delayed clearance of specific polymeric IgA immune complexes. Clin Exp Immunol 54:194, 1983

133. Sato M, Idewa T, Koshikowa S: Experimental IgA nephropathy in mice. Lab Invest 54:377, 1986

134. Scharschmidt LA, Lianos E, Dunn MJ: Arachidonate metabolites and the control of glomerular function. Fed Proc 42:3058, 1983

135. Schena FP, Mastrolitti G, Fracasso AR, Pastore A, Ladisa N: Increased immunoglobulin-secreting cells in the blood of patients with active idiopathic IgA nephropathy. Clin Nephrol 26:163, 1986

136. Schena FP, Pastore A, Sinico RA, Ladisa N, Montinaro V, Fornasieri A: Studies on the mechanism producing solubilization of immune precipitates in the serum of patients with primary IgA nephropathy. Semin Nephrol 7:336, 1987

137. Schena PF, Pastore A, Sinico RA, Montinaro V, Fornasieri A: Polymeric IgA decreases the capacity of serum to solubilize circulating immune complexes in patients with primary IgA nephropathy. J Immunol 141:125, 1988

138. Schlondorff D, Satriano JA, Hagege J, Perez J, Baud L: Effect of platelet-activating factor and serum-treated zymosan on prostaglandin E_2 synthesis, arachidonic acid release, and contraction of cultured rat mesangial cells. J Clin Invest 73:1227, 1984

139. Schreiner GF, Unanue ER: Origin of the rat mesangial phagocyte and its expression of luekocyte common antigen. Lab Invest 51:515, 1984

140. Sedor JR, Carey SW, Emancipator SN: Immune complexes bind to cultured rat glomerular mesangial cells to stimulate superoxide release: evidence for an Fc receptor. J Immunol 138:3751, 1987

141. Sinico RA, Fornasieri A, Oreni N, Benuzzi S, D'Amico G: Polymeric IgA rheumatoid factor in idiopathic IgA mesangial nephropathy (Berger's disease). J Immunol 137:536, 1986

142. Sinico RA, Fornasieri A, Paterna L, Maldifassi P, Benuzzi S: Studies on IgA antiglobulins in IgA nephropathy. Semin Nephrol 7:325, 1987

143. Sissons JGP, Woodrow DF, Curtis JR, Evans DJ, Gower PE, Sloper JC, Peters DK: Isolated glomerulonephritis with mesangial IgA deposits. Br Med J 3:611, 1975

144. Smith SM, Tung KSK: Incidence of IgA-related nephritides in American Indians in New Mexico. Human Pathol 16:181, 1985

145. Snapper CM, Paul WE: B cell stimulator factor-1 (interleukin 4) prepares resting murine B cells to secrete IgG1 upon subsequent stimulation with bacterial lipopolysaccharide. J Immunol 139:10, 1987

146. Socken DJ, Simms ES, Nagy BR, Fisher MM, Underdown BJ: Secretory component-dependent hepatic transport of IgA antibody-antigen complexes. J Immunol 127:316, 1981

147. Stork JE, Dunn MJ, Emancipator SN: Identification of complement receptor (CR1) on rat glomerular cells: effects of complement on prostaglandin synthesis (abstr). Clin Res 33:589, 1985

148. Syre G: IgA mesangial glomerulonephritis: significance and pathogenesis of segmental-focal glomerular lesions. Virchow's Arch [A] 402:11, 1983

149. Takahashi M, Czop J, Ferriera A, Nussenzweig V: Mechanism of solubilization of immune aggregates by complement: implications for immunopathology. Transplant Rev 32:121, 1976

150. Tojo S, Hatano M, Honda N, Miyahara T, Sugino N, Narita M, Sakai H: Natural history of IgA nephropathy in Japan. Semin Nephrol 7:386, 1987

151. Tolkoff-Rubin NE, Cosimi AB, Fuller T, Rubin RH, Colvin RB: IgA nephropathy in HLA-identical siblings. Transplantation

26:430, 1978
152. Tomino Y, endoh M, Nomoto Y, Sakai H: Immunoglobulin A₁ in IgA nephropathy. N Engl J Med 305:1159, 1981
153. Tomino Y, Endoh M, Nomoto Y, Sakai H: Specificity of eluted antibody from renal tissues of patients with IgA nephropathy. Am J Kidney Dis 1:276, 1982
154. Tomino Y, Sakai H: Exacerbating factors in patients with IgA nephropathy. Semin Nephrol 7:315, 1987
155. Tomino Y, Sakai H, Endoh M, Kaneshige H, Nomoto Y: Detection of immune complexes in polymorphonuclear leukocytes by double immunofluorescence in patients with IgA nephropathy. Clin Immunol Immunopathol 24:63, 1982
156. Tomino Y, Sakai H, Endoh M, Suga T, Miura M, Kaneshige H, Nomoto Y: Cross reactivity of IgA antibodies between renal mesangial areas and nuclei of tonsillar cells in patients with IgA nephropathy. Clin Exp Immunol 51:605, 1983
157. Tomino Y, Sakai H, Hashimoto K, Tanaka S: Antigenic heterogeneity in patients with IgA nephropathy. Semin Nephrol 7:294, 1987
158. Tomino Y, Sakai H, Miura M, Endoh M, Nomoto Y: Detection of polymeric IgA in glomeruli from patients with IgA nephropathy. Clin Exp Immunol 49:419, 1982
159. Tomino Y, Sakai H, Suga T, Miura M, Kaneshige H, Endoh M, Nomoto Y: Impaired solubilization of glomerular immune deposits by sera from patients with IgA nephropathy. Am J Kidney Dis 3:48, 1983
160. Trejdosiewicz LK, Malizia G, Badr-el-Din S, Smart CJ, Oakes DJ, Southgate J, Howdle PD, Janossy G, Poulter LW, Losowsky MS: T cell and mononuclear phagocyte populations of the human small and large intestine. Adv Exp Biol Med 216:465, 1987
161. Tsai CC, Giangiancomo JJ, Zuckner J: Dermal IgA deposits in Henoch-Schoenlein purpura and Berger's nephritis. Lancet 1:347, 1975
162. van de Putte LBA, Brutel de la Riviere G, van Breda Vriesman PJC: Recurrent or persistent hematuria: sign of mesangial immune-complex deposition. N Engl J Med 290:1165, 1974
163. van der Woude FJ, Hoedemaeker PJ, van der Giessen M, de Graeff PA, de Monchy J, The TH, van der Hem GK: Do food antigens play a role in the pathogenesis of some cases of human glomerulonephritis? Clin Exp Immunol 51:587, 1983
164. Velo M, Lozano L, Egido J, Gutierrez-Millet V, Hernando L: Natural history of IgA nephropathy in patients followed for more than ten years in Spain. Semin Nephrol 7:346, 1987
165. Velosa JA, Shah SV, Ou SL, Abboud HE, Dousa TP: Activities of lysosomal enzymes in isolated glomeruli: alterations in experimental nephrosis. Lab Invest 45:522, 1981
166. Waldherr R, Seelig HP, Rambausek M, Andrassy K, Ritz E: Deposition of polymeric IgA in idiopathic mesangial IgA glomerulonephritis. Klin Wochenschr 61:911, 1983
167. Waldo FB, Mestecky J, Kohaut EC: Mixed IgG-IgA aggregates as a model of immune complexes (IC) in IgA nephropathy (IgAN) (abstr). Kidney Int 33:326, 1988
168. Waxman FJ, Hebert LA, Cosio FG, Smead WL, VanAman ME, Taguiam JM, Birmingham DJ: Differential binding of immunoglobulin A and immunoglobulin G1 immune complexes to primate erythrocytes in vivo. J Clin Invest 77:82, 1986
169. Werber HI, Emancipator SN, Tykocinski ML, Sedor JR: The interleukin 1 gene is expressed by rat glomerular mesangial cells and is augmented in immune complex glomerulonephritis. J Immunol 138:3207, 1987
170. Williams DG, Perl SJ, Knight JF, Harada T: Immunoglobulin production in vitro in IgA nephropathy and Henoch Schonlein purpura. Semin Nephrol 7:322, 1987
171. Woo KT, Ghiang GSC, Lau YK, Lim CH: IgA nephropathy in Singapore: clinical, prognostic indices and treatment. Semin Nephrol 7:379, 1987
172. Woodroffe AJ, Gormly AA, McKenzie PE, Wootton AM, Thompson AJ, Seymour AE, Clarkson AR: Immunologic studies in IgA nephropathy. Kidney Int 18:366, 1980
173. Wyatt RJ, Julian BA, Woodford SY, McLean RH, Thompson JS: Immunogenetic markers as prognostic features in patients from Kentucky with IgA nephropathy. Semin Nephrol 7:389, 1987
174. Young KR, Reynolds HY: Bronchoalveolar washings: proteins and cells from normal lungs. In Immunology of the Lung and Upper Respiratory Tract, edited by Bienenstock J, p 157. New York, McGraw-Hill, 1984

Biology of Disease
Goodpasture Syndrome: Molecular Architecture and Function of Basement Membrane Antigen

BILLY G. HUDSON, JÖRGEN WIESLANDER, BILLIE J. WISDOM JR., AND MILTON E. NOELKEN

Department of Biochemistry and Molecular Biology, University of Kansas Medical Center, Kansas City, Kansas and Department of Nephrology, University of Lund, Lund, Sweden

Introduction
Molecular Identity of GBM Antigen
    Properties of collagenase-solubilized Goodpasture antigen
    Identity of membrane Goodpasture antigen
    Specificity of Goodpasture antibodies
Molecular Architecture of Membrane Goodpasture Antigen
    Protomer structure
    Supramolecular structure
    Organization of protomer subtypes
    Cryptic properties of Goodpasture determinant(s)
Possible Functions of Goodpasture Antigen
Diagnosis and Treatment
Conclusions and Perspectives

INTRODUCTION

In studies of victims from the influenza pandemic of 1918–1919, Ernest Goodpasture described the coexistence of fatal pulmonary hemorrhage and proliferative glomerulonephritis in a young man (25). The term Goodpasture syndrome was coined by Stanton and Tange in 1958 to describe cases characterized by the coexistence of these manifestations (73). The syndrome is now defined as an autoimmune disorder consisting of the triad of glomerulonephritis, lung hemorrhage, and antiglomerular basement membrane antibody formation, and it includes a broad spectrum of clinical features, ranging from massive pulmonary hemorrhage with little overt evidence of renal disease to fulminant crescentic glomerulonephritis and little overt evidence of pulmonary hemorrhage (24). Although the etiology of this syndrome remains unknown, profound advances have been made during the last 25 years in delineating the pathogenesis of the glomerulonephritis.

The nephritis is mediated by auto-antibodies that bind to an intrinsic structural constituent(s) of glomerular basement membrane (GBM) (Fig. 1). The pathogenic role of antibodies targeted to GBM was discovered in 1962 by Steblay, who induced fatal glomerulonephritis in sheep by repeated injections of isolated heterologous GBM (74). Characteristic linear binding of sheep immunoglobulin along GBM was observed by immunofluorescence. Glomerulonephritis could be induced in healthy sheep by passive transfer of serum antibodies from nephritic sheep (41) and by cross-circulation (75). The possible involvement of auto-antibodies mediating nephritis in humans was noted by Scheer and Grossman (68) who observed the binding of antibodies along GBM in two patients with Goodpasture syndrome. Subsequently, a landmark study by Lerner *et al.* (42) demonstrated the pathogenic role of anti-GBM auto-antibodies in mediating glomerulonephritis in humans by finding that subhuman primates developed renal failure with the passive transfer of human antibodies. The immunopathogenicity of the antibodies was further confirmed in this study when glomerular injury was accidentally induced in a renal homograft that was transplanted into a patient who had circulating anti-GBM antibodies after preparatory nephrectomy. More recently, this role was further confirmed by the finding that upon therapy, clinical improvement was correlated with reduction of antibody titer (32, 33, 44–46, 58, 61, 66). Because of these findings, the term Goodpasture syndrome is now commonly used in a more restricted sense, referring only to those cases in which there is evidence for the presence of anti-GBM antibody (23, 94) along with glomerulonephritis and lung hemorrhage.

In the last decade, searches for the identity of the basement membrane constituent to which the anti-GBM antibodies are targeted have culminated in the elucidation of both the molecular identity and architecture of the Goodpasture antigen. Information about the antigen is fundamental in delineating the molecular basis of Goodpasture syndrome and in designing diagnostic tests as well as specific therapy. Our recent studies have yielded substantial evidence that the major antigenic determinant(s) for Goodpasture antibodies is localized to the noncollagenous (NC1) domain of type IV collagen (Fig. 1D). Furthermore, the studies have led to the discovery of a new chain (α3) of the collagen IV molecule that bears the Goodpasture determinant(s) and to a new concept about the supramolecular structure of basement membrane collagen (9, 11, 39, 65, 86, 91, 92). Recent studies of Alport-type familial nephritis implicate a crucial role of the α3 chain in GBM function (30–32, 34, 37, 50, 54). This review describes the molecular relationship between the Goodpasture antigen and the collagen IV constituents of GBM, the molecular architecture and possible functions of the membrane Goodpasture antigen, and modes of diagnosis and treatment of Goodpasture syndrome.

MOLECULAR IDENTITY OF GBM ANTIGEN

Type IV collagen was recently identified as the GBM constituent that contains the major reactivity with Goodpasture antibodies (65, 86). This identification is based on information derived from three lines of study that pertain to 1) chemical and immunochemical properties of collagenase-solubilized Goodpasture antigen, 2) the molecular relationship between the collagenase-solubilized Goodpasture antigen and the known intrinsic constituents of basement membrane, and 3) specificity of the anti-GBM antibodies. In particular, knowledge of the structural features and properties of the collagenous constituent of GBM provided the requisite information for the identification.

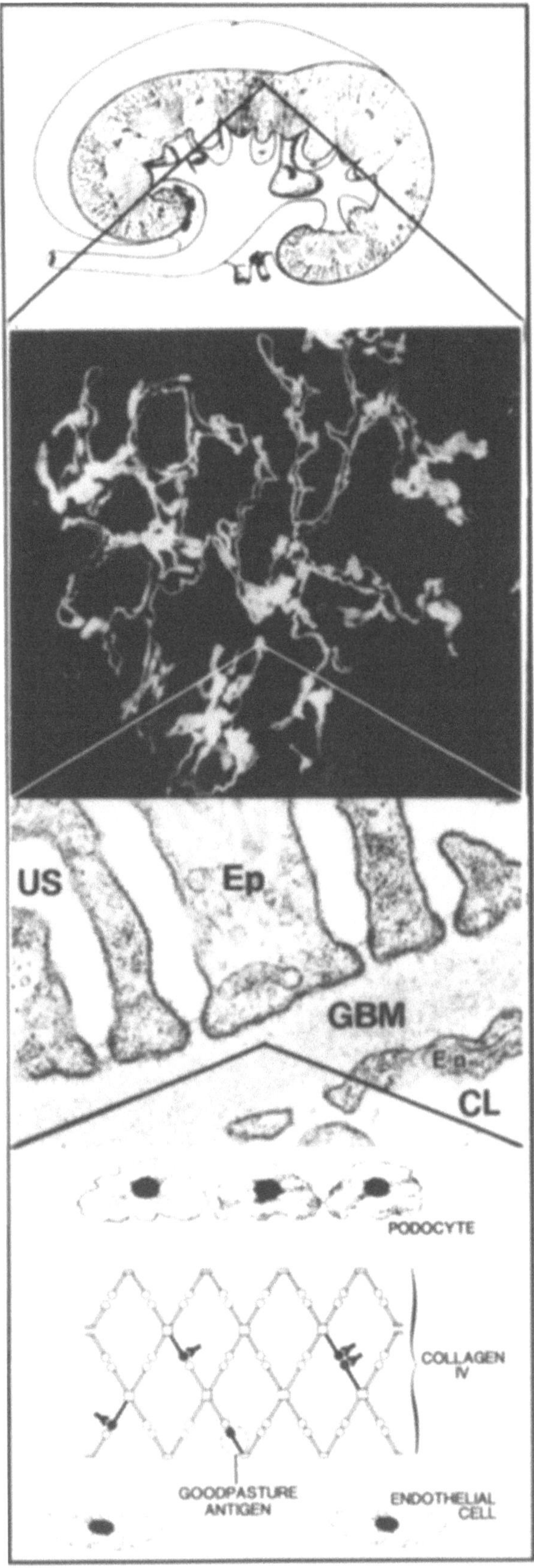

FIG. 1. Flow diagram depicting localization of Goodpasture antigen from tissue (organ) level to molecular level. A, depicts the kidney as one major target of pathogenic anti-GBM auto-antibodies in Goodpasture syndrome. B, typical linear staining of Goodpasture antibodies bound to GBM (immunofluorescence). C, electron micrograph of a section of glomerular capillary wall. D, diagram of collagen IV supramolecular structure showing Goodpasture antibodies bound to a specific subtype of collagen IV protomer (building block unit) that contains the α3 chain and Goodpasture determinant(s). Electron micrograph was provided by Dr. D. R. Abrahamson (University of Alabama) and adapted from reference 1. CL, capillary lumen; En, endothelium; Ep, epithelial podocytes; GBM, glomerular basement membrane; US, urinary space.

PROPERTIES OF COLLAGENASE-SOLUBILIZED GOODPASTURE ANTIGEN

Initial studies focused on the solubilization and characterization of GBM components that contain the antigenic determinants reacting with Goodpasture antibodies. Several investigators found that the Goodpasture determinant can be solubilized from GBM by treatment with purified bacterial collagenase (11, 21, 28, 29, 47, 49, 51, 52, 86, 88, 91, 95, 98), rendering it amenable to studies of its chemical and immunochemical properties. These studies culminated with the finding that the Goodpasture determinant(s) in the collagenase digest resides with two noncollagenous polypeptides, which exist in monomer (M_r = 26,000) and dimer (M_r = 50,000) forms (28, 88),

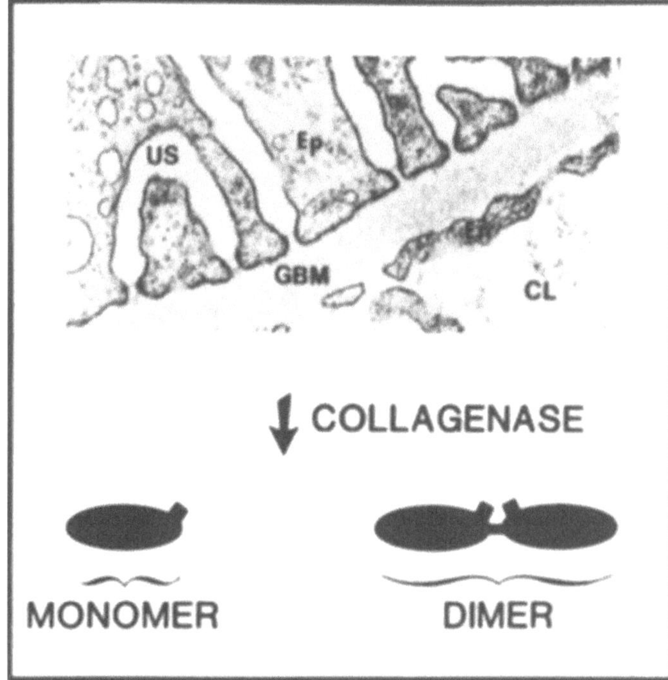

FIG. 2. Solubilization of Goodpasture antigen by collagenase digestion of GBM. GBM is first isolated from glomerular capillary wall (electron micrograph) and then subjected to collagenase digestion. Collagenase-solubilized antigen occurs in monomer and dimer form; these were subsequently designated M2* and D2*, respectively (11). Electron micrograph was provided by Dr. D. R. Abrahamson (University of Alabama) and adapted from reference 1. Abbreviations as in Figure 1.

as depicted in Figure 2. Each contains a disulfide bond that is essential for antibody reactivity (88). These soluble forms are commonly referred to as the Goodpasture antigen, but, as described below, they are proteolytic fragments derived from an insoluble collagenous precursor embedded in the GBM matrix.

IDENTITY OF MEMBRANE GOODPASTURE ANTIGEN

In recent studies, we discovered that these Goodpasture fragments, in the membrane matrix, are subunits of the NC1 domain of type IV collagen as depicted in Figure 3. The initial clue for this localization came from the apparent structural relatedness of the monomer form of the collagenase-solubilized Goodpasture antigen with that of the collagenase-resistant polypeptide that is derived from the NC1 domain of the α1 chain of collagen IV (16). Evidence for this structural relatedness was then obtained, as summarized in Table 1, which led to the conclusion that the Goodpasture antigen is localized to the NC1 domain of collagen IV (35, 85, 86).

Subsequently, additional evidence was obtained which indicates that the collagenase-solubilized Goodpasture antigens are integral subunits of the NC1 domain (9, 65, 92). This evidence, as summarized in Table 2, is based on extensive studies of the physical, chemical, and immunochemical properties of the hexamer form of the NC1 domain from GBM. The NC1 hexamer is a hallmark of collagen IV as described later. It is derived by collagenase digestion of two adjoining triple-helical molecules, and it is comprised of subunits that are derived from the carboxy-terminal regions of the respective collagen chains.

In the case of GBM, the hexamer is comprised of four distinct subunits with highly related structures, two of which, α1(IV) NC1 and α2(IV) NC1 (designated as M1 in earlier studies), are derived from the classical α1 and α2 chains of collagen IV (9). The other two, M2* and M3, are derived from two novel chains, designated α3 and α4, respectively (9). In the presence of detergent, the hexamer dissociates into its monomer and dimer subunits, as depicted by the electrophoretic patterns shown in Figure 4A. This pattern is basically the same as that reported by others who showed the monomer and dimer forms of the Goodpasture antigen (28, 88). However, the pattern is much more complex than originally suspected. Subsequent investigations (9, 11, 65, 92) revealed the

COLLAGEN IV

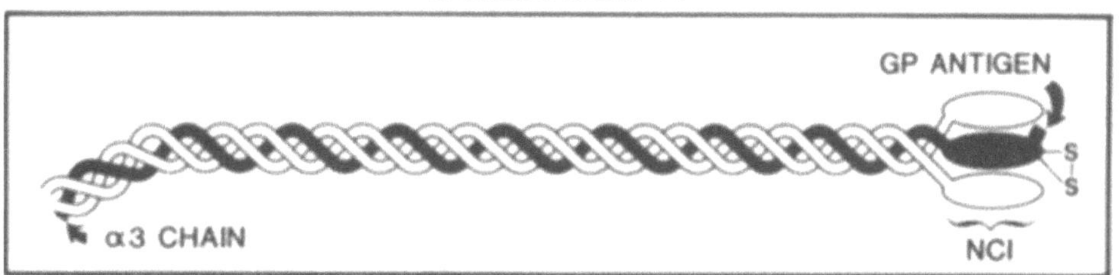

FIG. 3. Proposed molecular structure of membrane Goodpasture antigen. Collagenase-solubilized Goodpasture antigen (monomer form) depicted in Figure 2 is the NC1 domain of an α3 chain of a collagen IV protomer. Goodpasture determinant(s) require a disulfide bond(s) for binding to Goodpasture antibody. Structure of collagenous domain of α3 chain is assumed to be related to that of α1 and α2 chains of collagen IV because of the high degree of structural relatedness among NC1 domains of α1, α2, and α3 chains, as summarized in text. Protomers form a supramolecular structure in the GBM matrix as described in Figures 6 and 8. The possible kinds of protomers are described in Figure 7. Goodpasture antigen was localized to the NC1 domain of collagen IV by Wieslander *et al.* (86) and specifically to the α3 chain by Butkowski *et al.* (9) and Saus *et al.* (65).

TABLE 1. EVIDENCE FOR LOCALIZATION OF GOODPASTURE ANTIGEN TO NONCOLLAGENOUS DOMAIN OF COLLAGEN IV

GP antigen is released from GBM by collagenase digestion.
Native collagen IV from GBM:
  1) inhibits the binding of GP antibodies to purified GP antigen
  2) yields monomers and dimers upon collagenase digestion that react with GP antibodies.
Reduced collagen IV chains, after collagenase digestion, yield monomers of similar size to GP antigen.
Amino acid composition of the NC1 domain of collagen IV is similar to that of GP antigen.

Results are from reference 86.

TABLE 2. EVIDENCE THAT M2* IS AN INTEGRAL COMPONENT OF NONCOLLAGENOUS HEXAMER OF COLLAGEN IV

Collagenase-solubilized GP antigen (monomer M2* and dimer D2*) exists as part of a hexamer structure under nondenaturing conditions.
Subunits M1 (identified as $\alpha1(IV)NC1$ and $\alpha2(IV)NC1$) and subunit M2* also exist as part of a hexamer structure.
Hexamer contains a heterodimer comprised of M2* and M1.
In the presence of denaturants, the hexamer dissociates into its constituents, all of which exist in both monomer and dimer forms.
M2* coprecipitates with subunits $\alpha1(IV)NC1$ and $\alpha2(IV)NC1$ upon immunoprecipitation with antibodies directed toward any of these subunits.
Reactivity of M2* with GP antibodies is concomitant with hexamer dissociation, and the reactivity is reversibly lost upon reassociation of subunits.

Results are from references 9, 65, and 92.

existence of additional monomer and dimer subunits (Fig. 4B). Subunits designated M2* and D2* correspond to the monomer and dimer forms, respectively, of the collagenase-solubilized Goodpasture antigen as shown in Figure 2.

Subunit M2* exhibits physical and chemical properties that are identical or strikingly similar to those of subunits $\alpha1(IV)$ NC1 and $\alpha2(IV)$ NC1. Namely, all exist in a monomer-dimer relationship with similar molecular weights (11), all display similar denaturation-renaturation curves (92), all subunits reassociate to form hexamer even after extensive denaturation (92), and all contain Gly-X-Y triplets at the amino terminus (9). In a recent study, we obtained additional sequence data that show a further structural similarity between these subunits. Namely, the amino acid sequence of the amino-terminal region (residues 1–28) of M2* is highly related to that of a region of the $\alpha1$ and $\alpha2$ chains of collagen IV (65); this region includes the terminal sequence of the collagenous domain and the beginning sequence of the NC1 domain of the $\alpha1$ and $\alpha2$ chains. Moreover, the $\alpha1(IV)$ and $\alpha2(IV)$ domains and M2* all contain hydroxyproline in positions 6 and 12, reflecting further similarities in their primary structure.

These findings have led us to designate M2* as the NC1 domain of the $\alpha3$ chain of type IV collagen (65). This identity is based on 1) the sequence similarity between M2* and the NC1 domains of $\alpha1$ and $\alpha2$ chains of collagen IV, 2) the integral nature of M2* as a subunit of the NC1 hexamer of collagen IV, and 3) the multiple

similarities in the physical and chemical properties of M2* in comparison with those of the NC1 domains of the $\alpha1$ and $\alpha2$ chains of collagen IV. This identity of M2* then localizes the Goodpasture determinant(s) to the NC1 domain of the $\alpha3(IV)$ chain, as presented in Figure 3.

SPECIFICITY OF GOODPASTURE ANTIBODIES

Armed with knowledge of the identity of the membrane Goodpasture antigen, the specificity of circulating anti-GBM antibodies from Goodpasture syndrome patients can now be interpreted with respect to the known constituents of basement membranes. Over the years, several investigators reported studies showing the specificity of circulating antibodies from numerous Goodpasture syndrome patients to the collagenase-solubilized Goodpasture antigen (M2* and D2*). Others extended these studies to other membrane constituents. Also, the specificity of tissue-bound anti-GBM antibodies from an experimental animal model of antibody-mediated nephritis (Steblay nephritis) has recently been examined, and the specificity compared with that of circulating human Goodpasture antibodies. These findings revealed that collagen IV is the major target constituent.

The major titer of circulating Goodpasture antibodies is directed against the NC1 domain of collagen IV. Holdsworth et al. (28), presumably using the collagenase-solubilized antigens M2* and D2* from human GBM, identified anti-GBM antibodies in sera of over 500 patients and kidney eluates of 64 patients with anti-GBM disease. In a study of 22 Goodpasture syndrome patients, Wieslander and Heinegård (90) found that all had circulating antibodies to the collagenase-solubilized Goodpasture antigen (M2* and D2*). Eleven patients, as well as one control, had a high titer of antibodies to laminin, and one patient had antibodies to the 7S domain of the collagen IV. Pusey et al. (59) found that all 42 patients with Goodpasture syndrome or anti-GBM nephritis had antibodies that react with the collagenase-solubilized Goodpasture antigen. In a recent study of 17 Goodpasture syndrome patients, Bygren and Wieslander (unpublished data) found the major titer of antibodies is against the NC1 subunits, whereas in some patients, low titers against laminin, 7S domain, and entactin were found (Fig. 5). These findings demonstrate that all Goodpasture patients have, in common, antibodies directed against M2* and that some patients have additional antibodies directed against other basement membrane constituents and/or other collagen IV domains. Conceivably, the broader specificity of circulating antibodies occurring in some patients reflects a secondary response in which additional antibodies are produced against other antigens that are released from GBM as the nephritis progresses.

The specificity of circulating Goodpasture antibodies, with respect to the NC1 domains of each collagen IV alpha chain, is mainly directed against that of the $\alpha3$ chain. This specificity is evident from the Western blot analyses of human NC1 (91) and bovine NC1 domains, wherein M2* and D2* subunits contain the determinant(s) (11). This specificity is also supported by the monoclonal antibody studies reported by Pusey et al. (59). They concluded that Goodpasture antibodies have

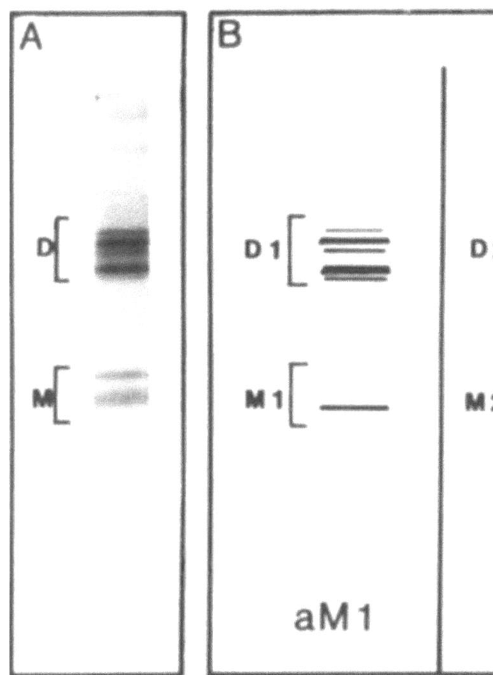
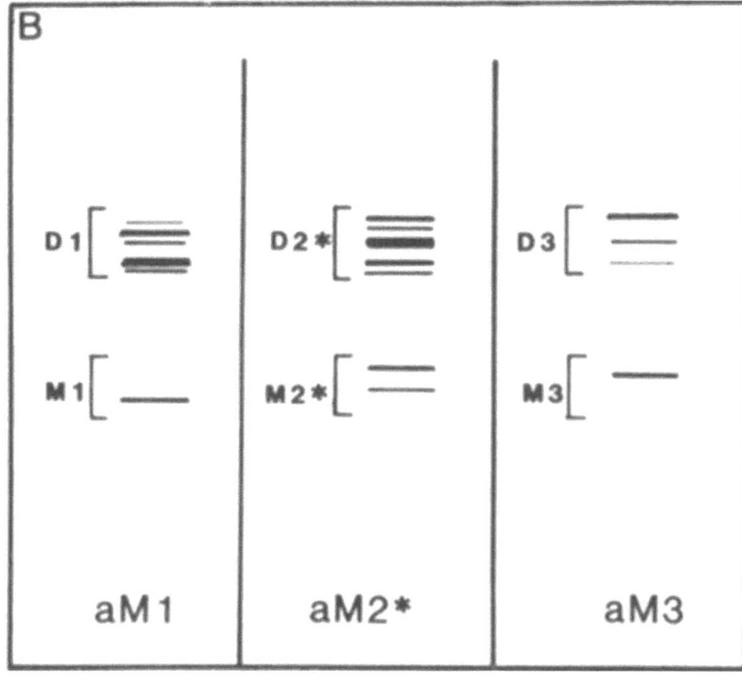

FIG. 4. Subunit composition of the NC1 hexamer from GBM. *A*, typical sodium dodecyl sulfate-polyacrylamide gel electrophoresis pattern of the NC1 hexamer from GBM. *B*, schematic diagram of Western blotting analysis using antibodies raised against each subunit of the NC1 hexamer (11). Each antibody preparation, anti-M1 (aM1), anti-M2* (aM2*), and anti-M3 (aM3), stains a distinct monomer and dimer set of subunits. The molecular basis of the multiplicity of dimers for each subunit type remains obscure. Pattern obtained for anti-M2* antibodies is identical to that for Goodpasture antibodies. Symbols M and D, monomer and dimer subunits, respectively. This figure was adapted from reference 40.

a highly restricted specificity in that a monoclonal antibody binds to the monomer and dimer forms of the collagenase-solubilized Goodpasture antigen and that preincubation with monoclonal antibody blocks the subsequent binding of human antibodies in six of six Goodpasture syndrome patients from 58 to 89%. Kleppel *et al.* (38) also found that the main Goodpasture reactivity for human NC1 is against a M28+++ monomer, whereas some reactivity is to other subunits. Butkowski and co-workers (unpublished data) subsequently showed that M28+++ is structurally identical, except for a single amino acid substitution, to the M2* subunit and that the other monomers correspond to the NC1 domains of the α1 and α2 chains of collagen IV. The latter reactivity may reflect a population of antibodies that crossreact with each NC1 domain because there is high sequence homology among the domains (65), or it may reflect the presence of additional antibodies reacting with distinct determinants on each respective domain in this patient.

The specificity of tissue-bound anti-GBM antibodies produced in experimental nephritis in sheep (Steblay's nephritis) was compared with that of circulating human Goodpasture antibodies in a recent study (13). The tissue-bound antibodies, when eluted from the diseased kidney, reacted with high titers against the NC1 subunits and with considerably lower titers against the 7S domain of collagen IV and laminin. Moreover, the major titer of eluted antibodies reacted with M2* and with low titers to M1 and M3, which correspond to the NC1 domains of the other α-chains of collagen IV. They concluded that a major population of antibodies in eluates from kidneys of nephritic sheep recognize the same antigen, M2*, present in both human and sheep GBM, as did serum antibodies from patients with Goodpasture syndrome; hence, the results strongly indicate the major nephritogen in Steblay nephritis and human Goodpasture syndrome is the M2* subunit. The finding of Fouser *et al.* (22) is in agreement with this conclusion. They found

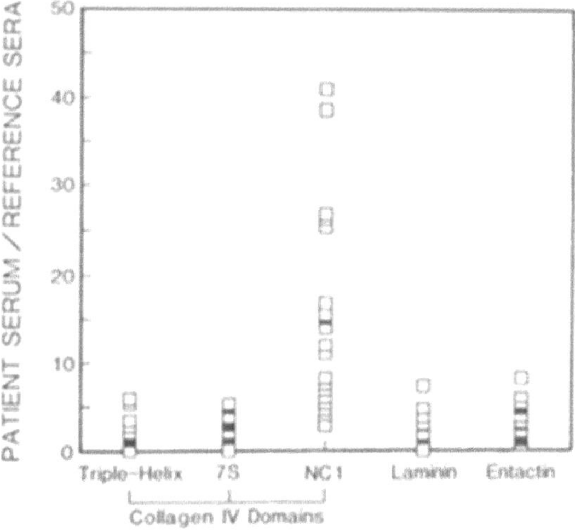

FIG. 5. Specificity of circulating antibodies from 17 patients with Goodpasture syndrome. Direct-binding enzyme-linked immunosorbent assays (ELISA) were used to determine the reactivity of Goodpasture antibodies with collagen IV domains and other components from bovine GBM (Bygren & Wieslander, unpublished data). Values are expressed as ratio of absorbance value found for patient sera to absorbance value found for normal serum. The major titer of Goodpasture antibodies is to the NC1 hexamer of collagen IV. Low titers of antibodies are to the 7S and triple-helical domain of collagen IV and to other basement membrane components (laminin and entactin).

that sheep immunized with purified human NC1 domains developed antibodies reactive with the M28 monomer. Furthermore, immunization of mice with mouse NC1 domains induced the production of anti-GBM antibodies that caused a Goodpasture syndrome-like disease (80, 84); and immunization of rabbits with dissociated human NC1 hexamer induced both lung hemorrhage and glomerulonephritis (82).

Overall, these studies indicate that the circulating anti-GBM antibodies from Goodpasture syndrome patients and the tissue-bound anti-GBM antibodies from diseased kidney of Steblay nephritic sheep are mainly directed to the NC1 domain of collagen IV and specifically to the NC1 domain (M2*) of the $\alpha3$(IV) chain. The low titers of antibodies to other domains of the collagen IV molecule [triple-helical, NC1 of $\alpha1$(IV) and $\alpha2$(IV), and 7S] and to other basement membrane constituents (laminin and entactin) probably reflect a secondary response to other antigens that are released from GBM as the nephritis progresses. Therefore, we conclude that the primary target molecule for the Goodpasture antibodies is type IV collagen of GBM and that the Goodpasture determinant(s) resides within the NC1 domain of the $\alpha3$ chain; hence, the primary Goodpasture antibody is termed anti-collagen-$\alpha3$(IV).

MOLECULAR ARCHITECTURE OF MEMBRANE GOODPASTURE ANTIGEN

Identification of the Goodpasture antigen as the new $\alpha3$ chain of collagen IV provides novel insights into the molecular architecture of both Goodpasture antigen and basement membrane collagen. The classical protomer or building block unit of collagen IV is a triple-helical molecule comprised of three polypeptide chains. Protomers are then interconnected, forming a supramolecular network in the membrane matrix. The $\alpha3$ chain comprises a new type of protomer that reflects novel features of the supramolecular structure of collagen IV in GBM.

PROTOMER STRUCTURE

The protomer is characterized by three distinct structural domains (Fig. 6, lower panel): the 7S domain at the amino-terminus, the triple-helical domain in the middle region, and the NC1 domain at the carboxy terminus (18, 78). The classical protomer of collagen IV contains two $\alpha1$(IV) chains and one $\alpha2$ chain. The $\alpha1$ (IV) chain contains 1642 total amino acid residues with 1413 residues residing in the collagenous domain (70), within which there are 21 interruptions of the Gly-X-Y sequence that vary in length between 2 and 11 residues. The last 229 residues are noncollagenous and are folded into a compact globular domain, termed NC1. In comparison, the $\alpha2$(IV) chain contains an additional 43 amino acids, 21 of which form a disulfide-bridged loop within the triple helix (6). The new $\alpha3$(IV) chain comprises another distinct protomer as described in a later section.

SUPRAMOLECULAR STRUCTURE

Several key ways are known in which protomers interact to form a supramolecular structure in the membrane matrix. Two distinct modes of end-to-end interactions between protomers have been elucidated. The protomers associate in a head-to-head (NC1-to-NC1) fashion to form dimers, i.e., -●●- (4, 78), and in a tail-to-tail (7S-to-7S) fashion to form tetramers (78), as presented in the model shown in Figure 6 (upper panel). These end-to-end associations initially proceed through noncovalent interactions, but they are later stabilized by disulfide bonds and, in mammalian membranes, by aldehyde-derived crosslinks. In an extension of this model, lateral associations occur between protomers and give rise to irregular polyhedral structures and a tighter collagen IV matrix (99, 100). Although these are fundamental ways

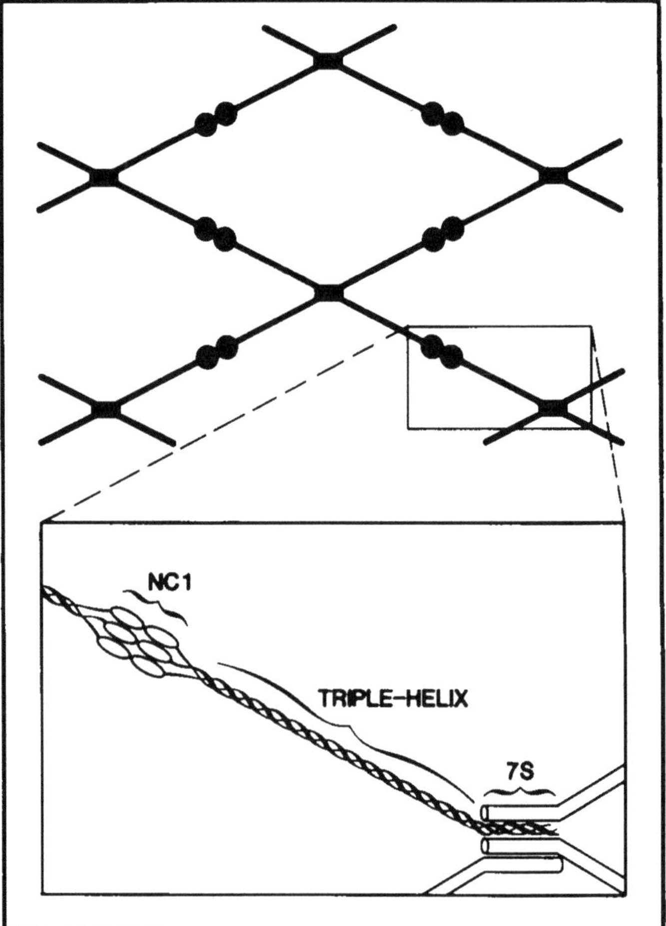

FIG. 6. Network model of supramolecular structure of collagen IV. Model is based on studies of basement membrane-like matrix produced by mouse Engelbreth-Holm-Swarm tumor (4, 78). Several lines of evidence indicate that the model applies to GBM, as reviewed in reference 40. *Boxed area (lower panel)*, enlargement of a region to show structure of collagen IV protomer and ways in which it is connected in matrix. Protomer is a triple-helical molecule comprised of three polypeptide chains. Protomer has three distinct structural domains: 7S domain at the amino-terminus, triple-helical domain in the middle region, and NC1 domain at the carboxy-terminus. Protomers associate in a head-to-head (NC1-to-NC1) fashion to form dimers and in a tail-to-tail (7S-to-7S) fashion to form tetramers. These end-to-end associations are stabilized by disulfide bonds and aldehyde-derived crosslinks.

in which the protomers are connected to form a functional matrix, the three-dimensional structure of the collagen IV matrix remains largely unknown.

ORGANIZATION OF PROTOMER SUBTYPES

The presence of the new $\alpha3$ and $\alpha4$ chains in GBM, together with the two classical chains ($\alpha1$ and $\alpha2$), reflects new features about the supramolecular structure of collagen IV. The chains comprise at least two distinct protomer subtypes, which differ in chain composition. The various protomer subtypes can be interconnected in different arrangements, have different topographical distributions, and differ in relative abundance in basement membranes of various tissues. Hence, a description of the organization of the Goodpasture antigen must include these features.

Several protomer subtypes are possible because of the existence of four distinct chains (Fig. 7). The classical protomer made of $\alpha1$ (IV) and $\alpha2$ (IV) chains, as described above, is termed subtype A. Several kinds of protomers are possible that contain the $\alpha3$ chain. These are designated subtype B in Figure 7. Up to 20 protomer subtypes are possible, but the actual number is unknown.

The existence of more than one protomer subtype introduces the possibility of several distinct arrangements in which protomers are interconnected and distributed about the supramolecular structure. Different subtypes can be interconnected through their NC1 domains, forming dimers, and through their 7S domains, forming tetramers. Evidence was obtained for the NC1-to-NC1 arrangements (A-A, B-B, and A-B) shown in Figure 8 from immunoprecipitation studies of the NC1 hexamer that is released on collagenase digestion (65). Specific connections of subtypes through their 7S domains are unknown.

Moreover, subtypes can have distinct topographical distributions within the supramolecular structure. As illustrated in Figure 9, subtypes A and B can be distributed in a regional or random fashion. A recent study using polyclonal and monoclonal antibodies suggests that subtype A has an endothelial/mesangial distribution, whereas subtype B has a more epithelial distribution (10). In addition, the relative abundance of subtypes varies among basement membranes from different tissues of origin, with GBM containing the largest quantity of subtype B relative to subtype A of the basement membranes thus far examined (39). By assuming that all $\alpha3$ chains exist in subtype B1 protomers (Fig. 7), then the ratio of B:A is about 1:4 in GBM, 1:30 in anterior lens capsule basement membrane, and 1:100 in placenta basement membrane.

On the basis of these considerations we conclude that protomer B, which contains the Goodpasture antigen ($\alpha3$ chain), is positioned in the collagen IV matrix in a specific way with respect to the classical protomer (subtype A). Conceivably, these modes of interactions and distributions of subtypes may be important in the assembly of a functional basement membrane as described below.

CRYPTIC PROPERTIES OF GOODPASTURE DETERMINANT(S)

The NC1 domain can be excised from the supramolecular structure by cleavage of GBM with bacterial collagenase as depicted in Figure 10. The excised domain exists as a hexamer under nondenaturing conditions, and it is comprised of subunits that are derived from the NC1 regions of the respective collagen chains of the two adjoining protomers. Protomers containing the $\alpha3$ chain (subtype B) yield hexamer containing the Goodpasture determinant(s). Excision of the hexamer does not in itself make the Goodpasture determinant(s) available for binding to Goodpasture antibodies. Thus, the determinant(s) is buried within the NC1 hexamer; *i.e.*, it has cryptic properties. This property may be of pivotal importance in the events that lead to the initial production of the pathogenic anticollagen-$\alpha3$(IV) antibody.

Exposure of the determinant(s) requires dissociation of the hexamer into its subunits, as portrayed in Figure 10. The hexamer can be made reactive to Goodpasture antibodies by treatment with dissociating agents such as 6 M guanidine-HCl or dilute acid (92). By using dilute

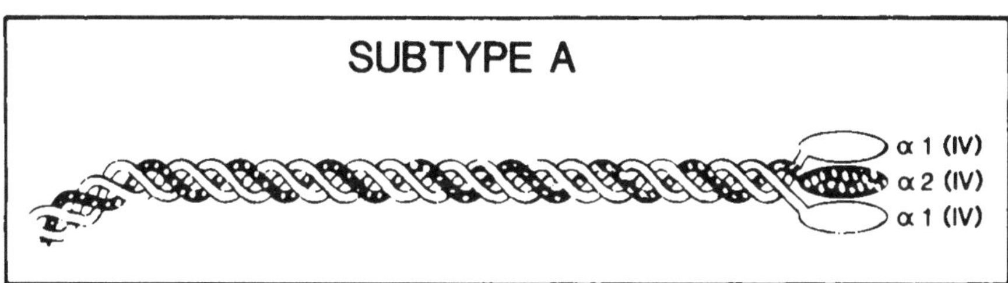

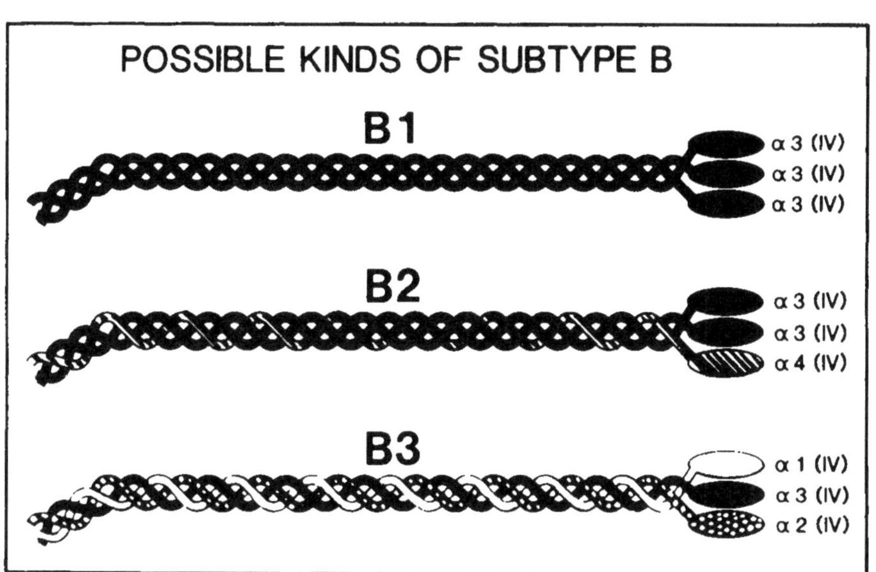

FIG. 7. Structure of protomer subtypes of collagen IV. Subtype A designates classical collagen protomer that is comprised of two $\alpha1$(IV) chains and one $\alpha2$(IV) chain (a heterotrimer). Subtype B protomer designates any protomer containing an $\alpha3$(IV) chain. Those comprised of $\alpha3$(IV) only are designated B1, those comprised of $\alpha3$(IV) and $\alpha4$(IV) as B2, and those comprised of $\alpha3$(IV) together with $\alpha1$(IV) and/or $\alpha2$(IV) chains as B3. Up to 20 protomer subtypes are possible based on the existence of four distinct chains.

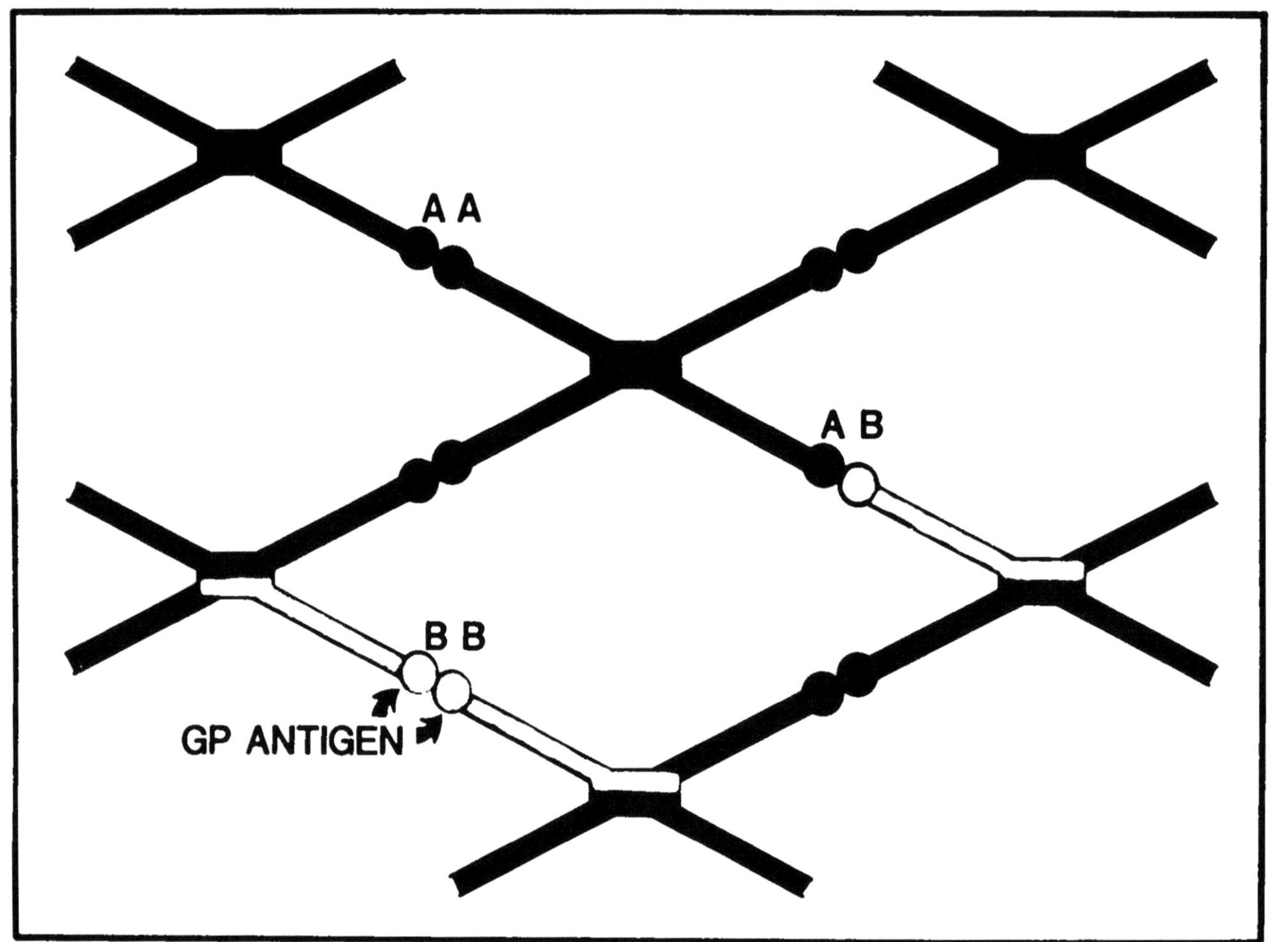

Fig. 8. End-to-end connections of protomer subtypes in collagen IV supramolecular structure. Several different arrangements are possible in which the subtypes are interconnected through their 7S and NC1 domains in collagen IV matrix. Evidence was obtained for NC1-to-NC1 arrangements A-A, B-B, and A-B (65). *Black*, classical protomer (subtype A); *white*, protomers (subtypes B) containing the Goodpasture determinant(s).

acid, maximal reactivity is obtained at pH ~3.0. The process is reversible, because reactivity is completely eliminated by adjusting the pH to 7.5 and reinduced by adjusting the pH back to 3.0. Rotary-shadowing electron microscopy studies demonstrated that activation at acid pH is accompanied by dissociation of the NC1 hexamer and that reversal of the activation is accompanied by reassociation of the hexamer. Circular dichroism studies showed that partial unfolding accompanies acid-induced dissociation and activation, but the unfolding is also reversible. By using 6 M guanidine-HCl as the dissociating agent, unfolding of subunits is minimal, activation is maximal, and activation can be reversed by removal of the agent. Thus, the determinant(s) appears to be sequestered between the subunits of the NC1 hexamer. These results suggest that exposure of the Goodpasture determinant(s) is a reversible process that requires dissociation of the NC1 hexamer but does not require unfolding of the $\alpha 3$ (IV) NC1 domain.

Conceivably, infection or exposure to toxic agents that normally precede the autoimmune response could expose the otherwise sequestered Goodpasture determinant(s) and thereby initiate antibody production in genetically predisposed individuals. In this connection, both lung hemorrhage and glomerulonephritis was induced in rab-

bits by immunization with the dissociated NC1 hexamer, suggesting that determinant(s) exposure is critical to the immune response affecting both lung and kidney (82). However, total sequestration of the Goodpasture determinant(s) *in situ* is unlikely because Goodpasture antibodies bind to the region of the lamina rara interna of the GBM (69) and mediate the inflammatory response, and a small amount of unsequestered determinant(s) was observed in the preparation of NC1 hexamer (92). The latter could reflect partial dissociation of the NC1 hexamer during isolation or the presence of a small amount of protomer B that is not crosslinked into the supramolecular structure.

POSSIBLE FUNCTIONS OF GOODPASTURE ANTIGEN

The supramolecular structure of collagen IV confers tensile strength to basement membrane and provides a scaffolding upon which other membrane components bind forming a functional matrix. These components include laminin, heparan sulfate proteoglycan, entactin, fibronectin, and other yet uncharacterized macromolecules. In addition, various cell types bind to the collagen matrix, including hepatocytes (62), endothelial cells (56), and certain tumor cells (3, 17, 55). The discovery of the

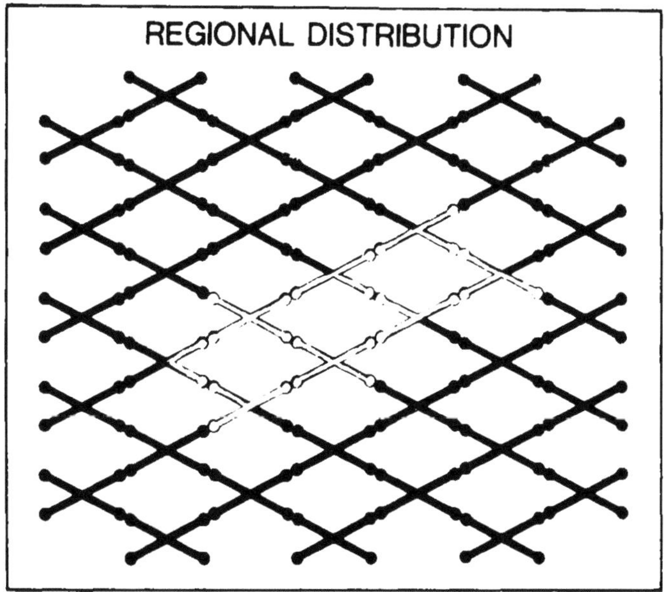

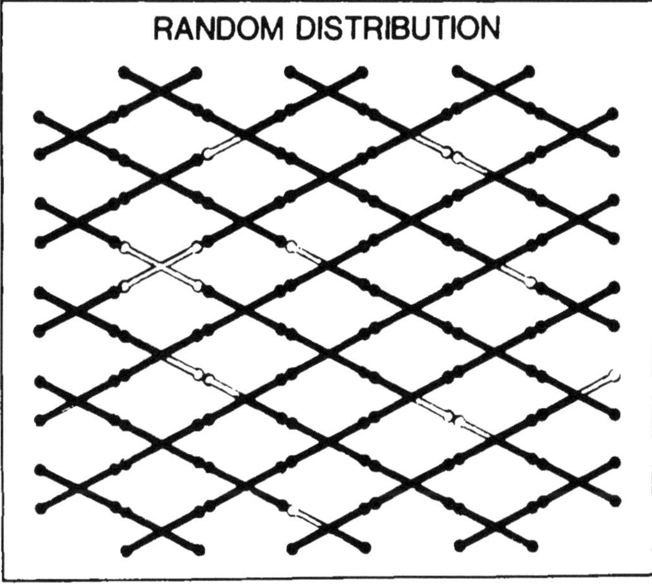

FIG. 9. Topographical distribution of protomer subtype A and B in collagen IV supramolecular structure. Existence of more than one protomer subtype introduces possibility of distinct distribution of a subtype within the matrix. A regional (*upper panel*) and random (*lower panel*) distribution for subtype A (*black*) and B (*white*) is illustrated. Relative abundance of subtypes can vary among basement membranes from different tissues of origin.

Goodpasture antigen as a new $\alpha 3$ chain brings a new dimension to the structure-function relationship of collagen IV. Conceivably, protomers containing this chain may confer specific functions to the membrane and/or be important in the assembly and maintenance of a functional membrane. In this connection, recent studies of patients with Alport-type familial nephritis implicate the $\alpha 3$ chain as a requirement for normal function of GBM.

Alport-type familial nephritis (FN) is an X-linked heritable disorder affecting various organs but predominantly characterized by sensorineural hearing loss and glomerulonephritis (26). Frequently, the initial symptom is either recurrent or persistent hematuria in childhood with progression of the disease to end-stage renal failure. Ultrastructural abnormalities in the GBM accompany the disorder that are characterized by thinning, diffuse splitting, and multilamination of the lamina densa (27, 53, 60, 63, 72, 97). Several investigators found that binding of Goodpasture antibodies to GBM is frequently absent in these patients, as determined by indirect immunofluorescence of tissue sections (30, 31, 34, 50, 54). The absence or reduced binding of a monoclonal antibody directed to the Goodpasture antigen was found in renal biopsy tissue from 10 patients (67). These findings provide circumstantial evidence for the existence of a biochemical abnormality in the GBM. Such an abnormality was postulated by Spear in 1973 (71). In a recent study, Kleppel *et al.* (37) obtained both immunochemical and chemical evidence for the absence of the collagenase-solubilized human Goodpasture antigen, the 28-kDa monomer, in the GBM from three males with Alport-type FN. These studies provide strong evidence for the absence of the membrane Goodpasture antigen in patients with Alport-type FN, indicating a specific structural abnormality in the GBM, and point to the importance of this component in conferring normal function to the GBM.

Knowledge of the molecular identity and architecture of the membrane Goodpasture antigen provides a conceptual framework to interpret these findings about Alport-type FN. Since the Goodpasture determinant(s) is located in the $\alpha 3$ chain, it follows that protomers of collagen IV containing this chain, subtype B (Fig. 7), are absent in these patients. Conceivably, these protomers are key in the fusion of epithelial and endothelial basement membranes during embryonic development of GBM (2, 64). As presented in Figure 11, the GBM initially develops by the fusion of the dual basement membranes that are positioned between the endothelium and epithelium. Possibly, subtype B protomers are distributed in both membranes or exclusively in one or the other. In either case, the absence of subtype B protomers could alter the molecular properties of the mature GBM causing the thinning, splitting, and mutilamination that are characteristic features of GBM in Alport-type FN. Since the defective gene for this disorder is located in the middle of the long arm of the X chromosomes (7), the gene for the $\alpha 3$ chain may be at the same locus.

DIAGNOSIS AND TREATMENT

Goodpasture syndrome is a medical emergency with a case fatality rate of 75–90% if not treated (58, 81). The three essential elements of diagnosis are 1) glomerulonephritis, commonly of the rapidly progressive or crescentic variety, 2) pulmonary hemorrhage, and 3) anti-GBM antibody formation (24). The presence of circulating anti-GBM antibodies permits differentiation of the syndrome from other causes of pulmonary hemorrhage and glomerulonephritis. Early diagnosis is paramount in the management and prognosis of Goodpasture syndrome patients because aggressive therapy to remove the pathogenic antibodies may substantially improve the outcome. Toward this end, several radioimmunoassays

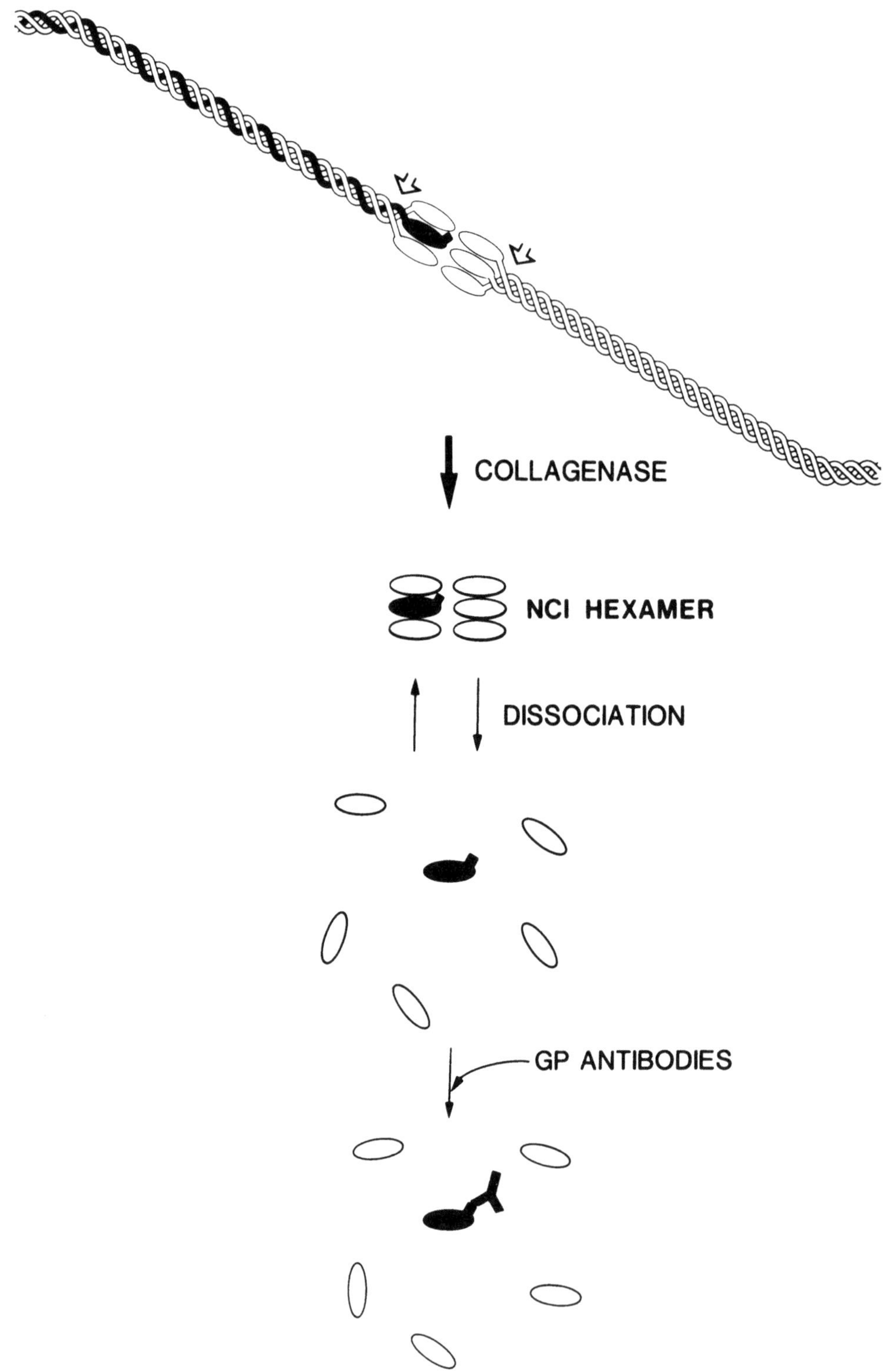

FIG. 10. Schematic showing release of the NC1 hexamer from GBM and mechanism of unmasking Goodpasture determinant(s). NC1 hexamer is released from collagen IV matrix upon collagenase digestion. It is derived from NC1 domains of two adjoining protomers, and it is comprised of six subunits (three from each protomer) that are derived from carboxyl-terminal regions (NC1) of respective chains. For emphasis, Goodpasture antigen (α3 chain) is shown in *red*, and Goodpasture determinant(s) is shown in *black*. Goodpasture determinant(s) is sequestered in NC1 hexamer.

(5, 8, 43, 48, 57, 93, 96) and enzyme-linked immunosorbent assays (20, 83, 89) have been developed to detect circulating anti-GBM antibodies.

Although these assays are useful tools, the specificity of antibodies detected is very broad. The measurements reflect the titer of anti-GBM antibodies that bind to a mixture of antigens that are solubilized by collagenase digestion or guanidine-HCl or urea extraction of GBM. Therefore, measurements reflect the collective presence of anti-GBM antibodies directed against various GBM constituents (collagen IV, laminin, entactin, and heparan sulfate proteoglycan) as well as different domains of

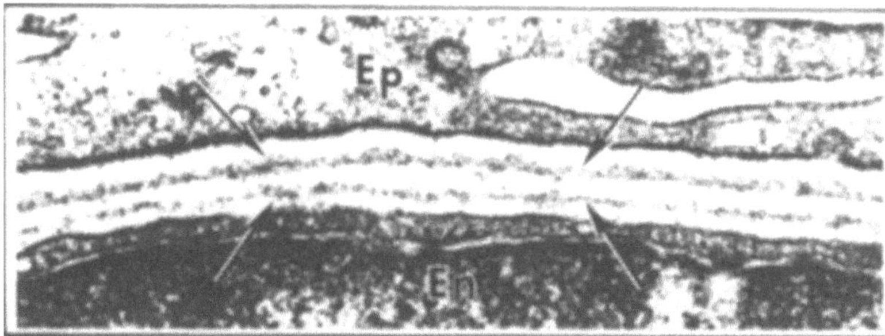

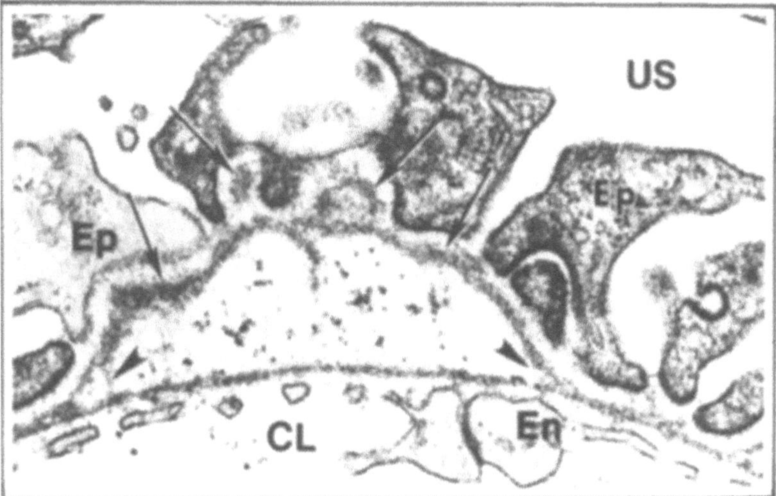

FIG. 11. Electron micrographs of newborn rat kidney glomerular capillary wall at early (*upper panel*) and later (*lower panel*) stages of development. In the early rat kidney glomerulus the GBM is formed by fusion of basement membrane from both endothelial and epithelial cells. Later, as kidney matures, most basement membrane biosynthesis is performed by epithelial cells. As seen in *lower panel*, new epithelial basement membrane (*arrows*) appears as a loop as it is inserted into existing fused basement membrane (*arrowheads*). Abbreviations as in Figure 1. Both electron micrographs were provided by Dr. D. R. Abrahamson (University of Alabama) and are reproduced with permission of the *Journal of Pathology* (1).

collagen IV (each NC1 subunit, triple-helix, and 7S). In the case of patients with Goodpasture syndrome, the assays would reflect antibodies to the Goodpasture antigen as well as secondary antibodies that occur in some patients, as described above. Moreover, patients with other forms of nephritis, such as lupus erythematosus nephritis and IgA nephropathy, have antibodies against GBM antigens (87). In particular, several patients with poststreptococcal glomerulonephritis have circulating antibodies against heparan sulfate proteoglycan (19), laminin, and the 7S domain of collagen IV (36), and patients with IgA nephropathy have immune complexes containing fibronectin and IgA that bind to the triple helical domain of collagen IV (14). Also, patients with Chagas disease have circulating antibodies to laminin (79). Hence, assays using a crude collagenase digest may give false positive results for the detection of antibodies that are specific for Goodpasture syndrome. Thus, only assays that measure antibodies directed against the Goodpasture antigen can be used for a specific diagnosis of Goodpasture syndrome. The identification of the $\alpha3$ chain of collagen IV as the Goodpasture antigen and the localization of the Goodpasture determinant(s) to the NC1 domain provide the necessary knowledge to design assays for measurement of the specific Goodpasture antibody, anticollagen-$\alpha3$(IV).

Currently, Goodpasture syndrome patients are treated by plasmapheresis in combination with the administration of steroids and immunosuppressive drugs (32, 33, 44–46, 58, 61, 66). The efficacy of this treatment combination was reviewed by Glassock *et al.* (24) who concluded that the protocol promotes the disappearance of pulmonary hemorrhage and improvement of renal func-

tion. In a recent review, Couser (15) concluded that optimal outcomes may be achieved in anti-GBM nephritis when therapy is directed at patients with mild but rapidly progressive disease before oliguria or severe azotemia.

Recently, Bygren *et al.* (12) have described the use of a new immunoadsorption technique that involves adsorption of IgG to staphylococcal protein A. The benefit of this process is that large volumes of plasma can be processed without plasma protein substitution because the patient's processed plasma can be safely reinfused. Furthermore, continuous depletion of plasma antibodies may facilitate the release of tissue bound anti-GBM antibodies.

CONCLUSIONS AND PERSPECTIVES

The extraordinary advances of the last decade in understanding the molecular architecture of basement membrane components, as depicted in Figure 12, have provided the requisite knowledge to identify the intrinsic GBM component that binds the anti-GBM antibodies of patients with Goodpasture syndrome. The major titer of antibodies, common to all these patients, is targeted to collagen IV and specifically to the NC1 domain of the $\alpha3$ chain. In certain patients, low titers of antibodies are also directed against laminin and entactin and to other domains of collagen IV, which presumably reflects a secondary immune response as the nephritis progresses. The evidence *in toto* strongly indicates that collagen IV ($\alpha3$ chain) is the Goodpasture antigen of basement membrane, and that anti-collagen-$\alpha3$(IV) is the primary pathogenic antibody in all patients with Goodpasture syndrome. Therefore, we conclude that the third essen-

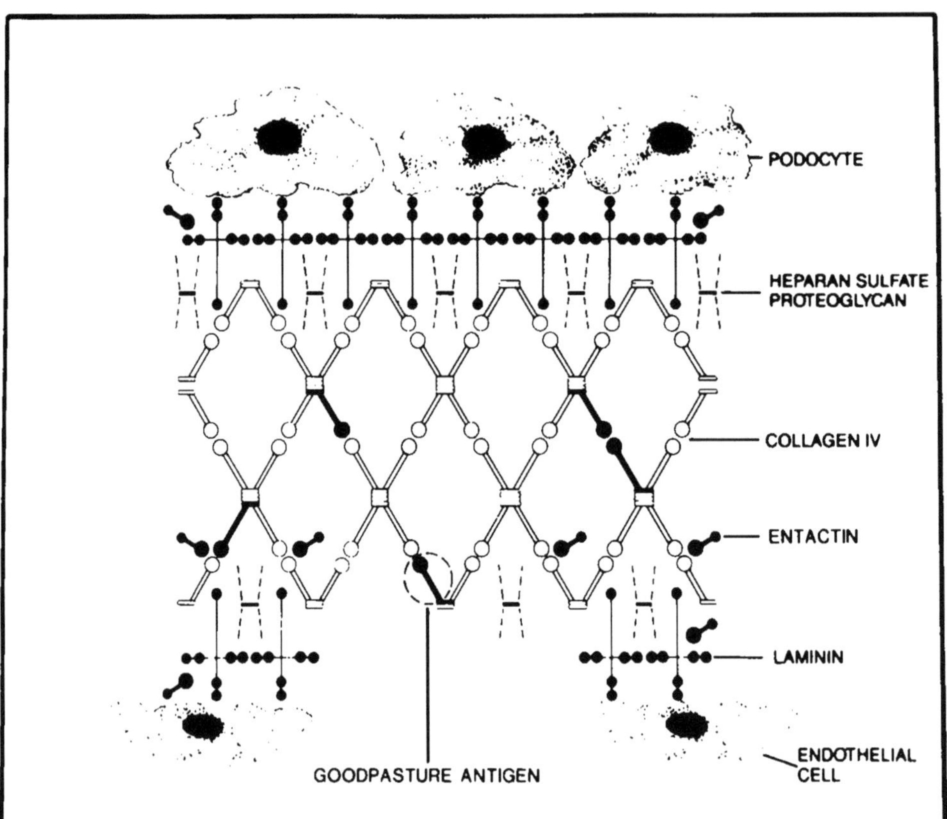

FIG. 12. Schematic depicting the structural relationship between Goodpasture antigen and other intrinsic components of GBM. Supramolecular structure of collagen IV serves as a scaffolding upon which other components (laminin, heparan sulfate proteoglycan, and entactin) bind to form a functional matrix (77). Collagen IV is compromised of at least two protomer subtypes (building block units) (9, 39, 65). Protomer is a triple-helical molecule, comprised of three α-chains, with a terminal globular domain. Classical promoter (subtype A) contains $\alpha1$ and $\alpha2$ chains and is represented by the undarkened protomers. Protomers (subtype B) containing $\alpha3$ chain, the Goodpasture antigen, are represented by the darkened protomers. In GBM, ratio of protomers A to B is 1 to 4 (39). Protomers may have distinct topographical distributions within matrix. Molecular dimensions of various components are not drawn to scale. Distribution of components represented within matrix is preferential (but not exclusive) (76).

tial element of diagnosis of Goodpasture syndrome should be revised to reflect this antibody specificity. Hence, the three essential elements of diagnosis are 1) glomerulonephritis, 2) pulmonary hemorrhage, and 3) anti-collagen-$\alpha3$(IV) antibody formation.

The molecular identity and architecture of the Goodpasture antigen also reflects novel structure-function relationships of basement membrane. Namely, the existence of at least two protomer subtypes of collagen IV, their arrangements and distributions to form a functional matrix (Fig. 12), their tissue-specific distributions, and their functions. Moreover, the novel protomer subtype, containing the $\alpha3$ chain and the Goodpasture determinant(s), is absent in patients with Alport-type familial nephritis, which implicates this subtype as a requirement for normal GBM function. It may confer specific functions to the membrane and/or be important in the assembly and maintenance of a functional membrane.

Although the contributions cited in this article reflect considerable progress in understanding the pathogenesis of Goodpasture syndrome, many important questions remain unanswered about the molecular architecture and function of the Goodpasture antigen: the structure of Goodpasture determinant(s); the primary structure of the $\alpha3$ chain; the kinds of protomer subtypes; modes of assembly and interactions of protomer subtypes; specific functions of protomer subtypes; modes of protomer subtype interaction with laminin, heparan sulfate proteoglycan, and entactin to form a three-dimensional structure; and regulation of protomer subtype biosynthesis. The answers will ultimately contribute to a better understanding of basement membrane structure and function, the etiology of Goodpasture syndrome and Alport-type familial nephritis, and the design of specific therapy.

Acknowledgments: We thank Drs. Pablo Bejarano, Pete Cuppage, Jared Grantham, Michael Sarras and Gary Wood and Julie Welch for critical reading of the manuscript. We also thank Parvin Todd for technical assistance, Dianne Basta and Mark Hudson for editorial assistance, Bill Page and Lisbeth Hotchkiss for artwork, and Dr. Dale R. Abrahamson for the electron micrographs.

Contributions from the authors' laboratory were supported by National Institutes of Health Grant DK 18381, Speas Trust Grant, Swedish Medical Research Grants 6481 and 6797, American Heart Association-Kansas Affiliate Fellowship, Ministry of Education and Science (Spain) Fulbright Fellowship, Council of Education and Science of Valencia (Spain) Fellowship, University of Kansas Medical Center, and the Instituto de Investigaciones Citologicas-Kansas University Medical Center International Center of Cell Biology.

Manuscript submitted November 29, 1988.

Address reprint requests to: Billy G. Hudson, Department of Biochemistry and Molecular Biology, University of Kansas Medical Center, 39th and Rainbow Blvd., Kansas City, KS 66103.

REFERENCES

1. Abrahamson DR: Recent studies on the structure and pathology of basement membrane. J Pathol 149:257, 1986
2. Abrahamson DR: Structure and development of the glomerular capillary wall and basement membrane. Am J Physiol 22:F783, 1987
3. Aumailley M, Timpl R: Attachment of cells to basement membrane collagen type IV. J Cell Biol 103:1569, 1986
4. Bächinger HP, Fessler LI, Fessler JH: Mouse procollagen IV: Characterization and supramolecular association. J Biol Chem 257:9796, 1982
5. Bowman C, Lockwood CM: Clinical application of a radioimmunoassay for auto-antibodies to glomerular basement membrane. J Clin Lab Immunol 17:197, 1985
6. Brazel D, Pollner R, Oberbäumer I, Kühn K: Human basement membrane collagen (type IV): The amino acid sequence of the

$\alpha 2(IV)$ chain and its comparison with the $\alpha 1(IV)$ chain reveals deletions in the $\alpha 1(IV)$ chain. Eur J Biochem 172:35, 1988

7. Brunner H, Schröder C, van Bennekom C, Lambermon E, Tuerlings J, Menzel D, Olbing H, Monnens L, Wieringa B, Ropers H-H: Localization of the gene for X-linked Alport's syndrome. Kidney Int 34:507, 1988

8. Buffaloe GW, Evans JE, McIntosh RM, Glassock RJ, Tracie B, Tavel TB, Terman DS: Antibodies to human glomerular basement membrane: Modified methodology for detection in human serum. Clin Exp Immunol 39:136, 1980

9. Butkowski RJ, Langeveld JPM, Wieslander J, Hamilton J, Hudson BG: Localization of the Goodpasture epitope to a novel chain of basement membrane collagen. J Biol Chem 262:7874, 1987

10. Butkowski RJ, Wieslander J, Kleppel M, Michael AF, Fish AJ: Basement membrane collagen in the kidney: Regional localization of novel chains related to collagen IV. Kidney Int 35:1195, 1989

11. Butkowski RJ, Wieslander J, Wisdom BJ, Barr JF, Noelken ME, Hudson BG: Properties of the globular domain of type IV collagen and its relationship to the Goodpasture antigen. J Biol Chem 260:3739, 1985

12. Bygren P, Freiburghaus C, Lindholm T, Simonsen O, Thysell H, Wieslander J: Goodpasture's syndrome treatment with *staphylococcal* protein A immunoadsorption. Lancet II:1295, 1985

13. Bygren P, Wieslander J, Heinegärd D: Glomerulonephritis induced in sheep by immunization with human glomerular basement membrane. Kidney Int 31:25, 1987

14. Cederholm B, Wieslander J, Bygren P, Heingård D: Circulating complexes containing IgA and fibronectin in patients with primary IgA nephropathy. Proc Natl Acad Sci USA 85:4865, 1988

15. Couser WG: Rapidly progressive glomerulonephritis: Classification, pathogenetic mechanisms, and therapy. Am J Kidney Dis XI:449, 1988

16. Dean DC, Barr JF, Freytag JW, Hudson BG: Isolation of type IV procollagen-like polypeptides from glomerular basement membrane. J Biol Chem 258:590, 1983

17. Dennis J, Waller C, Timpl R, Schirrmacher V: Surface sialic acid reduces attachment of metastatic tumor cells to collagen IV and fibronectin. Nature 300:274, 1982

18. Fessler LI, Fessler JH: Identification of the carboxyl peptides of mouse procollagen IV and its implications for the assembly and structure of basement membrane procollagen. J Biol Chem 257:9804, 1982

19. Fillit H, Damle SP, Gregory JD, Volin C, Poon-King T, Zabriskie J: Sera from patients with poststreptococcal glomerulonephritis contain antibodies to glomerular heparan sulfate proteoglycan. J Exp Med 161:277, 1985

20. Fish AJ, Kleppel M, Jeraj K, Michael AF: Enzyme immunoassay of anti-glomerular basement membrane antibodies. J Lab Clin Med 105:700, 1985

21. Fish AJ, Lockwood MC, Wong M, Price RG: Detection of Goodpasture antigen in fractions prepared from collagenase digests of human glomerular basement membrane. Clin Exp Immunol 55:58, 1984

22. Fouser LS, Michael AF, Kleppel MM, Vernier RL, Fish AJ: Nephritogenicity in sheep of the NC1 domain of type IV collagen from human glomerular basement membrane (hGBM) (abstr). Kidney Int 31:319, 1987

23. Glassock RJ: Clinical aspects of acute, rapidly progressive and chronic glomerulonephritis. In Diseases of the Kidney, Ed 3, edited by Early LE, Gottschalk CW, p 691–763. Boston, Little, Brown and Company, 1979

24. Glassock RJ, Cohen AH, Adler SG, Ward HJ: Secondary Glomerular Diseases. In The Kidney, Ed 3, edited by Brenner BM, Rector FC, pp 1014–1083. Philadelphia, WB Saunders, 1986

25. Goodpasture EW: The significance of certain pulmonary lesions in relation to the etiology of influenza. Am J Med Sci 158:863, 1919

26. Grünfeld J-P: The clinical spectrum of hereditary nephritis. Kidney Int 27:83, 1985

27. Hinglais N, Grünfeld J-P, Bois E: Characteristic ultrastructural lesion of the glomerular basement membrane in progressive hereditary nephritis (Alport's syndrome). Lab Invest 27:473, 1972

28. Holdsworth SR, Golbus SM, Wilson CB: Characterization of collagenase solubilized human glomerular basement membrane antigens reacting with human antibodies (abstr). Kidney Int 16:797, 1979

29. Hunt JS, Macdonald PR, McGiven AR: Characterization of human glomerular basement membrane antigenic fractions isolated by affinity chromatography utilising anti-glomerular basement membrane autoantibodies. Biochem Biophys Res Commun 104:1025, 1982

30. Jenis EH, Valeski JE, Calcagno PL: Variability of anti-GBM binding in hereditary nephritis. Clin Nephrol 15:111, 1981

31. Jeraj K, Kim Y, Vernier RL, Fish AJ, Michael AF: Absence of Goodpasture's antigen in male patients with familial nephritis. Am J Kidney Dis II:626, 1983

32. Johnson JP, Moore J, Austin HA III, Barlow JE, Antonovych TT, Wilson CB: Therapy of antiglomerular basement membrane antibody disease: Analysis of prognostic significance of clinical pathologic and treatment factors. Medicine 64:219, 1985

33. Johnson JP, Whitman W, Briggs WA, Wilson CB: Plasmapheresis and immunosuppressive agents in antibasement membrane antibody-induced Goodpasture's syndrome. Am J Med 64:354, 1978

34. Kashtan C, Fish AJ, Kleppel M, Yoshioka K, Michael AF: Nephritogenic antigen determinants in epidermal and renal basement membrane of kindreds with Alport-type familial nephritis. J Clin Invest 78:1035, 1986

35. Kefalides NA, Ohno N, Wilson CB: Antigenic components of bovine lens capsule that cross-react serum from Goodpasture's syndrome (abstr). Fed Proc 43:779, 1984

36. Kefalides NA, Pegg MT, Ohno N, Poon-King T, Zabriskie J, Fillit H: Antibodies to basement membrane collagen and to laminin are present in sera from patients with poststreptococcal glomerulonephritis. J Exp Med 163:588, 1986

37. Kleppel MM, Kashtan CE, Butkowski RJ, Fish AJ, Michael AF: Alport familial nephritis: Absence of 28 kilodalton noncollagenous monomers of type IV collagen in glomerular basement membrane. J Clin Invest 80:263, 1987

38. Kleppel MM, Michael AF, Fish AJ: Antibody specificity of human glomerular basement membrane type IV collagen NC1 subunits: Species variation in subunit composition. J Biol Chem 261:16547, 1986

39. Langeveld JPM, Wieslander J, Timoneda J, McKinney P, Butkowski RJ, Wisdom BJ, Hudson BG: Structural heterogeneity of the noncollagenous domain of basement membrane collagen. J Biol Chem 263:10481, 1988

40. Langeveld JPM, Yem AWT, Timoneda J, Saus J, Wisdom BJ, Jr, Hudson BG: Molecular structure of collagen IV of glomerular basement membrane. In Renal Basement Membranes in Health and Disease, edited by Price RG, Hudson BG, p 25–39. London, Academic, 1987

41. Lerner RA, Dixon FJ: Transfer of ovine experimental allergic glomerulonephritis (EAG) with serum. J Exp Med 124:431, 1966

42. Lerner RA, Glassock RJ, Dixon FJ: The role of antiglomerular basement membrane antibody in the pathogenesis of human glomerulonephritis. J Exp Med 126:989, 1967

43. Lockwood CM, Amos N, Peters DK: Goodpasture's syndrome: Radioimmunoassay for measurement of circulating anti-GBM antibody (abstr). Kidney Int 16:93, 1979

44. Lockwood CM, Boulton-Jones JM, Lowenthal RM, Simpson IJ, Peters DK, Wilson CB: Recovery from Goodpasture's syndrome after immunosuppressive treatment and plasmapheresis. Br Med J 2:252, 1975

45. Lockwood CM, Bowman C, Bakes D, Pressey A, Dash A: Autoimmunity and Glomerulonephritis. Adv Nephrol 16:291, 1987

46. Lockwood CM, Pussell B, Wilson CB, Peters DK: Plasma exchange in nephritis. Adv Nephrol 8:383, 1979

47. Mahieu P, Dardenne M, Bach JF: Detection of humoral and cell-mediated immunity to kidney basement membranes in human renal diseases. Am J Med 53:185, 1972

48. Mahieu P, Lambert PH, Miescher PA: Detection of antiglomerular basement membrane antibodies by a radioimmunological technique. Clinical application in human nephropathies. J Clin Invest 54:128, 1974

49. Marquardt H, Wilson CB, Dixon FJ: Human glomerular basement membrane. Selective solubilization with chaotropes and chemical and immunologic characterization of its components. Biochemistry 12:3260, 1973

50. McCoy RC, Johnson HK, Stone WJ, Wilson CB: Absence of nephritogenic GBM antigen(s) in some patients with hereditary nephritis. Kidney Int 21:642, 1982

51. McIntosh RM, Griswold W: Antigen identification in Goodpasture's syndrome. Arch Pathol 92:329, 1971

52. McPhaul JJ, Dixon FJ: The presence of anti-glomerular basement membrane antibodies in peripheral blood. J Immunol 103:1168, 1969

53. Milliner DS, Pierides AM, Holley KE: Renal transplantation in Alport's syndrome: Anti-glomerular basement membrane glomerulonephritis in the allograft. Mayo Clin Proc 57:35, 1982

54. Olson DL, Anand SK, Landing BH, Heuser E, Grushkin CM, Lieberman E: Diagnosis of hereditary nephritis by failure of glomeruli to bind anti-glomerular basement membrane antibodies. J Pediatr 96:697, 1980

55. Palotie A, Peltonen L, Risteli L, Risteli R: Effect of the structural components of basement membranes on the attachment of teratocarcinoma-derived endodermal cells. Exp Cell Res 144:31, 1983

56. Palotie A, Tryggvason K, Peltonen L, Seppä H: Components of subendothelial aorta basement membrane: Immunohistochemical localization and role in cell attachment. Lab Invest 49:362, 1983

57. Papaioannou DF, Klassen J: An improved solid-phase immunoassay for anti-GBM antibodies. J Immunol Meth 53:195, 1982

58. Peters DK, Rees AJ, Lockwood CM, Pusey CD: Treatment and prognosis in antibasement membrane antibody-mediated nephritis. Transplant Proc 14:513, 1982

59. Pusey CD, Dash A, Kershaw MJ, Morgan A, Reilly A, Rees AJ, Lockwood CM: A single autoantigen in Goodpasture's syndrome identified by a monoclonal antibody to human glomerular basement membrane. Lab Invest 56:23, 1987

60. Rome L, Cuppage FF, Vertes V: Familial hematuric nephritis. Pediatrics 38:808, 1966

61. Rosenblatt SG, Knight W, Bannayan GA, Wilson CB, Stein JH: Treatment of Goodpasture's syndrome with plasmapheresis. A case report and review of the literature. Am J Med 66:689, 1979

62. Rubin K, Höök M, Öbrink B, Timpl R: Substrate adhesion of rat hepatocytes: Mechanism of attachment to collagen substrates. Cell 24:463, 1981

63. Rumpelt H-J: Hereditary nephropathy (Alport syndrome): Correlation of clinical data with glomerular basement membrane alterations. Clin Nephrol 13:203, 1980

64. Sariola H, Timpl R, von der Mark K, Mayne R, Fitch JM, Linsenmayer TF, Ekblom P: Dual origin of glomerular basement membrane. Dev Biol 101:86, 1984

65. Saus J, Wieslander J, Langeveld JPM, Quinones S, Hudson BG: Identification of the Goodpasture antigen as the $\alpha3(IV)$ chain of collagen IV. J Biol Chem 263:13374, 1988

66. Savage COS, Pusey CD, Bowman C, Rees AJ, Lockwood CM: Antiglomerular basement membrane antibody mediated disease in the British Isles, 1980-4. Br Med J 292:301, 1986

67. Savage COS, Pusey CD, Kershaw MJ, Cashman SJ, Harrison P, Hartley B, Turner DR, Cameron JS, Evans DJ, Lockwood CM: The Goodpasture antigen in Alport's syndrome: Studies with a monoclonal antibody. Kidney Int 30:107, 1986

68. Scheer RL, Grossman MA: Immune aspects of the glomerulonephritis associated with pulmonary hemorrhage. Ann Int Med 60:1009, 1964

69. Sisson S, Dysart NK, Fish AJ, Vernier RL: Localization of the Goodpasture antigen by immunoelectron microscopy. Clin Immunol Immunopathol 23:414, 1982

70. Soininen R, Haka-Risku T, Prockop DJ, Tryggvason K: Complete primary structure of the α_1-chain of human basement membrane (type IV) collagen. FEBS Lett 225:188, 1987

71. Spear GS: Alport's syndrome: A consideration of pathogenesis. Clin Nephrol 1:336, 1973

72. Spear GS, Slusser RJ: Alport's syndrome: Emphasizing electron microscopic studies on the glomerulus. Am J Pathol 69:213, 1972

73. Stanton MC, Tange JD: Goodpasture's syndrome (pulmonary haemorrhage associated with glomerulonephritis). Austr Ann Med 7:132, 1958

74. Steblay RW: Glomerulonephritis induced sheep by injections of heterologous glomerular basement membrane and Freund's complete adjuvant. J Exp Med 116:253, 1962

75. Steblay RW: Transfer of nephritis from sheep with autoimmune nephritis to recipient sheep by artery-to-artery cross circulation (abstr). Fed Proc 23:449, 1964

76. Timpl R: Recent advances in the biochemistry of glomerular basement membrane. Kidney Int 30:293, 1986

77. Timpl R, Dziadek M: Structure, development and molecular pathology of basement membranes. Int Rev Exp Pathol 29:1, 1986

78. Timpl R, Wiedemann H, Van Delden V, Furthmayr H, Kühn K: A network model for the organization of type IV collagen molecules in basement membranes. Eur J Biochem 120:203, 1981

79. Towbin H, Rosenfelder G, Wieslander J, Avila JL, Rojas M, Szarfman A, Esser K, Nowack H, Timpl R: Circulating antibodies to mouse laminin in Chagas disease, American cutaneous leishmaniasis, and normal individuals recognize terminal galactosyl(α1-3)-galactose epitopes. J Exp Med 166:419, 1987

80. von der Mark H, Oberbäumer I, Timpl R, Kemler R, Wick G: Immunochemical and autoantigenic properties of the globular domain of basement membrane collagen (type IV). Eur J Biochem 146:555, 1985

81. Walker RG, Scheinkestel C, Becker GJ, Owen JE, Dowling JP, Kincaid-Smith P: Clinical and morphological aspects of the management of crescentic anti-glomerular basement membrane antibody (anti-GBM) nephritis/Goodpasture's syndrome. Q J Med 54:75, 1985

82. Weber M, Sorger K-H, zum Büschenfelde M, Köhler H: A Goodpasture-like syndrome in rabbits induced by the dissociated human NC1 molecule (abstr). Kidney Int, in press

83. Wheeler J, Sussman M: Enzyme-linked immunosorbent assay for circulating anti-glomerular antibodies. Clin Exp Immunol 45:271, 1981

84. Wick G, Von der Mark H, Dietrich H, Timpl R: Globular domain of basement membrane collagen induces autoimmune pulmonary lesions in mice resembling human Goodpasture disease. Lab Invest 55:308, 1986

85. Wieslander J, Barr JF, Butkowski RJ, Edwards SJ, Bygren P, Heinegård D, Hudson BG: Autoimmune disease of basement membranes: Localization of Goodpasture's antigen to type IV collagen (abstr). Fed Proc 43:1005, 1984

86. Wieslander J, Barr JF, Butkowski RJ, Edwards SJ, Bygren P, Heinegård D, Hudson BG: Goodpasture antigen of the glomerular basement membrane: Localization to noncollagenous regions of type IV collagen. Proc Natl Acad Sci USA 81:3838, 1984

87. Wieslander J, Bygren P, Heinegård D: Antiglomerular basement membrane antibody: Antibody specificity in different forms of glomerulonephritis. Kidney Int 23:855, 1983

88. Wieslander J, Bygren P, Heinegård D: Isolation of the specific glomerular basement membrane antigen involved in Goodpasture syndrome. Proc Natl Acad Sci USA 81:1544, 1984

89. Wieslander J, Bygren PG, Heinegård D: Anti-basement membrane antibody: Immunoenzymatic assay and specificity of antibodies. Scand J Clin Lab Invest 41:763, 1981

90. Wieslander J, Heinegård D: The involvement of type IV collagen in Goodpasture syndrome. Ann NY Acad Sci 460:363, 1985

91. Wieslander J, Kataja M, Hudson BG: Characterization of the human Goodpasture antigen. Clin Exp Immunol 69:332, 1987

92. Wieslander J, Langeveld J, Butkowski R, Jodlowski M, Noelken M, Hudson BG: Physical and immunochemical studies of the globular domain of type IV collagen: Cryptic properties of the Goodpasture antigen. J Biol Chem 260:8564, 1985

93. Wilson CB: Radioimmunoassay for anti-glomerular basement membrane antibodies. In Manual for Clinical Immunology, edited by Rose NR, Friedman H, p 376. Washington, American Society for Microbiology, 1980

94. Wilson CB, Dixon FJ: Anti-glomerular basement membrane antibody-induced glomerulonephritis. Kidney Int 3:74, 1973

95. Wilson CB, Holdsworth SR, Neale TJ: Anti-basement membrane antibodies in immunologic renal disease. Aust New Zealand J Med 11:94, 1981

96. Wilson CB, Marquardt H, Dixon FJ: Radioimmunoassay (RIA) for circulating antiglomerular basement (GBM) antibodies (abstr). Kidney Int 6:114a, 1974

97. Yoshikawa N, Cameron AH, White RHR: The glomerular basal lamina in hereditary nephritis. J Pathol 135:199, 1981

98. Yoshioka K, Kleppel M, Fish AJ: Analysis of nephritogenic antigens in human glomerular basement membrane by two-dimensional gel electrophoresis. J Immunol 134:3831, 1985

99. Yurchenco PD, Ruben GC: Basement membrane structure in situ: Evidence for lateral associations in the type IV collagen network. J Cell Biol 105:2559, 1987

100. Yurchenco PD, Tsilibary EC, Charonis AS, Furthmayr H: Models for the self-assembly of basement membrane. J Histochem Cytochem 34:93, 1986

From: *Pathology Reviews • 1990* Edited by: E. Rubin and I. Damjanov Copyright © 1990 The Humana Press Inc., Clifton, NJ

Biology of Disease

Pathogenesis of Anti-Basement Membrane Glomerulopathy and Immune-Complex Glomerulonephritis: Dichotomy Dissolved

JAN A. BRUIJN, PHILIP J. HOEDEMAEKER, AND GERT JAN FLEUREN

Department of Pathology, University of Leiden, Leiden, The Netherlands

Introduction
Etiologic Factors in Immunologically Mediated Glomerulonephritis
Animal Models: A Brief Review
  Immunization
  Polyclonal B cell stimulation
Pathogenetic Mechanisms
Recent Observations
Anti-Basement Membrane Antibodies and Dense Aggregate Formation
Clinical Significance
Concluding Remarks

INTRODUCTION

In the last few decades the understanding of pathogenic mechanisms in renal disease has increased considerably. Immunofluorescence studies led to the discovery that most forms of glomerulonephritis in humans are immunologically mediated. Clinically, glomerular diseases are classified on the basis of light and immunofluorescence microscopical patterns, since these provide indications concerning pathogenesis. It has been shown unequivocally that antibodies are involved in the pathogenesis of such diseases as lupus nephritis, membranous nephritis, IgA nephritis, and anti-glomerular basement membrane (GBM) nephritis, but in most cases the pathogenetic antigen involved is not known with certainty. It has become increasingly evident that extracellular matrix and cell-surface antigens can be of pathogenic importance. Recently developed biochemical, immunochemical, and molecular biological techniques open the way to further identification of the pathogenic antigens as well as the mechanisms involved in their interaction with the corresponding antibodies. This paper will analyze recent studies on pathogenic aspects of antiGBM glomerulopathy and immune complex glomerulonephritis. First, etiologic factors are described that are known to operate in animal models of human immunologically mediated glomerulonephritis. Then, a brief review of the earlier work in such animal models is given, followed by a discussion of the meaning of recent observations, which shed new light on existing theories concerning the pathogenesis of immunologically mediated glomerulonephritis

ETIOLOGIC FACTORS IN IMMUNOLOGICALLY MEDIATED GLOMERULONEPHRITIS

Immunologically mediated renal diseases can occur spontaneously [*e.g.*, idiopathic systemic lupus erythematosus-like nephropathy as seen in humans and New Zealand B/W mice] or may be evoked by various factors that can be divided into three groups: (1) passive immunization, causing glomerular disease in animals (*e.g.*, nephrotoxic serum nephritis, passive Heymann nephritis, anti-Thy 1.1 antibody-induced nephritis); (2) active immunization (experimental allergic nephritis, active Heymann nephritis, serum sickness, accelerated nephrotoxic serum nephritis); and (3) mechanisms leading to polyclonal B cell activation (graft-*versus*-host reactions, exposure to therapeutic and toxic agents, infection with microorganisms).

Originally, exogenous antigens, such as bacterial components, were thought to be involved in the pathogenesis of glomerulonephritis, and research on the role of such external antigens made use of passive or active immunization. These studies have been extensively reviewed elsewhere (52, 61). Later, when it was recognized that a considerable proportion of these diseases are probably caused by immune reactions to autoantigens, animal models were developed in which polyclonal or restricted polyclonal stimulation of B cells was induced, and studies were performed in animal strains in which autoimmunity occurred spontaneously. In these models, the production of a wide repertoire of antibodies, including autoreactive antibodies giving rise to circulating immune complexes and antibody- and immune-complex–mediated tissue damage, is of pathogenic importance. Polyclonal B cell activation can be induced by B cell-stimulating factors such as microorganisms, lipopolysaccharides, and drugs or can occur in the course of certain parasitic diseases such as malaria and African trypanosomiasis. Autoantibodies have been shown to be directed against a wide variety of autoantigens, such as double-stranded DNA, nonDNA nuclear antigens, RNA, immunoglobulin G, GBM antigens, endogenous murine leukemia retrovirus glycoprotein (gp70), and cell-surface glycoproteins such as gp330 and gp90. How this polyclonal B cell activation is governed and restricted is still not fully understood. B cells, both allo- and autoreactive, are normally under the control of suppressor mechanisms, *e.g.*, suppressor T cells and anti-idiotypic antibodies. In experimentally induced murine graft-*versus*-host disease the injection of parental T cells into F1 hybrids results under certain conditions in polyclonal B cell activation. In this model an allogeneic or noncognitive T-B cell cooperation was proposed as an underlying mechanism (3). Furthermore, it was postulated that in SLE as well, polyclonal B cell activation may occur as a result of a noncognitive cooperation between T and B cells (110). Noncognitive T-B cooperation can be due to a loss of suppressor cells or damage to major histocompatibility complex encoded cell-surface molecules known to be important in physiologic T-B cooperation. Such modulating damage can be induced by interaction of lymphocytes with molecules that either bind to the cell surface or are expressed in the vicinity of major histocompatibility complex encoded molecules (50). Alternatively, haptens such as drugs may bind to self-constituents, triggering a cross-reactive immune response directed against the hapten itself or against the hapten-modified autoantigen. Induction of immune complex glomerulonephritis by mercury salts in certain strains of rats may have a similar pathogenesis. Recent findings in rats seem to indicate that mercury induces noncognitive T-B cooperation through the activation of autoreactive T helper cells, probably anti-Ia, that then stimulate self-Ia-bearing B cells (91, 92). Furthermore, a loss of suppressor cell function has been reported (114). In this and other models the autoimmunity disappears spontaneously, probably by the down-regulative action of anti-idiotypic antibodies (26) or T suppressor cells (91).

ANIMAL MODELS: A BRIEF REVIEW

IMMUNIZATION

Nephrotoxic serum nephritis (Masugi nephritis) is induced by injection of heterologous antiGBM antibodies (for review, see 83). The heterologous and autologous phases of this disease, which has been studied mainly in rats and rabbits, are characterized by a linear pattern of binding of antibodies along the GBM, glomerular accumulation of leukocytes, and endothelial cell damage.

Other organs are affected in this model—including the placenta, lung, aorta, brain, and liver—due to a reaction of the antibodies against basement membrane antigens present in these organs as well (13, 101). In experimental allergic glomerulonephritis (Steblay nephritis) immunization of sheep with basement membrane preparations led to the formation of autoantibodies binding in a similarly linear fashion to the GBM (102). Transfer and absorption studies proved the pathogenetic potential of the anti-GBM antibodies in this model (75, 98). The nature of the GBM antigens involved in these diseases is still unknown. Isolation of various types of basement membrane molecules and identification of the different domains of these molecules led to the finding that antiGBM nephritis can be induced by antibodies directed against the noncollagenous 1 (NC1) domain of type IV collagen (45, 72, 116).

Heymann nephritis, which is regarded as a model for human membranous nephritis, has become one of the most extensively investigated models of immunologically mediated glomerular disease. In the active model, glomerulonephritis appears 6 weeks after intraperitoneal immunization of rats with homologous kidney homogenates in Freund's adjuvant (58, 59). Passive Heymann nephritis is induced by injection of heterologous antibodies directed against rat brush-border antigens (10, 11, 40, 60, 62). IgG is deposited in a granular pattern along the glomerular basement membrane; electron-dense aggregates are seen subepithelially, and the GBM shows irregular thickening and formation of spikes. The formation of the aggregates arises from *in situ* binding (108) of the antibodies to antigens occurring on the surface of the glomerular epithelial cells. A glycoprotein with a molecular weight of 330 kDa (gp330) was identified as the principal pathogenetic antigen (68).

In what are called serum sickness models, foreign serum proteins such as bovine serum albumin are administered as a single inoculation or in repeated injections. For acute (one-shot) serum sickness in rabbits, a single intravenous injection of 250–500 mg/kg bovine serum albumin is given. A variable percentage of the animals develop acute but usually reversible diffuse glomerulonephritis characterized by glomerular hypercellularity due mainly to infiltration of mononuclear macrophages (30, 47, 64, 65). Electron microscopical and immunofluorescence findings differ according to the antigen and immunization protocol used. Granular deposits of IgG, C3, and antigens have been found by some workers (41) but not others (33), and electron-dense aggregates have been found in both subendothelial (64) and epimembranous localizations (41). Studies on the temporal relationship between the development of lesions and the presence of immune complexes depending on the concentrations of antigen and antibody in the circulation (31, 47), as well as studies in mice and rats given intravenous injections of soluble immune complexes (82), led to the concept that the lesions in acute serum sickness develop as a result of immune complex formation in the circulation followed by deposition in the glomerulus. In antibody excess or equivalence, large immune complexes are formed that are either removed from the circulation by the mononuclear phagocytic system or deposited in the mesangium. Under antigen excess, small complexes are formed and deposited in the glomerular capillary wall (48).

In chronic serum sickness models in rabbits or rats, repeated intravenous injections of a foreign serum protein are given over 2–3 months. To obtain small soluble immune complexes the antigen injections are adjusted to the antibody concentrations measured. Depending upon the protocol used and the level of circulating complexes, the animals may develop severe chronic glomerular lesions (15, 30, 49, 119). Early mesangial hypercellularity and mesangial deposition of IgG, C3, and bovine serum albumin are later followed by the formation of subendothelial and subepithelial aggregates along the glomerular capillary wall, glomerular hypercellularity, infiltration by neutrophils, and glomerular sclerosis (5, 63, 119).

POLYCLONAL B CELL STIMULATION

Glomerulonephritis caused by allogeneic disease is an experimental renal disorder due to a graft-*versus*-host reaction induced by the injection of lymphocytes belonging to one of the parental strains and transferred to an F1 hybrid (51) or originating from a host-*versus*-graft reaction induced in chimeras by neonatal transfer of F1 lymphocytes into a neonate parental animal (2, 57). Lewis *et al.* (77) studied (Balb/c × A/JAX)F1 hybrid mice given an injection of Balb/c spleen cells and found that about one-third of the animals developed renal pathology resembling idiopathic membranous glomerulonephritis in humans. With the use of cell transfers in other parental-hybrid strain combinations, the graft-*versus*-host model was developed further by Gleichmann's group (51) and by us (16, 17, 21).

In another model of immunologically mediated glomerulonephritis, polyclonal B cell stimulation is obtained by repeated subcutaneous injection of mercuric chloride into rats, mice, or rabbits. The resulting immune complex glomerulonephritis is preceded in some strains by an antiGBM antibody-mediated phase (12, 91, 95, 99, 100). Findings made with this model have led to the suggestion that antinuclear antibodies and anti-basement membrane antibodies play a pathogenetic role (7, 14, 113).

Exposure to microorganisms may be related to the development of autoimmunity and renal disease. In mice, endogenous leukemia retroviruses and their gene products may be involved in the pathogenesis of immune-mediated nephritis. The retroviral envelope glycoprotein gp70 is found in sera of mice suffering from autoimmune disease, and gp70 is deposited in diseased glomeruli together with host immunoglobulin and complement (28, 66, 74, 76, 104, 122). Parasitic infections such as trypanosomiasis and malaria can lead to increased immunoglobulin production due to a genetically controlled nonspecific polyclonal stimulation (53, 54) and to the development of postinfectious glomerular disease (34–39, 90).

Spontaneous murine models of systemic lupus erythematosus concern several inbred strains of mice that develop disease late in life. These strains include New Zealand B/W, BXSB, and MRL/1, which have been extensively studied by several groups (for reviews, see 103, 105, 106). The animals develop immune complex nephritis, which has been suggested to be associated with circulating anti-gp70 and antiDNA antibodies. In the kidneys, thickening of the glomerular basement membrane and glomerular hypercellularity are observed, eventually followed by the development of glomerulosclerosis and end-stage renal failure.

PATHOGENETIC MECHANISMS

The above-mentioned work on the etiological factors involved in immune-mediated renal disorders and the animal models developed for these illnesses has greatly contributed to our understanding of pathogenic mechanisms involved in such renal diseases. Immunofluorescence techniques have allowed determination of the site and pattern of localization of antibodies in the glomerulus. On the basis of the immunofluorescence pattern, immunologically mediated renal diseases were originally divided into two main groups: one with a linear immunofluorescence pattern (antiGBM disease) and the other with granular deposits of antibodies (immune complex glomerulonephritis).

In anti-GBM disease, antibodies directed against constituents of the GBM may bind linearly along the glomerular capillary wall. Light microscopical findings are variable. In some patients, remission or a mild, protracted course develops (118), whereas others show extensive crescent formation leading to rapidly progressive renal insufficiency. In more than half of the cases of antiGBM disease, antitubular basement membrane (TBM) antibodies are found as well (118), and these antibodies are related to interstitial inflammation and tubular damage (9). In antiGBM disease, autoantibodies have been found to be directed against the noncollagenous NC1 domain of type IV collagen, which is a globular region situated at the carboxyl terminus of the molecule (117).

In immune complex glomerulonephritis, immunoglobulins, complement, and the corresponding antigens are located in a granular pattern along the glomerular capillary wall. Much has been learned from the various models about the mechanisms that are involved in the accumulation of immune complexes in glomeruli. It is believed that immune complexes can accumulate either by deposition of circulating complexes or by formation *in situ* when antibodies react with antigens that are planted or normally present in glomeruli (42, 43, 108) or by a combination of these two mechanisms (44). Complexes formed in the circulation are partially cleared by the macrophage-phagocytic system. The amount and site of deposition of complexes in the glomeruli are influenced by the antigen-antibody ratio in the circulation. When antigen is in large excess, very small complexes are formed and may be deposited in the glomeruli. The rate of formation and the localization of the immune complexes depend further on such factors as the amount, size, and charge of the complexes, the class and avidity of the antibodies, and the affinity of the antigen for glomerular structures. *In situ* formation (42, 43, 108) may arise from binding of antibodies to intrinsic glomerular antigens or to circulating antigens previously planted in glomeruli, such as foreign proteins or products originating from viruses, bacteria, or parasites. In animal models, several intrinsic glomerular antigens that may act as target have been recognized, such as the 330 kDa rat Heymann antigen (gp330) (68, 69, 97) and the mouse and rat plasma membrane enzyme dipeptidyl peptidase (gp90) (6, 96, 109; for review see 111). These antigens appear on the brush border of proximal tubular epithelial cells and on the surface of glomerular epithelial cells. *In vitro* studies by Camussi and coworkers (22, 23) suggested that after binding of antibodies to the antigens on the glomerular epithelial cell surface, antigenic redistribution and clustering occur, leading to immune-complex shedding, trapping in the subepithelial space, and epimembranous electron-dense aggregate formation (70). In immune complex glomerulonephritis, electron-dense aggregates can be found not only subepithelially but also in the mesangium or under the endothelium. The latter localizations of aggregates are believed by some to result from nonspecific trapping of circulating complexes (27), although *in situ* formation of pathogenic immune complexes on the endothelial cell membrane and in the mesangium has been suggested by others (8, 80, 81, 86).

These models are relevant for immunologically mediated renal diseases in humans for several reasons. A genetic control of susceptibility is present in both animal models and humans; the genetic makeup of an individual may determine whether a given agent will induce (auto)-immunity or immunosuppression (25, 29, 67, 73, 89, 91, 93, 94, 120). As to the renal pathogenetic antigens involved, in human glomerulonephritis a pathogenic role has been established more firmly for basement-membrane components than for cell-surface antigens, such as extracellular matrix cell binding epitopes and their receptors, precursor molecules, or renal tubular epithelial antigens. Recent data suggest that brush-border proteins similar to those found in the animal models are present in humans as well, but their nephritogenic role remains to be investigated (88, 111).

RECENT OBSERVATIONS

As indicated in this survey, in human and in animal models of immunologically mediated renal disease a distinction is generally made between immune complex nephritis and antiGBM disease. However, recent observations indicate that the line of demarcation between these two groups of diseases may not be as sharp as has been assumed. In the experimental models studied, autoantibodies directed against basement membrane components proved to be an important category of nephritogenic antibodies. Although such antibodies were assumed to bind and remain bound to the GBM in a linear fashion, data obtained with the models showed that the early linear fluorescence pattern these antibodies induce may be followed by the formation of immune aggregates. This phenomenon was observed in murine graft-*versus*-host disease (16), mercuric chloride-induced glomerulonephritis in rats (7, 99), and Heymann nephritis in the rat (62), a phase of linear binding of autoantibodies along the GBM preceding the formation of dense aggregates. A population of anti-brush border antibodies used to induce passive Heymann nephritis was shown to contain antiGBM antibodies, which are responsible for the observed early linear binding pattern occurring before the granular phase (62). Trypanosomiasis in the rat (19, 20) is accompanied by an antiGBM glomerulopathy. In this model antibodies are found in a nonlinear irregular pattern along the glomerular capillary wall 7 weeks after infection. These findings are consistent with earlier observations in humans showing that in late stages of antiGBM disease, the autoantibodies may occur in an irregular pattern due to extensive destruction of the GBM and distortion of the glomerular architecture. As early as 1976 it was suggested that antibodies directed against GBM occur more frequently than is generally thought and may be involved in more types of glomerulonephritis than the few clearly recognized forms of antiGBM nephritis mentioned above (84).

ANTI-BASEMENT MEMBRANE ANTIBODIES AND DENSE AGGREGATE FORMATION

What then would explain the transition from a linear to a granular immunofluorescence pattern? An answer may lie in the character of the GBM, which should not be seen as a static skeleton to which cells are attached but rather as a dynamic equilibrium between molecules. Modern techniques such as biochemical analysis and immunoelectron microscopy have provided insight into the molecular composition of the extracellular matrix and the patterns of antibody binding to the molecular constituents (18). At least three mechanisms might explain the concurrent presence of antiGBM antibodies and the development of dense aggregates (Fig. 1). First, after linear binding of antibodies directed against antigens occurring within the GBM, formation of electron-dense aggregates might occur by rearrangement and condensation of the bound antibodies and antigens (16, 79, 115) (Fig. 1, *top*). The process of condensation and growth of the complexes might be enhanced by combination of the bound antibodies with anti-idiotypic antibodies (26, 79, 123) or rheumatoid factors or, in the passive models, with endogenous antibodies during the autologous phase. So far, the presence of GBM components in granular aggregates has not been demonstrated. This could be due to an excess of antibodies or to the limited resolution of immunofluorescence microscopy (46). Antibodies directed against laminin (1), type IV collagen (121), and proteoglycans (78) can induce formation of electron-dense aggregates. Fukatsu *et al.* (46) mentioned the importance of the length of time spent by the antibodies in the circulation as one factor determining the type of renal disease and immunofluorescence pattern that develops. According to Miettinen *et al.* (87), the exact pattern also depends on the molecular specificity of the antibodies, *i.e.*, on the basement membrane component to which the antibodies are directed. The process of molecular rearrangement may be associated with a disturbance of extracellular matrix turnover induced by binding of the antibodies. Miettinen *et al.* (87) showed that injection and binding of antiheparan sulfate proteoglycan antibodies in rats triggers an accelerated basement membrane production by glomerular epithelial cells, which in turn leads to a gradual displacement of the old basement membrane layers with the bound antibodies toward the endothelium. The results of earlier

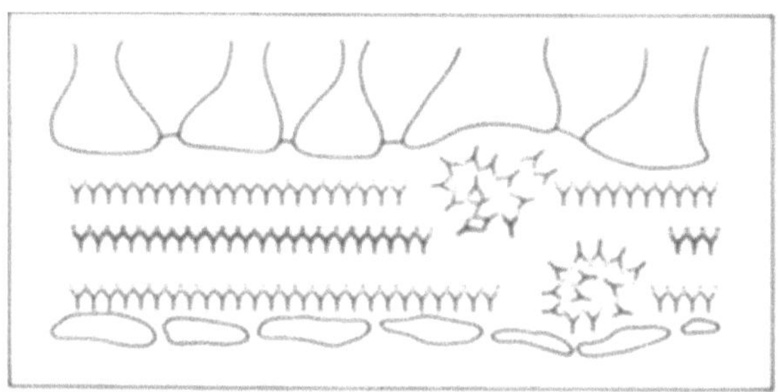

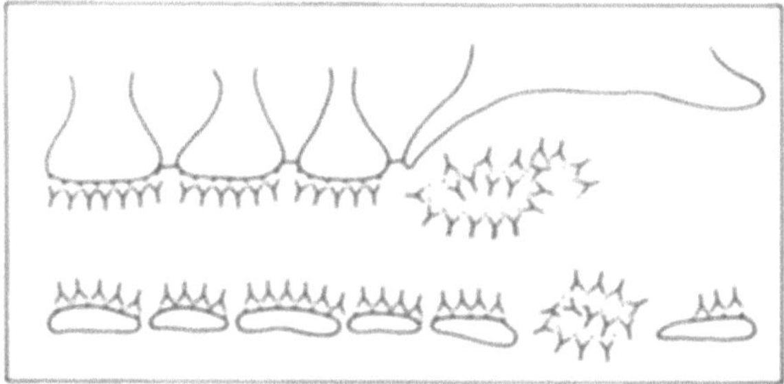

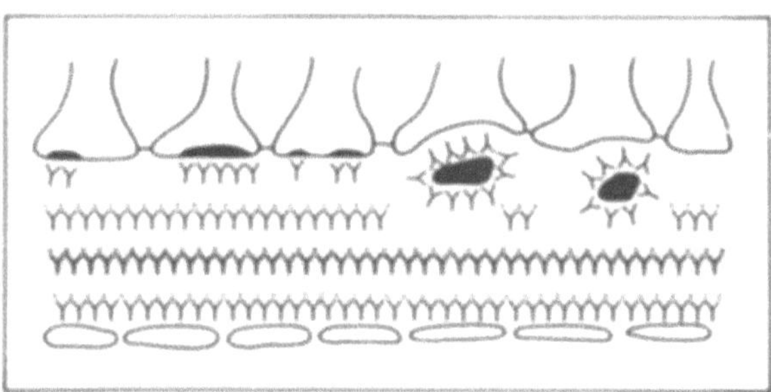

FIG. 1. Relationship between antiGBM antibodies and dense aggregate formation. *Top*, formation of immune complexes by linear binding of antibasement membrane antibodies (*left*), followed by rearrangement and condensation of the complexes and formation of dense aggregates (*right*). *Middle*, combination of antibodies with cell binding epitopes of basement membrane components or basement membrane precursor molecules occurring on the surface of epithelial and endothelial cells (*left*), followed by shedding and condensation of the complexes (*right*). *Bottom*, binding of antiGBM antibodies and binding of antibodies directed against antigens occurring in coated pits of epithelial cells (*left*), followed by dense aggregate formation after capping and shedding of the latter (*right*). See text for further explanation.

studies with silver nitrate labeling suggested that deposits may later be cleared from the peripheral capillary wall by gradual translocation into the mesangium (112).

Recent findings seem to indicate that the epitope specificity of the antibodies influences their binding pattern and the type of renal disease they induce. For example, when antibodies are directed against precursor forms or cell-binding epitopes of basement membrane components, they may bind to the area bordering the surface of epithelial or endothelial glomerular cells, a situation depicted in Figure 1 (*middle*). Observations by Fukatsu *et al.* (46) and Aten *et al.* (7) indicated that such antibodies may be involved in pathogenesis of mercury-induced membranous glomerulopathy. These autoantibodies initially bind in a linear fashion along the GBM.

Later, subepithelial granular aggregates are formed (Fig. 1, *middle*), at least partially due to shedding of immune complexes into the subepithelial space in a manner similar to that described for gp330-anti-gp330 complexes (70). Furthermore, antibodies may bind to basement membrane components newly secreted and shed by the visceral epithelial cells (46). It is unclear why epithelial cell detachment does not always occur, but its absence may be regarded as an argument against a cell binding nature of the target epitopes.

A third condition under which there could be an association between the presence of antiGBM antibodies and the formation of electron-dense aggregates would be the concurrent activity of both antiGBM antibodies and antibodies with other specificities (Fig. 1, *bottom*). In this situation the binding of antiGBM antibodies may cause damage to the GBM, facilitating the access of antibodies with other specificities (*e.g.*, anti-gp330 or anti-gp90) to their target antigen and induce the formation of electron-dense aggregates. Such mechanisms have been discussed for murine chronic graft-*versus*-host disease (16) and Heymann nephritis (62). The existence in autoimmune diseases of both antibasement membrane antibodies and antibodies directed against brush-border antigens such as gp330 and gp90 is in itself not surprising. Recent findings have shown a role played by both gp90 (56) and gp330 (85) in the attachment of cells to basement membrane proteins, indicating a functional receptor-ligand relationship between basement membrane components and cell-surface antigens. Common epitopes might be present on these two groups of antigens, both of which are expressed by epithelial cells and may derive from a supergene family (4, 32, 62, 71). In models in which experimental induction occurs by passive or active immunization, *e.g.*, Heymann nephritis, a role may be played by copurification of the basement membrane components with firmly bound brush-border antigens used for the immunization (18, 62).

Extensive research should be performed to throw more light on the functional and structural relationships between cell-surface antigens and basement membrane components. Finally, mention should be made of the recent discovery that pathological conditions may be accompanied by a neo-expression of epitopes not normally present or a modification of normal epitopes leading to a change in their antigenicity (24, 55, 107). This may explain why it is often so difficult to detect and purify nephritogenic autoantigens when use is made of normal kidney tissue.

CLINICAL SIGNIFICANCE

The distinction between antiGBM nephropathy and immune complex glomerulonephritis is still maintained by both pathologists and clinicians as a basis for the diagnosis and treatment of immunologically mediated renal disease. AntiGBM disease itself, as in Goodpasture's syndrome, is a clearly defined and well-characterized disease that is not subject to discussion. However, as discussed above, recent findings indicate that antibodies directed against GBM components may also be involved in the formation of electron-dense aggregates and the development of a granular immunofluorescence pattern. In our opinion, therefore, the exclusion of a pathogenic role of antiGBM antibodies on the basis of a nonlinear immunofluorescence pattern is not justified. In patients suffering from immune-complex glomerulonephritis, antiGBM autoantibodies should be considered as a pathogenic factor. Glomerular diseases characterized by a nonlinear immunofluorescence pattern can apparently be induced by antibodies directed against both GBM components and regions of the extracellular matrix that are not considered structural components of the GBM, such as cell-binding epitopes, precursor molecules, or receptor molecules present on cell surfaces. In sum, our findings indicate that antiGBM disease and immune complex nephritis should not be considered two separate disease entities but rather two poles demarcating a range of diseases. Eventually, this new insight into the pathogenetic mechanisms may lead to changes in the therapeutic approach of these diseases, although it seems too early to draw conclusions in that direction.

CONCLUDING REMARKS

Originally it was believed that the pathogenesis of immunologically mediated glomerulonephritis was largely determined by either circulating immune complexes—formed under conditions of antigen excess—or antiGBM antibodies. About a decade ago it became clear that besides the deposition of preformed complexes, *in situ* formation of glomerular deposits is also an important pathogenetic mechanism. Recent findings have only complicated the picture, showing that antiGBM disease and immune complex glomerulonephritis are not to be looked upon as separate disease entities but rather as the poles of a range of immunologically mediated renal diseases. The final outcome in a particular case is determined by a large number of partially related factors, including the physicochemical characteristics and epitope specificity of the antibodies, their time spent in the circulation, the relationship between different antibody populations with respect to concentration and time in polyclonal immune reactions or polyclonal antisera, and genetic influences.

However confusing these findings may seem, prospects for further research have also been provided by recent scientific developments. The use of newly developed methods for biochemical dissection of the extracellular matrix, the development of antibodies against isolated matrix components, and the application of DNA sequencing methods to analyze protein composition and structure have opened new perspectives for further study of the role of autoantigens at the molecular and epitope levels. Continued efforts in this field of research are necessary to complete the elucidation of mechanisms involved in the development and perpetuation of immune-mediated renal diseases as well as to improve preventive and therapeutic measures for this group of disorders.

Address reprint requests to: Jan A. Bruijn, Department of Pathology, University of Leiden, P.O. box 9603, 2300 RC Leiden, The Netherlands.

REFERENCES

1. Abrahamson DR, Caulfield JP: Proteinuria and structural alterations in rat glomerular basement membranes induced by intravenously injected anti-laminin immunoglobulin G. J Exp Med 156:128, 1982
2. Abramowicz D, Bruyns C, Goldman M: Chimerism and CTL unresponsiveness after neonatal injection of spleen cells in mice: Effects of T-cell depletion and of the semi or full allogeneic nature of the inoculum. Transplantation 44:696, 1987
3. Allison AC, Denman AM, Barnes RD: Hypothesis. Cooperating and controlling functions of thymus-derived lymphocytes in relation to autoimmunity. Lancet 2:135, 1971
4. Alpers CE, Cotran RS: Neoplasia and glomerular injury. Kidney Int 30:465, 1986
5. Arisz L, Noble B, Milgrom M, Brentjens JR, Andres GA: Experimental chronic serum sickness in rats. A model of immune complex glomerulonephritis and systemic immune complex deposition. Int Arch Allergy Appl Immunol 60:80, 1979
6. Assmann KJM, Tangelder MM, Lange WPJ, Tadema TM, Koene RAP: Membranous glomerulonephritis in the mouse. Kidney Int 24:303, 1983
7. Aten J, Bruijn JA, Veninga A, De Heer E, Weening JJ: Anti-laminin autoantibodies and mercury induced glomerulopathy. Kidney Int 33:309, 1988
8. Bagchus WM: Specificity of nephritogenic antibodies. An experimental study. Thesis, University of Groningen, Groningen, 1986
9. Bannister KM, Ulich TR, Wilson CB: Induction, characterization, and cell transfer of autoimmune tubulointerstitial nephritis. Kidney Int 32:642, 1987
10. Barabas AZ, Lannigan R: Induction of an autologous immune-complex glomerulonephritis in the rat by intravenous injection of heterologous anti-rat kidney tubular antibody. I. Production of chronic progressive immune-complex glomerulonephritis. Br J Exp Pathol 55:47, 1974
11. Barabas AZ, Lannigan R: Induction of an autologous immune complex glomerulonephritis in the rat by intravenous injection of heterologous anti-rat kidney tubular antibody. II. Early glomerular lesions. Br J Exp Pathol 55:282, 1974
12. Bariéty J, Druet P, Laliberté F, Sapin C: Glomerulonephritis with gamma- and beta-1C-globulin deposits induced in rats by mercuric-chloride. Am J Pathol 65:293, 1971
13. Baxter JH, Goodman HC: Nephrotoxic serum nephritis in rats. I. Distribution and specificity of the antigen responsible for the production of nephrotoxic antibodies. J Exp Med 104:467, 1956
14. Bellon B, Capron M, Druet E, Verroust P, Vial MC, Sapin C, Girard JF, Foidart JM, Mahieu P, Druet P: Mercuric chloride induced autoimmune disease in Brown-Norway rats: Sequential search for anti-basement membrane antibodies and circulating immune complexes. Eur J Clin Invest 12:127, 1982
15. Brentjens JR, O'Connell DW, Albini B, Andres GA: Experimental chronic serum sickness in rabbits that received daily multiple and high doses of antigen: A systemic disease. Ann NY Acad Sci 254:603, 1975
16. Bruijn JA, Hogendoorn PCW, Corver WE, Van den Broek LJCM, Hoedemaeker PhJ, Fleuren GJ: Pathogenesis of experimental lupus nephritis: a role for anti-basement membrane and anti-tubular brush border antibodies in murine chronic graft-versus-host disease. Clin Exp Immunol, in Press 1989
17. Bruijn JA, Van Elven EH, Corver WE, Oudshoorn-Snoek M, Fleuren GJ: Genetics of experimental lupus nephritis: non-H-2 factors determine susceptibility for renal involvement in murine chronic graft-versus-host disease. Clin Exp Immunol 76:284, 1989
18. Bruijn JA, Hogendoorn PCW, Hoedemaeker PhJ, Fleuren GJ: The extracellular matrix in pathology; a review. J Lab Clin Med 111:140, 1988
19. Bruijn JA, Oemar BS, Ehrich JHH, Fleuren GJ: Immune complex formation in the kidney: Recent observations in experimental trypanosomiasis. Ann Soc Belge Med Trop 68:11, 1988
20. Bruijn JA, Oemar BS, Ehrich JHH, Foidart JM, Fleuren GJ: Anti-basement membrane glomerulopathy in experimental trypanosomiasis. J Immunol 139:2482, 1987
21. Bruijn JA, Van Elven EH, Hogendoorn PCW, Corver WE, Hoedemaeker PhJ, Fleuren GJ: Murine chronic graft-versus-host

disease as a model for lupus nephritis. Am J Pathol 130:639, 1988

22. Camussi G, Brentjens JR, Noble B, Kerjaschki D, Malavasi F, Roholt OA, Farquhar MG, Andres G: Antibody-induced redistribution of Heymann antigen on the surface of cultured glomerular visceral epithelial cells: Possible role in the pathogenesis of Heymann glomerulonephritis. J Immunol 135:2409, 1985

23. Camussi G, Noble B, Van Liew J, Brentjens J, Andres G: Pathogenesis of passive Heymann nephritis (HN): Chlorpromazine (CL) inhibits antibody-mediated redistribution of cell surface antigens and prevents development of the disease. Kidney Int 99:268, 1986

24. Castronovo V, Mahieu P, Bracke M, Mareel M, Colin C, Lambotte R, Foidart JM: Role of laminin and α-galactosyl cell surface residues in tumour invasion and metastasis. Eur J Cell Biol 44 Suppl 20:3, 1987

25. Celada A, Barras C, Benzonama G, Jeannet M: Increased frequency of HLA-DRw3 in systemic lupus erythematosus. New Engl J Med 301:1398, 1979

26. Chalopin JM, Lockwood CM: Autoregulation of autoantibody synthesis in mercuric chloride nephritis in the Brown Norway rat. II. Presence of antigen-augmentable plaque-forming cells in the spleen is associated with humoral factors behaving as auto-anti-idiotypic antibodies. Eur J Immunol 14:470, 1984

27. Couser WG: Mechanisms of glomerular injury in immune-complex disease. Kidney Int 28:569, 1985

28. Croker BP, Del Villano BC, Jensen FC, Lerner RA, Dixon FJ: Immunopathogenicity and oncogenicity of murine leukemia viruses. I. Induction of immunologic disease and lymphoma in (Balb/c × NZB)F1 mice by Scripps leukemia virus. J Exp Med 140:1028, 1974

29. Datta SK, Tsichlis P, Schwartz RS, Chattophadhyay SK, Melief CJM: Genetic differences unrelated to H-2 in H-2-congenic mice. Immunogenetics 7:359, 1978

30. Dixon FJ, Feldman JD, Vazquez JJ: Experimental glomerulonephritis: The pathogenesis of a laboratory model resembling the spectrum of human glomerulonephritis. J Exp Med 113:899, 1961

31. Dixon FJ, Vazquez JJ, Weigle WO, Cochrane CG: Pathogenesis of serum sickness. Am Med Assoc Arch Pathol 65:18, 1958

32. Eagen JW, Lewis EJ: Glomerulopathies of neoplasia. Kidney Int 11:297, 1977

33. Easley JR, Halliwell WH: Relationship of proteinuria to glomerular basement membrane deposits in serum-sickness glomerulonephritis in rabbits. Vet Pathol 14:482, 1977

34. Ehrich JHH, Beck EJ, Haberkorn A, Meister G: Causes of death in lethal rat malaria. Trop Parasitol 35:127, 1984

35. Ehrich JHH, Horstmann RD: Origin of proteinuria in human malaria. Trop Med Parasitol 36:39, 1985

36. Ehrich JHH, Oemar BS, Bruijn JA, Wonigeit K, Fleuren GJ: Postinfectious glomerulonephritis in a rat model: Genetic control and susceptibility to a cyclosporin A treatment. In Recent Advances in Pediatric Nephrology, edited by K. Murakami et al., p 605. Amsterdam, Elsiever, 1987

37. Ehrich JHH, Oemar BS, Kerb W, Fleuren GJ, Bruijn JA, Wonigeit K: Cyclosporin A inhibits the trypanosomiasis-induced nephrotic syndrome. Kidney Int 29:1256, 1986

38. Ehrich JHH, Oemar BS, Wonigeit K, Bruijn JA, Fleuren GJ: Genetic control and cyclosporin A treatment of experimental glomerulonephritis. Pediatr Nephrol 1:19, 1987

39. Ehrich JHH, Sterzel RB, Deicher HRG, Foellmer HG: Rat malarial glomerulonephritis. An experimental model of post-infectious glomerular injury. Virchows Arch Cell Pathol 37:343, 1981

40. Feenstra K, Van der Lee R, Greben HA, Arends A, Hoedemaker PhJ: Experimental glomerulonephritis in the rat induced by antibodies directed against tubular antigen. I. The natural history: A histologic and immunohistologic study at the light microscopic and the ultrastructural level. Lab Invest 32:235, 1975

41. Fish AJ, Michael AF, Vernier RL, Good RA: Acute serum sickness nephritis in the rabbit (an immune deposit disease). Am J Pathol 49:997, 1966

42. Fleuren GJ, Grond J, Hoedemaeker PhJ: In situ formation of subepithelial glomerular immune complexes in passive serum sickness. Kidney Int 17:631, 1980

43. Fleuren GJ, Grond J, Hoedemaeker PhJ: The pathogenic role of free circulating antibody in autologous immune complex glomerulonephritis. Clin Exp Immunol 41:205, 1980

44. Ford PM, Kosatka I: The effect of in situ formation of antigen-antibody complexes in the glomerulus on subsequent glomerular localization of passively administered immune complexes. Immunology 39:337, 1980

45. Fouser LS, Michael AF, Kleppel MM, Vernier RL, Fish AJ: Nephritogenicity in sheep of the NC1 domain of type IV collagen from human gomerular basement membrane (hGBM). Kidney Int 31:319, 1987

46. Fukatsu A, Brentjens JR, Killen PD, Kleinman HK, Martin GR, Andres GA: Studies on the formation of glomerular immune deposits in Brown Norway rats injected with mercuric chloride. Clin Immunol Immunopathol 45:35, 1987

47. Germuth FG Jr: A comparative histologic and immunologic study in rabbits of induced hypersensitivity of serum sickness type. J Exp Med 97:257, 1953

48. Germuth FG, Rodriquez E: Immunopathology of the Renal Glomerulus. Boston, Little Brown, 1973

49. Germuth FG, Taylor JJ, Siddiqui SY, Rodriquez E: Immune complex disease. VI. Some determinants of the varieties of glomerular lesions in the chronic bovine serum albumin-rabbit system. Lab Invest 37:162, 1977

50. Gleichmann H: Studies on the mechanism of drug sensitization: T-cell-dependent popliteal lymph node reaction to diphenylhydantoin. Clin Immunol Immunopathol 18:203, 1981

51. Gleichmann E, Gleichmann H: Pathogenesis of graft-versus-host reactions (GVHR) and GVH-like diseases. J Invest Dermatol 85:115, 1985

52. Goldman M, Baran D, Druet P: Polyclonal activation and experimental nephropathies. Kidney Int 34:141, 1988

53. Greenwood BM: Possible role of a B-cell mitogen in hypergammaglobulinemia in malaria and trypanosomiasis. Lancet 1:435, 1974

54. Greenwood BM, Whittle HC: The pathogenesis of sleeping sickness. Trans R Soc Trop Med Hyg 6:716, 1980

55. Hakomori SI: Tumor-associated carbohydrate antigens. Annu Rev Immunol 2:103, 1984

56. Hanski C, Huhle T, Reutter W: Involvement of plasma membrane dipeptidyl peptidase IV in fibronectin-mediated adhesion of cells on collagen. Biol Chem Hoppe-Seyler 366:1169, 1985

57. Hard RC, Kullgren B: Etiology, pathogenesis and prevention of a fatal host-versus-graft syndrome in parent/F1 mouse chimeras. Am J Pathol 59:203, 1970

58. Heymann W, Hackel DB, Harwood S, Wilson SGF, Hunter JLP: Production of nephrotic syndrome in rats by Freund's adjuvant and rat kidney suspensions. Proc Soc Exp Biol Med 100:660, 1959

59. Heymann W, Lund HZ: Nephrotic syndrome in rats. Pediatrics 7:691, 1951

60. Hoedemaeker PhJ: Een Vorm van experimentele Immuun-complex-glomerulonephritis. Ned Tijdschr Geneeskd 116:1802, 1972

61. Hoedemaeker PhJ, Fleuren GJ, Weening JJ: Experimental models of the nephrotic syndrome. In The Nephrotic Syndrome, edited by Cameron JS, Glassock RJ, p 89. New York, Dekker, 1988

62. Hogendoorn PCW, Bruijn JA, Van den Broek LJCM, De Heer E, Foidart JM, Hoedemaeker PhJ, Fleuren GJ: Antibodies to purified renal tubular epithelial antigens contain activity against laminin, fibronectin, and type IV collagen. Lab Invest 58:278, 1988

63. Hogendoorn PCW, Bruijn JA, Gelok EWA, Van den Broek LJCM, Fleuren GJ: Development of progressive glomerulosclerosis in experimental chronic serum sickness. Nephrol Dial Transplant, in press 1989

64. Holdsworth SR, Neale TJ, Wilson CB: The participation of macrophages and monocytes in experimental immune complex glomerulonephritis. Clin Immunol Immunopathol 15:510, 1980

65. Hunsicker LG, Shearer TP, Plattner SB, Weisenburger D: The role of monocytes in serum sickness nephritis. J Exp Med 150:413, 1979

66. Izui S, McConahey PJ, Theofilopoulos AN, Dixon FJ: Association of circulating retroviral gp70-anti-gp70 immune complexes with murine systemic lupus erythematosus. J Exp Med 149:1099, 1979

67. Kashiwabara H, Shishido H, Tomura S, Tuchida H, Miyajima T: Strong association between IgA nephropathy and HLA-DR4 antigen. Kidney Int 22:377, 1982

68. Kerjaschki D, Farquhar MG: The pathogenic antigen of Heymann nephritis is a membrane glycoprotein of the renal proximal tubule brush border. Proc Natl Acad Sci USA 79:5557, 1982

69. Kerjaschki D, Farquhar MG: Immunocytochemical localization of the Heymann nephritis antigen (gp330) in glomerular epithelial cells of normal Lewis rats. J Exp Med 157:667, 1983

70. Kerjaschki D, Miettinen A, Farquhar MG: Initial events in the formation of immune deposits in passive Heymann nephritis. J Exp Med 166:109, 1987

71. Kerjaschki D, Noronha-Blob L, Sacktor B, Farquhar MG: Micro domains of distinctive glycoprotein composition in the kidney proximal tubule brush border. J Cell Biol 98:1505, 1984

72. Kleppel MM, Michael AF, Fish AJ: Antibody specificity of human glomerular basement membrane type IV collagen NC1 subunits. J Biol Chem 261:16547, 1986

73. Klonda PT, Acheson EJ, Golby FS, Lawler W, Manos J, Dyer PA, Harris R, Mallick NP, Williams G: Strong association between idiopathic membranous nephropathy and HLA-DRW3. Lancet 2:770, 1979

74. Lambert PH, Dixon FJ: Pathogenesis of glomerulonephritis in NZB/W mice. J Exp Med 127:507, 1968

75. Lerner RA, Dixon FJ: Transfer of ovine experimental allergic glomerulonephritis (EAG) with serum. J Exp Med 124:431, 1966

76. Lerner RA, Wilson CB, Del Villano BC, McConahey BJ, Dixon FJ: Endogenous oncornaviral gene expression in adult and fetal mice: Quantitative, histologic and physiologic studies of the major viral glycoprotein gp70. J Exp Med 143:151, 1976

77. Lewis RM, Armstrong MYK, André-Schwartz J, Muftuoglu A, Beldotti L, Schwartz RS: Chronic allogeneic disease. I. Development of glomerulonephritis. J Exp Med 128:653, 1968

78. Makino H, Lelongt B, Kanwar YS: Nephritogenicity of proteoglycans. II. A model of immune complex nephritis. Kidney Int 34:195, 1988

79. Mannik M, Agodoa LYC, David KA: Rearrangement of immune complexes in glomeruli leads to persistence and development of electron-dense deposits. J Exp Med 157:1516, 1983

80. Matsuo S, Caldwell PRB, Brentjens JR, Andres G: Nephrotoxic serum glomerulonephritis induced in the rabbit by anti-endothelial antibodies. Kidney Int 27:217, 1985

81. Mauer SM, Sutherland DER, Howard RJ, Fish AJ, Najarian JS, Michael AF: The glomerular mesangium. III. Acute immune mesangial injury: A new model of glomerulonephritis. J. Exp Med 137:553, 1973

82. McCluskey RT, Benacerraf B, Miller F: Passive acute glomerulonephritis induced by antigen-antibody complexes solubilized in hapten excess. Proc Soc Exp Biol Med 111:764, 1962

83. McCluskey RT, Vassalli P: Experimental glomerular diseases. In The Kidney, edited by Rouiller C, Muller A. New York, Academic, 1969

84. McPhaul JJ Jr, Mullins JD: Glomerulonephritis mediated by antibody to glomerular basement membrane. Immunological, clinical and histopathological characteristics. J Clin Invest 57:351, 1976

85. Mendrick DL, Chung DC, Smith DM, Rennke HG: Anti-gp330 monoclonal antibody interferes with cell adhesion in proximal tubule cell cultures. Kidney Int 31:175, 1987

86. Mendrick DL, Rennke HG: Immune deposits formed in situ by a monoclonal antibody recognizing a new intrinsic rat mesangial matrix antigen. J Immunol 137:1517, 1986

87. Miettinen A, Stow JL, Mentone S, Farquhar MG: Antibodies to basement membrane heparan sulfate proteoglycans bind to the laminae rarae of the glomerular basement membrane (GBM) and induce subepithelial GBM thickening. J Exp Med 163:1064, 1986

88. Natori Y, Hayakawa I, Shibata S: Heymann nephritis in rats induced by human renal tubular antigens: Characterization of antigen and antibody specificities. Clin Exp Immunol 69:33, 1987

89. Noel LH, Descamps B, Hors J, Dausset J: HLA antigen in three types of glomerulonephritis. Clin Immunol Immunopathol 10:19, 1978

90. Oemar BS, Ehrich K, Büngener W, Hackbarth HJ, Deicher HRG, Ehrich JHH: Genetic control of nephrotic syndrome in rat trypanosomiasis. Eur J Pediatr 140:187, 1983

91. Pelletier L, Hirsch F, Rossert J, Druet E, Druet P: Experimental mercury-induced glomerulonephritis. Springer Semin Immunopathol 9:359, 1987

92. Pelletier L, Pasquier R, Hirsch F, Sapin C, Druet P: Induction of T cells in mercury-induced autoimmune disease. In vitro demonstration. J Immunol 137:2548, 1986

93. Rees AJ, Peters DK, Compston DAS, Batchelor JR: Strong association between HLA-DRW2 and antibody-mediated Goodpasture's syndrome. Lancet 1:966, 1978

94. Reinertsen JL, Klippel JH, Johnson AH, Steinberg AB, Decker JL, Mann DL: B-lymphocyte alloantigens associated with systemic lupus erythematosus. New Engl J Med 299:515, 1978

95. Roman-Franco AA, Turellic M, Cilbini B, Ossi E, Millgram F, Andres GA: Anti-basement membrane antibodies and antigen-antibody complexes in rabbits injected with mercuric chloride. Clin Immunol Immunopathol 9:464, 1978

96. Ronco P, Allegri L, Melcion C, Pirotsky E, Appay MD, Bariéty J, Pontillon F, Verroust P: A monoclonal antibody to brush border and passive Heymann nephritis. Clin Exp Immunol 55:319, 1984

97. Ronco P, Neale TJ, Wilson CB, Galceran M, Verroust P: An immunopathologic study of a 330 kd protein defined by monoclonal antibodies and reactive with anti-Rtea antibodies and kidney eluates from active Heymann nephritis. J Immunol 136:125, 1986

98. Rudofsky U, Steblay RW: Studies on autoimmune nephritis in sheep. II. Passive transfer of nephritis in sheep by plasma. Fed Proc 25:659, 1966

99. Sapin C, Druet E, Druet P: Induction of anti-glomerular basement membrane antibodies in the Brown-Norway rat by mercuric chloride. J Clin Exp Immunol 28:173, 1977

100. Savige JA, Lockwood CM: Factors affecting the glomerular protein leak after polyclonal activation in the HgCl$_2$-induced model of anti-GBM disease in the Brown Norway rat. Clin Exp Immunol 70:619, 1987

101. Seegal BC, Loeb EN: The production of chronic glomerulonephritis in rats by the injection of rabbit anti-rat-placenta serum. J Exp Med 84:211, 1946

102. Steblay RW: Glomerulonephritis induced in sheep by injections of heterologous basement membrane and Freund's complete adjuvant. J Exp Med 116:253, 1962

103. Steinberg AD, Huston DP, Taurog JD, Cowderg JS, Raveche ES: The cellular and genetic basis of murine lupus. Immunol Rev 55:121, 1981

104. Strand M, August JT: Oncornavirus envelope glycoprotein in serum of mice. Virology 75:130, 1976

105. Theofilopoulos AN, Dixon FJ: Etiopathogenesis of murine SLE. Immunol Rev 55:179, 1981

106. Theofilopoulos AN, McConahey PJ, Izui S, Eisenberg RA, Pereira AB, Creighton WD: A comparative immunologic analysis of several murine strains with autoimmune manifestations. Clin Immunol Immunopathol 15:258, 1980

107. Towbin H, Rosenfelder G, Wieslander J, Avila JL, Rojas M, Szarfman A, Esser K, Nowack H, Timpl R: Circulating antibodies to mouse laminin in Chagas disease, American cutaneous Leishmaniasis, and normal individuals recognize terminal galactosyl(α1-3)-galactose epitopes. J Exp Med 166:419, 1987

108. Van Damme BJC, Fleuren GJ, Bakker WW, Vernier RL, Hoedemaeker PhJ: Experimental glomerulonephritis in the rat induced by antibodies directed against tubular antigens. V. Fixed glomerular antigens in the pathogenesis of heterologous immune complex glomerulonephritis. Lab Invest 38:502, 1978

109. Van Leer EHG, Moullier Ph, Ronco P, Verroust P: Lymphocyte expression of a gp90 kD brush border antigen. Clin Exp Immunol 67:572, 1987

110. Van Rappard-van der Veen FM: Murine graft-versus-host disease as a model for SLE. Thesis, University of Amsterdam, Amsterdam, 1983

111. Verroust P, Ronco P, Chatelet F: Antigenic targets in membranous glomerulonephritis. Springer Semin Immunopathol 9:341, 1987

112. Walker F: The origin, turnover and removal of glomerular basement membrane. J Pathol 110:233, 1973

113. Weening JJ, Fleuren GJ, Hoedemaeker PhJ: Demonstration of antinuclear antibodies in mercuric-chloride glomerulopathy in the rat. Lab Invest 39:405, 1978

114. Weening JJ, Hoedemaeker PhJ, Bakker WW: Immunoregulation and anti-nuclear antibodies in mercury-induced glomerulopathy in the rat. Clin Exp Immunol 45:64, 1981

115. Wener MH, Mannik M: Mechanisms of immune deposit formation in the renal glomeruli. Springer Semin Immunopathol 9:219, 1986

116. Wick G, von der Mark H, Dietrich H, Timpl R: Globular domain

of basement membrane collagen induces autoimmune pulmonary lesions in mice resembling Goodpasture disease. Lab Invest 55:308, 1986

117. Wieslander J, Heinegard D: The involvement of type IV collagen in Goodpasture's syndrome. Ann NY Acad Sci 460:363, 1985

118. Wilson CB: Immunopathology of antibasement membrane antibodies. In Mechanisms of Immunopathology, edited by Cohen S, Ward PA, McCluskey RT. New York, Wiley, 1979

119. Wilson CB, Dixon FJ: Quantitation of acute and chronic serum sickness in the rabbit. J Exp Med 134:7s, 1971

120. Wooley PH, Griffin J, Panayi G, Batchelor JR, Welsh JR, Gibson TJ: HLA-DR antigens and toxic reaction to sodium aurothiomalate and D-penicillamine in patients with rheumatoid arthritis. N Engl J Med 303:300, 1980

121. Yaar M, Foidart JM, Brown KS, Rennard SI, Martin GR, Liotta L: The Goodpasture-like syndrome in mice induced by intravenous injections of anti-type IV collagen and anti-laminin antibody. Am J Pathol 107:79, 1982

122. Yoshiki T, Mellors RC, Strand M, August JT: The viral envelope glycoprotein of murine leukemia virus and the pathogenesis of immune complex glomerulonephritis in New Zealand mice. J Exp Med 140:1011, 1974

123. Zanetti M, Wilson CB: Participation of auto-anti-idiotypes in immune complex glomerulonephritis in rabbits. J Immunol 131:2781, 1983

Section III

Tumor Biology

Biology of Disease
Molecular Mechanisms of Oncogenesis

THOMAS A. SEEMAYER, AND WEBSTER K. CAVENEE

Departments of Pathology, Pediatrics and Medicine, McGill University Faculty of Medicine, The Montreal Children's Hospital and Ludwig Institute for Cancer Research (Montreal Branch), Royal Victoria Hospital

INTRODUCTION

A review of the literature of the past several years shows hundreds of reports describing oncogene identification, expression, deregulation, amplification and mutation, chromosomal alterations and molecular events in experimental and naturally occurring cancer. It is our intention here to focus on concepts and principles and to present an overview of the molecular events thought to be important in cancer. We discuss the history and nature of oncogenes and then consider cytogenetic and molecular mechanisms which may be operative in neoplasia. Because many contributions originate from analyses of relatively rare pediatric cancers, particular emphasis will be accorded cancers arising in children. Since the molecular events uncovered in the childhood cancers appear to be operative in adults, we will consider a few of these diseases as well.

ONCOGENES

EARLY DISCOVERIES

The notion that cancer can be attributed to discrete genetic elements was first supported experimentally in 1911 when Rous (141) reported that an unusual sarcoma in chickens could be induced by cell-free filtrates. The significance of this work, recognized some decades later, was that some neoplasms could be virally-induced. This landmark observation was fully appreciated years hence (he eventually received the Nobel Prize) with the discovery of the retroviral enzyme reverse transcriptase (9, 169) and a unique gene, v-*src* (one of four genes in the Rous sarcoma virus), which endowed the retrovirus (RV) with oncogenic properties (112). Further work with cloned viral oncogene (v-*onc*) segments as probes showed that genes of similar structure were present not only in normal chickens but many other species, including man (164). From this evolved the concept that retroviral oncogenes (v-*onc*) had been acquired by the virus through infection of the host (transduction) and, once in the virus, fell under the control of strong viral promoters sufficient to render the virus oncogenic. It is now thought that the ability of these genes to transform cells may also require a small mutational change in their nucleotide sequence, usually at the 3' end (17). Hence, by the mid-1970s, the concept of "cancer genes," *i.e.*, oncogenes, as predicted by Huebner and Todaro in 1969, (74) had been given a good measure of experimental support.

ONCOGENES AS GROWTH AND DIFFERENTIATION GENES

At present, some 40 proto (cellular) oncogenes (c-*onc*) have been identified and, in most instances, assigned to specific chromosomal regions by *in situ* hybridization to metaphase chromosomes or by segregation in somatic cell hybrids. Twenty retroviral oncogenes are known. In general, RV oncogenes (v-*oncs*) differ from c-*oncs* in consisting of exons alone, being devoid of intervening sequences. Ten DNA viruses have been found to contain oncogenes. Oncogenes are designated by a three-letter abbreviation accorded either from the animal or tumor in which they were first identified. Cellular oncogenes have been found in all species examined. Their presence in yeast (two c-*ras* genes) is essential for spore germination and cell growth (85). Indeed, the conservation of c-*oncs* throughout a billion years of evolution strongly implies that these genes serve critical functions necessary for survival. In this regard, it is now known that many c-*oncs* are expressed at specific times and in selective tissues during growth and differentiation (106). The fact that this expression is highly regulated has led some to propose that a mechanism operative in neoplasia may be an inappropriate timing and/or amount of c-*onc* gene product expression (102).

Since c-*onc* expression appears to be important for growth and differentiation, numerous investigators have undertaken studies to determine their normal protein products and sites of action. It appears that c-onc gene products reside within the nucleus, cytosol,and plasma membrane (174). Four biochemical functions have been ascribed to oncogene proteins: regulation of DNA replication; control of gene transcription; metabolic regulation of proteins that bind guanosine triphosphate (GTP); and, protein phosphorylation at the level of the plasma membrane (17). Consequently, the function or malfunction of these vital cellular genes can have dramatic effects on DNA synthesis, transcription, adenyl cyclase regulation, and expression of growth factors and growth factor receptors. Taken together, the life of a cell is intimately linked to oncogene function.

Shortly after the discovery that v-*src* codes for a protein (pp60) (25) which phosphorylates tyrosine (76) (an astonishing finding at the time, since most protein kinases until then were known to preferentially phosphorylate serine or threonine), seven additional v-*oncs* were found to code for protein kinases which phosphorylate tyrosine. Although the targets of such activities are not well described, one particularly provocative target appears to be vinculin at sites of adhesion plaques. Since one effect of triggering the receptor for growth factors is an increase of intracellular phosphotyrosine, such oncogene proteins, if improperly regulated, could also usurp the process of signal transduction. Oncogene proteins have also been shown to have homology with growth factors (*e.g.*, c-*sis* with platelet-derived growth factor) (40) and growth factor receptors (*e.g.*, c-erb-B with epidermal growth factor receptor) (41). In the latter instance, the receptor produced is truncated, devoid of the EGF-binding region, yet has an intact transmembrane segment and catalytic intracellular domain. Other oncogene proteins, those related to the ras family (c-Ha-*ras*, c-Ki-*ras*, c-N-*ras*), code for guanine nucleotide binding proteins (p21) (78) which may function in an analogous fashion to "G" or "N" proteins which regulate transmembrane information exchange. Finally, other oncogenes, c-*myc*, c-*myb*, c-*fos*, and c-*ski*, exert their function through gene products which act in the nucleus by affecting DNA replication and transcription. Among these, c-*fos* may function as a "master switch" by serving as a regulatory gene which turns on other genes (176).

ONCOGENES AND THE NEOPLASTIC STATE

Since c-*oncs* are part of the essential genetic dowry of eukaryotes, through what manner are these genes subverted in cancer? One mechanism operative in animals and known as promoter insertion, comes about after the imposition of a RV upstream, within, or downstream to a c-*onc* in the infected animal (17). In this model, the c-*onc* is driven by strong viral promoters, with or without mutations of an adjacent cellular gene, presumably sufficient to result in neoplasia. Five different oncogenes (c-erb-B, c-*mos*, c-*myc*, c-*myb*, and c-Ha-*ras*) have been implicated in this particular type of oncogenesis. In some instances, it is not necessary that oncogenes be shuffled contiguous to strong viral promoters in order to elicit cancer. Indeed, studies of transgenic mice have shown that the juxtaposition of c-*myc* genes next to enhancer segments for heavy or light chain immunoglobulin genes is sufficient to induce lymphoma within a few months of birth (1).

A second mechanism by which oncogenes may contribute to the neoplastic state is by a point mutation, the net effect being an altered gene product. In an elegant series of experiments, Weinberg and colleagues used DNA from methylcholanthrene-induced sarcomas to transduce transformed cell properties (155) in an approach derived from prior studies on pneumococcus (7) and polyoma virus (178). Utilizing nontransformed NIH/3T3 fibroblasts as targets in this DNA-mediated gene transfer experiment (DNA transfection), they were able to show that the transforming potential of the chemically induced tumor resided in a small segment of DNA. Furthermore, change of a single nucleotide in c-Ha-ras-1 at position 12 (thymidine substituted for guanosine) in a human bladder carcinoma cell line resulted in a single amino acid substitution, which elicited highly efficient cell transformation capability (26, 132). The pivotal role of mutation of the 12th codon in another *ras* family member, c-Ki-*ras*, has been demonstrated recently in another human cancer, colorectal adenocarcinoma. Fully one-third of such tumors, as well as adenomas associated with the cancers, have been shown to manifest a single amino acid alteration stemming from genetic changes at this codon (20, 52). Moreover, evidence for *ras* mutational activation was obtained in premalignant villous adenomas (52). Collectively, these latter data suggest that mutagenic events and oncogene activation can precede the development of cancer, as diagnosed histologically. Finally, by combining *in vitro* gene amplification by the polymerase chain reaction and detection of mutations by RNAase A mismatch cleavage, c-Ki-*ras* mutations at codon 12 were consistently detected in ductal pancreatic adenocarcinomas (4). Similar point mutations have been identified in human adenocarcinoma of the lung (138), the myelodysplastic syndrome (73) and experimental cancers (145, 167). As additional cancers are studied, particularly after gene amplification by the polymerase chain reaction, it may turn out that oncogene mutations are common events in the oncogenic process.

One property which distinguishes malignant from benign neoplasms is the ability of the former to metastasize. If oncogenes are operative in the cascade of events central to cancer, one might anticipate a role for such genes in conferring metastatic potential to a neoplasm. In this regard, a group of transforming oncogenes which codes for protein kinases (c-*ras*, c-*mos*, c-*raf*, c-*src*, c-*fes*, c-*fms*) have been shown to confer metastatic potential to fibroblastic cell lines (46).

Other genetic mechanisms thought to be operative in human cancers include chromosomal translocations, inversions or deletions, and gene, particularly oncogene, amplification. In these, cytogenetic aberrations are often manifest in karyotypic studies of the neoplasm, hence microscopically visible chromosomal alterations appear to be the central theme in these human cancers. In the next section, we shall explore these aspects of the oncogenic process.

The Summing Up

Discovered at the early part of the century but recognized little more than 10 years ago, oncogenes have come to assume a pivotal place in thinking regarding diverse cancers. Known to be expressed in a highly regulated fashion in growth and differentiation, the aberrant expression of such genes may, in some way, contribute to the neoplastic state. At this writing, mutant oncogenes have not been shown to be inherited. Although much is known about these putative "cancer genes," their exact role, if any, in the chain of events leading to neoplasia continues to be a matter of intense debate. Most of the

available evidence suggests that oncogenes are more likely to contribute to the progression, rather than initiation of cancer. The coming decade should bring resolution of this issue.

Many excellent overviews of oncogenes have appeared in the past several years. For the interested reader, the following readings are suggested (15–17, 65, 77, 82, 86, 87, 99, 156, 174, 180, 181, 183, 190).

CYTOGENETIC ABERRATIONS IN CANCER

Early Discoveries

The concept that cancer stems from an alteration in the genetic material originated with the zoologist Boveri in 1914 (21) and continued with the studies of Muller (in 1927) on radiation mutagenicity in fruitflies and Auerbach (in 1946) with nitrogen mustard mutagenicity. It is now believed that the oncogenic process is not the result of a single mutagenic event, but rather one which stems from sequential genetic alterations, one of which may be manifested cytogenetically. In fact, it has been noted that the majority of cancers have a demonstrable cytogenetic defect (196). This is particularly the case in leukemias and lymphomas analyzed with extended banding (400 to 1200 bands) techniques (195). Of notable interest is the recurrent identification of a given cytogenetic lesion for certain cancers. Hence, the majority of patients with chronic myeloid leukemia manifest a reciprocal translocation between chromosomes 9 and 22 [t(9;22) (q34;q11)]. In like fashion, most Burkitt lymphomas feature a reciprocal translocation (111) between chromosomes 8 and 14 [t(8;14) (q24;q32)]; those tumors lacking this translocation feature reciprocal genetic exchanges of chromosomes 2p13 or 22q11 with chromosome 8. The significance of these genetic shufflings assumed even greater significance when it was shown that important genes were situated at the sites of the chromosomal breaks.

The Philadelphia Chromosome

The chronic myeloid leukemia-associated Philadelphia chromosome was identified in 1960 by Nowell and Hungerford (124) and interpreted to represent a deletion of the short arm of chromosome 22. Subsequently, Rowley (142) showed that a reciprocal translocation of genetic information between chromosomes 9 and 22 constituted the fundamental lesion. The breakpoint on chromosome 9 (q34) assumed additional relevance with the discovery that c-abl locus which normally codes for a 145 kilodalton protein with tyrosine kinase activity maps to the same chromosomal position. Through the translocation process, c-*abl* is placed in juxtaposition to a region on chromosome 22 known as the breakpoint cluster region (bcr). The two regions unite in a head-to-tail configuration to produce a hybrid gene (5' bcr segment and truncated c-*abl* gene lacking the first exon) which codes for an 8.5 kb transcript which encodes an aberrant protein (p210) with increased tyrosine kinase activity (13). Whether this abnormal gene product is central to oncogenesis in this disease is not as yet clear, particularly since recent studies indicate that the p210 gene product is unable to effect transformation of NIH/3T3 fibroblasts (36). More recently, it has been found that the Philadelphia chromosome positive form of acute lymphocytic leukemia may be associated with yet another aberrant gene product (p190) (30, 98). Finally, rearrangement of the bcr gene may represent an additional important event in the development of this leukemia, even in settings devoid of the Philadelphia chromosome (42). Thus, in chronic myeloid leukemia, a strong association exists between cytogenetic aberrations and oncogene expression, one characterized by abnormal oncogene products and gene rearrangements. The relationship of these alterations to the neoplastic process remains, as yet, unestablished.

Burkitt Lymphoma

The relevance of reciprocal translocations in Burkitt lymphoma also seems to be linked to oncogene expression, albeit in a different fashion. In many of these tumors, the oncogene protein appears to be qualitatively normal, but its production is deregulated (amount and/or timing) as a result of the translocation. The common denominator in all three translocations found in Burkitt lymphomas has been chromosome 8q24, a region (37) which codes for a nuclear protein, c-myc, that affects DNA replication and transcription. As a result of the particular translocation, c-myc genes are brought in close association with genes (joining, constant, variable regions) which are pivotal to B cell differentiation (#14 heavy chain, #2 κ light chain, #22 λ light chain) (35). Presumably as a consequence of these, and possibly other genetic interchanges, a dominant clone of B cells emerges, driven relentlessly to proliferate as a monoclonal B cell neoplasm. The mechanism which brings about the activation of c-myc in Burkitt lymphomas is controversial and, as yet, unresolved. Moreover, studies in transgenic mice indicate clearly that myc activation in itself is insufficient to induce malignancy (101).

Follicular Lymphoma

A somewhat analogous situation applies to other B cell lymphomas. In one such condition, follicular lymphoma, a reciprocal translocation (t14;18) brings about the juxtaposition of heavy chain immunoglobulin genes on chromosome 14 with genes (bcl-2) which reside on chromosome 18. This translocation results in the accumulation of high levels of bcl-2 gene messenger RNA (171). The bcl-2 gene may represent a novel oncogene, as no known retroviral counterpart has been identified. Its protein product has been demonstrated immunohistochemically in neoplastic cells of follicular lymphomas, but not in normal or non-neoplastic germinal centers (122). Molecular abnormalities have been identified in regions near or within the bcl-2 locus in 100% of these lymphomas. The oncogenic potential of bcl-2 has been further demonstrated in gene transfer experiments with NIH3T3 cells (133). Similar molecular changes have been identified in 28% of diffuse large cell B lymphomas, as well (182).

T Cell Neoplasia

Much the same scenario can be portrayed for diverse T cell leukemias and lymphomas. These neoplasms, as with chronic myeloid leukemia and Burkitt lymphoma, may affect children as well as adults, and present either as leukemia or as a thymic or nodal mass. In many, the neoplasm arises *de novo*, although in ataxia telangiectasia, T cell neoplasia appears to represent the terminal event of a genetically determined immune deficiency and chromosomal instability syndrome. As with B cell neoplasms, the focal point of many of these T-cell cancers involves a specific, albeit different, chromosomal region, 14q11-13, that encompasses the locus which codes for the alpha chain of the T-cell receptor (115). Translocations [t(8;14) t(11;14)] and inversions involving this region are common in some T-cell neoplasms. As in the case of B cell maturation, an assortment of gene segments is shuffled during T cell ontogeny. In leukemias/lymphomas associated with t(8;14 (q24;q11), the breakpoint on chromosome 14 is 36kb 5′ to the alpha chain of the T cell receptor gene, while the breakpoint on chromosome 8 is 3kb 3′ of the c-myc gene. As a result, the constant region of the α-chain T cell receptor gene is translocated 3′ to the c-myc locus on 8q24 (51). In the common T cell acute lymphoblastic leukemia of childhood, [t(11;14 (p13;q11)], the breakpoint on chromosome 14 is within the locus for the α-chain of the T cell receptor. At this writing, the corresponding breakpoint on chromosome 11 is not known to be associated with an oncogene.

The β-chain genes for the T cell receptor have been mapped to the 7q32-q34 region. As many as nine chromosomal regions involving reciprocal translocations of this segment have been described in T cell lymphomas and leukemias (32). Thus, T cell neoplasia, in general demonstrates a strong association with genes which code for the T cell antigen polypeptide chains.

Fragile Sites

While these specific translocations are illustrative of the B and T cell neoplasms cited, more recent study of diverse B cell lymphomas reveals that similar chromosomal sites (#11, 14 18) are associated with an assortment of lymphoid neoplasms (31, 35, 125). The number of chromosomal alterations and sites associated with cancer appears to be rather limited and found in high frequency either with known oncogene loci or heritable fragile sites (100, 118, 125, 197). The latter appear as nonstaining gaps on both chromatids and are inherited in a codominant Mendelian fashion. In cells grown in media deficient in folic acid and thymidine, 17 such sites (16 autosomal, 1 X) have been identified. Current data indicate a striking degree of linkage between such fragile sites and chromosomal breakpoints associated with cancer.

Ewing's Tumor

Ewing's sarcoma is one solid tumor which has recently been shown to bear a reciprocal translocation, [t(11;22) (q24;q12)] (6, 172). The initial description of this alteration came from several centers in France and was followed shortly thereafter by a report of an identical translocation in peripheral neuroepithelioma (185). The proto-oncogene, c-*sis*, located at 22q13, while translocated to chromosome 11 in the process, is neither rearranged nor activated as a result of the translocation. Thus, identical cytogenetic lesions have been observed in two discrete neoplasms, if, in fact, they are indeed different. One of us reported a similar cytogenetic event in a neoplasm originally interpreted to be Ewing's sarcoma, yet subsequently found to contain neuron-specific enolase and neurosecretory granules (150). In this, double minute chromosomes were seen on direct tumor preparations. Such structures are an index of gene amplification, especially common amongst tumors derived from the neural crest (131). These findings collectively suggest that at least some neoplasms thought to be Ewing's sarcoma may be of neuroectodermal origin, a view consonant with other studies on the osseous variant of this tumor (80).

GENE AMPLIFICATION

In two childhood cancers (retinoblastoma, neuroblastoma) karyotypic study of the neoplasms may reveal evidence of gene amplification in the form of either homogeneously staining regions (HSRs) or double minute (DM) chromosomes (11). The former alteration, first noted in drug-resistant Chinese hamster ovary cell lines, (126) appears as pale chromosomal regions devoid of a banding pattern. The latter manifests as small paired chromatin bodies devoid of chromocenters which segregate randomly at cell division (11). In neuroblastomas and cultured cell lines thereof, the HSRs may be found on diverse chromosomes, yet take origin from chromosome 2 (p23–24), the region which codes for N-*myc* (166). N-*myc* has been shown to have significant genomic, messenger and protein product homology to c-*myc* (93, 157). In contrast to c-*myc*, N-*myc* lacks a retroviral homologue. With cloned gene probes and *in situ* hybridization, such regions have been shown to contain repetitive segments coding for N-*myc* (91, 146). Further studies of neuroblastoma and retinoblastoma cell lines demonstrated enhanced expression of N-*myc* mRNA consequent to genomic amplification. *In situ* hybridization established that the primitive neuroblastic cells, as opposed to the larger, more differentiated cells, were responsible for enhanced N-*myc* transcription (61, 147). Equally important, N-*myc* expression was not detected during the process of cytodifferentiation as these tumors matured over time (61). Moreover, enhanced N-*myc* expression appeared to correlate with a poor clinical prognosis (61, 147). Hence, gene amplification constitutes still another mechanism whereby oncogene expression may contribute to oncogenesis; in this instance, most evidence suggests that the impact of such expression on cancer biology is that of tumor promotion rather than initiation.

Recent studies have established that N-*myc* is amplified in neuroblastomas of children who present at an advanced clinical stage (III or IV) (24, 92). Moreover, these findings have been confirmed using DNA recovered from paraffin blocks (170) with methods described by Goelz (60) and Dubeau (44). Usually, N-*myc* DNA amplification is associated with increased transcription, as well. Of particular interest is the fact that in very young children who present with neuroblastoma stage IV-S, a distinct form of neuroblastoma associated with a good prognosis and tendency for the tumor to undergo spontaneous maturation and/or regression, N-*myc* is not amplified (149). This suggests that such tumors may not have incurred the ultimate lesions required for carcinogenesis. In this context, only a single gene copy of N-*myc* has been detected in ganglioneuromas, *i.e.*, neuroblastomas which have matured (cytodifferentiated) (149). Hence, the magnitude of amplification of a particular oncogene (N-*myc* in the case of neuroblastoma) appears to correlate well with both clinical stage and prognosis. Since N-*myc* amplification has been shown to cause down-modulation of class I major histocompatibility antigen (MHC) expression in neuroblastomas, it is conceivable that tumors with amplified N-*myc* may more easily escape T cell surveillance if MHC-restricted mechanisms are central to their elimination (14). What remains unclear is the relationship, if any, between N-*myc* amplification (locus 2p23-24), the chromosomal deletion (lp31p36) observed in over 70% of neuroblastomas successfully studied, and the activation of the N-*ras* oncogene which resides proximal but not adjacent to the breakpoint on chromosome 1.

SMALL CELL CARCINOMA OF THE LUNG

Oncogenes of the *myc* family (c-*myc*, L-*myc*, N-*myc*) are often amplified in small cell carcinomas of the lung. The amplification of genomic segments (109, 120, 191) and mRNA (120) in these tumors presents striking parallels with neuroblastoma. A recent study employing c-RNA riboprobes and *in situ* hybridization reveals that in a given small cell carcinoma, only one of the myc genes is amplified; additionally, no morphologic differences were apparent between tumors that expressed c-*myc*, N-*myc* or L-*myc* mRNA (64). N-*myc* expression, while usually associated with neuroectodermal tumors, has been reported in Wilms' tumor and hepatoblastoma (123). These data suggest that overexpression of this oncogene may represent a marker for neoplasms derived from primitive cell precursors.

CARCINOMA OF THE BREAST

Oncogene amplification has been demonstrated in mammary carcinomas. The HER-2/neu oncogene (also called c-erbB-2), originally identified as an oncogene activated by a point mutation in chemically-induced rat neuroblastomas, has been implicated in the oncogenic process in this common cancer. Amplification of this oncogene has been reported to be associated with tumors of advanced stage (199) and with a heightened clinical recurrence rate and poor survival (158). The HER-2/neu genomic amplification correlates with expression of its protein product, as demonstrated immunohistochemically within intraductal and invasive ductal mammary carcinoma in frozen tissue sections (175). In another study, the p21 gene product of c-Ha-*ras* has been demonstrated to be consistently increased in the invasive and metastatic components of mammary carcinoma (97).

The prognostic significance of c-erbB-2 amplification in breast cancers has been questioned recently. In a collaborative study of mammary cancers, a second group of investigators failed to confirm the importance of c-erbB-2 amplification in predicting overall survival or time to relapse (2). The possible bases for these conflicting data were addressed in a concurrent response (159). It is likely that this important issue will be resolved only after study of a large series of patients with long-term clinical follow-up.

DIVERSE CARCINOMAS AND SARCOMAS

Finally, there may exist a significant association of molecular alterations of oncogenes in diverse malignant solid tumors of epithelial or mesenchymal origin (192). Deletions or amplifications of c-*myc*, c-Ha-*ras*, c-*myb*, or c-Ki-*ras* have been observed in more than one-third of such neoplasms and appeared to correlate with clinical behavior.

RECESSIVE MUTATIONS AND CANCER

Knudson lists the number of hereditary cancers at about 50 (89). In this setting, the tendency to develop cancer is inherited in a Mendelian dominant fashion, a factor modulated by gene penetrance. If oncogenes are central to the oncogenic process, they function, presumably, in the heterozygous state. In the past several years, the concept has arisen that predisposition to some cancers is a consequence of a recessive mutation whose effect is observed after the tumor-specific loss of its normal homologue. From this emerged the notion of tumor-suppressor genes and "antioncogenes" (62, 89), the latter an extension of a theory proposed earlier by Comings (34). Pediatric neoplasms which may arise through such a mechanism include retinoblastoma, Wilms' tumor, hepatoblastoma, osteosarcoma and certain variants of rhabdomyosarcomas. The elucidation of this recessive mutational mechanism was made possible by study of hereditary cancer families with recombinant DNA technology which exploited highly polymorphic sites within the genome of these informative individuals.

THE BASIS FOR THE RECESSIVE ONCOGENE CONCEPT

The idea that cancer might arise as a sequel to recessive mutations evolved following incisive experiments by Harris which demonstrated that malignancy could be averted when malignant cells were fused with benign cells (70). From this came forth the concept that recessive mutations could be manifest by genetic events that resulted in the absence or functional allelic loss (of the unaffected gene) on the homologous chromosome (127). Shortly thereafter, the two "hit" hypothesis of Knudson was proposed as a general mechanism of cancer induction to explain the epidemiologic features peculiar to retinoblastoma (88). In this hypothesis, the induction of cancer requires two mutagenic events, *i.e.*, "hits," to a cell. The first such "hit" may be visited either on the germ or

somatic cell. If the former, all bodily cells bear this genomic alteration (constitutional) and are rendered especially vulnerable to a second "hit." The second mutational event always occurs to a somatic cell. Thus, the pivotal event is the cell affected by the first mutational change. When the germ cell is affected (either transmitted through the germ line or following a new mutation), tumors would be predicted (by this model) to be bilateral, multifocal, and to arise precociously. It now appears that the model is correct, at least for some retinoblastomas.

The existence of tumor-suppressor genes has been established in studies of Drosophila melanogaster in which at least 24 such genes have been identified. Since these genes appear to be required in normal development, the loss of function of both alleles causes cell growth to becomes unrestricted. That a single copy of a normal gene can avert the malignant transformation has been shown after insertion of a segment of the cloned lethal (2) giant larvae gene into flies deficient in the gene (79).

For those interested in additional reading material regarding the development of the recessive oncogene concept, the following references (57, 67, 71, 90, 130, 143, 165) are suggested.

RETINOBLASTOMA AND OSTEOSARCOMA

Retinoblastoma is an ancient disease, having been identified in Mayan sculptures from 2000 B.C. (139). It represents the most common intraocular neoplasm of childhood, one which accounts for 1% of childhood cancer deaths in the United States. Over the past half-century, the incidence has doubled (1/16,000 live births) due to an increasing number of survivors, which increases the gene pool. Based on morphology, the photoreceptor cell has long been regarded as the cell of origin for the tumor. Recent molecular studies with probes for the rod and cone cell α subunits of transducin suggest that the tumor is of cone cell lineage (19).

About 25% of tumors are bilateral stemming from germ cell mutations, although only 5 to 10% of children present with a positive family history. In either situation in which a child inherits a germ line mutation, the mutation is fully penetrant and transmitted in an autosomal dominant fashion. These latter children are at particular risk for second neoplasms, (over 20 types have been identified) the overwhelmingly most common being osteosarcoma, even in sites not subjected to irradiation. This prompted the notion that the putative retinoblastoma mutation is pleiotropic and that the retinoblastoma (Rb) locus might have broader effects. It now appears likely that the locus is the site of a cancer suppressor gene; the loss or inactivation of this genetic material appears central to the induction of diverse cancers.

The first clue to the location of the locus responsible for retinoblastoma came from a case study of an affected child who also had multiple nonocular congenital anomalies, mental retardation and a karyotypic lesion affecting the 13th chromosome (107). The specific chromosomal alteration was later shown by extended banding techniques to be a deletion, 13q14 (194). Further support incriminating this chromosomal site followed in family studies which revealed close linkage between the retinoblastoma gene and an enzyme, esterase-D, which had been mapped to 13q14 (162). The 13q14 constitutional deletion is uncommonly found in children with retinoblastoma (8); other cytogenetic aberrations (absence of one chromosome 13, isochromosome 6p, extra copies of chromosome 1q) have also been identified (139). Given the rare chromosomal deletion form of retinoblastoma and the linkage of the autosomal dominant form to esterase-D, the hypothesis was advanced that the tumor arose by a loss of genetic material at 13q14 too minute to be detected by existing banding techniques (163). Bear in mind that an average chromosome consists of 100,000 kilobases and an average gene contains 40 kilobases. Since one chromosome (with high resolution banding) may have 40 visible bands, one band (2,500 kilobases) contains about 60 genes.

These studies provided the basis for a series of studies in which cloned DNA fragments from specific regions of chromosome 13 were used to determine chromosomal complements in normal and tumor tissue from retinoblastoma patients (27). Studying at first tumor cells from nonhereditary cases, evidence was obtained in support of the notion that nondisjunctional loss of the "wild-type" nondeleted chromosome and reduplication of the abnormal chromosome might represent a mechanism central to oncogenesis. Alternatively, mitotic recombination resulting from a break and cross-over event may have been responsible. In either case, homozygosity for a mutant allele at 13q14 (homozygosity defined as the loss of activity of both normal alleles) appeared to be required for the induction of retinoblastoma. Other analyses of esterase-D isozymes in normal and retinoblastoma cells provided data which was interpreted as somatic inactivation of genes near the esterase-D locus, including the remaining normal gene at the retinoblastoma locus in oncogenesis (59). Furthermore, in hereditary cases it was demonstrated that the chromosome 13 homologues retained in the tumor contained the predisposing germline mutation, not the normal "wild-type" allele of the retinoblastoma locus (28). Shortly thereafter, a similar mechanism involving chromosome 13 was found in osteosarcomas, both those arising in retinoblastoma patients and sporadic forms (66).

These studies provided the conceptual and methodologic basis for identification of the chromosome carrying the predisposing mutant allele in families. An obvious extension is the use of DNA genotyping in families to determine relative risk for development of the disease. In 1986, the first such report described five families in which the fetus at risk, both parents (one with retinoblastoma) and a previously affected child (or a normal child if one parent had bilateral retinoblastomas) were examined. An assortment of probes for chromosome 13 and different restriction enzymes (13 different probe-enzyme combinations) were used to analyze genomic DNA; as well, isozymic forms of esterase-D were determined in cell lysates. In two cases, the likelihood of developing the tumor was predicted; in the other three, no tumor was expected to develop. With informative loci flanking the retinoblastoma locus, the calculated predictive accuracy in some cases was as high as 94% (29).

The search for the retinoblastoma gene produced astonishing results within the past 3 years. One of the first reports revealed that a 1.5 kb human DNA sequence derived from a human chromosome 13 λ phage library could detect deletions involving 13q14 in some retinoblastomas (43). This was soon followed by the description of an isolated cDNA clone, termed p4.7R, which detected a locus spanning at least 70 kb on 13q14, all or part of which is deleted in some retinoblastomas and osteosarcomas, yet which is present in adenovirus-12 immortalized retinal cells and other tumors (53). Furthermore, although the gene was expressed in many neoplasms, no 4.7 kb transcripts were detected in retinoblastomas or osteosarcomas. Several months later, the retinoblastoma gene was further characterized, cloned and sequenced (104). Nucleotide sequencing and structural analysis of the genomic locus disclosed an extremely large gene composed of at least 12 exons spanning a region of over 100 kb that codes for mRNA of 4.6 to 4.7 kb. Analysis of this gene and its expressed mRNA in retinoblastomas showed various structural alterations as well as missing or aberrant transcripts in many instances (54). Subsequently, more subtle mutations of the gene have been detected by the ribonuclease protection assay (45). The consistency with which mutations in this region are detected supports the identification of 4.7R as the retinoblastoma gene. Since the gene has been cloned, it now becomes possible to detect restriction fragment length polymorphisms within the gene itself and thereby determine with heightened precision the risk for developing retinoblastoma in patients with the appropriate hereditary setting (188).

The protein product of the retinoblastoma locus is a nuclear phosphoprotein of 110,000 kilodaltons (pp110) which is associated with DNA binding activity (105). Since the inactivation of the gene (both alleles) is followed by uncontrolled cell growth as manifest by retinoblastoma, it is likely that the gene product in some way functions to suppress cell division. The transforming proteins from two DNA viruses, E1A of adenovirus (186) and large T antigen of SV40 virus (39), have been shown to bind to the retinoblastoma gene product. These data suggest that the ability of these oncogenic viruses to transform and immortalize cells may come about through blocking the action of the retinoblastoma protein. These studies provide the first direct linkage between an oncogene and an antioncogene.

WILMS' TUMOR

Wilms' tumor, the most common renal neoplasm of children, accounts for 6% of all pediatric cancers. The neoplasm is unique in having a uniform worldwide incidence, 1 case/10,000 children. Very few cases (<1%) demonstrate a familial tendency, even though 4.8% of individuals present with bilateral neoplasms. The first report which indicated a genetic basis for Wilms' tumor was in 1964 when Miller et al. (117) described six patients with Wilms' tumor and aniridia, two conditions unlikely to occur together by chance alone. The significance of this association was enhanced with the discovery of an

11p(13-15.1) interstitial deletion in three children with the WAGR syndrome of Wilms' tumor, aniridia, genitourinary abnormalities and motor/mental retardation (137). Although data are scanty regarding cytogenetic aberrations in conventional Wilms' tumor, scattered reports describing the deletion (83) as well as normal tumor karyotypic findings (84) have appeared. It is also worth noting that gonadoblastoma has been described in association with aniridia and an 11p11-13 deletion (5). As with retinoblastoma, a closely linked gene coding for an enzyme, catalase, has been assigned to a region (11p13) close to the Wilms' tumor locus (81).

Using DNA from seven primary Wilms' tumors and corresponding normal DNA (leukocytes, renal tissue) and four probes mapped to 11p15, a RFLP study revealed molecular mechanisms similar to those described above for retinoblastoma and osteosarcoma in five of the seven cases (95). Once again, recessive mutational events appeared to be expressed after abnormal chromosomal segregation during mitosis. Hence, loss of the two normal alleles at a locus predisposed to the neoplasm. Similar results were reported concurrently (47, 129). About this time, an equally important molecular analysis of sporadic Wilms' tumors suggests that the initial mutagenic event is visited upon the paternal chromosome which is retained and that the subsequent nonrandom loss of the protective maternal allele at this locus paves the way for the emergence of the neoplasm (144). The manner by which this could be explained is genomic imprinting, as hypothesized by Wilkins (189). Indeed, there is considerable evidence that gene expression is regulated according to inheritance, be it maternal or paternal. It is possible that in Wilms' tumor, genomic imprinting renders inactive a transforming gene on the maternally derived chromosome 11, leaving a functional transforming Wilms' gene on the paternal chromosome 11. This hypothesis implies that chromosome 11 contains at least one transforming gene which is under the regulatory control of the Wilms' gene.

Related studies have described the loss of the c-Ha-*ras*-1 allele in sporadic Wilms' tumor, (134) indicating a close proximity between the locus for this oncogene and the Wilms' tumor gene. For those cases in which RFLP analysis failed to reveal a homozygous tumor pattern, the mechanisms thought to prevail included point mutation, gene conversion, minute deletions or inversions which could not be detected by these techniques. More recent work focused on regions contiguous to 11p13 revealed type 1 insulin-like growth factor receptors in Wilms' tumors (56), enhanced transcription for insulin-like growth factor II (11p15.1) (135) and deletion of the locus for the B-subunit of follicle stimulating hormone (58) in some patients with Wilms' tumor and those with the aniridia-Wilms' tumor complex. Finally, DNA probes have identified a cytogenetically undetected deletion associated with a balanced translocation in a patient with familial aniridia but not Wilms' tumor. As well, two new anonymous DNA segments were defined which physically isolate the aniridia and Wilms' tumor loci (38).

A series of experiments have been reported in which normal human chromosomes (#11, 13, X) were introduced into a Wilms' tumor cell line by the microcell transfer technique. Tumorigenicity in nude mice remained in cell lines which received either the X or 13th chromosome. In contrast, no tumors developed in mice injected with cell lines which had received a normal chromosome 11. Thus, as with retinoblastoma, important regulatory information appears to be contained on chromosome 11; inactivation (absence) of this genetic sequence presumably is central to the induction of Wilms' tumor (184). However, the direct applicability of the retinoblastoma model to this disease may not be as straightforward as these data suggest. Two groups (63, 75) have analyzed families segregating predisposition to Wilms' tumor for genetic linkage to chromosome 11p loci. In no case was such association observed. This may suggest that the gene in the WAGR locus in 11p13 is the target of the predisposing gene or that familial forms of Wilms' tumor are genetically distinct from their corresponding sporadic cases.

BECKWITH-WIEDEMANN SYNDROME

Two reports in the 1960s described children with visceromegaly, umbilical hernia, macroglossia, hemihypertrophy and general gigantism (12, 187). Soon thereafter, a striking incidence (>10%) of neoplasms in these children was described with tumors arising in the kidneys (Wilms'), liver (hepatoblastoma), adrenal cortex (carcinoma), and from diverse sites (rhabdomyosarcoma) (161). Abnormalities involving chromosome 11 (duplication p13 ter region), (duplication 11q23-24) (179) and (trisomy 11p15) have been reported in some of these children (173). In this "overgrowth" syndrome, recent work has revealed that the 11p region often implicated contains genes which code for insulin (69) and insulin-like growth factor II (23). In familial Beckwith-Wiedemann syndrome, genetic linkage has been demonstrated for 11p15 markers (A. Koufos, manuscript submitted for publication), as would be expected from the somatic chromosomal aberrations discussed above. Further, the placement of chromosomal interchanges occurring in mitosis has indicated a locus localized to 11p15.5 in the genesis of rhabdomyosarcoma and Wilms' tumor. (148) Whether the defect eliciting the developmental syndrome is the same as that for the tumors is an area of active research.

OTHER CHILDHOOD CANCERS

Study of RFLP's from patients with hepatoblastoma and certain types of rhabdomyosarcomas utilizing 11p probes revealed non-disjunctional loss of the wild-type chromosome with reduplication of the mutant allele, rather than simple deletion or loss of the normal chromosome (96). The chromosomal localization of the human rhabdomyosarcoma locus, more closely identified with additional 11p probes, has been assigned to a region between 11p15.5 and 11pter. As well, mitotic recombination appears to represent a common molecular event central to the induction of this tumor (148). Thus, the mechanisms operative in tumor induction for these two embryonal neoplasms appear similar to that reported for Wilms' osteosarcoma and retinoblastoma.

NEUROFIBROMATOSIS

Much of the preceding discussion has related to relatively uncommon neoplasms. A more common condition is neurofibromatosis, an autosomal dominant disease associated with a high mutation rate. Two forms of neurofibromatosis are known to exist. The least common, bilateral acoustic neurofibromatosis (BANF), features centrally located acoustic neuromas, nerve root neurofibromas, brain and spinal cord gliomas and spinal meningiomas. More frequent is von Recklinghausen's disease which is characterized by multiple neurofibromas involving the skin, peripheral and spinal nerves. Apart from producing, on occasion, massive overgrowth of tissue, malignant transformation is one possible outcome in those who inherit this gene.

Within the past year, the map position of the locus for each condition has been identified; moreover, recessive mutations appear to be central to the induction of the neoplastic state. After detecting loss of genes on chromosome 22 in acoustic neuromas from some patients with either the sporadic or hereditary form of the disease (151), Seizinger and colleagues studied blood lymphocytes and tumor tissue (3 acoustic neuromas, 3 cervical neurofibromas, and one meningioma) from patients with BANF utilizing polymorphic probes for loci on the long arm of chromosome 22. Specific allelic loss was detected in each, indicating that loss of essential genetic information was pivotal to the genesis of these neoplasms (152). Furthermore, genetic linkage analysis placed the gene for BANF in the center of the long arm of chromosome 22, probably in the region 22q11.1-22q13.1 (140).

The locus for the more common form of neurofibromatosis, von Recklinghausen's disease, has been localized to the 17th chromosome by linkage analysis of 15 kindreds. This latter study also indicated that, in many cases, neurofibromas stem from a mutation at a single locus (10). Of additional interest is the fact that genetic linkage has been established between von Recklinghausen's neurofibromatosis and the gene encoding nerve growth factor receptor (153).

COLORECTAL CANCER AND FAMILIAL POLYPOSIS

The foregoing discussion demonstrates the power of molecular genetic approaches to the mechanisms of carcinogenesis. Many of the analyses were prompted by isolated case reports describing specific chromosomal aberrations in cancer patients. For an additional example, in colorectal cancers, the clue stemmed from a patient with colon carcinoma and large bowel polyposis associated with Gardner's syndrome in whom a constitutional interstitial deletion was detected on the long arm of chromosome 5 (72).

Two genetic conditions are known to predispose to colorectal cancer: familial adenomatous polyposis (FAP) and Gardner's syndrome. Linkage analysis established that the gene for FAP is on the fifth chromosome, most probably near 5q21-q22 (18, 108). A study of tumor and constitutional DNA in patients with sporadic colorectal carcinomas with a highly polymorphic minisatellite probe for 5q showed that at least 20% of these patients lost one of the alleles at this locus as compared with normal matched controls (160).

The molecular genetic aberrations in colorectal neoplasms are, however, complex. It has previously been noted that point mutations of the ras oncogene occur in some 40–50% of these malignancies (20, 52). In addition, cytogenetic and molecular studies have demonstrated that many such malignancies incur losses of genetic material on chromosomes 17, 18 and 22 (49, 119, 128, 136). Vogelstein *et al.* (177) undertook the molecular study of a large number of colorectal neoplasms to determine the temporal sequence of genetic alterations in these conditions. Their data suggest that *ras* gene mutations are often early, but not obligate events in tumorigenesis; additional aberrations (allelic loss) on chromosomes 5, 17 and/or 18 are also required. From this emerged the hypothesis that colorectal cancers (perhaps others, as well) require mutational activation of one allele of an oncogene, followed by the loss of both parental alleles at other chromosomal sites which code for tumor suppressor genes (177).

OTHER CANCERS

In an effort to uncover the molecular mechanisms central to the development of mammary cancer an assortment of probes for loci on different chromosomes have been used. By comparing tumor and normal tissues, somatic loss of constitutional heterozygosity in chromosome 13 was demonstrated with premenopausal, low differentiation state ductal breast tumors in some patients. Mitotic chromosomal loss was proposed as the most likely mechanism for the loss of normal 13 alleles (110).

However, the specificity of chromosome 13 for mammary carcinoma is not altogether certain. A second report has described a reduction to homozygosity of a gene segment on chromosome 11 in 20% of postmenopausal patients with breast cancers who were heterozygous at multiple loci on chromosome 11. Moreover, the loss of heterozygosity appeared to be associated with aggressive tumors, devoid of estrogen and progesterone receptors, and distant metastases (3).

The findings of molecular alterations on chromosome 13 in some mammary carcinomas prompted several groups to determine whether the retinoblastoma site might be involved. In the first report, Lee and colleagues showed that the retinoblastoma gene is inactivated in 2/9 human breast cancer cell lines. In each, the corresponding transcript was aberrant and the pp110 gene product was nondetectable (103). These findings were confirmed by T'Ang *et al.* (168), both in breast cancer cell lines and some primary noncultured tumors. The DNA alterations included homozygous internal deletions and total deletion of the locus; transcripts were accordingly absent or truncated. These data support the notion that the retinoblastoma mutation has pleiotropic effects on certain types of tissues.

Amplification of *myc*-related oncogenes and point mutations of the ras oncogenes have been described in lung cancer, particularly in the most virulent form, small cell carcinoma. The importance of these data is enhanced by molecular genetic findings from several laboratories that demonstrate a very high frequency of loss of heterozygosity for loci on chromosomes 3p (121), 13q12-13q33 and 17p (193) in small cell carcinoma; as well, 3p alterations were discovered in a significant proportion of other cell types of lung cancer (22, 94). Furthermore, the molecular events occurring on 3p and 13q in small cell carcinomas antedated N-*myc* amplification (193).

The demonstration of molecular aberrations at 13q in small cell lung carcinoma is further highlighted by the demonstration of cytogenetic abnormalities involving the retinoblastoma locus (68). With the use of several cDNA probes which span over 180 kb of DNA and represent the 4.7 kb retinoblastoma transcript, a significant incidence of structural rearrangements and abnormalities of the gene was detected along with a lack of Rb mRNA expression in some small cell cancers (primary tumors and cell lines) and cell lines derived from pulmonary carcinoids; in contrast, these aberrations were not identified in other types of lung cancer or normal lung.

Molecular alterations (DNA and/or RNA) involving the retinoblastoma gene have been reported additionally in several soft tissue (non-osseous) sarcomas (54, 116). Thus, abnormalities in the retinoblastoma gene have been identified in retinoblastoma, osteosarcoma, several types of soft tissue sarcoma, mammary carcinoma, small cell carcinoma of the lung and pulmonary carcinoids.

Somatic loss of genetic sequences on 11p in five of twelve patients with urinary bladder carcinoma (48) has been described.

Loss of alleles for loci on chromosome 3 has been documented in sporadic renal cell carcinoma (198). These studies were prompted by the description (33) of a balanced translocation, t(3;8) (p21;q24) in patients with hereditary renal cell carcinoma. More recently, genetic linkage analysis has placed the gene for Von Hippel-Lindau disease (which may include renal cell carcinoma as one of its manifestations) to a nearby (3p25) region (154).

An assortment of autosomal dominant syndromes manifest as variations of multiple endocrine neoplasia. One such form, designated MEN2, is associated with medullary thyroid carcinoma and pheochromocytoma. Until recently the molecular basis for the syndrome was unknown. With the assistance of minisatellite probes for chromosome 1, gene deletions on the short arm of this chromosome were demonstrated in seven of fourteen tumors, including both medullary thyroid carcinoma and pheochromocytoma (114). Studies in a variant of this syndrome, MEN2A, describe a close association with this condition and the genetic region 10p11.2-q11.2 (113).

roles in growth and development. Both in development and the neoplastic state, c-oncs appear to collaborate rather than function independently. Cellular oncogenes are activated in the neoplastic process by four (nonviral) mechanisms; (a) chromosomal translocations; (b) gene amplifications; (c) point mutations; and (d) DNA rearrangements. The timing of c-onc gene product expression may be as important in oncogenesis as the level of expression. At this writing, mutant oncogenes have not been shown to be inherited. Oncogene amplification, if important in oncogenesis, is more likely to be involved with tumor progression rather than initiation.

Chromosomal/molecular aberrations tend to be characteristic for a given type of cancer. These genetic alterations are often situated near heritable fragile sites, tumor-suppressor gene loci and/or oncogene loci. Similar molecular mechanisms involving translocations and inversions may underly the common T and B cell neoplasms. The loss/inactivation of both normal alleles at a locus thought to encode for tumor-suppressing activities (antioncogenes) may represent an event common to many childhood and adult neoplasms. The consistency and cell specificity with which this has been identified is consistent with a role for such genes in cellular differentiation. At this writing, the paradigm for such a controlling locus is 13q14, the site of the retinoblastoma gene. Based on recent studies in familial and sporadic Wilms' tumor which suggest etiological heterogeneity, theoretical modifications of the carcinogenesis model which has been central to understanding retinoblastoma may soon be forthcoming to explain molecular mechanisms operative in other cancer. The role of genomic imprinting in carcinogenesis is only recently being explored. Further study of this process may prove to be a fruitful area of future research.

CONCLUDING REMARKS

This review has focused on three aspects of human neoplasia: oncogenes, chromosomal aberrations and molecular mechanisms common to diverse neoplasms. Progress in these areas has been substantial, particularly in recent years. While much of this information has been made possible by DNA technology, in particular the exploitation of highly polymorphic sites scattered throughout the genome, important index clues have often been forthcoming from the clinical study of cancer patients. As demonstrated in a number of neoplasms, multiple sites within the genome have been identified to manifest aberrations within a given cancer. From these data, it is apparent that oncogenesis is a process much more complex than originally envisioned. Yet, given the power of present technology and the pace of discoveries, one can anticipate the dissection of the genome to a level at which the complex interplay of genes responsible for human cancers will be identified.

Dr. Seemayer is the recipient of the McPherson, Fraser Monat McGill University Associateship and the Research Scientist Award of the McGill University-Montreal Children's Hospital Research Institute.

SUMMARY

Cellular oncogenes (c-oncs) have been highly conserved throughout evolution and subserve important

REFERENCES

1. Adams JM, Harris AW, Pinkert CA, Corcoran LM, Alexander WS, Cory S, Palmiter RD, Brinster RL: The c-myc oncogene driven by immunoglobulin enhancers induces lymphoid malignancy in transgenic mice. Nature (London) 318:533, 1985
2. Ali IU, Campbell G, Lidereau R, Callahan R: Amplification of c-erbB-2 and aggressive human breast tumors? Science 240:1795, 1988
3. Ali IU, Lidereau R, Theillet C, Callahan R: Reduction to homozygosity of genes on chromosome 11 in human breast neoplasia. Science 238:185, 1987
4. Almoguera C, Shibata D, Forrester K, Martin J, Arnheim N, Perucho M: Most human carcinomas of the exocrine pancreas contain mutant c-K-ras genes. Cell 53:549, 1988
5. Andersen SR, Geertinger P, Larsen HW, Mikkelsen MN, Parbing A, Vestermark S, Warburg M: Aniridia, cataract and gonadoblastoma in a mentally retarded girl with deletion of chromosome 11. Ophthalmologia 176:171, 1978
6. Aurias A, Rimbaut C, Buffe D, Dubousset J, Mazabraud A. Chromosomal translocations in Ewing's sarcoma. N Engl J Med 309:496, 1983
7. Avery OT, MacLeod CM, MacCarty A: Studies on the chemical nature of the substances inducing transformation of pneumococcal types. J Exp Med 79:133, 1944
8. Balaban G, Gilbert F, Nichols W, Meadows AT, Shields J: Abnormalities of chromosome 13 in retinoblastomas from individuals with normal constitutional karyotypes. Cancer Genet Cytogenet 6:213, 1982
9. Baltimore D: RNA-dependent DNA polymerase in virions of RNA tumor viruses. Nature (London) 226:1209, 1970
10. Barker D, Wright E, Nguyen K, Cannon L, Fain P, Goldgar D, Bishop DT, Carey J, Baty B, Kivlin J, Willard H, Waye JS, Greig G, Leinwand L, Nakamura Y, O'Connell P, Leppert M, Lalouel J-M, White R, Skolnick M: Gene for von Recklinghausen neurofibromatosis is in the pericentromeric region of chromosome 17. Science 236:1100, 1987
11. Barker PE: Double minutes in human tumor cells. Cancer Genet Cytogenet 5:81, 1982
12. Beckwith JB: Macroglossia, omphalocele, adrenal cytomegaly, gigantism, and hyperplastic visceromegaly. Birth Defects Series V, pp 188–196. New York, National Foundation-March of Dimes, 1969
13. Ben-Neriah Y, Daley GQ, Mes-Masson AM, Witte ON, Baltimore D: The chronic myelogenous leukemia-specific p210 protein is the product of the bcr/abl hybrid gene. Science 233:212, 1986
14. Bernards R, Dessain SK, Weinberg RA: N-myc amplification causes down-modulation of MHC Class I antigen expression in neuroblastoma. Cell 47:667, 1986
15. Bishop JM: Oncogenes. Sci Am 246:80, 1982
16. Bishop JM: Viral oncogenes. Cell 42:23, 1985
17. Bishop JM: The molecular genetics of cancer. Science 235:305, 1987
18. Bodmer WF, Bailey CJ, Bodmer J, Bussey HJR, Ellis A, Gorman P, Lucibello FC, Murday VA, Rider SH, Scambler P, Sheer D, Solomon E, Spurr NK: Localization of the gene for familial adenomatous polyposis on chromosome 5. Nature (London) 328:614, 1987
19. Bogenmann E, Locherie MA, Simon MI: Cone cell-specific genes expressed in retinoblastoma. Science 240:76, 1988
20. Bos JL, Fearon ER, Hamilton SR, Verlaan-de Vries M, van Boom JH, van der Eb AJ, Vogelstein B: Prevalence of ras gene mutations in human colorectal cancers. Nature (London) 327:293, 1987
21. Boveri T: Zur Frage der Entstehung Malinger Tumoren. Jena, Germany, Fisher, 1914
22. Brauch H, Johnson B, Hovis J, Yano T, Gazdar A, Pettengill OS, Graziano S, Sorenson GD, Poiesz BJ, Minna J, Linehan M, Zbar B: Molecular analysis of the short arm of chromosome 3 in small-cell and non-small-cell carcinoma of the lung. N Engl J Med 317:1109, 1987
23. Brissenden JE, Ullrich A, Francke U: Human chromosomal mapping of genes for insulin-like growth factors I and II and epidermal growth factor. Nature (London) 310:781, 1984
24. Brodeur GM, Seeger RC, Schwab M, Varmus HE, Bishop MJ: Amplification of N-myc in untreated human neuroblastomas correlates with advanced disease stage. Science 224:1121, 1984
25. Brugge JS, Eirkson RL: Identification of a transformation-specific antigen induced by an avian sarcoma virus. Nature (London) 269:346, 1977
26. Capon DJ, Chen EY, Levinson AD, Seeburg PH, Goeddel DV: Complete nucleotide sequences of the T24 human bladder carcinoma oncogene and its normal homologue. Nature (London) 302:33, 1982
27. Cavenee WK, Dryja TP, Phillips RA, Benedict WF, Godbout R, Gallie BL, Murphree AL, Strong LC, White RL: Expression of recessive alleles by chromosomal mechanisms in retinoblastoma. Nature (London) 305:779, 1983
28. Cavenee WK, Hansen MF, Nordenskjold M., Kock E, Maumenee I, Squire JA, Phillips RA, Gallie BL: Genetic origin of mutations predisposing to retinoblastoma. Science 228:501, 1985
29. Cavenee WK, Murphree AL, Shull MM, Benedict WF, Sparkes RS, Kock E, Nordenskjöld M: Prediction of familial predisposition to retinoblastoma. N Engl J Med 314:1201, 1986
30. Chan LC, Karhi KK, Rayter SI, Heisterkamp N, Eridani S, Powles R, Lawler SD, Groffen J, Foulkes JG, Greaves MF, Wiedemann LM: A novel abl protein expressed in Philadelphia chromosome positive acute lymphoblastic leukaemia. Nature (London) 325:635, 1987
31. Cleary ML, Galili N, Sklar J: Detection of a second t(14;18) breakpoint cluster region in human follicular lymphomas. J Exp Med 164:315, 1986
32. Cleary ML: Oncogenes and translocations in the pathogenesis of T-cell neoplasia. Am J Surg Pathol 12:163, 1988
33. Cohen AJ, Li FP, Berg S, Marchetto DJ, Tsai S, Jacobs SC, Brown RS: Hereditary renal-cell carcinoma associated with a chromosomal translocation. N Engl J Med 301:592, 1979
34. Comings DE: A general theory of carcinogenesis. Proc Natl Acad Sci USA 70:3324, 1973
35. Croce CM, Tsujimoto Y, Erikson J, Nowell PC: Chromosomal translocations and B cell neoplasia. Lab Invest 51:258, 1984
36. Daley GQ, McLaughlin J, Witte ON, Baltimore D: The CML-specific p210 bcr/abl protein, unlike v-abl, does not transform NIH/3T3 fibroblasts. Science 237:532, 1987
37. Dalla-Favera R, Bregni M, Erikson J, Patterson D, Gallo RC, Croce CM: Human c-myc onc gene is located on the region of chromosome 8 that is translocated in Burkitt lymphoma cells. Proc Natl Acad Sci USA 79:7824, 1982
38. Davis LM, Stallard R, Thomas GH, Couillin P, Junien C, Nowak NJ, Shows TB: Two anonymous DNA segments distinguish the Wilms' tumor and aniridia loci. Science 241:840, 1988
39. DeCaprio JA, Ludlow JW, Figge J, Shew J-Y, Huang C-M, Lee W-H, Marsilo E, Paucha R, Livingston DM: SV40 large tumor antigen forms a specific complex with the product of the retinoblastoma susceptibility gene. Cell 54:275, 1988
40. Doolittle RF, Hunkapiller MW, Hood LE, Devare SG, Robbins KC, Aaronson SA, Antoniades HN: Simian sarcoma virus onc gene, v-sis, is derived from the gene encoding a platelet-derived growth factor. Science 221:275, 1983
41. Downward J, Yarden Y, Mayes E, Scrace G, Totty N, Stockwell P, Ullrich A, Schlessinger J, Waterfield MD: Close similarity of epidermal growth factor receptor and v-erb-B oncogene protein sequences. Nature (London) 307:521, 1984
42. Dreazen O, Rassool F, Sparkes RS, Klisak I, Goldman JM, Gale RP: Do oncogenes determine clinical features in chronic myeloid leukaemia? Lancet 1:402, 1987
43. Dryja TP, Rapaport JM, Joyce JM, Petersen RA: Molecular detection of deletions involving band q14 of chromosome 13 in retinoblastomas. Proc Natl Acad Sci USA 83:7391, 1986
44. Dubeau L, Chandler LA, Gralow JR, Nichols PW, Jones PA: Southern blot analysis of DNA extracted from formalin-fixed pathology specimens. Cancer Res 46:2694, 1986
45. Dunn JM, Phillips RA, Becker AJ, Gallie BL: Identification of germline and somatic mutations affecting the retinoblastoma gene. Science 241:1797, 1988
46. Egan SE, Wright JA, Jarolim L, Yanagihara K, Bassin RH, Greenberg AH: Transformation by oncogenes encoding protein kinases induces the metastatic phenotype. Science 238:202, 1987
47. Fearon ER, Vogelstein B, Feinberg AP: Somatic deletion and duplication of genes on chromosome 11 in Wilms' tumor. Nature (London) 309:176, 1984

48. Fearon ER, Feinberg AP, Hamilton SH, Vogelstein B: Loss of genes on the short arm of chromosome 11 in bladder cancer. Nature (London) 318:377, 1985

49. Fearon ER, Hamilton SR, Vogelstein B: Clonal analysis human colorectal tumors. Science 238:193, 1987

50. Feinberg AP, Vogelstein B, Droller MJ, Baylin SB, Nelkin BD: Mutation affecting the 12th amino acid of the c-Ha-ras oncogene product occurs infrequently in human cancer. Science 220:1175, 1983

51. Finger LR, Harvey RC, Moore RCA, Showe LC, Croce CM: A common mechanism of chromosomal translocation in T- and B-cell neoplasia. Science 234:982, 1986

52. Forrester K, Almoguera C, Han K, Grizzle WE, Perucho M: Detection of high incidence of K-ras oncogenes during human colon tumorigenesis. Nature (London) 327:298, 1987

53. Friend SH, Bernards R, Rogelj S, Weinberg RA, Rapaport JM, Albert DM, Dryja TP: A human DNA segment with properties of the gene that predisposes to retinoblastoma and osteosarcoma. Nature (London) 323:643, 1986

54. Friend SH, Horowitz JM, Gerber MR, Wang X-F, Bogenmann E, Li FP, Weinberg RA: Deletions of a DNA sequence in retinoblastomas and mesenchymal tumors: Organization of the sequence and its encoded protein. Proc Natl Acad Sci USA 84:9059, 1987

55. Fung Y-K T, Murphree AL, T'Ang A, Qian J, Hinrichs SH, Benedict WF: Structural evidence for the authenticity of the human retinoblastoma gene. Science 236:1657, 1987

56. Gansler T, Allen KD, Burant CF, Inabnett T, Scott A, Buse MG, Sens DA, Garvin AJ: Detection of type 1 insulinlike growth factor (IGF) receptors in Wilms' tumors. Am J Pathol 130:431, 1988

57. Gateff E: Malignant neoplasms of genetic origin in Drosophila melanogaster. Science 200:1448, 1978

58. Glaser T, Lewis WH, Bruns GAP, Watkins PC, Rogler CE, Shows TB, Powers VE, Willard HF, Goguen JM, Simola KOJ, Housman DE: The B-subunit of follicle-stimulating hormone is deleted in patients with aniridia and Wilms' tumour, allowing a further definition of the WAGR locus. Nature (London) 321:882, 1986

59. Godbout R, Dryja TP, Squire J, Gallie BL, Phillips RA: Somatic inactivation of genes on chromosome 13 is a common event in retinoblastoma. Nature (London) 304:451, 1983

60. Goelz SE, Hamilton SR, Vogelstein B: Purification of DNA from formaldehyde fixed and paraffin embedded human tissue. Biochem Biophys Res Commun 130:118, 1985

61. Grady-Leopardi EF, Schwab M, Ablin AR, Rosenau W: Detection of N-myc oncogene expression in human neuroblastoma by in situ hybridization and blot analysis: relationship to clinical outcome. Cancer Res 46:3196, 1986

62. Green AR, Wyke JA: Anti-oncogenes: a subset of regulatory genes involved in carcinogenesis. Lancet 2:475, 1985

63. Grundy P, Koufos A, Morgan K, Li FP, Meadows AT, Cavenee WK: Familial predisposition to Wilms' tumor does not map to the short arm of chromosome 11. Nature (London) 336:374, 1988

64. Gu J, Linnoila RI, Seibel NL, Gazdar AF, Minna JD, Brooks BJ, Hollis GF, Kirsch IR: A study of myc-related gene expression in small cell lung cancer by in situ hybridization. Am J Pathol 132:13, 1988

65. Hamlyn P, Sikora K: Oncogenes. Lancet 2:326, 1983

66. Hansen MF, Koufos A, Gallie BL, Phillips RA, Fodstad O, Brogger A, Gedde-Dahl T, Cavenee WK: Osteosarcoma and retinoblastoma: a shared chromosomal mechanism revealing recessive predisposition. Proc Natl Acad Sci USA 82:6212, 1985

67. Hansen MF, Cavenee WK: Genetics of cancer predisposition. Cancer Res 47:5518, 1987

68. Harbour JW, Lai S-L, Whang-Peng J, Gazdar AF, Minna JD, Kaye FJ: Abnormalities in structure and expression of the human retinoblastoma gene in SCLC. Science 241:353, 1988

69. Harper ME, Ullrich A, Saunders GF: Localization of the human insulin gene to the distal end of the short arm of chromosome 11. Proc Natl Acad Sci USA 78:4458, 1981

70. Harris H, Miller OJ, Klein G, Worst P, Tachibana T: Suppression of malignancy by cell fusion. Nature (London) 223:363, 1969

71. Harris H: The genetic analysis of malignancy. J Cell Sci 4 (Suppl):431, 1986

72. Herrera L, Kakati S, Givas L, Pietrzak E, Sandberg AA: Gardner syndrome in a man with an interstitial deletion of 5q. Am J Med Genet 25:473, 1986

73. Hirai H, Kobayashi Y, Mano H, Hagiwara K, Maru Y, Omine M, Mizoguchi H, Nishida J, Takaku F: A point mutation at codon 13 of the N-ras oncogene in myelodysplastic syndrome. Nature (London) 327:430, 1987

74. Huebner RJ, Todaro GJ: Oncogenes of RNA tumor viruses as determinants of cancer. Proc Natl Acad Sci USA 64:1087, 1969

75. Huff V, Compton DA, Chao L-Y, Strong LC, Gieser CF, Saunders GF: Lack of linkage of familial Wilms' tumour to chromosomal band 11p13. Nature (London) 336:377, 1988

76. Hunter T, Sefton BM: Transforming gene product of Rous sarcoma virus phosphorylates tyrosine. Proc Natl Acad Sci USA 77:1311, 1980

77. Hunter T: The proteins of oncogenes. Sci Am 251:70, 1984

78. Hurley JB, Simon MI, Teplow DB, Robinshaw JD, Gilman AG: Homologies between signals transducing G proteins and ras gene products. Science 226:860, 1984

79. Jacob L, Opper M, Metzroth B, Phannavong B, Mechler BM: Structure of the 1(2)gl gene of Drosophila and delimitation of its tumor suppressor domain. Cell 50:215, 1987

80. Jaffe R, Santamaria M, Yunis EJ, Tannery NH, Agostini RM, Medina J, Goodman M: The neuroectodermal tumors of bone. Am J Surg Pathol 8:885, 1984

81. Junien C, Turleau C, DeGrouchy J, Said R, Rethore MO, Tenconi RK, Darfier JL: Regional assignment of catalase (CAT) gene to band 11p13:association with the aniridia-Wilms' tumor-gonadoblastoma (WAGR) complex. Annales de Genetique 23:165, 1980

82. Kaczmarek L: Protooncogene expression during the cell cycle. Lab Invest 54:365, 1986

83. Kaneko Y, Egues MC, Rowley JD: Interstitial deletion of short arm of chromosome 11 limited to Wilms' tumor cells in a patient without aniridia. Cancer Res 41:4577, 1981

84. Kaneko Y, Kondo R, Rowley JD, Moohr JW, Maurer HS: Further chromosome studies on Wilms' tumor cells of patients without aniridia. Cancer Genet Cytogenet 10:191, 1983

85. Kataoka T, Powers S, Cameron S, Fasano O, Goldfarb M, Broach J, Wigler M: Functional homology of mammalian and yeast RAS genes. Cell 40:19, 1985

86. Klein G, Klein E: Oncogene activation and tumor progression, Carcinogenesis 5:429, 1984

87. Klein G, Klein E: Conditioned tumorigenicity of activated oncogenes. Cancer Res 46:3211, 1986

88. Knudson AG: Mutation and cancer:statistical study of retinoblastoma. Proc Natl Acad Sci USA 68:820, 1971

89. Knudson AG: Hereditary cancer, oncogenes, and antioncogenes. Cancer Res 45:1437, 1985

90. Knudson AG: Genetics of human cancer. Ann Rev Genet 20:231, 1986

91. Kohl NE, Kanada N, Schreck RR, Bruns G, Latt SA, Gilbert F, Alt FW: Transposition and amplification of oncogene-related sequences in human neuroblastomas. Cell 35:359, 1983

92. Kohl NE, Gee CE, Alt FW: Activated expression of N-myc gene in human neuroblastomas and related tumors. Science 226:1335, 1984

93. Kohl NE, Legouy E, DePinho RA, Nisen PD, Smith RK, Gee CE, Alt FW: Human N-myc is closely related in organization and nucleotide sequence to c-myc. Nature (London) 319:73, 1986

94. Kok K, Osinga J, Carritt B, Davis MB, van der Hout AH, van der Veen AY, Landsvater RM, de Leij LFMH, Berendsen HH, Postmus PE, Poppema S, Buys CHCM: Deletion of a DNA sequence at the chromosomal region 3p21 in all major types of lung cancer. Nature (London) 330:578, 1987

95. Koufos A, Hansen MF, Lampkin BC, Workman ML, Copeland NG, Jenkins NA, Cavenee WK: Loss of alleles at loci on human chromosome 11 during genesis of Wilms' tumour. Nature (London) 309:170, 1984

96. Koufos A, Hansen MF, Copland NG, Jenkins NA, Lampkin BC, Cavenee WK. Loss of heterozygosity in three embryonal tumours suggests a common pathogenetic mechanism. Nature (London) 316:330, 1985

97. Kromowitz FB, Viola MV, Chao S, Oravez S, Mishriki Y, Finkel G, Grimson R, Lundy J: Ras p21 expression in the progression of breast cancer. Hum Pathol 18:1268, 1987

98. Kurzrock R, Shtalrid M, Romero P, Kloetzer WS, Talpas M, Trujillo M, Blick M, Beran M, Gutterman JU: A novel c-abl protein product in Philadelphia-positive acute lymphoblastic leu-

kaemia. Nature (London) 325:631, 1987

99. Land H, Parada LF, Weinberg RA: Cellular oncogenes and multistep carcinogenesis. Science 222:771, 1983

100. LeBeau MM: Chromosomal fragile sites and cancer-specific rearrangements. Blood 67:849, 1986

101. Leder A, Pattengale PK, Kuo A, Stewart TA, Leder P: Consequences of widespread deregulation of the c-myc gene in transgenic mice: Multiple neoplasms and normal development. Cell 45:485, 1988

102. Leder P, Battey J, Lenoir G, Moulding C, Murphy R, Potter H, Stewart T, Taub R: Translocations among antibody genes in human cancer. Science 222:765, 1983

103. Lee EY-HP, To H, Shew J-Y, Bookstein R, Scully P, Lee W-H: Inactivation of the retinoblastoma susceptibility gene in human breast cancers. Science 241:218, 1988

104. Lee W-H, Bookstein R, Hong F, Young L-J, Shew J-Y, Lee EY-HP: Human retinoblastoma susceptibility gene: cloning, identification and sequence. Science 235:1394, 1987

105. Lee W-H, Shew J-Y, Hong FD, Sery TW, Donoso LA, Young L-J, Bookstein R, Lee EY-HP: The retinoblastoma susceptibility gene encodes a nuclear phosphoprotein associated with DNA binding activity. Nature (London) 329:642, 1987

106. Leibowitz RM: Oncogenes as mediators of cell growth and differentiation. Lab Invest 55:249, 1986

107. Lele KP, Penrose LS, Stallard HB: Chromosome deletion in a case of retinoblastoma. Am J Human Genet 27:171, 1963

108. Leppert M, Dobbs M, Scambler P, O'Connell P, Nakamura Y, Stauffer D, Woodward S, Burt R, Hughes J, Gardner E, Lathrop M, Wasmuth J, Lalouel J-M, White R: The gene for familial polyposis coli maps to the long arm of chromosome 5. Science 238:1411, 1987

109. Little CD, Nau MM, Carney DN, Gazdar AF, Minna JD: Amplification and expression of the c-myc oncogene in human lung cancer cell lines. Nature (London) 306:194, 1983

110. Lundberg C, Skoog L, Cavenee WK, Nordenskjold M: Loss of heterozygosity in human ductal breast tumors indicates a recessive mutation on chromosome 13. Proc Natl Acad Sci USA 84:2372, 1987

111. Manolov G, Manolova Y: Marker band in one chromosome 14 from Burkitt lymphomas. Nature (London) 237:33, 1972

112. Martin GS: Rous sarcoma virus: a function required for the maintenance of the transformed state. Nature (London) 227:1021, 1970

113. Mathew CGP, Smith BA, Thorpe K, Wong Z, Royle NJ, Jeffreys AJ, Ponder BAJ: Depletion of genes on chromosome 1 in endocrine neoplasia. Nature (London) 328:524, 1987

114. Mathew CGP, Chin KS, Easton DF, Thorpe K, Cater C, Liou GI, Fong S-L, Bridges CDB, Haak H, Nieuwenhuijzen Kruseman AC, Schifter S, Hansen HH, Telenius H, Telenius-Berg M, Ponder BAJ: A linked genetic marker for multiple endocrine neoplasia type 2A on chromosome 10. Nature (London) 328:527, 1987

115. McKeithan TW, Shima EA, LeBeau MM, Minowada J, Rowley JD, Diaz MO: Molecular cloning of the breakpoint junction of a human chromosomal 8;14 translocation involving the T-cell receptor alpha-chain gene and sequences on the 3' side of MYC. Proc Natl Acad Sci USA 83:6636, 1986

116. Mendoza AE, Shew J-Y, Lee EY-HP, Bookstein R, Lee W-H: A case of synovial sarcoma with abnormal expression of the human retinoblastoma gene. Human Pathol 19:487, 1988

117. Miller RW, Fraumeni JF, Manning MD: Association of Wilms' tumor with aniridia, hemihypertrophy and other congenital malformations. N Engl J Med 270:922, 1964

118. Mitelman F: Restricted number of chromosomal regions implicated in aetiology of human cancer and leukemia. Nature (London) 310:325, 1984

119. Muleris M, Salmon RJ, Zafrani B, Girodet J, Dutrillaux B: Consistent deficiencies of chromosome 18 and of the short arm of chromosome 17 in eleven cases of human large bowel cancer: a possible recessive determinism. Ann Genet (Paris) 28:206, 1985

120. Nau MM, Brooks Jr BJ, Carney DN, Gazdar AF, Battey JF, Sausville EA, Minna JD: Human small-cell lung cancers show amplification and expression of the N-myc gene. Proc Natl Acad Sci USA 83:1092, 1986

121. Naylor SL, Johnson BE, Minna JD, Sakaguchi AY: Loss of heterozygosity of chromosome 3p markers in small-cell lung cancer. Nature (London) 329:451, 1987

122. Ngan B-Y, Chen-Levy Z, Weiss LM, Warnke RA, Cleary ML: Expression in non-Hodgkin's lymphoma of the bcl-2 protein associated with the t(14;18) chromosomal translocation. N Engl J Med 318:1638, 1988

123. Nisen PD, Zimmerman KA, Cotter SV, Gilbert F, Alt FW: Enhanced expression of the N-myc gene in Wilms' tumors. Cancer Res 46:6217, 1986

124. Nowell PC, Hungerford DA: A minute chromosome in human chronic granulocytic leukemia. Science 132:1497, 1960

125. Nowell PC, Croce CM: Chromosomes, genes, and cancer. Am J Pathol 125:8, 1986

126. Nunberg JK, Kaufman RJ, Schimke RT, Urlaub G, Chasin LA: Amplified dihydrofolate reductase genes are localized to a homogenously staining region of a single chromosome in a methotrexate-resistant Chinese hamster ovary cell line. Proc Natl Acad Sci USA 75:5553, 1978

127. Ohno S: Genetic implication of karyological instability of malignant somatic cells. Physiol Rev 51:496, 1971

128. Okamoto M, Sasaki M, Sugio K, Sato C, Iwama T, Ikeuchi T, Tonomura A, Sasazuki T, Miyaki M: Loss of constitutional heterozygosity in colon carcinoma from patients with familial polyposis coli. Nature (London) 331:273, 1988

129. Orkin SH, Goldman DS, Sallan SE: Development of homozygosity for chromosome 11p markers in Wilms' tumour. Nature (London) 309:172, 1984

130. Ponder B. Gene losses in human tumours. Nature (London) 335:400, 1988

131. Potluri VR, Gilbert F, Helson L: Neuroectodermal tumors: chromosomal changes and gene amplification. Am J Hum Genet 36:345, 1984

132. Reddy EP, Reynolds RK, Santos E, Barbacid M: A point mutation is responsible for the acquisition of transforming properties by the T24 human bladder cancer oncogene. Nature (London) 300:149, 1982

133. Reed JC, Cuddy M, Slabiak T, Croce M, Nowell PC: Oncogenic potential of bcl-2 demonstrated by gene transfer. Nature (London) 336:259, 1988

134. Reeve AE, Housiaux PJ, Gardner RJM, Chewings WE, Grindley RM, Millow LJ: Loss of a Harvey ras allele in sporadic Wilms' tumour. Nature (London) 309:174, 1984

135. Reeve AE, Eccles MR, Wilkins RJ, Bell GI, Millow LJ: Expression of insulin-like growth factor-II transcripts in Wilms' tumour. Nature (London) 317:258, 1985

136. Reichmann A, Martin P, Levin B: Chromosomal banding patterns in human large bowel cancer. Int J Cancer 28:431, 1981

137. Riccardi VM, Sujansky E, Smith AC, Francke U: Chromosomal imbalance in the aniridia-Wilms tumor association:11p interstitial deletion. Pediatrics 61:604, 1979

138. Rodenhuis S, van de Wetering ML, Mooi WJ, Evers SG, van Zandwijk N, Bos JL: Mutational activation of the K-ras oncogene. N Engl J Med 317:929, 1987

139. Rootman J, Carruthers JDA, Miller RR: Retinoblastoma. Perspect Pediatr Pathol 10:208, 1987

140. Rouleau GA, Wertelecki W, Haines JL, Hobbs WJ, Trofatter JA, Seizinger BR, Martuza RL, Superneau DW, Conneally PM, Gusella JF: Genetic linkage of bilateral acoustic neurofibromatosis to a DNA marker on chromosome 22. Nature (London) 329:246, 1987

141. Rous P: A sarcoma of the fowl transmissible by an agent separable from the tumor cells. J Exp Med 13:397, 1911

142. Rowley JD: A new consistent chromosomal abnormality in chronic myelogenous leukaemia identified by quinacrine fluorescence and giemsa staining. Nature (London) 243:290, 1973

143. Sager R: Genetic suppression of tumor formation: A new frontier in cancer research. Cancer Res 46:1573, 1986

144. Schroeder WT, Chao L-Y, Dao DD, Strong LC, Pathak S, Riccardi V, Lewis WH, Saunders GF: Nonrandom loss of maternal chromosome 11 alleles in Wilms tumours. Am J Human Genet 40:413, 1987

145. Schwab M, Alitalo K, Varmus HE, Bishop MJ, George D: A cellular oncogene (c-Ki-ras) is amplified, overexpressed, and located within karyotypic abnormalities in mouse adrenocortical tumour cells. Nature (London) 303:497, 1983

146. Schwab M, Alitalo K, Klempnauer K-H, Varmus HE, Bishop JM,

Gilbert F, Brodeur G, Goldstein M, Trent J: Amplified DNA with limited homology to myc cellular oncogene is shared by human neuroblastoma cell lines and a neuroblastoma tumour. Nature (London) 305:245, 1983

147. Schwab M, Ellison J, Busch M, Rosenau W, Varmus HE, Bishop JM: Enhanced expression of the human gene N-myc consequent to amplification of DNA may contribute to malignant progression of neuroblastoma. Proc Natl Acad Sci USA 81:4940, 1984

148. Scrabble HJ, Witte DP, Lampkin BC, Cavenee WK: Chromosomal localization of the human rhabdomyosarcoma locus by mitotic recombination mapping. Nature (London) 329:645, 1987

149. Seeger RC, Brodeur GM, Sather H, Dalton A, Siegel SE, Wong KY, Hammond D: Association of multiple copies of the n-myc oncogene with rapid progression of neuroblastomas. N Engl J Med 313:1111, 1985

150. Seemayer TA, de Chadarévian J-P, Vekemans M: Histological and cytogenetic findings in a malignant tumor of the chest wall and lung (Askin tumor). Virchows Arch [A] 408:289, 1985

151. Seizinger BR, Martuza RL, Gusella JF: Loss of genes on chromosome 22 in tumorigenesis of human acoustic neuroma. Nature (London) 322:644, 1986

152. Seizinger BR, Rouleau G, Ozelius LJ, Lane AH, St George-Hyslop P, Huson S, Gusella JF, Martuza RL: Common pathogenetic mechanism for three tumour types in bilateral acoustic neurofibromatosis. Science 236:317, 1987

153. Seizinger BR, Rouleau GA, Ozelius LJ, Lane AH, Faryniarz AG, Chao MV, Huson S, Korf BR, Parry DM, Pericak-Vance MA, Collins FS, Hobbs WJ, Falcone BG, Iannazzi JA, Roy JC, St George-Hyslop PH, Tanzi RE, Bothwell MA, Upadhyaya M, Harper P, Goldstein AE, Hoover DL, Bader JL, Spence MA, Mulvihill JJ, Aylsworth AS, Vance JM, Rossenwasser GOD, Gaskell PC, Roses AD, Martuza RL, Breakefield XO, Gusella JF: Genetic linkage of von Recklinghausen neurofibromatosis to the nerve growth factor receptor gene. Cell 49:589, 1987

154. Seizinger BR, Rouleau GA, Ozelius LJ, Lane AH, Farmer GE, Lamiell JM, Haines J, Yuen JWM, Collins D, Majoor-Krakauer D, Bonner T, Mathew C, Rubenstein A, Halperin J, McConkie-Rosell A, Green JS, Trofatter JA, Ponder BA, Eierman L, Bowmer MI, Schimke R, Oostra B, Aronin N, Smith DI, Drabkin H, Waziri MH, Hobbs WJ, Martuza RL, Conneally PM, Hsia YE, Gusella JF: Von-Hippel-Lindau disease maps to the region of chromosome 3 associated with renal cell carcinoma. Nature (London) 332:268, 1988

155. Shih C, Shilo BZ, Goldfarb MP, Dannenberg A, Weinberg RA: Passage of phenotypes of chemically transformed cells via transfection of DNA and chromatin. Proc Natl Acad Sci USA 76:5714, 1979

156. Slamon DJ, deKernion JB, Verma IM, Cline MJ: Expression of cellular oncogenes in human malignancies. Science 224:256, 1984

157. Slamon DJ, Boone TC, Seeger RC, Keith DE, Chazin V, Lee HC, Souza LM: Identification and characterization of the protein encoded by the human N-myc oncogene. Science 232:768, 1986

158. Slamon DJ, Clark GM, Wong SG, Levin WJ, Ullrich A, McGuire WL: Human breast cancer: correlation of relapse and survival with amplification of the HER-2/neu oncogene. Science 235:177, 1987

159. Slamon DJ, Clark GM: Response. Science 240:1796, 1988

160. Solomon E, Voss R, Hall V, Bodmer WF, Jass JR, Jeffreys AJ, Lucibello FC, Patel I, Rider SH: Chromosome 5 allele loss in human colorectal carcinomas. Nature (London) 328:616, 1987

161. Sotelo-Avila C, Gooch WM: Neoplasms associated with the Beckwith-Wiedemann syndrome. In Perspectives in Pediatric Pathology, Vol 3, edited by Rosenberg HS, Bolande RP, pp 255–272. Chicago, Year Book Medical Publishers, 1976

162. Sparkes RS, Sparkes MD, Wilson MA, Towner JW, Benedict W, Murphree AL, Yunis JJ: Regional assignment of genes for human esterase-D and retinoblastoma to chromosome band 13q14. Science 208:1042, 1980

163. Sparkes RS, Murphree AL, Lingua RW, Sparkes MD, Field LL, Funderburk SJ, Benedict WF: Gene for hereditary retinoblastoma assigned to human chromosome 13 by linkage to esterase-D. Science 219:971, 1983

164. Spector D, Varmus HE, Bishop JM: Nucleotide sequences related to the transforming gene of ASV are present in DNA of uninfected vertebrates. Proc Natl Acad Sci USA 75:4102, 1978

165. Stanbridge EJ: Suppression of malignancy in human cells. Nature (London) 260:17, 1976

166. Stanton LW, Schwab M, Bishop JM: Nucleotide sequence of the human N-myc gene. Proc Natl Acad Sci USA 83:1772, 1986

167. Suhumar S, Notario V, Martin-Zanca D, Barbacid M: Induction of mammary carcinomas in rats by nitroso-methylurea involves malignant activation of H-ras-1 locus by single point mutations. Nature (London) 306:658, 1983

168. T'Ang A, Varley JM, Chakraborty S, Murphree AL, Fung Y-KT: Structural rearrangement of the retinoblastoma gene in human breast carcinoma. Science 242:263, 1988

169. Temin HM, Mizutani S: RNA-dependent DNA polymerase in virions of Rous sarcoma virus. Nature (London) 226:1211, 1970

170. Tsuda H, Shimosato Y, Upton MP, Yokota J, Terada M, Ohira M, Sugimura T, Hirohashi S: Retrospective study on amplification of N-myc and c-myc genes in pediatric solid tumors and its association with prognosis and tumor differentiation. Lab Invest 59:321, 1988

171. Tsujimoto Y, Cossman J, Jaffe E, Croce CM: Involvement of the bcl-2 gene in human follicular lymphoma. Science 228:1440, 1985

172. Turc-Carel C, Philip I, Berger M-P, Philip T, Lenoir GM: Chromosomal translocations in Ewing's sarcoma. N Engl J Med 309:497, 1983

173. Turleau C, De Grouchy J, Chavin-Colin F, Martelli H, Voyer J, Charlas R: Trisomy 11p15 and Beckwith-Wiedemann syndrome: a report of two cases. Human Genet 67:219, 1984

174. Varmus HE: The molecular genetics of cellular oncogenes. Ann Rev Genet 18:553, 1984

175. Venter DJ, Kumar S, Tuzi NL, Gullick WJ: Overexpression of the c-erbB-2 oncoprotein in human breast carcinomas: immuno-histological assessment correlates with gene amplification. Lancet 2:69, 1987

176. Verma IM: Proto-oncogene fos: a multifaceted gene. Trends in Genetics 2:93, 1986

177. Vogelstein B, Fearon ER, Hamilton SR, Kern SE, Preisinger AC, Leppert M, Nakamura Y, White R, Smits AMM, Bos JL: Genetic alterations during colorectal-tumor development. N Engl J Med 319:525, 1988

178. Vogt M, Dulbecco R: Steps in the neoplastic transformation of hamster embryo cells by polyoma virus. Proc Natl Acad Sci USA 49:171, 1963

179. Waziri M, Patil SR, Hanson JW, Bartley JA: Abnormality of chromosome 11 in patients with features of Beckwith-Wiedemann syndrome. J Pediatr 102:873, 1983

180. Weinberg RA: A molecular basis for cancer. Sci Am 249:126, 1983

181. Weinberg RA: Oncogenes and the mechanisms of carcinogenesis. Sci Am Med Section 12, II pp 1–10, 1984

182. Weiss LM, Warnke RA, Sklar J, Cleary ML: Molecular analysis of the t(14;18) chromosomal translocation in malignant lymphomas. N Engl J Med 317:1185, 1987

183. Weiss RA, Marshall CJ: Oncogenes. Lancet 2:1138, 1984

184. Weissman BE, Saxon PJ, Pasquale SR, Jones GR, Geiser AG, Stanbridge EJ: Introduction of a normal human chromosome 11 into a Wilms' tumor cell line controls its tumorigenic expression. Science 236:175, 1987

185. Whang-Peng J, Triche TJ, Knutsen T, Miser J, Douglass EC, Israel MA: Chromosomal translocation in peripheral neuroepithelioma. N Engl J Med 311:584, 1984

186. Whyte P, Buchkovich KJ, Horowitz JM, Friend SH, Raybuck M, Weinberg RA, Harlow E: Association between an oncogene and an anti-oncogene: The adenovirus E1A proteins bind to the retinoblastoma gene product. Nature (London) 334:124, 1988

187. Wiedemann HR: Complexe malformatif familial avec hernie ombilicale et macroglossie: un "syndrome nouveau?" J Genet Hum 13:223, 1964

188. Wiggs J, Nordensjöld M, Yandell D, Rapaport J, Grondin V, Janson M, Werelius B, Petersen R, Craft A, Riedel K, Liberfarb R, Walton D, Wilson W, Dryja TP: Prediction of the risk of hereditary retinoblastoma, using DNA polymorphisms within the retinoblastoma gene. N Engl J Med 318:151, 1988

189. Wilkins RJ: Genomic imprinting and carcinogenesis. Lancet 1:329, 1988

190. Williman CL, Fenoglio-Preiser CM: Oncogenes, suppressor genes, and carcinogenesis. Hum Pathol 18:895, 1987

191. Wong AJ, Ruppert JM, Eggleston J, Hamilton SR, Baylin SB,

Vogelstein B: Gene amplification of c-myc and N-myc in small cell carcinoma of the lung. Science 233:461, 1986

192. Yokota J, Tsunetsugu-Yokota Y, Battifora H, LeFevre C, Cline MJ: Alterations of myc, myb, and ras-Ha proto-oncogenes in cancers are frequent and show clinical correlation. Science 231:261, 1986

193. Yokota J, Wada M, Shimosato Y, Terada M, Sugimura T: Loss of heterozygosity on chromosomes 3, 13 and 17 in small-cell carcinoma and on chromosome 3 in adenocarcinoma of the lung. Proc Natl Acad Sci USA 84:9252, 1987

194. Yunis JJ, Ramsay N: Retinoblastoma and subband deletion on chromosome 13. Am J Dis Child 132:161, 1978

195. Yunis JJ, Bloomfield CD, Ensrud K: All patients with acute nonlymphocytic leukemia may have a chromosomal defect. N Engl J Med 305:135, 1981

196. Yunis JJ: The chromosomal basis of human neoplasia. Science 221:227, 1983

197. Yunis JJ: Fragile sites and predisposition to leukemia and lymphoma. Cancer Genet Cytogenet 12:85, 1984

198. Zbar B, Brauch H, Talmadge C, Linehan M: Loss of alleles of loci on the short arm of chromosome 3 in renal cell carcinoma. Nature 327:721, 1987

199. Zhou D, Battifora H, Yokota J, Yamamoto T, Cline MJ: Association of multiple copies of the c-erbB-2 oncogene with spread of breast cancer. Cancer Res 47:6123, 1987

Biology of Disease

DNA Repair and Its Pathogenetic Implications

VILHELM A. BOHR, MICHELE K. EVANS, AND ALBERT J. FORNACE JR.

Division of Cancer Therapy, Laboratory of Molecular Pharmacology, Radiation Oncology Branch, National Cancer Institute, Bethesda, Maryland

Introduction
DNA Repair Mechanisms in Mammalian Cells
  DNA damage and repair
  DNA repair genes
  Measurements of DNA repair
  Recombinational repair and post-replication repair mechanisms
Chromatin Organization and DNA Repair
Heterogeneity of DNA Repair. Preferential DNA Repair in Mammalian Cells
Inducible Responses to DNA Damage
DNA Repair Deficient Disorders
  Xeroderma pigmentosum
  Bloom's syndrome
  Fanconi's anemia
  Cockayne's syndrome
Conditions Suspect for DNA Repair Deficiency
  Ataxia telangiectasia
  Nevoid basal cell carcinoma syndrome
  Dysplastic nevus syndrome
  Gardner's syndrome
  Dyskeratosis congenita
  Trichothiodystrophy
  Retinoblastoma
  mer⁻ phenotype
Perspectives
  Aging
  Risk of cancer
  DNA repair and neurodegenerative diseases
  Role of DNA damage in atherosclerosis
  Role of DNA repair and DNA damage-inducible responses in chemoresistant tumor cells
Concluding Remarks

INTRODUCTION

The environment in which we live poses continuous threats to our genetic material. Ionizing radiation, ultraviolet light from the sun, and a multitude of chemical agents cause alterations of DNA that would be detrimental, were it not for the constant cellular monitoring and repair of most defects as they occur. In addition, cellular DNA is subject to spontaneous damage and loss of bases as well as changes in base sequence due to infidelity of replication or recombination. There are many endogenous chemical reactions that damage DNA. They arise from normal chemical reactions at 37°C such as depurination or the deamination of cytosine. If such damages were not repaired, as many as 10% of the bases in the

DNA of an average cell of an elderly human would be altered (117). Such an accumulation of damage is not compatible with life as we know it unless very effective mechanisms exist to repair damaged DNA.

The DNA repair processes are the cellular responses associated with the restoration of the normal nucleotide sequence of DNA after damage. These processes must be regarded, along with processes such as replication and recombination, as essential transactions of the genetic material in all life forms. In a sense, DNA repair can be viewed as a kind of immune system at the DNA level. Just as the immune system provides protection for the organism against many foreign objects, the DNA repair machinery can find and deal differentially with many types of damage to the DNA in its restoration of normal function. As with the immune system, stimulation or regulation of DNA repair may become a therapy against disease.

The field of DNA repair has grown considerably and attracted renewed interest in recent years. It now has many interactions with other areas of research. A comprehensive textbook has recently appeared (36) that reflects the wide scope and importance of DNA repair processes. In the present review we can only deal with a few aspects of DNA repair, and we have chosen some that seem of particular relevance to pathology and cancer research. We will discuss some recent advances or approaches in the molecular understanding of DNA repair that we expect to have future implications. One example is that we can now study DNA repair at subcellular levels not previously possible. Such studies have shown that the function and organization of the repair processes is diversified in mammalian cells. This intragenomic heterogeneity of DNA damage and repair will be detailed in this review since it has importance for the molecular biology of DNA repair and implications for human disease and risk assessment. We will also discuss recent findings that DNA damage can directly induce certain mammalian genes. DNA damage inducible genes may be important in genotoxic stress responses. Since there have been many reviews dealing with the major human DNA repair diseases we will describe them only briefly and

focus more on less well-recognized human diseases that are DNA damage sensitive and are suspect for DNA repair of deficiency.

DNA REPAIR MECHANISMS IN MAMMALIAN CELLS

DNA DAMAGE AND REPAIR

Many compounds and agents are known to cause direct damage to DNA. This damage can give rise to malignant transformation, in part via mutations at specific sites in certain oncogenes. Some common types of damage to the DNA are shown in Figure 1. They include changes or alterations of the bases, intrastrand or interstrand cross-links, strand breaks, and the formations of bulky adducts. Most carcinogens or types of radiation give rise to more than one of these modifications. Ionizing radiation causes strand breaks and base modifications. Ultraviolet (254 nm) irradiation induces many different types of damage (photoproducts) in DNA of which the most common is the pyrimidine dimer; this is a covalent linkage between two adjacent pyrimidines. Another less common photoproduct after ultraviolet irradiation is a 6-4 linkage between adjacent pyrimidines, the so-called 6-4 photoproduct.

When our cells are exposed to damage, they confront

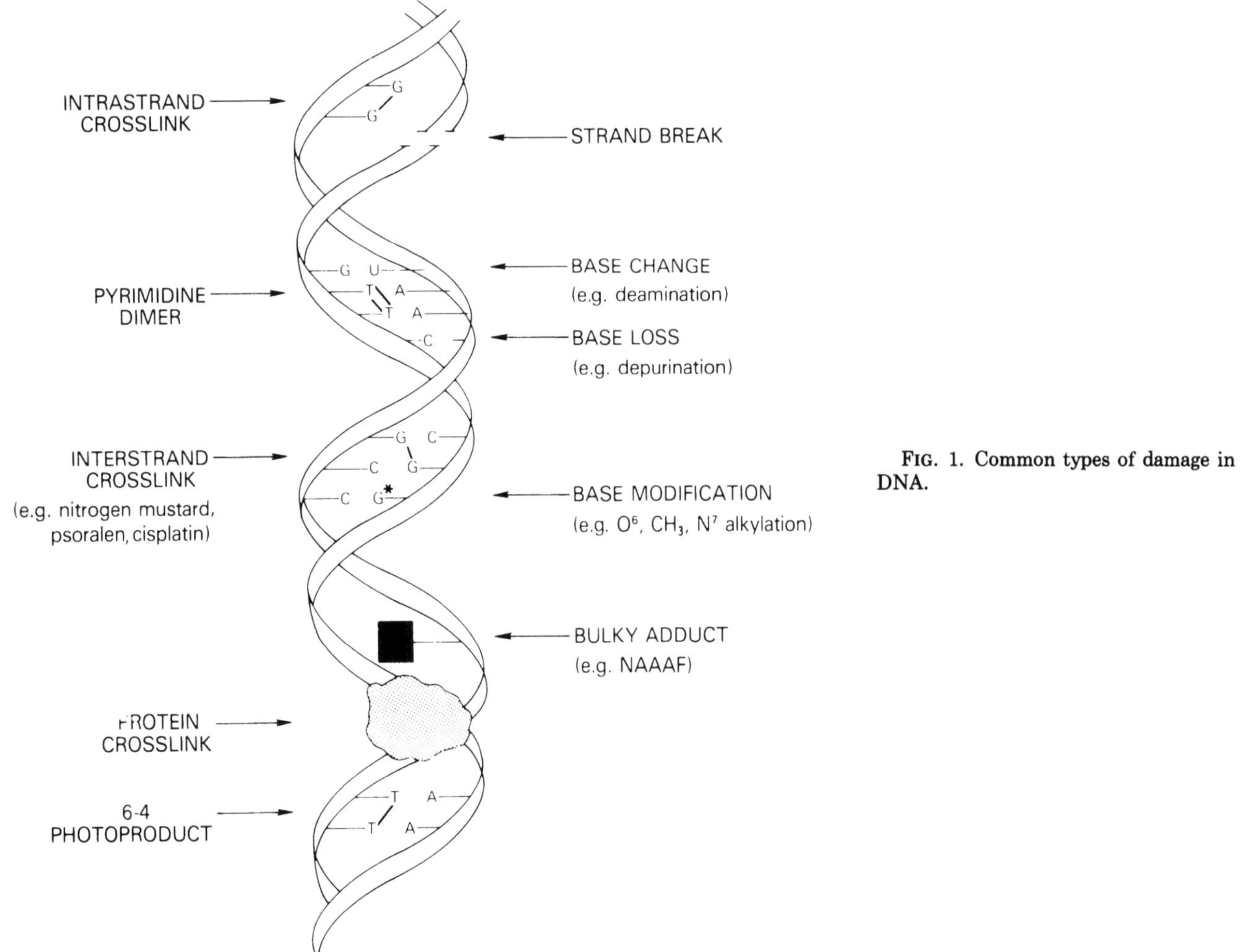

FIG. 1. Common types of damage in DNA.

it in different ways, schematized in Table 1. Damage can in some cases be tolerated by cells. This is an important pathway that is still poorly understood and that in many cases involves damage bypass replication and introduction of errors in daughter DNA. As indicated in Table 1, some forms of damage can be directly reverted, but most are excised by the more elaborate excision repair pathways. These are the pathways that are usually termed the DNA repair mechanism. As will be discussed, recombination processes can be categorized both under tolerance and repair pathways (Table 1).

The enzymatic pathways involved in DNA repair appear to vary considerably with the type of damage introduced, but the most general and well-characterized mechanism is the nucleotide excision repair process responsible for the removal of ultraviolet-induced damage and bulky chemical adducts (Fig. 2). The sequential steps in nucleotide excision repair include 1) preincision recognition of damage, 2) incision of the damaged DNA strand near site of the defect, 3) excision of the defective site and localized degradation of the affected strand, 4) repair replication to replace the excised region with a corresponding stretch of normal nucleotides, and finally 5) ligation to join the repair patch at its 3' end to the contiguous parental DNA.

The enzymes involved in DNA repair can be classified according to their role in the steps outlined above. Recognition of the damage and incision may be performed by the same enzyme. An example of this is the pyrimidine dimer specific endonuclease, T4 endonuclease V, from bacteriophage T4 infected *Escherichia coli* that has a combined glycosylase and AP endonuclease activity resulting in cleavage of the DNA strand at sites of pyrimidine dimers (Fig. 2). In *E. coli* the repair process can also be conducted by the ABC excinuclease enzyme complex that consists of three high molecular weight gene products. The ABC excinuclease enzymes recognize many bulky adducts in DNA (111). Since it recognizes a spectrum of different adducts, it probably detects a general structural change in the DNA upon damage. The enzyme complex nicks the DNA strand at both sides of the adduct and in most cases removes a stretch of 12 bases containing the adduct. It is possible, but not yet established, that a similar enzyme complex to ABC excinuclease is present in eukaryotic cells. Whereas in bacteria many enzymes involved in DNA repair have been characterized (111), only few of those involved in mammalian repair are known. The repair replication step

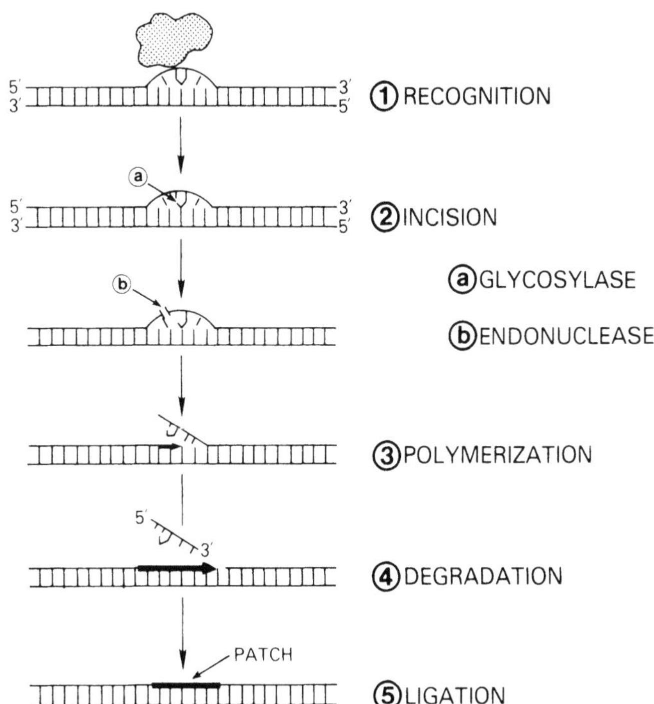

FIG. 2. Steps in nucleotide excision repair; *a* and *b*, activities of pyrimidine dimer specific endonuclease, T4 endonuclease V.

is performed by a DNA polymerase, and whereas there are two polymerases in bacteria, there are four (α, β, γ and δ) in mammalian cells. The notion has prevailed that the α and β polymerases (and possibly the δ enzyme) are mainly responsible for the repair polymerization. The final step in the process is the ligation. In mammalian cells, at least two types of ligases are known, ligase I and II, and the latter appears to be specifically involved in DNA repair.

DNA REPAIR GENES

At least 30 gene products involved in DNA repair are known from studies in yeast (35), and the number is likely higher in mammalian cells. The genetic disease xeroderma pigmentosum (XP) demonstrates the association between defective repair of DNA lesions and cancer. The patients develop frequent skin cancer and often also a higher incidence of internal cancers. It was established two decades ago (24) that cells from patients with this disorder were defective in their repair of ultraviolet-induced damage. Complementation group analysis performed on XP cell strains and on repair deficient rodent cell lines has suggested that at least nine and possibly more than 13 genes are involved in early steps of the excision of ultraviolet-light-induced DNA lesions in mammalian cells. Two of these genes have been cloned, and others are in advanced stage of cloning. One cloned gene, ERCC-1, has been characterized at the molecular level (131). It is homologous with excision repair genes in yeast and in *E. coli* which could indicate that the excision repair system is conserved during evolution. It is likely that the cloning and characterization of prokaryotic and eukaryotic repair genes will pave the way to a deeper understanding of mammalian repair systems and their association with cancer.

TABLE 1. CELLULAR RESPONSES TO DNA DAMAGE

Tolerance	Repair
By-pass replication	Direct Reversal
Replication arrest	Enzymatic photoreversal
Translesion DNA synthesis	Purine insertase
	Ligation
	Methyl transferase
	Excision Repair Processes
	Base excision repair
	Nucleotide excision repair
Recombination	

MEASUREMENTS OF DNA REPAIR

Many different approaches to measuring DNA repair have been developed over the years. Since the methodology obviously provides the basis for the interpretation and understanding of the results obtained we have listed some examples of the more classic approaches to studying DNA repair in Table 2 (see 29, 36). A simple method for measuring DNA repair involves determination of the loss of radioactively labeled adducts. The adducts in DNA can also be directly identified by some techniques listed in Table 2. DNA repair activity after ultraviolet damage has been determined by many different techniques measuring one or more of the aforementioned steps of the repair process. The repair can be measured as the ligation of DNA strand breaks, for example by using alkaline elution or alkaline sucrose gradient analysis of DNA or by methods that assess the unwinding of DNA caused by formation of strand breaks. The polymerization step of the repair process may be measured by unscheduled DNA synthesis or repair replication. It is often important to distinguish for analysis effects in the parental DNA from those in replicated DNA. Also, DNA replicated after damage is presumably free of damage and could erroneously be assayed as repaired DNA in the assays. The separation of repaired and replicated DNA can be accomplished by use of replication inhibitors

TABLE 2. EXAMPLES OF METHODS TO STUDY DNA REPAIR

DNA Strand breaks
  Single strand breaks
    Alkaline elution
    Alkaline sucrose gradients
    Alkaline unwinding assay
    Nucleoid sedimentation (strand breaks in supercoiled DNA)
  Double strand breaks
    Neutral elution
Adducts in DNA
  Radioactively labeled adduct
    Extract and scintillation count DNA
  Antibodies, monoclonal or polyclonal
    Pyrimidine dimers
    Photoproducts, various carcinogens
  Direct identification
    Thin layer chromatography, pyrimidine dimers
    HPLC, various adducts
  Indirect identification
    Enzymatic probes
      T4 endonuclease V for pyrimidine dimers
      ABC excinuclease for various adducts
    Electrophoresis
      Cross-links (psoralen, protein)
DNA repair synthesis
  Unscheduled DNA synthesis
  Repair replication
    Metabolic inhibitors
    BrdUrd incorporation
Errors in genetic code
  DNA sequencing
  High performance liquid chromatography
Other related biological parameters
  Replication
  Colony forming ability, cellular resistance
  Sister chromatid exchanges
  Chromosome breaks

or by prelabeling the DNA with the heavy thymidine analogue bromodeoxyuridine (BrdUrd) and separating the replicated DNA from the parental by CsCl gradient equilibrium centrifugation. Immunological methods have been developed that assay the formation and removal of adducts by monoclonal antibodies to specific adducts (147) or to BrdUrd incorporated into DNA repair patches (25, 69).

RECOMBINATIONAL REPAIR AND POST-REPLICATION REPAIR MECHANISMS

A major problem any organism faces is how to replicate its DNA when the template (parent strand DNA) contains DNA damage. A similar problem occurs in the repair of double strand lesions, such as interstrand cross-links or double strand breaks (*cf.* Fig 1). In both cases the cell is faced with the dilemma that there is no intact template to direct the polymerase in the synthesis of daughter strand DNA during semiconservative synthesis or the synthesis of a gapped DNA during repair synthesis. Certain simple types of damage, like methylation at the 0^6 position of guanine by nitrosoureas, may cause point mutations in daughter strand DNA by the polymerase mistakenly inserting a thymine rather than a cytosine opposing the methylated guanine. However, many types of DNA damage are blocks to replication. For example, ultraviolet-induced pyrimidine dimers are absolute blocks to *E. coli* polymerases I and III *in vitro* (134) and blocks to replication in mammalian cells (5). Alterations of polymerase proofreading capability, such as suppression of the 3' to 5' exonuclease activity, may allow some error-prone replication past such blocks (11), but considering that mammalian cells survive ultraviolet irradiation where more than 10^5 dimers/cell are produced, this would be a very inefficient and error-prone way to handle such damage. In the case of interstrand cross-links, replication would be blocked since strand separation could not occur. In both bacteria and eukaryotes exposed to ultraviolet damage, transient gaps occur in daughter strand DNA, presumably opposing the template DNA containing the dimers (36, 108). With time (several hours in mammalian cells) the gaps have been replaced by intact uninterrupted DNA even though the parental DNA still contains the damage. This has commonly been referred to as post-replication repair, although replication on a damaged template may be a more accurate description. In bacteria these gaps are removed by recombination events mediated by the recA protein (and other related proteins) that involve the gapped DNA and the intact sister duplex DNA (43). Accurate replication occurs because the damaged template has been substituted with undamaged DNA via a recombinational mechanism.

A reasonable model (but not the only) for this process is shown in Figure 3A and will be discussed in some detail. In step I, semiconservation DNA synthesis is shown proceeding normally until the polymerase encounters damage on one parent strand. In step II, the replication fork has proceeded past this damage, but a gap now exists in one daughter strand. The single-stranded parental DNA (heavy solid line) is homologous (same polarity) to the daughter strand DNA (light dashed line)

Fig. 3. *A*, DNA replication on a damaged template: possible recombination events. Scheme of DNA synthesis on a damaged template is shown with parent strand DNA (*solid lines*) and daughter strand DNA (*dashed lines*). Polarity of strands is indicated by + or −. In steps I and II DNA replication proceeds past a region in the parental DNA containing DNA damage. In II, a gap exists in daughter strand DNA opposing this damage (*heavy lines*). Recombination intermediates are shown in steps III and IV, and resolution of these intermediates with products A to D are shown in V (see text for further explanation). In *B*, the topological equivalent of left crossover point of step IV in *A* is shown. This crossover point or Holliday structure can be resolved into duplex DNA by nicking at positions p or positions r.

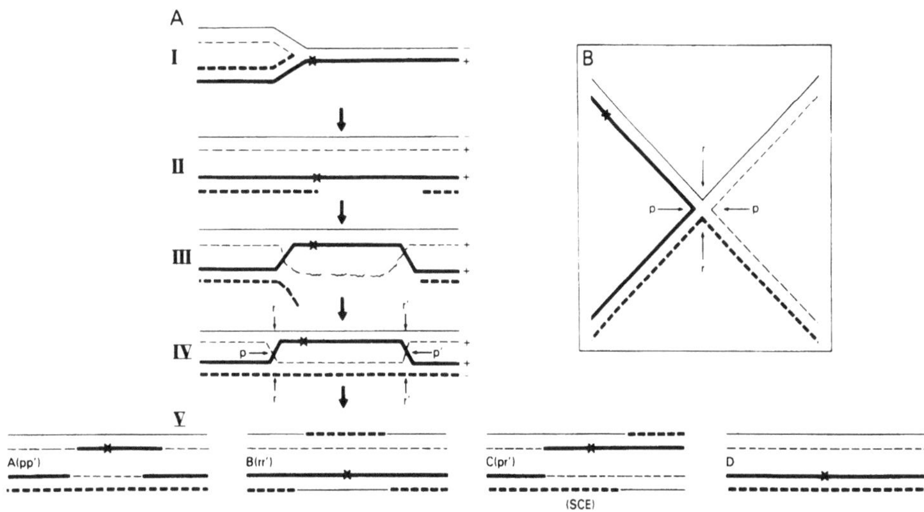

of the sister duplex DNA. RecA protein (143) is known to mediate the displacement of one strand in duplex DNA by homologous single-stranded DNA, and this is shown in step III between the single-stranded parent DNA (+ strand) and the intact sister duplex DNA (light lines) with a resultant D loop. The displaced intact daughter strand (light dashed line) is now free to base pair with the gapped daughter strand DNA and provides an intact undamaged template for polymerase to fill the gap. The result (after filling in the gap and ligation) is shown in step IV where symmetric D loops connect the two duplexes. The crossover or branch points, designated p and p′ in step III, need to be resolved. Such crossover points are frequently called Holliday structures after the investigator (49) who first proposed such an intermediate during recombination events between two homologous DNA duplexes (such as during gene conversion). A Holliday structure can be viewed as a transient connection between two DNA strands. There is good evidence that such structures can exist in bacteria and virus and are generated during recombination repair (43). A crossover point or Holliday structure is topologically equivalent to a four-sided structure such as shown in Figure 3*B*. By making nicks at positions p or positions r, this four-sided structure can be resolved into standard duplex DNA. The two Holliday structures of step IV in Figure 3*A* can be resolved by cutting the DNA at position p or positions r and by cutting at position p′ or positions r′. By cutting at positions p and p′ or positions r and r′ (product A or B of V), some parental DNA would remain in the daughter strand, and each strand would actually be a mosaic of fragments of parent and daughter strand DNA since similar events would occur at every damaged site. This is actually what has been observed in bacteria. The crossover points or Holliday structures are movable. They can slide along the DNA strands and migrate long distances in the DNA by branch migration in an energy-free manner since for every base pair that is disrupted another one forms (83). This is apparently the case in bacteria since the fragments of recombined parent and daughter DNA may be up to 20,000 nucleotides long (44). In addition to products A and B in Figure 3*A*, step V, cuts at p and r′ (or p′ and r) would result in a double

strand exchange or a sister chromatid exchange (SCE) (product C of V). If the two Holliday intermediates migrate toward each other by branch migration and meet, then product D would result. Since in bacteria ~50% of the pyrimidine dimers originally in parent strand DNA can be found in daughter strand DNA after postreplication repair (39), it is likely that products A, B, and C predominate in bacteria. In bacteria, the recA protein is also needed for the repair of double strand lesions, such as interstrand crosslinks and double strand breaks. Since growing bacteria frequently contain at least a portion of a second chromosome (S or G2 phase cells) (59), the recombination may occur between homologous chromosomes in the same cell. Bacteria deficient in recombination repair (recA⁻) show increased sensitivity, as measured by cell killing, to many DNA damaging agents. In mutants deficient in both recombination and nucleotide excision repair, there is very high sensitivity to DNA damaging agents (*e.g.*, ultraviolet-irradiation).

Evidence for recombination events, such as outlined in Figure 3, is not as strong in eukaryotes as for bacteria. For example, most pyrimidine dimers remain in the parent strand after postreplication repair. It has been proposed that mammalian DNA polymerases can insert a nucleotide (usually an adenine) when a noncoding base (DNA damage) is encountered in the template, although this would result in highly error-prone replication (36). In yeast, DNA repair mutants, such as RAD54, RAD52, RAD51, and RAD1 (35, 112), are deficient in mitotic and meiotic recombination. These mutants are also sensitive to DNA damaging agents that produce double strand lesions such as double strand breaks and interstrand crosslinks. The RAD52 protein from yeast can substitute for the T4 genes 46 and 47 in carrying out recombination and DNA repair in bacteria (23). This suggests that some components of the recombination mechanisms in bacteria and eukaryotes are similar. There are probably at least three different DNA repair pathways/systems in yeast: RAD3 (nucleotide excision), RAD52 (recombination), and RAD6 groups; all are probably involved in repair of double strand lesions in DNA (35, 51).

In mammalian cells there is also evidence for recombination events after DNA damage. At the cytogenetic level, SCEs can be visualized, and their frequency is increased after DNA damage, but this frequency is <0.1% of the frequency of damage to the DNA. Various recombination events are known to occur in mammalian cells. Viruses and transfected plasmids have been shown to recombine at higher levels when containing DNA damage (123). In mouse L cells, Wang *et al.* (138) have shown that various carcinogens, which are DNA damaging agents, can increase the frequency of homologous recombination. The exchange of pyrimidine dimers (31) from parent to daughter strand DNA has been observed in human and other mammalian cells. In contrast to bacteria, only 1–3% of the dimers were exchanged from parent to daughter strand. When human cells containing low levels of cross-links produced in G0/G1 replicated their DNA in the subsequent S phase, the level of cross-links was found to be equal in parent and daughter DNA (122). Detection of exchanged DNA in mammalian cells is very low compared with bacteria (43, 75). This may be due to much smaller regions of exchange in mammalian cells and perhaps also by the preponderance of products such as the one shown in Figure 3, *VD*. As discussed above and noted in Table 1, recombination events can be viewed both as tolerance and repair responses. Abnormalities in such processes may lead to disturbances in the fidelity of DNA synthesis and increased mutagenesis. At the cytogenetic level recombination events are probably involved in the production of SCE, and disturbances in recombination may be involved in the generation of chromosome abnormalities.

CHROMATIN ORGANIZATION AND DNA REPAIR

A mammalian nucleus contains almost 50 cm DNA, and the packaging of this into a 10-μm sphere requires a 50,000-fold reduction in length. It is well recognized that DNA in the nucleus of mammalian cells exists in the form of chromatin that is organized and packaged into higher order structures. This highly complex structural organization must affect all nuclear reactions including replication, transcription, recombination, and DNA repair. The mammalian genome contains on the order of 10^5 genes that constitute on the order of 1% of total DNA, the remainder being noncoding sequences. Later, we will discuss recent findings on DNA repair in individual genes.

To relate aspects of the DNA damage processes to this higher order structure of chromatin, we will briefly discuss how this structural hierarchy of the nuclear material might affect our thinking on DNA repair. Figure 4 shows some well-characterized levels of structural organization of DNA from the cell nucleus to the primary sequence. For many years determinations of DNA repair have been based on measurements (such as those listed in Table 2) in the total cellular DNA (Fig. 4A) that provide an average measurement over the entire genome. However, DNA repair in parts of the genome may now be measured. DNA repair has been examined in fractions of the genome that could be readily isolated for analysis. It was shown that ultraviolet damage is repaired with similar efficiency in repetitive α sequences and in bulk DNA but

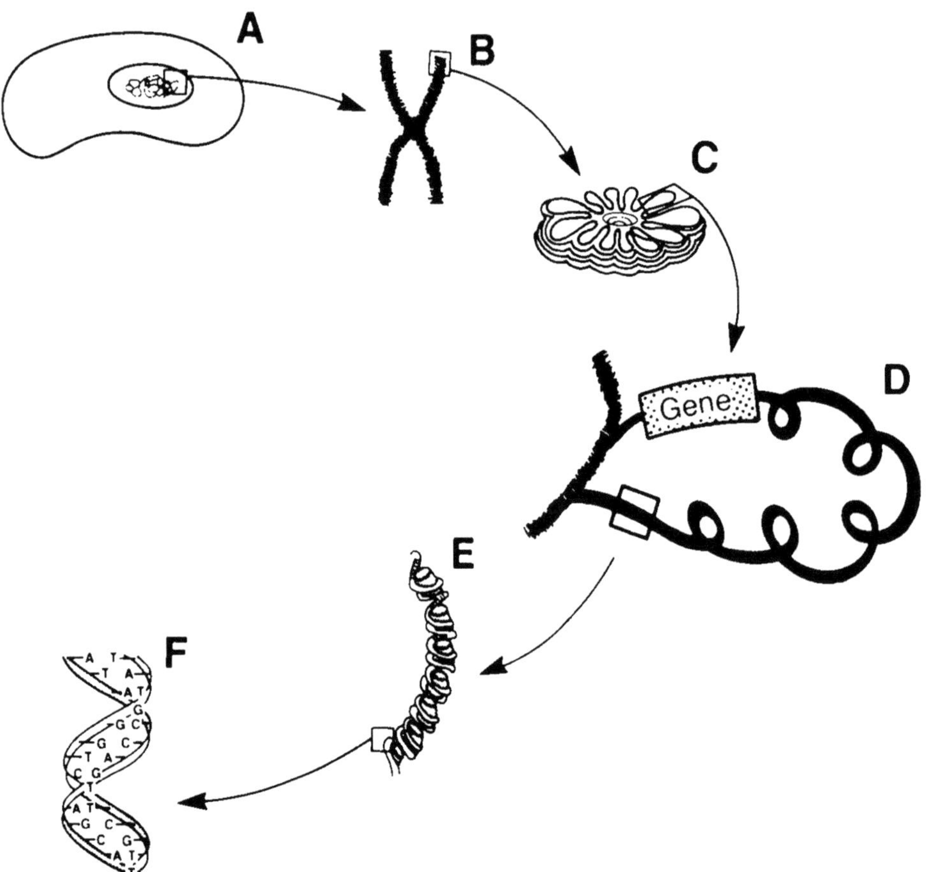

FIG. 4. Organization of DNA in mammalian nucleus. *A*, whole cell nucleus; *B*, chromosome; *C*, minibands on chromosome; *D*, higher order structure, loop, attached to nuclear matrix; *E*, core and linker, nucleosomes in chromatin; *F*, primary structure of DNA, base sequence. Reproduced with permission of *Trends in Biochemical Sciences.*

that the repair of certain carcinogen adducts was markedly deficient in α DNA (121). As shown in Figure 4*B*, the genome is further organized into individual chromosomes where cytogenetic or morphological methods such as karyotyping or analysis of sister chromatid exchanges are available to study damage, breaks, or recombination events. Although unscheduled DNA synthesis can be determined in individual chromosomes, more sophisticated DNA repair assays have not yet been developed at this level. With the use of pulse field electrophoresis very large DNA fragments can be visualized, and this approach should be promising.

As shown in Figure 4*C* and *D*, the DNA in chromosomes is further organized in higher order structures believed to be loops or domains extending from a central nuclear matrix or scaffold (98) (Fig. 4*D*). The sizes of these loops have been estimated by many different approaches to be in the order of 30–100 kb (95) and are believed to be functional domains for important DNA dependent enzymatic reactions in the nucleus. It is believed that genes are located within such loops, possibly in a dynamic manner, associated with the nuclear matrix at some times and dissociated at other times (98). Studies have demonstrated preferential repair of ultraviolet damage in matrix associated DNA (obtained by nuclease digestion) compared with total nuclear DNA in mammalian cells (85). Other approaches based on experiments using inhibitors have suggested that only one repair process can occur in a domain at a given time (reviewed in Ref. 15). As will be discussed in the next chapter, examination of repair in and around the dihydrofolate reductase (DHFR) gene in Chinese hamster ovary (CHO) cells has disclosed the existence of a 60–80-kb repair domain. The repair domain has the same size as the previously mentioned loops or domains in chromatin, and the DNA repair processes may be organized or regulated within such loops or domains. However, new approaches are needed to further clarify these notions.

Moving to the next level of structural hierarchy, work is being done to analyze DNA damage and repair processes at the level of nucleosomes (core and linker regions) (Fig. 4*E*). Approaches are based on differential nuclease sensitivity in core and linker regions of nucleosomes (120). Many bulky adducts have been shown to bind preferentially to linker regions. It appears that there is an initial reorganization of the nucleosomes during the repair process (148) and that the 5' and 3' ends of the nucleosome particle are repaired more efficiently than its central part (68).

Figure 4*F* shows the primary structure or nucleotide sequence of DNA. By many approaches it is possible to study the sequence specificity of damage in very small fragments (<1 kb) of DNA, but repair cannot be easily studied at this level since the doses of the damaging agent are too high for biological studies. Available techniques to study repair after ultraviolet exposure in specific sequences are limited to fragment sizes of >5 kb (11). New approaches are needed, for example, to study DNA repair processes in short stretches of nucleotides such as exons or regulator units of a gene or DNase I hypersensitive regions that all have lengths of <1 kb.

DNase I hypersensitive regions are believed to be sites of high accessibility, and they might be very accessible to DNA damage with bulky adducts and/or to the repair machinery. Also, many DNase hypersensitive sites are located in regulator regions of genes where repair might be particularly important. It would also be important to study DNA damage and repair in specific codons within genes such as those known to activate specific oncogenes.

HETEROGENEITY OF DNA REPAIR. PREFERENTIAL DNA REPAIR IN MAMMALIAN CELLS

Techniques have now been developed to study damage and repair in genes and other specific sequences (15, 17). DNA repair after ultraviolet damage can be studied in individual genes using the pyrimidine dimer specific T4 endonuclease V enzyme to cleave parental DNA at dimer sites. By quantitative Southern hybridization and probing for a sequence of interest, the number of damaged sites can be measured in specific restriction fragments (11). This technique is outlined in Figure 5. More recently, this methodology has been modified to measure agents other than ultraviolet (15), for example by the use of the ABC excision nuclease to cleave the DNA strand specifically at damaged sites (127) or by formation of strand breaks at sites of alkylation damage (113).

Most available results on repair in specific sequences have been obtained after ultraviolet damage to the cells. It was initially demonstrated that repair of ultraviolet damage in the essential gene for dihydrofolate reductase (DHFR) in CHO cells was much more efficient than the repair in the overall genome (16). This may provide an explanation for the paradox that rodent cells are deficient in overall genome DNA repair but are as resistant to ultraviolet damage as normal, repair-proficient human cells; they survive by selectively repairing the vital sequences. As with CHO cells, cell lines from patients with the human disorder XP repair only a small fraction of the induced pyrimidine dimers in the overall genome. However, the XP cells are much more sensitive to ultraviolet irradiation than CHO cells. It was demonstrated that at least one essential gene was not repaired in these cells (12), and it is possible that during repair in XP cells there is a lack of recognition of the essential genomic regions as is the case in normal human cells. It has been suggested that the determination of repair in essential genomic regions is an important feature for comparisons between DNA repair and cellular survival (12).

In normal, repair-proficient human cells, the whole genome is repaired during 24 hours after ultraviolet damage. However, essential genes are repaired faster than noncoding sequences in the genome (81). Some results from the gene-repair studies in hamster and human cells are summarized in Table 3. Repair has also been examined in many different genes and in cells of various different species. The data suggest that the preferential repair of active genes after ultraviolet damage is a general phenomenon in mammalian cells. The findings discussed here are based on the measurement of pyrimidine dimers, but the less common photoproduct 6-4 also appears to be preferentially repaired (in CHO cells)

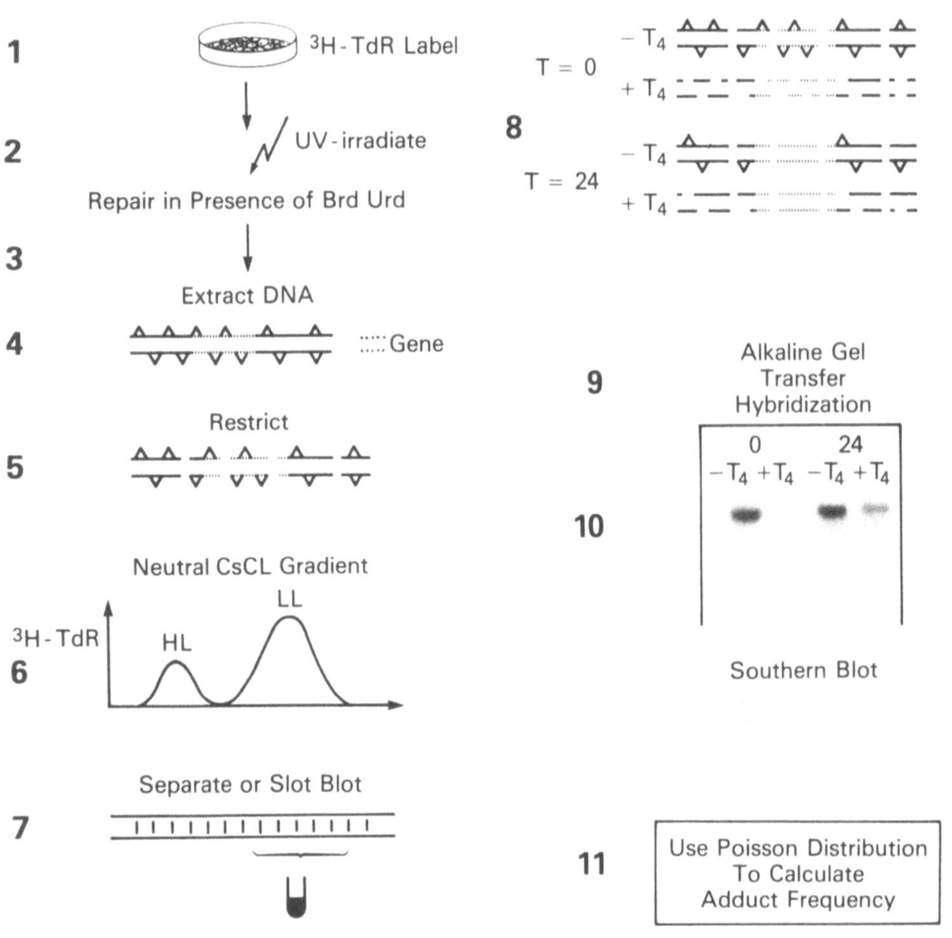

FIG. 5. DNA repair in a gene. Protocol for measuring frequency of pyrimidine dimers in a restriction fragment: 1, cells prelabeled; 2, cells ultraviolet irradiated; 3, repair; 4, DNA extraction; 5, restriction; 6, separation of replicated from parental DNA; 7, gradient fractionation; 8, reaction with pyrimidine dimer specific endonuclease (T4 endonuclease V); 9, alkaline gel electrophoresis; 10, Southern transfer and hybridization; 11, calculations.

TABLE 3. PREFERENTIAL DNA REPAIR IN MAMMALIAN CELLS AFTER ULTRAVIOLET DAMAGE

Cells	% Repair	
	After 8 hr	After 24 hr
CHO		
Bulk DNA		15
Noncoding regions		15
Active gene	50	75
Human		
Bulk DNA	35	80
Active gene	75	80
Mouse		
c-abl proto oncogene		80
c-mos proto oncogene		20

In rodent cells, active genes are efficiently repaired, whereas noncoding regions or inactive genes have minimal repair. In human cells, active genes are repaired much faster than bulk of genome or inactive genes.

(D. C. Thomas *et al.*, unpublished data). The preferential repair of the CHO DHFR gene is confined to a 60–80-kb region centered around the 5′ end of the gene (13), as shown in Figure 6. The initial frequency of pyrimidine dimers is similar in all fragments in and around the DHFR gene, whereas the repair differs considerably and is maximal at the 5′ end of the gene. This constitutes a repair domain, and its size is similar to a loop or higher order structure in chromatin. This may relate DNA repair processes to chromatin structure.

Different genes within the same cell can be repaired with different efficiencies. In a study on the repair of many proto-oncogenes in mouse cells it was found that the *c-abl* gene is repaired much more efficiently than the *c-mos* gene (76). Since the *c-abl* gene is actively transcribed in the cells, whereas the *c-mos* is not, these experiments indicate that a correlation exists between the level of transcription and the efficiency of repair for a gene. This was further supported by studies on the repair of ultraviolet damage in the metallothionein gene in CHO (86) and human cells (70). The repair in this gene is markedly more efficient when the gene is transcriptionally active than when it is not. These findings suggest that there is some cellular association between repair machinery and transcription machinery.

Several studies over the last decade have suggested that DNA damage and repair in the mammalian genome is governed by the openness or accessibility of chromatin (9, 15, 98, 130, 144). In support of this, we recently completed a study on preferential repair of the DHFR gene in wild-type CHO cells and ultraviolet-sensitive CHO cells, some of which were transfected with repair genes (14). The transfectants contained either the bacterial gene *den*V coding for the pyrimidine dimer specific repair enzyme T4 endonuclease V or the well-characterized human repair gene, ERCC-1 (131). The ultraviolet sensitive mutants did not repair ultraviolet damage, but

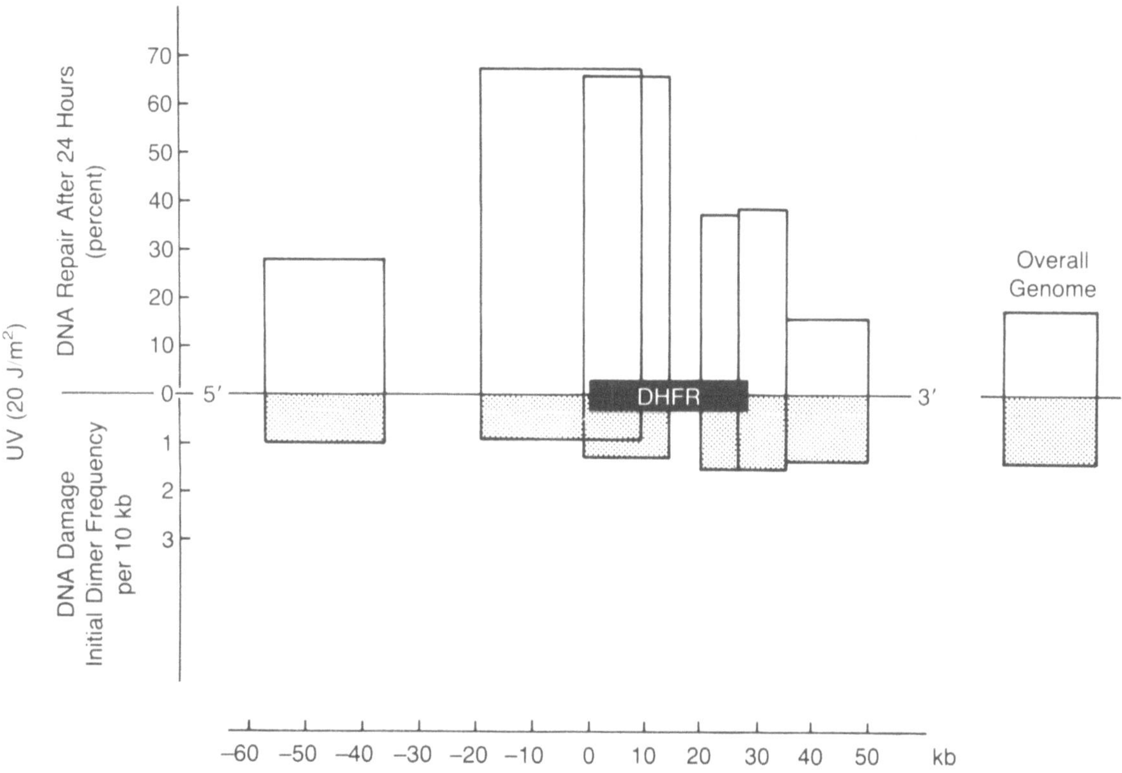

FIG. 6. A DNA repair domain. DNA damage and repair after ultraviolet (UV) damage (pyrimidine dimers) in DHFR gene locus in CHO cells. Percentage of DNA damage and repair is indicated for each restriction fragment studied. Reproduced with permission of *Trends in Biochemical Sciences*.

repair was restored in the transfectants. Cells containing the *denV* gene repaired all genomic sequences equally efficiently (8), whereas cells containing the human ERCC-1 gene repaired the active DHFR gene much more efficiently than the noncoding sequences. Apparently the ERCC-1 gene product reacts more like the expected enzyme involved in normal repair in mammalian cells. Since the T4 endonuclease V is a small 16-kDa enzyme half the estimated size of the ERCC-1 gene product, these repairs support that the preferential repair of active genes is related to chromatin accessibility. The ERCC-1 gene product may also be a part of a large enzyme complex responsible for excision. Incidentally, these transfected cell lines constitute an example of gene therapy for DNA repair. In the future we may be able to insert repair genes as a therapy in some cases of defective DNA repair.

Preferential repair of genes might be ascribed to the more open chromatin structure in actively transcribed genomic regions (discussed in Ref. 6). The recent demonstration that DNA repair shows strand specificity toward the transcribing strand (82), however, suggests that repair is directed toward certain sequences rather than just by chromatin accessibility. Further studies are needed to examine the relative importance of local chromatin structure, primary DNA sequence, and function of DNA for determination of efficiency and organization of DNA repair.

Certain molecules are key in locating vital sequences for the DNA repair machinery. Also local levels of methylation may be important. Ho *et al.* (48) recently reported

that demethylation of CHO cells by growth of the cells for many generations in azacytidine enhanced the overall genome DNA repair and changed the fine structure organization of the DNA repair domain in the DHFR gene. Another set of molecules that may be important in the regulation of preferential DNA repair is the topoisomerases. The topoisomerase I and II enzymes regulate the tension or stress in DNA. There have been many studies on the role of topoisomerase II in DNA repair at the level of the overall genome, some of them using new and more specific inhibitors, but the role of the enzyme is not yet clarified. At the level of the individual gene, one study showed that the topoisomerase II inhibitor novobiocin did not have any effect on repair of the DHFR gene in CHO cells after ultraviolet damage, whereas it inhibited repair of the overall genome (7). This supports the possibility that different repair mechanisms exist for repair in genes and for repair in the remainder or bulk of the genome. Repair of active genes could involve topoisomerase I, a possibility that is further attractive in light of recent data on the binding of topoisomerases to specific sequences. In particular, topoisomerase I appears to bind to actively transcribed regions (27, 41).

INDUCIBLE RESPONSES TO DNA DAMAGE

In bacteria such as *E. coli* (137), various adverse stimuli can lead to induction of stress regulons (a regulon is a group of coordinately regulated genes) such as the *recA* mediated SOS response (set of reactions in response to stress in *E. coli.*), the adaptive response to alkylating agents, and the *oxyR* mediated response to oxidative stress. Other regulons can be activated by stresses not directly related to DNA damage, such as the *htpR* mediated heat shock response, and responses to starvation, heavy metals, and other adverse stimuli. In the case of the SOS response (137), ~20 different genes, many coding for DNA repair enzymes and factors important in mutagenesis, are coordinately induced after DNA damage. DNA damage leads to activation of a specific proteinase function in the *recA* protein that cleaves a repressor protein, *lexA*. *LexA* protein binds to the regulatory region of SOS genes and, with its removal by activated *recA* protein, transcription of these genes is increased. Many SOS genes code for low abundance transcripts that are rapidly induced 2- to 10-fold by activated *recA* protein. Overexpression or constitutive expression of some SOS genes may be deleterious. Stress responses can be complex with some overlap between different regulons. For example, in *E. coli* many DNA damaging compounds induce the SOS regulon and certain heat shock genes (132).

The search for SOS-like responses in mammalian cells and most other eukaryotes has been limited since few DNA repair genes have been isolated. Recently, an increasing number of such genes have been isolated from yeast DNA repair mutants (35). In particular, the RAD2, RAD6, RAD51, RAD52, and RAD54 DNA repair genes have been found to be DNA damage inducible (35, 103). A good example of a specific DNA damage-inducible response is the RAD2 nucleotide excision repair gene that shares many characteristics of SOS genes: a role in DNA repair, low abundance RNA, rapid induction by DNA damage, and induction of 2- to 10-fold (103). The genes of certain other enzymes that are involved in DNA repair in yeast, such as DNA ligase (52) and DNA polymerase I (53), are also DNA damage-inducible. Cellular phenomena, such as induction of a recombinogenic function by DNA damaging agents in yeast (20), are suggestive of SOS-like functions. In addition to SOS-like genes, which are specifically induced by DNA damage, other DNA damage-inducible genes probably represent more general stress responses. For example, ubiquitin (129) and several other genes of unknown function (79) have been found to be induced by either DNA damage or by an unrelated type of stress, heat shock. Various other genes, many of unknown function, have been isolated on the basis of DNA damage inducibility (79, 107). Ruby and Szostak (107) have estimated that there may be 80 or more DNA damage-inducible genes; thus nearly 1% of the genes in yeast may play some role in the response to genotoxic stress.

Whether a SOS-like response is present in mammalian cells has been controversial for many years. Various cell survival studies support the assertion that pretreatment with a DNA damaging agent may provide some protection against a second later treatment. However, the magnitude of the protection is frequently much less than that seen in bacteria (91). Treatment of both marsupial and insect cells with protein synthesis inhibitors (which block inducible factors) immediately after DNA damage increased cytotoxicity (62, 87) and decreased mutagen-

icity (87). Such observations are also reminiscent of the SOS response in bacteria. Recent approaches, such as viral host reactivation experiments (91) and particularly transfection of plasmids containing DNA damage (96), indicate that prior exposure of the cells to DNA damage can increase repair and yield of undamaged plasmid or virus. One mammalian DNA repair gene, DNA polymerase-β, has been shown to be damage-inducible (33). This enzyme is presumed to be involved in the polymerization step of base excision repair such as after DNA damage by alkylating agents. Treatment of CHO cells with alkylating agents induced a rapid increase in DNA polymerase-β RNA, whereas other types of stress, such as heat shock, did not (33).

Another approach to study DNA damage-inducible responses in mammalian cells has been to isolate genes on the basis of level of increased expression after DNA damage. Based on results in bacteria and yeast, such an approach may identify genes involved in both specific or general stress responses. In human fibroblasts, Herrlich's group has isolated several cDNA clones coding for transcripts that are induced by DNA damage (2). Induction was mediated by an extracellular factor produced by cells treated with DNA damaging agents and by the tumor promoter 12-*O*-tetradecanoyl-phorbol-13-acetate, which is not a DNA damaging agent. Two induced genes have been identified as collagenase and metallothionein II, and similar results have been found for plasminogen (106). In human keratinocytes, transcripts coding for several different keratins, cystatin A, and glyceraldehyde phosphate dehydrogenase were induced 12 hours after cytotoxic doses of ultraviolet irradiation (54). The induction of these genes may represent general stress responses, and proteins such as collagenase and plasminogen activator may be involved in the response to tissue injury.

Recently, cDNA clones coding for over 20 different DNA damage-inducible transcripts have been isolated by hybridization subtraction in Chinese hamster ovary cells (32). The strategy of this study was to select transcripts that had some characteristics of SOS genes: low abundance, rapid induction, and induction of 2- to 10-fold. Many of these genes were rapidly induced by DNA damaging agents even at less cytotoxic doses than in earlier studies (2, 54, 106) in both rodent and human cells (32). The clones were divided into two general classes. In the first, induction only occurred after treatment with ultraviolet irradiation or other agents that produce DNA damage repaired by nucleotide excision repair. In the second class, induction also occurred after exposure to alkylating agents or H_2O_2, which is repaired by base excision mechanisms. Based on these results, the induction of these genes may represent stress responses that to some degree are specific for DNA damage.

DNA REPAIR DEFICIENT DISORDERS

This group of rare disorders will be dealt with only briefly here, for more comprehensive reviews see Refs. 3, 45, and 128. An overview of the symptoms, features, and deficiencies is given in Table 4.

TABLE 4. DNA DAMAGE SENSITIVE HUMAN HEREDITARY DISORDERS WITH ESTABLISHED OR POTENTIAL DNA REPAIR DEFICIENCY

Disorder	Risk of cancer	Clinical features	Characteristics
DNA repair deficiency			
Xeroderma pigmentosum	++++	Photosensitivity	Hypersensitive to UV.
		Neurological abnormalities	Defective excision repair.
		Mental impairment	9 complementation groups.
			Increased chromosome breakage and sister chromatid exchanges after UV.
Cockayne's syndrome	None	Dwarfism	Hypersensitivity to UV.
		Neurological abnormalities	Lack of preferential DNA repair.
		Mental retardation	Impaired post-UV DNA and RNA synthesis.
		Photosensitivity	
Bloom's syndrome	++++	Telangiectasia	Ligase I deficiency.
		Photosensitivity	Spontaneous chromosome breaks, aberrations and sister chromatid exchanges. Altered glycosylase.
		Immunodeficiency	
Probable Defect			
Fanconi's anemia	++++	Skeletal abnormalities	Spontaneous chromosome damage.
		Bone marrow hypofunction	Hypersensitivity to cross-linking agents.
		Mental deficiency	Possible deficiency in cross-link repair.
		Leukemia	
Ataxia telangiectasia	+++	Telangiectasia	Hypersensitivity to x-irradiation and some carcinogens.
		Cerebellar ataxia	Spontaneous chromosome rearrangements.
		Immunodeficiency	x-ray resistant DNA synthesis.
		Neurologic abnormalities	Possible deficiency in repair of strand breaks.
Suspected DNA repair defect			
Tricothiodystrophy (PIBID)	None	Telangiectasia	Possible defective excision repair.
		Sulfur deficient hair	
		Neurological abnormalities	
		Mental impairment	
Dyskeratosis congenita	++	Hyperpigmentation	Possible defective cross-link repair.
		Telangiectasia	
		Leukoplakia	
Nevoid basal cell carcinoma	+++	Skeletal abnormalities	Increased rate of spontaneous chromosome breaks and sister chromatid exchanges.
		Mental impairment	Possible deficiency in UV repair.
Gardner's syndrome	++++	Polyps in colon	Increased rate of sister chromatid exchanges after UV.
		Osteomas	
		Dental deformities	
No known repair defect			
Dysplastic nevus syndrome	++++	Dysplastic nevi	Hypersensitive to UV.
			Increased sister chromatid exchanges.
			Chromosomal rearrangements after UV.
Retinoblastoma	++++	Hypersensitive to ionizing irradiation	Hypersensitivity to ionizing irradiation.
		Ocular malignancy	Spontaneous chromosomal deletion.
		Dysmorphic features	

UV, ultraviolet irradiation.

XERODERMA PIGMENTOSUM

Clinical features of this disease include extreme photosensitivity associated with freckling, erythema, hypopigmented macules, telangiectasias, atrophy, scarring, and hyperpigmentation. Some of these features are seen in Figure 7A. Ultraviolet irradiation causes progressive skin damage leading to squamous cell carcinoma and multiple skin cancers including basal cell carcinomas and malignant melanoma in exposed skin areas. Some patients have developed internal malignancies including lung and a primary brain sarcoma at unusually young

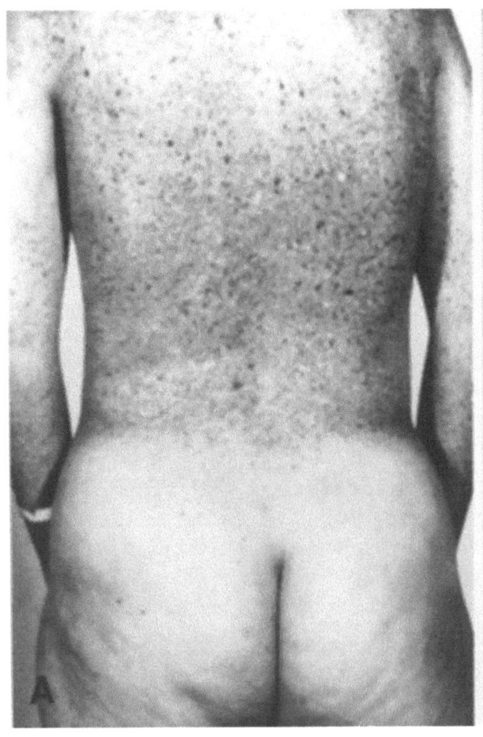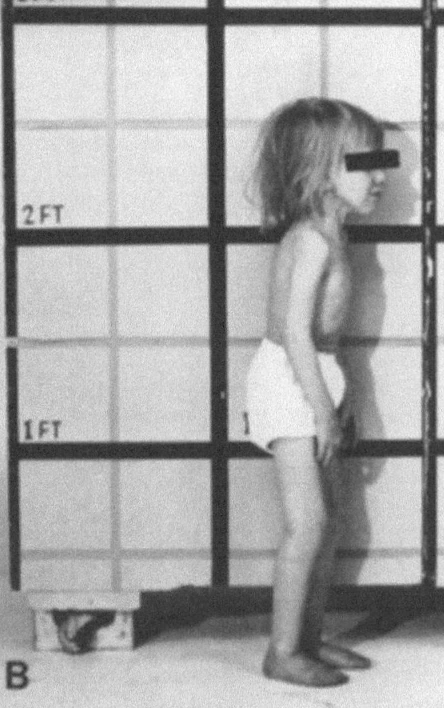

FIG. 7. Clinical features in xeroderma pigmentosum and Cockayne's syndrome. *A*, xeroderma pigmentosum. Note hypo- and hyperpigment macules and telangiectasia in sun-exposed areas. *B*, Cockayne's syndrome: 10-year female with CS. Note short stature, cachexia and dwarfism (photographs kindly obtained from J. H. Robbins).

ages (63). Multiple neurologic symptoms can be found in patients with this disease (64).

XP cells are hypersensitive to ultraviolet radiation, and many drugs and carcinogens cause abnormal biological responses including increased cell killing and an increased mutation rate (65). There are nine complementation groups of XP, indicating the involvement of at least nine genes in the repair process. Complementation group A has the lowest level of unscheduled DNA synthesis and the largest number of patients. Groups B and G have unscheduled DNA synthesis that is <10% of normal controls. Groups C, E, and F have levels of unscheduled DNA synthesis between 10 and 50% of normal (63). Although the variant class has normal unscheduled DNA synthesis, complementation group D has a unscheduled DNA synthesis level of ~25–50%.

A considerable research effort has been and is directed toward understanding the exact nature of the genetic defect in XP cells. For recent reviews, see Refs. 64, 65, 67. It appears that the repair deficiency is at an early step in the repair process such as recognition or incision (*cf.*, Fig. 2), but we still do not know which repair enzymes are deficient or lacking.

BLOOM'S SYNDROME

Clinical features include photosensitivity, butterfly rash across the malar region of the face, normally proportioned dwarfed body and moderate to severe immunodeficiency. Neurologic abnormalities are uncommon, but Bloom's syndrome patients have a very high risk for developing hemopoietic cancer. An estimated 20% of those affected will develop malignant disease by age 20 (40). Deficiencies in the immune system have been demonstrated in this disease (141). There are numerous cytogenetic abnormalities in most Bloom's syndrome patients such as a 15-fold increased rate of spontaneous

SCE as well as a high incidence of mitotic chiasmata. Mitotic crossing over, which is rare in normal human cells, is common in Bloom's syndrome cells. Nonhomologous translocations, allocyclic chromosomes, transverse breakage at centromeres are also frequent aberrations. Ultraviolet resistance appears to be decreased in some Bloom's syndrome fibroblasts (3). The considerable hypersensitivity in these cells may indicate a DNA repair deficiency, but most repair assays in these cells so far have been normal. However, Willis and Lindahl (145) and Chan (87) recently found that Bloom's syndrome lymphoblastoid cell lines have a deficiency of DNA ligase I, and evidence for an altered uracil DNA glycosylase in five Bloom's syndrome cell lines has recently been demonstrated (116, 135).

FANCONI'S ANEMIA

Fanconi's anemia is an autosomal recessive disease characterized by refractory anemia progressing to pancytopenia, congenital and developmental abnormalities, and an increased incidence of malignancy. Fanconi's anemia heterozygotes have been reported to have a threefold increased risk of developing malignancy over the United States white population. Studies of the cellular characteristics of Fanconi's anemia cells indicate a wide range of hypersensitivity. There is an increased incidence of spontaneous chromatid aberrations such as gaps, breaks, and chromosomal translocations. Further chromosomal aberrations are induced by cross-linking agents such as mitomycin C, nitrogen mustard, photoactivated psoralens, diepoxybutane, and cis-platinum diaminedichloride (37). Fujiwara found a defect in the ability to repair DNA interstrand cross-links after mitomycin C in some Fanconi's anemia cells (38), but other investigators have reported proficient cross-link repair in these cells.

COCKAYNE'S SYNDROME

Interestingly, there may now be a human disorder that is deficient specifically in the preferential DNA repair of active genes. Cockayne's syndrome (CS) is characterized by severe photosensitivity, dwarfism, cachexia, microcephaly, prognathism, and loss of facial adipose tissue (3) (Fig. 7B). Central nervous system manifestations of the syndrome however are the most disabling. These include mental retardation, spasticity, sensorineural deafness, cerebellar ataxia, dementia, incontinence, and normal pressure hydrocephalus. Most patients die before the third decade of progressive neurological degeneration. There appears to be no increased incidence of malignant disease in CS.

CS fibroblasts and lymphocytes demonstrate hypersensitivity to ultraviolet irradiation and certain carcinogens, although to a lesser degree than XP cells (136). Compared with normal cells, CS cells have a reduced capacity to reactivate ultraviolet irradiated adenoviruses (72) and to repair ultraviolet irradiated, transfected plasmid (58). Assays of DNA repair such as unscheduled DNA synthesis and repair replication have been normal. There is a lack of recovery of replicative DNA synthesis after ultraviolet damage in CS cells similar to that found in XP cells (72). It has also been demonstrated (77) that there is much less recovery of early RNA synthesis after ultraviolet damage in CS cells compared with normal human fibroblasts. Whereas no repair deficiency has been found at the level of the overall genome, it has been reported from different laboratories that CS cells appear to be deficient in the preferential DNA repair of active genes (78, M. K. Evans and V. A. Bohr, unpublished data). Many genes have been examined in different CS cell lines, and these genes are repaired with the same efficiency as the overall genome (which is repaired at a normal level). Also, the nuclear matrix associated DNA, which is preferentially repaired in normal human cells, is not preferentially repaired in CS cells (85). This disorder may thus have a mutation in some gene that normally is involved in the specific preferential repair of active regions. It is further possible that this specific DNA repair deficiency causes the disease, and it certainly warrants much study of this disorder.

CONDITIONS SUSPECT FOR DNA REPAIR DEFICIENCY

Although a repair deficiency has not yet been demonstrated, these disorders are hypersensitive to DNA damage and are often associated with high risk of cancer. The hypersensitivity to DNA damage in these diseases is, however, generally milder than that in the previously discussed diseases.

ATAXIA TELANGIECTASIA

Clinical manifestations include a progressive cerebellar ataxia with degeneration of Purkinje cells, oculocutaneous telangiectasias, progressive neurologic degeneration, premature graying, and skin atrophy. As with the other chromosome breakage syndromes (Fanconi's anemia and Bloom's syndrome), there is a significantly increased incidence of neoplastic disease (84). The considerable sensitivity of ataxia telangiectasia lymphocytes and cultured fibroblasts to the lethal effects of x-irradiation is a hallmark of the disease (89). This hypersensitivity extends to many other DNA-damaging agents (80). There does not appear to be a universal hypersensitivity to ultraviolet light or ultraviolet-mimetic chemicals in ataxia telangiectasia (73). Despite the proven x-irradiation hypersensitivity of ataxia telangiectasia cells, DNA synthesis is not inhibited in these cells. Whereas normal cells display inhibition of DNA synthesis after exposure to ultraviolet and x-irradiation ataxia telangiectasia cells have been found to have a radioresistant replication initiation and chain elongation mechanism (36, 89, 90). No definitive defect in DNA repair has been established in this syndrome.

NEVOID BASAL CELL CARCINOMA SYNDROME

Major clinical manifestations include multiple basal cell carcinomas, ectopic calcifications, multiple skeletal anomalies, kyphoscoliosis, ophthalmologic abnormalities, and in some cases mental retardation. There is a marked increased incidence of intracranial tumors. The basal cell carcinomas of nevoid basal cell carcinoma syndrome (NBCCS) differ from ordinary basal cell carcinomas in their histology and location. Approximately 65–75% of the affected individuals will develop malignant change in lesions.

Cytogenetic evaluation of the syndrome has been done by many investigators. Increased levels of spontaneous chromosome and chromatid breaks in fibroblasts and cultured lymphocytes (46) and increased levels of SCE in patients have been reported (105). Clonogenic survival studies (21) show that NBCCS cells are hypersensitive to x-irradiation, but there is no defective excision repair of x-irradiation-induced lesions. The effects of ultraviolet radiation on survival and repair efficiency of NBCCS was studied by Ringborg (99). Peripheral leukocytes of NBCCS patients when compared with normal controls demonstrated a 25% reduction in maximal DNA repair as measured by unscheduled DNA synthesis. There is still not enough evidence to establish a DNA repair defect in this disorder.

DYSPLASTIC NEVUS SYNDROME

Dysplastic nevus syndrome is an autosomal dominant disorder in which affected kindreds are at increased risk of developing hereditary cutaneous malignant melanoma. The dysplastic nevus is characterized by nuclear atypia and a disorderly growth pattern in melanocytes. Morphologically, they are characterized by irregularities in outline, pigmentation, and site of distribution. Greene et al. (42) have observed a cumulative lifetime probability of melanoma of ~56% in all blood line family members of patients with the dysplastic nevus syndrome. The risk is even higher in those family members with dysplastic nevi. Dysplastic nevus syndrome cells have been found to be hypersensitive to ultraviolet irradiation and to certain chemical carcinogens by some investigators (97). However, increased ultraviolet sensitivity is not a consistent finding in this syndrome. Alkaline elution measurements of DNA repair after chemical damage did not show any repair deficiency in dysplastic nevus syndrome cells (93).

GARDNER'S SYNDROME

Clinical stigmata include adenomatous polyps of the colon that arise between the ages of 15 and 25 years, concomitant sebaceous cysts, desmoid tumors, fibromas, osteomas, and dental deformities. Colon cancer appears in a very high percentage of Gardner's syndrome patients. Survival curves for some Gardner's syndrome cells showed intermediate survival between normal fibroblast curves and AT cells. Some Gardner's syndrome cells were also found to be more sensitive to ultraviolet irradiation than normal cells but not as sensitive as XP cells (56). Gardner's syndrome cells have been found to be hypersensitive to fluorescent light induced chromatid breaks (92). Gardner's syndrome cells showed no deficiency in unscheduled DNA synthesis but some deficiency in liquid holding recovery capacity, an indirect measurement of the repair of potentially lethal damage (74).

DYSKERATOSIS CONGENITA

Dyskeratosis congenita is a rare genodermatosis whose major clinical features include nail dystrophy, reticulated hyperpigmentation, and leukoplakia. In addition there is a severe atrophy of the skin on the fingers and toes, alopecia of eyebrows and eyelashes, growth retardation, telangiectasia, and mental retardation. Dyskeratosis congenita is also associated with an increased incidence of malignancy: approximately 16% of patients develop carcinomas (119).

The karyotype of dyskeratosis congenita cells is normal, but studies have demonstrated that some patients have abnormal rates of chromosome breakage (114). The rate of SCE in dyskeratosis congenita lymphocytes is twice as high as control values, whereas there is no increased chromosome breakage rate (18). Carter *et al.* (19) found that fibroblasts from two dyskeratosis congenita patients were slower to repair psoralen interstrand DNA cross-links than normal individuals. SCE rates of dyskeratosis congenita lymphocytes exposed to ultraviolet light and to psoralens were higher than those of normal individuals.

TRICHOTHIODYSTROPHY

Trichothiodystrophy is a broad-based term under which three similar syndromes are grouped. For a recent review, see Ref. 72. One syndrome, PIBIDS (photosensitivity, vulgar icthyosis, brittle sulfur deficient hair, impaired intelligence, diminished fertility, short stature), has been studied for its hypersensitivity and repair (26). These patients have noncongenital vulgar icthyosis, sulfur deficient brittle hair, decreased fertility, impaired intelligence, photosensitivity, central nervous system abnormalities, recurrent infections, and a DNA repair defect similar to that described in XP group D. There does not appear to be any increased risk of cancer associated with this disease. Several authors have investigated the DNA repair capacity of patients with PIBIDS. Stephanini *et al.* (124) found decreased levels of resistance and of unscheduled DNA synthesis in PIBIDS cells after ultraviolet irradiation, but normal repair after damage of the cells with many chemical agents. Fusion experiments with normal human cells and XPA cells resulted in the normalization of unscheduled DNA synthesis in PIBIDS cells (124). Lehman *et al.* (72) demonstrated impaired excision repair and a decreased RNA synthesis early after ultraviolet irradiation similar to those reported in CS cells in some trichothiodystrophy and PIBIDS cell lines. Although these previous investigations have suggested a DNA repair deficiency in trichothiodystrophy, recent studies show a considerable heterogeneity in the ultraviolet response among cells from trichothiodystrophy patients with some responses being normal (71).

RETINOBLASTOMA

Retinoblastoma is a rare childhood malignancy of the eye that occurs in a hereditary and a nonhereditary form. Patients with retinoblastoma who are carriers of the Rb gene are also at increased risk of developing osteosarcoma, Wilm's tumor, fibrosarcoma, and Ewing's sarcoma. A subset of patients with the hereditary type of retinoblastoma harbor a deletion in the long arm of chromosome 13. Studies in fibroblasts from retinoblastoma patients with this deletion have shown increased sensitivity to x-irradiation, whereas cells from patients without the deletion have normal sensitivity (142).

MER⁻ PHENOTYPE

This is not a hereditary disorder but a described DNA repair deficiency with probable important clinical implications. The mer⁻ phenotype was originally defined as a cellular deficiency in the ability to support the growth of adenovirus containing alkylation damage (28). This deficiency is due to a lack of functional O^6-alkylguanine-DNA alkyltransferase that can remove alkylation damage from the O^6 position of guanine in DNA (146). Although the mammalian gene has not been cloned and the protein not purified to homogeneity, the deficiency is probably due to a lack of this protein since expression of the bacterial gene with recombinant vectors restores normal sensitivity (109). The mer⁻ phenotype is found in ~10–20% of transformed human cell lines (28, 146); this includes both virus-transformed cell lines, chemically transformed cell lines, and tumor cell lines. Unlike hereditary diseases such as xeroderma pigmentosum, untransformed cells from the individual are normal, and often only one of several transformed lines are mer⁻. The frequency of the mer⁻ phenotype is far greater than would be expected from simple mutations. It is remarkably stable, and revertants are infrequent. Mer⁻ cells are hypermutable by many alkylating agents (146). Due to deficient repair the mer⁻ cells might accumulate more mutations in parts of the genome such as oncogenes than mer⁺ cells. This could play a role in malignant progression. Due to the increased cellular sensitivity to alkylating agents of mer⁻ tumor cells compared with a patient's normal untransformed cells, tumors with this phenotype might provide an opportunity for curative therapy with alkylating agents.

PERSPECTIVES

In the previous sections we have dealt with some pathogenetic aspects of DNA repair. We have reviewed features of these mechanisms and their role in human disease, and we have attempted to discuss some recent advances and approaches in this field. We should like to end with a brief discussion of some features we trust will be increasingly associated with DNA repair.

AGING

There has been much speculation and many experiments to clarify whether DNA repair was involved in the aging process. One prevalent theory suggests that these processes are a result of the accumulation of damage in the genome with the resulting loss of function of certain genes. It was, for example, found that mammals with longer life-spans had higher levels of nucleotide excision repair (110) and that cells of old rats contained approximately 800 DNA breaks more per genome than those of young rats (133). It has been postulated that during the aging process DNA repair mechanisms become increasingly error prone, resulting in an accumulation of DNA damage and eventually cell death (133). No conclusive evidence has, however, been presented to correlate DNA repair processes with aging. For a comprehensive review of the potential role of DNA repair in aging, see Ref. 139. Experiments so far have been based on DNA repair analyses in the overall genome, and with studies of DNA repair at the level of certain individual genes, some new interesting relationships may appear.

RISK OF CANCER

There have been studies correlating efficiencies of DNA repair with the risk of cancer. In a study in patients with familial polyposis and colorectal carcinoma Pero *et al.* (140) found a reduced level of unscheduled DNA synthesis in the lymphocytes of affected patients after N-acetoxy-$N2$-fluoroenyl-acetamide treatment. It has been proposed that DNA repair synthesis is a marker of predisposition to colorectal cancer (140). Kovacs and co-workers (60, 61) have studied unscheduled DNA synthesis after ultraviolet irradiation in lymphocytes from patients with cancer and in their first-degree relatives. Out of 41 patients with breast cancer 20 had decreased levels of thymidine incorporation compared with 3 of 27 in the normal control group. The second study was conducted on first-degree relatives of patients with breast cancer: 19 of 29 women who were daughters of women with breast cancer had reduced levels of unscheduled DNA synthesis; 17 of 25 women with sisters who were diagnosed with breast cancer had levels of DNA repair lower than control values. Furthermore, 9 of 10 women who had both mothers and sisters with breast cancer were found to have decreased levels of unscheduled DNA synthesis.

Bohr and Koeber (10) found decreased repair of strand breaks in patients with secondary cancer. Lower DNA repair capacities may be an important risk factor in the genesis of some of the most commonly occurring malignancies. It might be feasible to establish screening of DNA repair capacity as a part of preventive cancer screening.

DNA REPAIR AND NEURODEGENERATIVE DISEASES

Since patients with DNA repair disorders frequently have neurological manifestations, some research effort has been directed toward the role of DNA repair processes in neurological disease. Primary neuronal degeneration is common in XP patients, and in recent years some evidence has evolved to support the concept that XP neurons die because of the lethal accumulation of DNA damage (100, 102). A correlation exists between the age of the XP patient at the time of the onset of neurological symptoms and the relative sensitivity of his cells to ultraviolet damage (100). DNA repair defects may thus be involved in some neurological diseases, and this possibility has been investigated. Although no DNA repair defect has been established in neurologic diseases other than XP and Cockayne's syndrome, various hypersensitivities have been reported in several, listed in Table 5 (101, 115, 125). Huntington's chorea cells have been shown to be somewhat hypersensitive to the lethal effects of ionizing radiation and radiomimetic chemicals. Cell lines from patients with Alzheimer's and Parkinson's diseases were hypersensitive to x-irradiation damage, and cells from patients with Huntington's disease, familial dysautonomia, and Alzheimer's disease were hypersensitive to x-irradiation and alkylation damage. Sensitivity to both x-irradiation and alkylating agents has been reported in multiple system atrophy (idiopathic orthostatic hypotension). In Alzheimer's disease, studies have indicated a defect in the repair of alkylation damage (104), but other studies have not confirmed these findings (57). Thus many primary neuronal degenerations are hypersensitive to DNA damaging agents, and it may ultimately appear that DNA repair is important in neurological disease and that proficient DNA repair is necessary to maintain the integrity of the nervous system.

TABLE 5. HYPERSENSITIVITY TO DNA DAMAGE IN NEURODEGENERATIVE DISEASE

Disease	X-ray	UV
Xeroderma pigmentosum	−	+
Cockayne's syndrome	−	+
Ataxia telagiectasia	+	−
Huntington disease	+	−
Downs syndrome	+	−
Alzheimer's disease	+	−
Parkinson's disease	+	−
Usher's syndrome	+	−
Familial dysautonomia	+	−
Multiple system atrophy	+	−
Friedrich's ataxia	+	nt
Retinitis pigmentosum[a]	−	−
Amyotrophic lateral sclerosis[a]	−	nt
Spinal muscular atrophy[a]	nt	−
Multiple sclerosis[a]	−	−

UV, ultraviolet irradiation; +, hypersensitive; − not hypersensitive; nt, not tested. Table is based on Ref. 132 with modifications.

[a] Not primary neuronal degeneration.

ROLE OF DNA DAMAGE IN ATHEROSCLEROSIS

Evidence from various investigators has raised the possibility that DNA damage may be involved in etiology of atherosclerosis. Early atheromatous plaques have been found to be monoclonal which indicates that these lesions may be neoplastic (reviewed recently in Ref. 4). Altered expression of genes implicated in neoplastic growth, such as onc genes and growth factor genes, has been found in atheromatous plaques (118). It is well-known that most carcinogens (which initiate neoplastic transformation) are DNA damaging agents and mutagens. Cholesterol epoxides and other oxidation products of cholesterol, which may form *in vivo*, have been shown to be mutagenic (50, 118). Both oxidation products of cholesterol (50) and typical carcinogens, such as benzo(a)pyrene and 7, 12-dimethylbenz(a,h) anthracene (1), have been found to be atherogenic. Considering that mechanisms exist for the repair of DNA damage by these agents, DNA repair is probably important in modulating the effect of such damage in endothelial cells.

ROLE OF DNA REPAIR AND DNA DAMAGE-INDUCIBLE RESPONSES IN CHEMORESISTANT TUMOR CELLS

A serious problem in clinical oncology is the emergence of resistant tumor cells during chemotherapy. There appears to be multiple mechanisms for chemoresistance, including alterations in drug uptake and efflux, metabolism, binding to DNA, and DNA repair (47, 88). Lately, there have been suggestions that DNA repair may be important in resistance. For example, cis-diamminedichloroplatinum(II) (DDP) DNA adducts have been shown to be removed four-fold more rapidly in a DDP-resistant murine cell line compared with the parent line with normal sensitivity (30). Increased DNA repair, as measured by increased repair synthesis, has also been found in DDP-resistant human ovarian carcinoma cell lines (88). Elevated levels of DNA polymerase-β have been found in chemoresistant cell lines such as a DDP-resistant murine leukemia line (66). As discussed earlier, the DNA polymerase-β gene was recently found to be DNA damage-inducible (33), which raises the possibility that altered stress responses may have some role in chemoresistance. A similar argument can be made for metallothionein: metallothionein genes are DNA damage-inducible in both human (33) and rodent (34) cells. Increased expression of metallothionein has been found in chemoresistant tumor cells and has been associated with increased resistance to DNA damaging agents (55). Often chemoresistance appears multifactorial even in the same cell line (30, 47, 55, 88, 126) and cannot easily be explained by a mutation or other alteration in a single gene. However, if a regulatory factor that controlled the expression of a group (regulon) of stress response genes was altered in a chemoresistant cell, then this single change could produce various different effects.

As discussed, many factors may be involved in cellular chemoresistance. But it is becoming evident that induction of certain genes and DNA repair processes are important.

CONCLUDING REMARKS

As we have seen, DNA repair processes play a role in many aspects of pathogenetics and will likely be even more important as we gain more knowledge and can assess these processes at levels not previously possible. Aside from the discussed likely associations between DNA repair and cancer, neurological symptoms, and aging processes, many disorders that are either repair deficient or suspect are associated with frequent occurrence of immundeficiency. It is therefore possible that proficient DNA repair is necessary for maintenance of a normal immune system in humans.

At the very least we hope that the reader has become convinced that studies in DNA repair are important and worthwhile efforts in modern biomedical research.

Acknowledgments: We thank J. H. Robbins for photographs (Fig. 7) and critical reading of the manuscript.

REFERENCES

1. Albert RE, VanderLaan M, Burns FJ, Nishizumi M: Effect of carcinogens on chicken atherosclerosis. Cancer Res. 37:2232, 1977
2. Angel P, Poting A, Mallick U, Rahmsdorf HJ, Schorpp M, Herrlich P: Induction of metallothionein and other mRNA species by carcinogens and tumor promoters in primary human fibroblasts. Mol Cell Biol 6:1760, 1986
3. Arlett CF: Human repair defects. J Inherited Metab Disease 9 Suppl 1:69, 1986
4. Benditt, E. P. Origins of human atherosclerotic plaques: The role of altered gene expression. Arch Pathol Lab Med 112:997, 1988
5. Berger CA, Edenberg HJ: Pyrimidine dimers block SV40 replication forks. Mol Cell Biol 6:3443, 1986
6. Bohr VA: DNA repair and transcriptional activity in genes. J Cell Sci 90:175, 1988
7. Bohr VA, Hanawalt PC: Novobiocin does not affect DNA repair in an active gene. Carcinogenesis 7:1917, 1986
8. Bohr VA, Hanawalt PC: Enhanced repair of pyrimidine dimers in coding and non-coding genomic sequences in CHO cells expressing a prokaryotic DNA repair gene. Carcinogenesis 8:1333, 1987
9. Bohr VA, Hanawalt PC: Factor that affect the initiation of excision repair in chromatin. In DNA Repair and Its Inhibition, edited by Collins A, Johnson R, Downes C, p 109. Oxford, IRL Press, 1984
10. Bohr VA, Koeber L: DNA repair in lymphocytes from patients with secondary leukemia as measured by strand rejoining. Mutat Res DNA 146:219, 1985
11. Bohr VA, Okumoto DS: Analysis of frequency of pyrimidine dimers in specific genomic sequences. In DNA Repair: A Laboratory Manual, Vol. 3, edited by Friedberg EC, Hanawalt PC, p 347. New York, Marcel Dekker, 1988
12. Bohr VA, Okumoto DS, Hanawalt PC: Survival of UV-irradiated mammalian cells correlates with efficient DNA repair in an essential gene. Proc Natl Acad Sci USA 83:3830, 1986
13. Bohr VA, Okumoto DS, Ho L, Hanawalt PC: Characterization of a DNA repair domain containing the dihydrofolate reductase gene in CHO cells. J Biol Chem 261:16666, 1986
14. Bohr VA, Chu EYH, van Duin M, Hanawalt PC, Okumoto DS: Human repair gene restores normal pattern of preferential DNA repair in repair defective CHO cells. Nucl Acids Res 16:7397, 1988
15. Bohr VA, Phillips DH, Hanawalt PC: Heterogeneous DNA damage and repair in the mammalian genome. Cancer Res 47:6426, 1987
16. Bohr VA, Smith CA, Okumoto DS, Hanawalt PC: DNA repair in an active gene: Removal of pyrimidine dimers from the DHFR gene of CHO cells is much more efficient than the genome overall. Cell 40:359, 1985
17. Bohr VA, Wassermann K. DNA repair at the level of the gene. Trends Biochem Sci 13:429, 1988
18. Burgdorf W, Kurvink K, Cervenka J: Sister chromatid exchange

in dyskeratosis congenita lymphocytes. J Med Genet 14:256, 1977
19. Carter DM, Pan M, Gaynor A, McGuire JS, Sibrack L: Psoralen-DNA cross-linking photoadducts in dyskeratosis congenita: Delay in excision and promotion of sister chromatid exchange. J Invest Dermatol 73:97, 1979
20. Cundari E, Vellosi R, Galli A, Bronzetti G: Inducibility of gene conversion in Saccharomyces cerevisiae treated with MMS. Mutation Res 174:271, 1986
21. Chan G, Little JB: Cultured diploid fibroblasts from patients with nevoid basal cell carcinoma syndrome are hypersensitive to killing by ionizing radiation. Am J Pathol 3:50, 1982
22. Chan JYH, Becker FF, German J, Ray JH: Altered DNA ligase I activity in Bloom's syndrome cells. Nature 325:357, 1987
23. Chen DS, Bernstein H: Yeast gene RAD52 can substitute for page T4 gene 46 or 47 in carrying out recombination and DNA repair. Proc Natl Acad Sci USA 85:6821, 1988
24. Cleaver JE: Defective repair replication of DNA in xeroderma pigmentosum. Nature 218:652, 1968
25. Cohn SM, Lieberman MW: The use of antibodies to 5-bromo-2'-deoxyuridine for the isolation of DNA sequences containing excision repair sites. J Biol Chem 259:12456, 1984
26. Crovato A, Rabora F: PIBI(D)S syndrome trichothiodystrophy with xeroderma pigmentosum (Group D) mutation. J Am Acad Dermatol 16:940, 1987
27. Culotta V, Sollner-Webb B: Sites of topoisomerase I action on X. laevis ribosomal chromatin: Transcriptionally active rDNA has an ~200 bp repeating structure. Cell 52:585, 1988
28. Day RS III, Ziolkowski CHJ, Scudiero DA, Meyer SA, Lubiniecki AS, Girardi AJ, Galloway SM, Bynum GD: Defective repair of alkylated DNA by human tumour and SV40-transformed human cell strains. Nature 288:724, 1980
29. DNA Repair. A Laboratory Manual of Research Procedures, Vol 3, edited by Friedberg EC, Hanawalt PC, New York, Marcel Dekker, 1988
30. Eastman A, Schulte N: Enhanced repair as a mechanism of resistance to cis-diamminedichloroplatinum (II). Biochemistry 27:4730, 1988
31. Fornace AJ Jr: Recombination of parent and daughter strand DNA after UV-irradiation in mammalian cells. Nature 304:552, 1983
32. Fornace AJ Jr, Alamo I Jr, Hollander MC: DNA damage inducible transcripts in mammalian cells. Proc Natl Acad Sci USA 85:8800, 1988
33. Fornace AJ Jr, Hollander MC, Willson S: Induction of mammalian betapolymerase RNA by DNA damaging agents. Mol Cell Biol 9:851, 1989
34. Fornace AJ Jr, Schalch H, Alamo I Jr: Coordinate induction of metallothionein I and II in rodent cells by UV-irradiation. Mol Cell Biol 8:4716, 1988
35. Friedberg EC: DNA repair in the yeast Saccharomyces cerevisiae. Microbiol Rev 52:70, 1988
36. Friedberg EC: In DNA Repair. New York, WH Freeman, 1985
37. Fujiwara Y, Matsumoto A, Ishihashi M, Satoh Y: Heritable disorders of DNA repair: Xeroderma pigmentosum and fanconi's anemia. Curr Probl Dermatol 17:182, 1987
38. Fujiwara Y, Tatsumi M, Sasaki MS: Cross-link repair in human cells and its possible defect in Fanconi's anemia cells. J Mol Biol 113:635, 1977
39. Ganesan, AK: Persistence of pyrimidine dimers during post-replication repair in UV-irradiated E. coli K12. J Mol Biol 87:103, 1974
40. German J: Bloom's syndrome. VII. Progress report for 1978. Clin Genet 15:361, 1979
41. Gilmour DS, Pflugfelder G, Wang JC, Lis JT: Topoisomerase I interacts with transcribed regions in Drosophila cells. Cell 44:401, 1986
42. Greene M, Clark W, Tucker MA, Elder D, Kraemer K, Thompson J, Matozzo I, Fraser M: Aquired precursors of cutaneous malignant melanoma, the familial dysplastic nevus syndrome. New Engl J Med 312:19, 1985
43. Hall JD, Mount DW: Mechanisms of DNA replication and mutagenesis in UV-irradiated bacteria and mammalian cells. Prog Nucleic Acid Res 25:1, 1981
44. Hanawalt PC, Cooper PK, Ganesan AK, Smith CA: DNA repair in bacteria and mammalian cells. Ann Rev Biochem 48:783, 1979

45. Hanawalt PC, Sarasin A: Cancer-prone hereditary diseases with DNA processing abnormalities. Trends Genet May:124, 1986
46. Happle R, Hoehn: Cytogenetic studies on cultured fibroblast-like cells derived from basal cell carcinoma tissue. Clin Genet 4:17, 1973
47. Harris AL, Hickson ID: Drug resistance, DNA repair and growth factors. In Resistance to Antineoplastic Drugs, edited by Kessel D, p 234. Boca Raton, CRC Press, 1988
48. Ho L, Bohr VA, Hanawalt PC: Demethylation enhances removal of pyrimidine dimers from the overall genome and from specific DNA sequences in CHO cells. Mol Cell Biol 9:1594, 1989
49. Holliday R: A mechanism for gene conversion in fungi. Genet Res 5:282, 1964
50. Imai H, Werthessen NT, Subramanyam V, Lequesne PW, Soloway AN, Kanisawa M: Angiotoxicity of oxygenated sterols and possible precursors. Science 207:651, 1980
51. Jachyjmczyk WJ, von Borstel RC, Mowat MRA, Hastings PJ: Repair of interstrand cross-links in DNA of Saccharomyces cerevisiae requires 2 systems for DNA repair: The RAD3 and the RAD51 system. Mol Gen Genet 182:196, 1981
52. Johnson AL, Barker DG, Johnston LH: Induction of yeast DNA ligase genes in exponential and stationary phase cultures in response to DNA damaging agents. Curr Genet 11:107, 1986
53. Johnston LH, White JHM, Johnson AL, Lucchini G, Plevani P: The yeast DNA polymerase I transcript is regulated in both mitotic cell cycle and in meiosis and is also induced after DNA damage. Nucleic Acids Res 15:5017, 1987
54. Kartasova T, Ponec M, Van de Putte P: Induction of proteins and mRNAs after UV irradiation of human epidermal keratinocytes. Exp Cell Res 174:421, 1988
55. Kelley AL, Basu A, Teicher BA, Hacker MP, Hamer DH, Lazo JS: Overexpression of metallothionein confers resistance to anticancer cells. Science 241:1813, 1988
56. Kinsella TJ, Little JB, Nove J, Weichselbaum RR, Li FP, Meyer RJ, Marchetto DJ, Patterson WB: Heterogeneous response to X-Ray and UVL irradiations of cultured skin fibroblasts in two families with Gardner's syndrome. J Natl Cancer Inst 68:697, 1982
57. Kinsiella TJ, Dobson PP, Fornace Jr AJ, Barrett SF, Ganges MB, Robbins JH: Alzheimer's disease fibroblasts have normal repair of N-methyl-N-nitro-N-nitrosoguanine induced DNA damage determined by the alkaline elution technique. Biochem Biophys Res Commun 149:355, 1987
58. Klocker H, Schneider R, Burtscher HJ, Auer B, Hirsch-Kauffman M, Schweigher M: Transient expression of a plasmid gene, a tool to study Fanconi's anemia repair in human cells: Defect of DNA repair in Cockayne Syndrome one thymine cylcobutane dimer is sufficient to block transcription. Eur J Cell Biol 39:346, 1985
59. Kohn KW, Steigbigel NH, Spears CL: Cross-linking and repair of DNA in sensitive and resistant strains of E. coli treated with nitrogen mustard. Proc Natl Acad Sci USA 53:1154, 1965
60. Kovacs E, Almedral A: Reduced DNA repair synthesis in healthy women having first degree relatives with breast cancer. Eur J Can Clin Oncol 23:1051, 1987
61. Kovacs E, Stucki D, Weber W, Muller H: Impaired DNA repair synthesis in lymphocytes of breast cancer patients. Eur J Can Clin Oncol 22:863, 1986
62. Koval TM: Inducible repair of ionizing radiation damage in higher eukaryotic cells. Mutation Res 173:291, 1986
63. Kraemer KH: Heritable diseases with increased sensitivity to cellular injury. In Update: Dermatology in General Medicine, edited by Fitzpatrick TB, Eisen AZ, Wolff K, Freedberg IM, Austen KF, p 113. New York, McGraw Hill, 1983
64. Kraemer KH, Myung ML, Scotto MSJ: Xeroderma pigmentosum. Arch Dermatol 123:241, 1987
65. Kraemer KH, Slor H: Xeroderma pigmentosum. Clin Dermatol 3:1, 1985
66. Kraker AJ, Moore CW: Elevated DNA polymerase beta activity in a cis-diamminedichloroplatinum (II) resistant P388 murine leukemia cell line. Cancer Lett 38:307, 1988
67. Lambert WC, Lambert M: DNA repair deficiency and cancer in xeroderma pigmentosum. Cancer Rev 7:56, 1987
68. Lan KSY, Smerdon MJ: A nonuniform distribution of excision repair synthesis in nucleosome core DNA. Biochemistry 24:7771, 1985
69. Leadon SA: Differential repair of DNA damage in specific nucleo-

tide sequences in monkey cells. Nucleic Acids Res 14:8979, 1986
70. Leadon SA, Snowden MM: Differential repair of DNA damage in the human metallothionein gene family. Mol Cell Biol 8:5331, 1988
71. Lehmann AR, Arlett CF, Broughton BC, Harcourt SA, Steingrimsdottir H, Stefanini M, Taylor AMR, Natarajan AT, Green S, King MD, Mackie RM, Stephenson JBP, Tolmie JL: Trichothiodystrophy, a human DNA repair disorder with heterogeneity in the cellular response to UV light. Cancer Res 48:6090, 1988
72. Lehmann AR: Cockayne's syndrome and trichothiodystrophy: Defection repair without cancer. Cancer Rev 7:82, 1987
73. Lehmann AR, Kirk-Bell S, Arlett CF, Harcourt SA, de Weerd-Kastelein EA, Keijzer W, Hall-Smith P: Repair of UV damage in a variety of human fibroblast cell strains. Cancer Res 37:904, 1977
74. Little JB, Nove J, Weichselbaum RR: Abnormal sensitivity of diploid skin fibroblasts from a family with Gardner's syndrome to the lethal effects of x-irradiation, uv light and mitomycin-C. Mutation Res 70:241, 1980
75. Loveday KS, Latt SA: Search for DNA interchange corresponding to SCE in Chinese hamster ovary cells. Nucleic Acids Res 5:4087, 1978
76. Madhani HD, Bohr VA, Hanawalt PC: Differential DNA repair in transcriptionally active and inactive proto-oncogenes: c-*abl* and c-*mos*. Cell 45:417, 1986
77. Mayne LV, Lehmann AR: Failure of RNA synthesis to recover after UV irradiation: An early defect in cells from individuals with Cockayne's syndrome and xeroderma pigmentosum. Cancer Res 42:1473, 1982
78. Mayne LV, Mullender LHF, van Zeeland AA: Cockayne's syndrome: A UV sensitive disorder with a defect in the repair of transcribing DNA but normal overall excision repair. In Mechanisms and Consequences of DNA Damage Processing, UCLA Symposia on Molecular and Cellular Biology, New Series, vol 83, edited by Friedberg EC, Hanawalt PC, p 349, New York, Alan R. Liss Inc, 1988
79. McClanahan T, McEntee K: DNA damage and heat shock dually regulate genes in *Saccharomyces cerevisiae*. Mol Cell Biol 6:90, 1986
80. McKinnon PJ: Ataxia telangiectasia: An inherited disorder of ionizing radiation sensitivity in man. Hum Genet 75:197, 1987
81. Mellon IM, Bohr VA, Smith CA, Hanawalt PC: Preferential DNA repair of an active gene in human cells. Proc Natl Acad Sci USA 83:8878, 1986
82. Mellon I, Spivak G, Hanawalt PC: Selective removal of transcription-blocking DNA damage from the transcribed strand of the mammalian DHFR gene. Cell 51:241, 1987
83. Meselson M: Formation of hybrid DNA by rotary diffusion during genetic recombination. J Mol Biol 71:795, 1972
84. Morrell D, Cromartie E, Swift M: Mortality and cancer incidence in 263 patients with ataxia telangiectasia. J Natl Cancer Inst 77:89, 1986
85. Mullenders LHF, van Kesteren van Leeuwen AC, van Zeeland AA, Natarajan AT: Nuclear matrix associated DNA is preferentially repaired in normal human fibroblasts, exposed to a low dose of UV light but not in Cockayne's syndrome fibroblasts. Nucl Acids Res 16:10607, 1988
86. Okumoto DS, Bohr VA: DNA repair in the metallothionein gene increases with transcriptional activation. Nucl Acids Res 15:10021, 1987
87. Overberg R, Chandrasena G, Rupert CS: Radiation-induced recovery processes in cultured marsupial cells. Mutation Res 194:83, 1988
88. Ozols RF, Masuda H, Hamilton TC: Mechanisms of cross-resistance between radiation and antineoplastic drugs. Natl Cancer Inst Monogr 6:159, 1988
89. Painter RB: Ataxia Telangiectasia: Genetics, Neuropathology and Immunology of a Degenerative Disease of Childhood, edited by Gatti RA, Swift M. New York, Liss, p 167, 1985
90. Painter RB, Young BR: Radiosensitivity in Ataxia telangiectasia: A new explanation. Proc Natl Acad Sci USA 77:7315, 1980
91. Paoletti C: Inducible responses to DNA damages, CNRS symposium. Biochimie 64:541, 1982
92. Parshad R, Sanford KK, Jones GM: Chromatid damage induced by fluorescent light during G2 phase in normal and Gardner's syndrome fibroblasts. Interpretation in terms of deficient DNA repair. Mutat Res 151:57, 1985
93. Perera MIR, Um KI, Greene MH, Waters HL, Bredberg A, Kraemer KH: Hereditary dysplastic nevus syndrome: Lymphoid cell ultraviolet hypermutability in association with increased melanoma susceptibility. Cancer Res 46:1005, 1986
94. Pero RW, Markowitz M, Powell J, Johnson D, Lund-Pero M, Winawer S, Miller DG: DNA repair synthesis as a marker of predisposition to colorectal cancer. Prog Clin Biol Res 279:289, 1988
95. Pienta KJ, Coffey DS: A structural analysis of the role of the nuclear matrix and DNA loops in the organization of the nucleus and chromosome. J Cell Sci Suppl 1:123, 1984
96. Protic M, Roilides E, Levine AS, Dixon K: Enhancement of DNA repair capacity of mammalian cells by carcinogen treatment. Somat Cell Mol Genet 14:351, 1988
97. Ramsay RG, Chen P, Imray FP, Kidson C, Lavin MF, Hockey A: Familial melanoma associated with dominant UV radiation sensitivity. Cancer Res 42:2909, 1982
98. Reeves R: Transcriptionally active chromatin. Biochim Biophys Acta 782:343, 1984
99. Ringborg U, Lambert B, Landegren J, Lewensohn R: Decreased uv-induced DNA repair synthesis in peripheral leukocytes from patients with novoid basal cell carcinoma syndrome. J Invest Dermatol 76:268, 1981
100. Robbins JH: A childhood neurodegeneration due to defective DNA repair: A novel concept of disease based on studies of xeroderma pigmentosum. J Child Neurol, in press
101. Robbins JH, Brumback RA, Polinsky RJ, Wirtschafter JD, Tarone RE, Scudiero DA, Otsuka F: Hypersensitivity to DNA damaging agents in abiothrophies: A new explanation for degeneration of neurons, photoreceptors, and muscle in Alzheimers, Parkinson and Huntington diseases, Retinitis pigmentosa and Duchennes muscular dystrophy. In Molecular Biology of Aging, edited by Woodhead AD, Blackett AD, Hollaender A, p 315. New York, Plenum, 1985
102. Robbins JH, Polinsky RJ, Moshell AN: Evidence that lack of deoxyribonucleic acid repair causes death of neurons in xeroderma pigmentosum. Ann Neurol 13:682, 1983
103. Robinson GW, Nicolet CM, Kalainov D, Friedberg EC: A yeast excision-repair gene is inducible by DNA damaging agents. Proc Natl Acad Sci USA 83:1842, 1986
104. Robison SH, Munzer BS, Tandan RUP, Bradley WG: Alzheimers disease cells exhibit defective repair of alkylating agent-induced DNA damage. Ann Neurol 21:250, 1987
105. Romke C, Godde-Salz E, Grote W: Investigations of chromosomal stability in the Gorlin-Goltz syndrome. Arch Dermatol Res 277:370, 1985
106. Rotem N, Axelrod JH, Miskin R: Induction of urokinase-type plasminogen activator by UV light in human fetal fibroblasts is mediated through a UV-induced secreted protein. Mol Cell Biol 7:622, 1987
107. Ruby SW, Szostak JW: Specific *Saccharomyces cerevisiae* genes are expressed in response to DNA-damaging agents. Mol Cell Biol 5:75, 1985
108. Rupp WD, Howard-Flanders P: Discontinuities in the DNA synthesized in an excision-deficient strain of E. coli following UV irradiation. J Mol Biol 31:291, 1968
109. Samson L, Derfler B, Waldstein EA: Suppression of human DNA alkylation-repair defects by E. coli DNA-repair genes. Proc Natl Acad Sci USA 83:5607, 1986
110. Tice RR, Setlow RB: DNA repair and replication in aging organisms and cells. In Handbook of the Biology of Aging, edited by Finch CE, Schneider EL, p 173. New York, Von Nostrand Reinhold, 1985
111. Sancar A, Sancar GB: DNA repair enzymes. Ann Rev Biochem 57:29, 1988
112. Schiestl RH, Prakash S: RAD1, an excision repair gene of Saccharomyces cerevisiae, is also involved in recombination. Mol Cell Biol 8:3619, 1988
113. Scicchitano DA, Hanawalt PC: Repair of *N*-methyl purines in specific DNA sequences in Chinese hamster ovary cells: Absence of strand specificity in the dihydrofolate reductase gene. Proc Natl Acad Sci USA 86:3050, 1989
114. Scoggins RB, Prescott KJ, Asher GH, Blaylock WK, Bright RW: Dyskeratosis congenita with fanconi type anemia: Investigations

of immunologic and other defects. Clin Res 19:409, 1971

115. Scudiero DA, Polinsky RJ, Brumback RA, Tarone RE, Nee LE, Robbins JH: Alzheimer disease fibroblasts are hypersensitive to the lethal effects of a DNA-damaging chemical. Mutat Res 159:125, 1986

116. Seal G, Brech K, Karp SJ, Cool BL, Sirover MA: Immunological lesions in human uracil DNA glycosylase: Association with Bloom Syndrome. Proc Natl Acad Sci USA 85:2339, 1988

117. Setlow RB: Thory presentation. A background summary. In Modern Biological Theories of Aging, edited by Warner HR, Butler RN, Sprott RL, Sneider EL, p 177. New York, Raven, 1987

118. Sevanian A, Peterson AR: Cholesterol epoxide is a direct acting mutagen. Proc Natl Acad Sci USA 81:4198, 1988

119. Sirinavin C, Trowbridge A: Dyskeratosis congenita: Clinical features and genetic aspects. J Med Genet 12:339, 1975

120. Smerdon MJ, Lieberman MW: Nucleosome rearrangements in human chromatin during UV-induced DNA repair synthesis. Proc Natl Acad Sci USA 75:4238, 1978

121. Smith CA: DNA repair in specific sequences in mammalian cells. J Cell Sci Suppl 6:225, 1987

122. Sognier MA, Hittelman WN: Mitomycin-induced chromatid breaks in HeLa cells: A consequence of incomplete DNA replication. Cancer Res 46:4032, 1986

123. Song K-Y, Chekuri L, Rauth S, Ehrlich S, Kucherlapati R: Effect of double-strand breaks on homologous recombination in mammalian cells and extracts. Mol Cell Biol 5:3331, 1985

124. Stefanini M, Lagomarsini P, Arlett CF, Marinoni S, Barrone C, Crovato F, Trevisan, Cordone G, Nuzzo F: Xeroderma pigmentosum (complementation group D) mutation is present in patients affected by trichothiodystrophy with photosensitivity. Hum Genet 74:107, 1986

125. Tarone RE, Otsuka F, Robbins JH: A sensitive assay for detecting hypersensitivity to ionizing irradiation in lymphoblastoid lines from patients with Duchenne muscular dystrophy and primary neuronal degenerations. J Neurol Sci 65:367, 1984

126. Teicher BA, Holden SA, Kelley MJ, Shea TC, Cucchi CA, Rosowsky A, Henner WD, Frei E, III: Characterization of a human squamous carcinoma cell line resistant to cis-diamminedichloroplatinum (II). Cancer Res 47:388, 1987

127. Thomas DC, Morton AG, Bohr VA, Sancar A: A general method for quantitating bulky aducts in mammalian genes. Proc Natl Acad Sci USA 85:3723, 1988

128. Timme TL, Moses RE: Diseases with DNA damage processing defects. Am J Med Sci 295:40, 1988

129. Treger JM, Heichman KA, McEntee K: Expression of the yeast UBI4 gene in response to DNA-damaging agents and in meiosis. Mol Cell Biol 6:1132, 1988

130. van Zeeland AA, Smith CA, Hanawalt PC: Sensitive determination of pyrimidine dimers in DNA of UV-irradiated mammalian cells. Mutat Res 82:173, 1981

131. van Duin M, de Wit J, Odijik H, Westerveld A, Yasui A, Koken MHM, Hoeymakers JHJ, and Bootsma D: Molecular characterization of the human excision repair gene ERCC-1: cDNA cloning and aminoacid homology with the yeast DNA repair gene RAD 10. Cell 44:913, 1986

132. VanBogelen RA, Kelley PM, Neidhardt FC: Differential induction of heat shock, SOS, and oxidation stress regulons and accumulation in E. coli. J Bacteriol 169:26, 1987

133. Vijg J, Knook DL: DNA repair in relation to the aging process. J Am Geriatr Soc 35:532, 1987

134. Villani G, Boiteux S, Radman M: Mechanism of UV-induced mutagenesis: Extent and fidelity of in vitro DNA synthesis on irradiated templates. Proc Natl Acad Sci USA 75:3037, 1978

135. Vollberg TM, Seal G, Sirover MA: Monoclonal antibodies detect conformational abnormality of uracil DNA glycosylase in Bloom syndrome cells. Carcinogenesis 8:1725, 1987

136. Wade MH, Chu EHY: Effects of DNA damaging agents on cultured fibroblasts derived from patients with cockayne syndrome. Mutation Res 59:49, 1979

137. Walker GC: Mutagenesis and inducible responses to DNA damage in E. coli. Microbiol Rev 48:60, 1984

138. Wang Y, Maher VM, Liskay RM, McCormick JJ: Carcinogens can induce homologous recombination between duplicated chromosomal sequences in mouse L cells. Mol Cell Biol 8:196, 1988

139. Warner H, Butler R, Spott R, Schneider E, eds: Modern Biological Theories of Aging, Vol 31. New York, Raven, 1987

140. Pero RW, Miller DG, Lipkin M: Reduced capacity for DNA repair synthesis in patients with or genetically predisposed to colorectal cancer. J Natl Cancer Inst 70:867, 1983

141. Weemaes CMR: Immune responses in 4 patients with bloom syndrome. Clin Immunol Immunopathol 12:12, 1979

142. Weichselbaum RR, Nove J, Little JB: Skin fibroblasts from a D-deletion type retinoblastoma patients are abnormally X-ray sensitive. Nature 266:726, 1977

143. West SC, Cassuto E, Howard-Flanders P: recA protein promotes homologous-pairing and strand-exchange reactions between duplex DNA molecules. Proc Natl Acad Sci USA 78:2100, 1981

144. Wilkins RJ, Hart RW: Preferential DNA repair in human cells. Nature 247:35, 1974

145. Willis AE, Lindahlt: DNA ligase I deficiency in Bloom's syndrome. Nature 325:355, 1987

146. Yarosh DB: The role of 06-methylguanine-DNA methyltransferase in cell survival, mutagenesis and carcinogenesis. Mutat Res 145:1, 1985

147. Yuspa SH, Poirier MC: Chemical carcinogenesis: From animal models to molecular models in one decade. Adv Cancer Res 50:25, 1988

148. Zolan ME, Smith CA, Calvin NM, Hanawalt PC: Rearrangement of mammalian chromatin structure following excision repair. Nature 299:462, 1982

From: *Pathology Reviews • 1990* Edited by: E. Rubin and I. Damjanov Copyright © 1990 The Humana Press Inc., Clifton, NJ

Biology of Disease
Molecular Diagnosis of Human Cancer

MARTIN J. CLINE

School of Medicine, Center for Health Sciences, University of California, Los Angeles, California

INTRODUCTION

The discovery of oncogenes introduced an era in which it is possible to identify genetic elements involved in the initiation and progression of malignant diseases (9, 10, 36, 61, 75, 126, 167). In some cases, these genetic elements can be used as molecular markers of human cancers.

Proto-oncogenes were originally defined as normal genes similar in structure to cancer-causing genes of certain retroviruses (10). This definition is too restrictive, and it is now known that cancer-related genes exist that have never been found in retroviruses. A better definition of a proto-oncogene is a normal cellular gene involved in cell proliferation and differentiation, which has the potential of contributing to development of a malignancy when its structure or expression is altered (9, 75). Many activated proto-oncogenes act dominantly to produce malignancy; however, increasing evidence suggests that other normal gene sequences act to suppress the malignant phenotype and that malignancy is fully expressed only when these cancer suppressor genes are lost or inactivated (19, 79).

Proto-oncogenes have been classified according to the location or biological activity of their products: secretory, cell surface, cytoplasmic, or nuclear proteins. The secreted and external cell surface oncogene proteins are of two types: growth factors such as *c-SIS* and cell surface receptors such as *c-ERBB-1* and *c-FMS*. The growth factor receptors have a tripartite structure consisting of an external domain that interacts with the soluble growth factor, a lipid-soluble transmembrane domain, and an intracytoplasmic domain. The last is often a tyrosine kinase that transmits intracellular signals when activated by binding of ligand to the external domain. The known oncoproteins located at the inner cell membrane or in the cytoplasm also comprise two classes: protein kinases such as c-SRC and *c-ABL* and G proteins such as *c-Ha-RAS*. Both types are thought to be involved in intracellular signaling from the cell membrane. Several oncoproteins are primarily nuclear in location. Some of these such as *c-MYC* and *c-JUN* have been shown to bind DNA and are thought to be regulators of gene expression. The number of identified proto-oncogenes is increasing as new ones are identified by their biological activity or by structural homology with other known genes. About 50 proto-oncogenes are known; many have homologs among the viral oncogenes (9, 167). Table 1 lists the major families of proto-oncogenes and important examples.

Various structural changes can convert a normal proto-oncogene to a cancer gene; a process often called activation. Three types of activating events have been found in human tumors, examples of which are given in Table 2. Table 2 has been compiled from the recent literature and a study population examined in the author's laboratory consisting of 295 adenocarcinomas of breast, colon, lung, liver, stomach, kidney, and ovary, 28

TABLE 1. CLASSES OF PROTO-ONCOGENES

Examples	Proposed activity	Location	Ref.
Growth factors			
c-SIS	B chain PDGF	Secreted	8, 164
INT-2	Fibroblast growth factor	?	18, 151
HST	related		
Growth factor receptors			
c-ERBB-1	Receptor EGF	Membrane	34
c-ERBA	Receptor thyroid hormone	Cytoplasm	168
c-ERBB-2	Probable receptor	Membrane	26, 138
C-FMS	Receptor CSF-1	Membrane	139
c-MET, c-ROS-1	Probable receptors	?	31, 108
Protein kinases			
c-ABL, SRC	Protein kinases (tyrosine)	Inner membrane/ cytoplasm	60, 61
FES, TKL			
YES, FGF, etc.			
c-MIL, RAF	Protein kinases (serine/ threonine)	Cytoplasm	14
G proteins			
c-RAS-Ha	Signal transduction	Cytoplasm	63
c-RAS-Ki	GTP binding, GTPase		
N-RAS	?	?	16, 152
Nuclear			
c-MYC	DNA binding	Nucleus	29
N-MYC	?	Nucleus	104
c-MYB	?	Nucleus	92
p53	? regulator DNA polymerase-α	Nucleus	51
c-JUN, c-FOS	Transcription regulation	Nucleus	12
Undefined			
ETS-1, 2	Unknown		20
ERG			

PDGF, platelet-derived growth factor; EGF, epidermal growth factor.

TABLE 2. PROTO-ONCOGENES FREQUENTLY ALTERED IN HUMAN CANCER

Gene	Amplification		Rearrangement		Mutation		Tumors involved	Ref.
	No.	%	No.	%	No.	%		
c-MYC	447	4.3	329	0.9	—	?	B and T lymphomas Carcinomas Sarcomas	29, 80, 91
N-MYC	262	1.1	262	0	—	?	Neuroendocrine	134, 136
c-RAS-Ki	352	2.0	352	0	>100	50–95	Adenocarcinomas	18, 125
c-RAS-Ha	350	0.6	350	0	>100	<10	Adenocarcinomas	44, 119
N-RAS	230	0	230	0	>100	10–50	AML, T-ALL, MDS	57
c-ERBB-1	239	5.9	239	0	—	?	Squamous Ca	85
c-ERBB-2	428	7.1	338	0	—	?	Breast, gastric, renal	73, 132
p53	451	0.9	307	5.6	—	?	CML, osteosarcoma	1, 92
c-ABL	284	0	>100	>95	?	?	CML	53, 78
			>20	2–25			ALL	

Precise figures derive from a study population of 672 malignancies of various types. Approximate figures are derived both from study population and literature.

squamous cancers, 32 sarcomas, 24 neuroendocrine tumors, 265 hematological malignancies, and 28 miscellaneous cancers.

A mutation can cause a proto-oncogene to make an altered protein. This phenomenon has been best defined for genes of the *RAS* family (16, 22, 39, 44, 93, 97, 121) where mutations in critical codons change protein configuration so that function is altered (93). Proto-oncogenes can also be activated by gene duplication events that result in an amplified DNA fragment containing from 3 to more than 100 copies of the gene (91). Such amplified genes make very high levels of messenger RNA (mRNA) and oncogene protein. A third mechanism of proto-oncogene activation is by gene rearrangement often as a result of a chromosomal rearrangement. The rearranged oncogenes either make altered products or increased amount of normal product. Examples are the *bcr/c-ABL* rearrangement in chronic myelocytic leukemia (25, 35, 53, 78, 142) and the *c-MYC* rearrangement in Burkitt's lymphoma (21, 29, 114, 117, 153). Additional mechanisms of proto-oncogene activation probably exist in human tumors, since there are descriptions of alterations of transcription control regions by insertion of viral sequences in animal tumors and a recent case of a human breast cancer with disruption of the *c-MYC* gene by a mobile genetic element (100).

DETECTION SYSTEMS

At present most systems for detecting molecular changes in cancer genes are based on well-established nucleic acid hybridization techniques (89). Recently, however, antibodies to proteins of some normal and mutated proto-oncogenes have been described (46, 145, 160) and are commercially available. In general a good antibody is superior to *in situ* nucleic acid hybridization when the objective is to examine the distribution of oncogene product in individual cells or to identify overexpression of a gene in a subpopulation of cells in a tissue. However, for detecting a point mutation in a clone of malignant cells or detecting expression of an aberrant mRNA, hybridization techniques are more sensitive than conventional immunohistochemistry especially when hybridization is combined with methods of specific nucleic acid amplification such as the polymerase chain reaction (PCR). The PCR utilizes synthetic oligodeoxynucleotide primers and thermostable DNA polymerase to enzymatically amplify specific gene fragments. A 100,000-fold amplification can be achieved in a few hours, and DNA can be analyzed from a single hair follicle (56) or even a single cell. Crude cell lysates can be used, thereby eliminating the need for DNA purification. PCR is also applicable to paraffin-embedded fixed tissues as well as fresh tissues (65). After DNA amplification by PCR, the presence of a mutation can be detected by use of specific hybridization probes containing the anticipated mutation (16, 124), by cleavage with the enzyme RNAase A of nucleic acid duplexes containing a single base mismatch (4), or by direct sequencing of the amplified DNA fragment (131).

Some gene rearrangements involve too large a piece of DNA to effectively utilize PCR, which is limited to fragments of DNA no longer than 1000–2000 base pairs. In such situations it may be more convenient to work with the mRNA transcribed from the rearranged gene. For example, the rearrangement of the breakpoint cluster region (*bcr*) and *c-ABL* genes in chronic myelocytic leukemia (CML) involves stretches of DNA of several thousand bases. However, the novel mRNA from the fusion of the two genes involves a small defined sequence at the fusion junction. One can therefore apply the following analytic strategy: 1) isolate mRNA, 2) make a DNA copy (cDNA) using the enzyme reverse transcriptase, 3) use this cDNA to amplify the region around the fusion point using PCR with appropriate primers, and 4) use hybridization probes or sequencing to detect the novel fusion point (72). Similar strategies have also been applied to rearrangements involving immunoglobulin and TCR genes. These amplification and hybridization techniques are already finding application in some clinical laboratories. Other novel techniques utilizing DNA blots of multiple genes and cDNA probes or antibodies and fluorescence-activated cell sorting are being explored for analysis of gene expression in tumor tissues.

In many cases the specific gene involved in tumor development is unknown, but its general chromosomal location has been defined by karyotype analysis. The location of the relevant gene can sometimes be more precisely pinpointed by analysis of linkage to genes whose chromosomal site is better defined. Such linkage analysis is often accomplished by examination of genes that have more than one form at a given locus (*i.e.*, are polymorphic). Such genetic polymorphisms are often identified by the way genes are cleaved by specific enzymes. Consequently the analysis of restriction fragment length polymorphisms (RFLP) is often used to define linkage to cancer genes or cancer-suppressor genes (107).

NUCLEAR ONCOPROTEINS AS CANCER MARKERS

N-MYC

Amplification (duplication) of genes is a common event in cultured mammalian cells *in vitro* (133) and in human cancers *in vivo* (92; Table 2). One of the first proto-oncogenes in which amplification was characterized was the *N-MYC* gene in a neuroblastoma cell line. This gene shares structural homology with the *c-MYC* oncogene (134). In fetal life *N-MYC* is expressed in cells of the nervous system. Appropriately, amplification of this gene occurs only in neuroendocrine tumors including neuroblastoma, retinoblastoma, carcinoid, and some small cell lung cancer cell lines (92, 109, 134, 136, 140). The protein product of the gene is nuclear in location and an antibody useful in histologic section has been described (145).

N-MYC amplification occurs in about 20% of neuroblastomas and shows correlation with advanced stage of disease and aggressive tumor behavior (136). From the standpoint of cancer diagnostics this gene appears to be a useful marker of prognosis. Availability of an antibody should allow detection of those rare tumors with N-MYC overexpression but without gene amplification.

c-*MYC* Gene

Burkitt's Lymphoma/Leukemias. Burkitt's lymphoma cells have a translocation involving chromosome 8 at band q24, the site of the c-MYC proto-oncogene. The reciprocal site in 90% of cases is chromosome 14q32, the locus of the Ig heavy chain gene (IgH). In the remaining 10% of cases, chromosome band 2p12 or 22q11 is involved. These are sites of the κ- and λ-light chain genes, respectively. In patients with the 8;14 translocation all or part of the c-*MYC* gene is translocated to the IgH locus (21, 29, 114, 117, 153). In the variant translocations, c-MYC remains on chromosome 8, and a portion of the light chain genes translocates to a region downstream (3') of c-*MYC* (29). Similar chromosomal translocations have been seen in other non-Burkitt's B cell lymphomas and in most cases of B cell acute lymphoblastic leukemia (B-ALL) and in some pre-B ALL cases (102). These karyotypic and molecular abnormalities appear to be specific for early B cell malignancies.

C-MYC consists of a first noncoding exon and two coding exons interrupted by two introns. On chromosome 8, breakpoints have been mapped at different sites relative to this gene: 1) in the sequences upstream (5') of the first exon, 2) in the first intron, 3) at an undefined distance 5' of c-*MYC*, and 4) at various locations in the 3' flanking sequences in the variant translocations (29, 80).

The Ig and T cell receptor (TCR) genes consist of variable (V), joining (J), diversity (D), and constant (C) regions that undergo somatic recombinations during B and T cell differentiation to generate the diversity characteristic of Ig and TCR molecules. These recombinations are thought to be catalyzed by a common recombinase system that recognizes DNA signal sequences of 7–9 base pairs opposed to each recombinant segment (170). In over half of Burkitt's cases, breaks on chromosome 14 involve a region responsible for the class switches that occur during the process of antibody production, raising speculation that the gene rearrangements in malignancy represent operation of a faulty switch mechanism. In the variant translocations, the breaks occur upstream from the J region segments. This and the presence of inserted nucleotides at the breakpoint suggest that these result from mistakes during the normal process of VDJ joining.

In those cases where the c-MYC gene is not decapitated by the rearrangement (*i.e.*, loses it first exon), there are often point mutations in the promoter or exon 1 and even within the coding regions of exon 2 and 3 (143). The end result of these rearrangements or mutations is the deregulation and overexpression of the abnormal c-MYC gene and decreased expression of the remaining normal gene. Several models have been proposed to explain this activation (29, 80, 114, 117).

T Cell Lymphomas. If the combination of c-*MYC* and Ig gene rearrangements is the hallmark of Burkitt's-like B cell malignancies, then rearrangements of the TCR genes are characteristic of certain T cell malignancies. Chromosome 14q11 is the site of the T cell α-receptor (TaR) gene. It is involved in at least four recurring chromosomal abnormalities observed in patients with T

cell ALL: 1) inv 14 (q11;q32); 2) t(8;14) (q24;q11); 3) t(11;14)(p13;q11); and 4) t(10;14)(q24;q11) (2). Therefore the TaR gene may be involved in the pathogenesis of some T cell ALLs analogous to that of Ig genes in B cell leukemias and lymphomas.

The t(8;14) (q24;q11) chromosomal translocation occurs in some T cell malignancies (41, 96). It results in juxtaposition of c-*MYC* and TaR genes. The breakpoint on chromosome 14 splits the TaR locus between V and C genes resulting in the translocation of C to chromosome 8 distal to the c-*MYC* gene and transcriptional deregulation of c-*MYC* as is the case in the corresponding B cell malignancies (41, 42, 96). From these data it is apparent that certain rearrangements of the c-*MYC* gene are pathognomonic of B and T cell malignancies and may serve as markers of disease. As discussed below, the specificity of these gene rearrangements may be applicable to the detection of minimal residual disease remaining after therapy.

Other Cancers. Rearrangements of the c-*MYC* gene occur but are rare except in B and T cell lymphomas and leukemias (91, 100); however, amplification of c-*MYC* with concomitant increased expression is common in a wide variety of human tumors (91, 172; Table 2). The frequency of amplification varies between about 0 and 15% and appears to be a function of tumor type. Amplification is rare in colon cancers and fairly common in sarcomas (91). Our initial observations suggested that amplification correlated with more advanced tumors and more aggressive behavior (172). Although this observation is probably correct, the phenomenon is not sufficiently specific to be used as a tumor marker for predicting prognosis.

p53 Gene Alterations in Osteogenic Sarcomas and CML

The human p53 gene is made up of 11 exons and encodes a nuclear protein of 53 kD. This protein binds to the transforming proteins of several DNA tumor viruses. Many observations suggest a role for the p53 gene in oncogenesis and regulation of the cell cycle (27, 97, 113, 122). Elevated levels of the p53 protein occur in most transformed cell lines. Protein encoded by the p53 gene can complement activated *RAS* genes in *in vitro* transformation of primary rodent cell cultures and can immortalize such cells (113). The synthesis of p53 increases in resting cells after stimulation with mitogen, and stimulated cells can be blocked from entering S phase by microinjection of p53-specific antibody (97). Although these studies indicate that expression of the p53 gene is associated with cell proliferation, lack of expression of the gene due in most cases to genomic rearrangements occurs in several transformed human and rodent cell lines, including HL-60 leukemic cells, osteogenic sarcoma cell lines (92), and mouse erythroleukemia cell lines transformed *in vivo* by Friend leukemia virus (127). My laboratory has observed rearrangements of the p53 gene uniquely in two human malignancies; osteogenic sarcoma (92) and the blast crisis of CML (1). Altered genes are detected by Southern blotting in 20–30% of these malignancies, but are rare in other common human cancers (1, 91, 92). No abnormalities are found in the chronic phase of CML, suggesting that p53 gene alteration is a frequent concomitant of the clonal evolution of disease to blast crisis. It is possible that hybridization signals using p53 gene probes may be useful as cancer markers for predicting transition from chronic to blast phase CML.

RAS ONCOGENE PROTEINS AS CANCER MARKERS

Genes of the *RAS* family are ancient; similar genes have been found in lower organisms including yeast. They encode 21 kDa GTP binding proteins with GTPase activity (16, 22, 39, 44, 63, 93, 97, 121). The proteins are localized to inner cell membranes and are similar to various G proteins that interact with hormone and neurotransmitter receptors to transduce information via second messengers such as cyclic AMP. Transcripts of *c-Ha-RAS* and *c-Ki-RAS* are expressed throughout fetal development (105, 145). Their proteins are found in brain, bone, epithelial, and hematopoietic tissues in growing animals, suggesting that the *RAS* family of genes are active in a wide range of normal proliferating cell types. Ectodermal, endodermal, and mesenchymal tumors also express *RAS* genes (148). Occasional reports suggest that increased expression of *RAS* genes may correlate with tumor behavior (88, 162); however, better documentation is needed before this phenomenon can be considered a molecular marker of cancer prognosis.

Altered versions of *RAS* genes are found in a wide variety of tumors but never in normal tissues. Amplified variants of *RAS* genes are rare in human tumors with the possible exception of ovarian adenocarcinomas (45, 91, 176). Deletions involving the chromosomal region (11p) containing *c-Ha-RAS* are common in many types of cancer (172); mutations in specific regions of the coding sequence of *Ki-RAS* are very common in certain adenocarcinomas (4, 44, 119, 121, 141), and mutations of *N-RAS* are common in leukemias (16, 17, 124, 152).

Twenty-one of 22 pancreatic cancers were shown to have a mutation at codon 12 of the *c-Ki-RAS* gene by PCR gene amplification and the RNAase A mismatch cleavage method (4). By use of oligonucleotide probes and PCR, 5 of 10 lung adenocarcinomas had similar mutations (125, 161). By both techniques, between 30 and 45% of colon cancers have a *c-Ki-RAS* mutation (17, 49). Interestingly, this mutation appears to be an early event in colon carcinogenesis since it is often detectable in premalignant adenomatous polyps. Subsequent progression apparently involves additional molecular events since changes in chromosomes 5, 17, and 18 are common in more advanced tumors (103, 150, 163). Interestingly, the gene for familial adenomatous polyposis was found by RFLP analysis to be located on the long arm of chromosome 5 (11). Clearly *c-Ki-RAS* mutations may be a useful marker in certain adenocarcinomas. One report also suggests that immunocytochemical assay for RAS protein may be useful in diagnosis of colon cancer (30).

The *N-RAS* gene is structurally homologous to *Ha-* and *Ki-RAS* genes. Many human leukemias and myelodysplastic syndromes have been shown to contain *RAS* oncogenes capable of transforming NIH 3T3 cells (57,

58, 67, 86). Other studies using hybridization probes specific for wild-type *N-RAS* genes or mutated alleles frequently identified mutations of codon 12 or 13 in varions hematologic malignancies including acute myeloid leukemia, common and T cell variants of ALL, CML, and myelodysplastic syndromes (16, 17, 43, 57, 58, 66, 67, 86). In myelodysplastic syndromes, the mutation may serve as a molecular marker of malignant progression; in the other malignancies it may be useful as a marker of minimal residual disease remaining after treatment. These gene mutations apparently alter the three-dimensional structure of the RAS proteins (33, 93).

ALTERED GENES FOR GROWTH FACTORS AND RECEPTORS

Several proto-oncogenes encode growth factors or cell surface receptors for growth factors (Table 1). Some of these may have potential utility as cancer markers.

c-ERBB-1

c-ERBB-1 encodes the gene for epidermal growth factor receptor. This receptor is a tyrosine kinase that is activated by binding of epidermal growth factor to its external domain. The *c-ERBB-1* locus was initially identified by its homology with the transforming gene, v-erbB, of avian erythroblastosis virus. Comparison of the predicted amino acid sequence of v-erbB with that of the receptor for EGF revealed homologies and suggested that *c-ERBB-1* was the gene coding for the receptor (34). Amplified and rearranged *c-ERBB-1* genes have been found in some primary squamous carcinomas and brain tumors (24, 62, 85, 98). In some squamous carcinoma cell lines, the *c-ERBB-1* gene is rearranged, and altered transcripts and protein are made. It has been suggested that amplification of this gene may be associated with more aggressive squamous tumors; however, the evidence is unconvincing, and this gene has not yet secured a firm place as a cancer marker.

c-ERBB-2

The *c-ERBB-1* gene is homologous to another gene, *c-ERBB-2*. The *c-ERBB-2* gene encodes a protein with the configuration of a transmembrane growth factor receptor similar to the epidermal growth factor receptor (138). Genes similar to *c-ERBB-2* have also been identified in the human genome by other investigators and called *HER-2* and the *v-ERBB*-related gene (26, 73). The *neu* oncogene, originally identified in a series of ethylnitrosourea-induced rat neuroblastomas, has also been found to be related to *v-ERBB* (132). Comparison of the nucleotide sequences of these *v-ERBB*-related genes reveals that they are all the same. In the literature, therefore, one finds this gene referred to as *c-ERBB-2*, *neu* and *HER-2*. This gene is sometimes amplified in adenocarcinomas but not in other tumor types (173), suggesting that it encodes a protein on glandular epithelium. Breast cancers and certain carcinomas of the stomach are the adenocarcinomas that most frequently show *c-ERBB-2* amplification (91). In 1987 a report by Slamon *et al.* (146) stated that amplification of *c-ERBB-2* was a useful marker for predicting recurrence of breast cancers after initial therapy. Because of the potential importance of this observation as defining a prognostically significant cancer marker, the subject was re-examined by several groups of investigators utilizing large numbers of cases. Unfortunately their results did not confirm the utility of *c-ERBB-2* as a prognostic marker; 698 breast cancers analyzed for *c-ERBB-2* have been reported (7, 23, 73, 146, 158–160, 174, 175). When the 509 cases in other series are compared with the 189 cases in the initial Slamon series (146) the incidence of *c-ERBB-2* amplification in the former is 15% and in the latter is 28%. Similarly, the incidence of amplification in primary tumors with axillary lymph nodes containing metastases is 15% (38/247) in the former compared with 40% (34/86) in the latter. The reasons for this discrepancy are unclear.

Data of several investigators suggest that alterations in several different proto-oncogenes including *c-MYC*, *c-ERBB-2*, and *c-INT*-related genes may be involved in the progression of breast cancers and that no one genetic mechanism dominates (23, 174). The observation that *c-ERBB-2*, amplification is restricted to some adenocarcinomas still stands, and the availability of a good antibody (160) should allow analysis of heterogeneity of gene expression in cancers.

Although most studies have concentrated on amplification of the *c-ERBB-2* gene in human tumors, there is evidence that in rodents the gene can also become activated by a single mutation altering the transmembrane domain of the receptor-like protein encoded by the gene (5, 106). One should therefore look for similar mutation in human tumors.

OTHER GROWTH FACTORS AND RECEPTORS

A small segment of the long arm of chromosome 5 contains multiple genes for growth factors or receptors related to hematopoiesis (115): CSF-1, a hematopoietic colony stimulating factor for growth and differentiation of mononuclear phagocytes; GM-CSF, a growth factor for granulocytes and mononuclear phagocytes; c-FMS, the gene for the CSF-1 receptor; the platelet derived growth factor receptor; and interleukin-3. Deletions of this chromosomal segment are frequently observed in therapy-related myelodysplastic syndromes and acute nonlymphocytic leukemia, as well as refractory anemia with abnormal megakaryocytes (referred to as the 5q-syndrome, 115). Because deletions of this region are common in therapy related acute nonlymphocytic leukemia and are relatively uncommon in *de novo* acute nonlymphocytic leukemia, it has been suggested that there is a genetic deletion that may be a marker of mutagen-induced leukemia (128). Efforts to clone this gene are underway.

Platelet-derived growth factor is composed of a dimer of structurally related peptide chains designate A and B (8, 69). The precursor of the B chain is encoded by the *c-SIS* gene on chromosome 22, and the A chain is encoded by a separate gene on chromosome 7. Some sarcoma and glioma cell lines express high levels of both A chain and B chain mRNA, whereas others express only A or only B (8). Gene amplification has not been reported

in these tumor lines. Altered forms of c-SIS have thus far been found in familial meningiomas (13) and may be considered a marker of this neoplasm.

ALTERED TYROSINE KINASES

Proto-oncogenes of the tyrosine kinase family were the first to be discovered and characterized (9, 10, 36, 61, 75, 126). This is a very numerous family, with some genes that are expressed in a cell lineage-specific manner and others that are widely expressed in cells of many types (60, 61). Although the c-SRC gene was identified first, it is the *c-ABL* proto-oncogene that has been best characterized in a human malignancy. The elucidation of its role in CML has become a model for the examination of the role of proto-oncogenes in neoplasia.

c-ABL AND CML

CML is a disease of pluripotent hematopoietic stem cells with a biphasic or triphasic clinical course. An initial chronic phase is followed either by an intermediate accelerated phase or directly by an acute blast crisis phase characterized by increasing cell proliferation, cellular maturation arrest, and development of additional karyotypic abnormalities (55).

Over 90% of CML cases have the Philadelphia (Ph^1) chromosome anomaly that is a result of a reciprocal translocation involving the long arms of chromosomes 9 and 22. This anomaly is characterized at the molecular level by a translocation of the *c-ABL* proto-oncogene from chromosome 9 to within a 5.8-kilobase segment of DNA known as the *bcr* on chromosome 22 (53). Although the breakpoints on both chromosomes are variable, the novel mRNA is a unique 8-kilobase *bcr/c-ABL* chimeric transcript that contains *bcr* sequences upstream of the breakpoint and *c-ABL* sequences downstream (25, 142). This transcript is translated into a 210-kDa phosphoprotein that unlike the normal 145 kDa protein possesses high levels of tyrosine kinase activity and is phosphorylated on tyrosine residues (35, 78). The promiscuous tyrosine kinase activity of p210 is probably important in the pathogenesis of CML, since some CML cases lack the pH^1 chromosome but still have molecular rearrangements of the *ABL* gene (35). The Ph^1 chromosome also occurs in 25–30% of adult and 2–10% of children with ALL (118). Their leukemic cells express novel *c-ABL* tyrosine kinases of 185–190 kDa as a result of a fusion of the putative first exon of the *bcr* gene with *c-ABL* (55). These molecular events may be used as molecular markers in confirming the diagnosis of CML and related diseases. With the commonly used probe from 3′ *bcr* sequences (Oncogene Scientific, Mineola, New York), gene rearrangements are seen in more than 90% of Ph^1 positive cases and in more than 95% with additional bcr probes Molecular probes are positive in a small percentage of cases where karyotype analyses for the Ph^1 chromosome are negative, indicating an unusual translocation of *bcr* and *ABL*. Hybridization analyses using Southern blotting are more rapid and less costly that karyotype anlysis. Furthermore, as discussed above, much more rapid analysis of the *bcr/ABL* fusion is now possible using PCR and reverse transcription of the fused mRNA (72). This will probably become the diagnostic procedure of choice.

HEMATOPOIETIC-SPECIFIC TYROSINE KINASES

Alterations of c-ABL appear to be uniquely associated with hematologic malignancies. There are other proto-oncogenes in the same family of tyrosine kinases whose expression appears to be restricted to hematopoietic cell. The *LCK* gene is one example that is primarily lymphoid (90). The *BMK* gene is expressed in lymphoid and myeloid cells and macrophages (59). C-KIT appears to be a membrane bound tyrosine kinase similar to the macrophage growth factor (CSF-1) receptor and to the receptor for platelet-derived growth factor (171). The *HCK* gene is expressed primarily in granulocytes (177), and *LTK* may encode a hematopoietic receptor (6). Abnormalities of structure or expression of these genes may exist in hematologic disorders and should be researched as possible markers.

OTHER TYROSINE KINASES

Human *c-RAF-1* sequences were identified in tumorigenic clones of NIH/3T3 cells transfected with DNA from a radiation-resistant human laryngeal carcinoma cell line (71). The transforming activity was associated with the tyrosine kinase domain of the gene, suggesting the possibility that altered forms of this gene may be implicated in the pathogenesis of this type of tumor. There are also preliminary reports of alterations of RAF and a related gene, *PKS*, in hematopoietic disorders.

BCL AND TCL GENE REARRANGEMENTS IN LYMPHOMAS/LEUKEMIAS

Modern cytogenetic techniques reveal chromosomal abnormalities in virtually all leukemias and lymphomas. In many instances, genes of possible relevance to evolution of malignancy are located at chromosomal breakpoints (28). Some of these have been molecularly cloned: 1) the *bcl-1* gene in the (11;14) (q13;q24) translocation seen in various B cell malignancies (157); 2) the *bcl-2* gene in the (14;18) (q32;q21) translocation characteristic of follicular lymphomas (155, 156); and 3) the *tcl-1, tcl-2, tcl-3* genes and various chromosomal translocations frequently seen in T cell malignancies (83, 101, 123, 155). In each of these abnormalities, the relevant gene is brought in close proximity to either the Ig genes in B cell malignancies or α- or β-TCR genes in T cell malignancies. Although the *bcl* and *tcl* genes have been cloned, their function is still largely unidentified. They are probably proto-oncogenes. They may serve as molecular markers of malignancy and in identifying clinically different subtypes of lymphomas.

The *bcl-1* locus on chromosome llq23 is rearranged in about 10% of CLL cases (64, 157). Some *bcl-2* (18q21) rearrangements are seen in various B cell malignancies at frequencies of 20% for small noncleaved cell lymphomas, 40% for diffuse large cell lymphomas, and over 70% for follicular lymphomas (28, 81). CLL also has a recurring translocation t(14;19)(q32;q13) involving the Ig heavy chain locus on chromosome 14. Efforts to clone the rearranged gene on chromosome 19 are ongoing (95).

The *bcl-2* gene encodes a 25 kDa protein expressed at high levels in lymphomas with the t(14;18) karyotype. Lymphomas with *bcl-2* rearrangements may have a more aggressive clinical course, but this observation must be confirmed by further studies. An antibody useful in detecting the protein in frozen tissue section should soon be generally available (110).

IMMUNOGLOBULIN AND TCR GENE REARRANGEMENTS

Rearrangements of the Ig and TCR genes have been used as markers of lineage, clonality, and stage of differentiation in B and T cell neoplasms. Ig gene rearrangements are an early and specific event in normal B cell differentiation. TCR molecules are structurally and functionally analogous to the Ig molecules of B cells and are T cell specific. Rearrangements of these genes may therefore (sometimes) provide a marker of tumor lineage. A particular rearrangement is specific for a given cell clone and therefore provides evidence of clonality. Finally, rearrangements of these genes occur in a hierarchial pattern in normal cell differentiation so that they have been used to define stage of differentiation of lymphoid tumors. In this way molecular analysis has been used to supplement analyses of immunologic markers and karyotype. Unfortunately molecular rearrangements are not always consistent with phenotypic markers since malignant cells are imperfect in their differentiation pattern. For example, Ig chain rearrangements may occur in a leukemia that otherwise has characteristics of myeloid differentiation, just as myeloid antigens are sometimes found on lymphoid blast cells (149). TCR a, b, γ, and δ gene rearrangements have also been used as markers of cell lineage and clonality in T cell malignancies (48, 130). Although the Ig and TCR genes are unquestionably valuable in the establishment of clonality, they must be used with caution in defining lineage and stage of differentiation. For instance, the complete (VDJ) rearrangement of IgH and TCR-β genes are good markers of B cell and T cell lineage, respectively; however, the first DJ rearrangement of IgH and TCR-β genes can be found in cells of either T or B lineage, and neither rearrangement of the TCR γ nor δ gene is lineage specific (154).

GENE DELETION AND ANTIONCOGENES

Early studies of the fusion of normal and malignant cells often resulted in a normal growth pattern suggesting that the normal phenotype, and therefore normal genes, may sometimes be dominant. Subsequent analysis of the inheritance pattern of familial and sporadic retinoblastoma suggested that the tumor phenotype was recessive and that tumor development required mutations of the allelic genes on both chromosomes (76). More recent analyses indicated that this is indeed the case and defined a region on chromosome 13 near band q14 that was frequently involved in this tumor (19, 79). Recently the involved gene has been cloned and designated Rb gene (50). It is now known that varions alterations including rearrangements, loss, and mutations can result in inactivation of the Rb gene leading to decreased expression of mRNA and protein and to development of osteosarcomas and retinoblastomas (19, 50, 74, 79, 165, 166). How the Rb gene acts as a tumor suppressor is unknown. It codes for a 105-kDa nuclear protein that apparently interacts with the transforming proteins of many DNA viruses (32). It has been suggested that these viruses may induce malignancy by complexing with and thereby inactivating the Rb protein.

Just as there are many oncogenes, there may be many antioncogenes. This concept is supported by the many observations of nonrandom chromosomal loss in specific neoplasms. Examples of loss of specific sequences include those on chromosome 11 in Wilms' tumors (111), chromosome 22 in acoustic neuroma (137), chromosomes 11 and 13 in breast cancers (3, 87), and chromosome 3 in lung cancers (77).

Loss of Rb gene sequences detected by RFLP analysis has already been used as a marker to predict familial predisposition to retinoblastoma (20, 169). Soon other tumor suppressor genes will probably be identified and used as cancer markers.

DNA TUMOR VIRUS GENES AS CANCER MARKERS

Certain DNA tumor viruses have been consistently associated with certain human malignancies. This subject has been well covered recently (82, 178) and is beyond the scope of this review; however, it is germaine to consider briefly the main classes of viruses and the techniques that have been employed in their detection.

HUMAN PAPILLOMA VIRUSES

Among the strongest evidence for an oncogenic potential of human papilloma virus (HPV) is the association of HPV-5 or -8 DNA with epidermodysplasia verruciformis, a disease characterized by disseminated flat warts that have a 30% probability of developing carcinomas on sun-exposed areas of skin (116). Other genotypes of HPV are less commonly associated. Since the early 1980s the association of HPV-16 and HPV-18 with female cervical cancer has been recognized (37, 178). Subsequently additional related HPV genotypes have been found, notably HPV-31 and HPV-33. Approximately 14 HPV types have now been found in the female genital tract, of which HPV-6 and -11 are most consistently associated with genital warts. HPV-16 DNA is found in approximately 50% of cervical vulvar and penile cancers and in smaller percentages of laryngeal, tongue, and lung cancers. One or another HPV type can be found in about 80% of genital tumors (178). Integration of viral DNA is characteristic of primary tumors, whereas precancerous lesions frequently have unintegrated viral DNA (38, 178). In most cervical cancer cell lines and primary tumors HPV DNA persists, and transcripts covering an open reading frame designated E6–E7 are present (135), suggesting a requirement for these viral gene sequences in maintenance of the malignant state.

Analysis of HPV genes in tumors has generally been by traditional hybridization techniques (112, 178). Recently, the sensitivity and rapidity of the PCR has been used in analysis (47). Oligonucleotide primers to the E6 region of HPV-11, -16, and -18 were used to amplify these gene sequences that can be detected in infected but not uninfected cells with sensitivity down to 10–20 copies of the virus in 10^4 cells. Such a technique could readily be applied to cervical swabs. Other approaches to viral detection include *in situ* hybridization and the use of monoclonal antibodies raised against the E6 protein (54).

EPSTEIN-BARR VIRUS

Epstein-Barr virus is classically associated with infectious mononucleosis and two malignant disorders: African Burkitt's lymphoma and nasopharyngeal carcinoma (40). More recently the virus has been associated with various polyclonal lymphoproliferative disorders and with rare tumors including thymic carcinoma (84) and an unusual T cell lymphoma with a chronic antecedent illness (70). Viral DNA has been detected in these various disorders in B lymphocytes, oropharyngeal epithelial carcinoma cells (84, 144), and the T lymphoma cells (70). There are some recent reports of Epstein-Barr virus markers in Hodgkin's disease lymph nodes. Conventional and *in situ* hybridization techniques have been used in detection.

USES OF MOLECULAR MARKERS IN CANCER DIAGNOSIS

Knowledge of the molecular mechanisms of cancer development is still primitive. Nevertheless, this growing body of information is rapidly being applied to the clinic in cancer diagnosis. Analysis of immunoglobulin and TCR genes are being used to discriminate certain malignant and nonmalignant disorders on the basis of the monoclonal or polyclonal nature of the proliferating cells. Within limits, these rearrangements may also be used to define the cell lineage of a lymphoid tumor. Antibody and nucleic acid probes are now being used with increasing ease and sophistication to define DNA viral participation in certain human cancers. Undoubtedly in the future they will be examined for potential use in predicting development of cancers such as those of the uterine cervix (99). Their application will be facilitated by the ease with which one can now perform assays for the presence of foreign DNA sequences in cells. Interestingly one of the first molecular analyses applied to malignant disease has been in the area of cancer susceptibility. The initial studies relate specifically to familial retinoblastoma and antioncogenes. With the appearance of the cancer-suppressor genes, and the extensive documentation of nonrandom gene loss in cancers, one anticipates that this field of prediction of susceptibility will rapidly expand to include the common cancers of lung, colon, and breast and the interesting hematologic neoplasms.

Molecular probes are already being used in the diagnosis of specific malignancies. It is easier to perform DNA hybridization with a *bcr* probe than karyotype analysis to define *CML*. Such analyses will be facilitated by the use of PCR coupled to reverse transcription of mRNA (72). It is also likely that the frequent mutations of the *c-RAS-Ki* gene in common adenocarcinomas will be used in making earlier diagnosis of colon, pancreatic, and lung cancers by using PCR-based analyses on exfoliated cells or minibiopsies.

Thus far the clinical application of molecular probes to predict tumor behavior (and therefore to dictate clinical intervention) has been largely restricted to the *N-MYC* gene and neuroblastomas. Efforts to utilize molecular analysis in prognostication have so far proved disappointing in breast, colon, prostate, and squamous cancers. Perhaps this situation will improve as we learn more about the multiple sequential mechanism involved in tumor progression (74, 75) and about the role of genes such as *bcl-2, tcl-1, -2, -3, c-ETS* (120), and *c-MAS* whose functions are largely undefined. Clearly molecular analyses are going to redefine how we treat diseases that spread through the blood and bone marrow. The sensitive analytic techniques will allow us to define disease remaining after chemotherapy or radiation. Let us take the CML cell containing fusion of the *bcr* and *c-ABL* genes as an example. By the new amplification and hybridization techniques (56, 65, 72, 129) one can now detect the fused gene product in one abnormal cell among 10^3 or 10^4 normal hematopoietic cells. This sensitivity may be increased to one neoplastic cell in 10^5 or 10^6. This approach is not restricted to CML. There are unique molecular markers for various B and T cell malignancies and for virus-associated neoplasms. The ability to detect minimal residual disease with molecular markers is likely to revolutionize the diagnosis and treatment of cancer.

Original observations were supported by a gift for research from R. J. Reynolds Tobacco and United States Public Health Service Grant CA 15619.

REFERENCES

1. Ahuja H, Bar-Eli M, Clarke P, Snyder D, Foreman S, Goldman J, Cline MJ: p53 gene alterations in blast crisis of chronic myelocytic leukemia. Proc Natl Acad Sci USA, in press
2. Ahuja H, Cline MJ: Genetic and cytogenetic changes in acute lymphoblastic leukemia. Med Oncol Tumor Pharmacol 5:211, 1988
3. Ali IU, Lidereau R, Theillet C, Callahan R: Reduction to homozygosity of genes on chromosome 11 in human breast neoplasia. Science 238:185, 1987
4. Almoguera C, Shibata D, Forrester K, Martin V, Arnheim N, Perucho M: Most human carcinomas of the exocrine pancreas contain mutant c-K-ras genes. Cell 53:549, 1988
5. Bargmann CI, Weinberg RA: Increased tyrosine kinase activity associated with the protein encoded by the activated neu oncogene. Proc Natl Acad Sci USA 85:5394, 1988
6. Ben-Neriah Y, Bauskin AR: Leukocytes express a novel gene encoding a putative transmembrane protein-kinase devoid of an extracellular domain. Nature 333:672, 1988
7. Berger MS, Locher GW, Saurer S, Gullick WJ, Waterfield M, Groner B, Hynes NE: Correlation of c-erbB-2 gene amplification and protein expression in human breast carcinoma with nodal status and nuclear grading. Cancer Res 48:1238, 1988
8. Betsholtz C, Johnsson A, Heldin CH, Westermark B, Lind P, Urdea MS, Eddy R, Shows TB, Philpott K, Mellor AL: cDNA sequence and chromosomal localization of human platelet-derived growth factor A-chain and its expression in tumor cell lines. Nature 320:695, 1986
9. Bishop JM: The molecular genetics of cancer. Science 235:305, 1987
10. Bishop JM: Cellular oncogenes and retroviruses. Annu Rev Biochem 52:301, 1983
11. Bodmer WF, Bailey CJ, Bodmer J, Bussey HJR, Ellis A, Gorman P, Lucibello FC, Murday VA, Rider SH, Scrambler P, Sheer D, Solomon E, Spurr NK: Localization of the gene for familial adenomatous polyposis on chromosome 5. Nature 328:614, 1987
12. Bohmann D, Bos TJ, Admon A, Nishimura T, Vogt P, Tijan R: Human proto-oncogene *c-jun* encodes a DNA binding protein with structural and functional properties of transcription factor AP-1. Science 238:1386, 1986
13. Bolger GB, Stamberg J, Kirsch IR, Hollis GF, Schwarz DF, Thomas GH: Chromosome translocation t(14;22) and oncogene (c-sis) variant in a pedigree with familial meningioma. New Engl J Med 312:564, 1985
14. Bonner T, O'Brien SJ, Nash WG, Rapp UR, Morton CC, Leder P: The human homologs of the *raf* (*mil*) oncogene are located on human chromosomes 3 and 4. Science 223:71, 1984
15. Bos JL, Fearon ER, Hamilton SR, Verlaan-de Vries M, van Boom JH, van der Eb AJ, Vogelstein B: Prevalence of ras gene mutation in human colorectal cancers. Nature 327:293, 1987
16. Bos JL, Toksoz D, Marshall CJ, Verlaan-de Vries M, Veeneman GH, Van der Eb AJ, van Boom JH, Janssen JWG, Steenvoorden ACM: Amino acid substitutions at codon 13 of the N-ras oncogene in human acute myeloid leukemia. Nature 315:726, 1985
17. Bos JL, Verlaan-de Vries M, van der Eb AJ, Janssen JWG, Delwel R, Lowenberg B, Colly LP. Mutations in N-ras predominate in acute myeloid leukemia. Blood 69:1237, 1987
18. Casey G, Smith R, McGillivray D, Peters G, Dickson C: Characterization and chromosome assignment of the human homolog of *int-2*, a potential proto-oncogene, Mol Cell Biol 6:502, 1986
19. Cavenee WK, Hansen MF, Nordenskjold M: Genetic origin of mutations predisposing to retinoblastoma. Science 228:501, 1985
20. Cavenee WK, Murphree AL, Shull MM, Benedict WF, Sparkes RS, Kock E, Nordenskjold M: Prediction of familial predisposition to retinoblastoma. New Engl J Med 314:1201, 1986
21. Cesarman E, Dalla-Favera R, Bentley D, Groudine MT: Mutations in the first exon are associated with altered transcription of *c-myc* in Burkitt lymphoma. Science 238:1272, 1987
22. Chang EJ, Furth ME, Scolnick EM, Lowy DR: Tumorigenic transformation of mammalian cells induced by a normal gene homologous to the oncogene of Harvey murine sarcoma virus. Nature 297:479, 1982
23. Cline MJ, Battifora H, Yokota J: Proto-oncogene abnormalities in human breast cancer: Correlations with anatomic features and clinical course of disease. J Clin Oncol 5:999, 1987
24. Coeley G, Smith JA, Gusterson B, Hendler F, Ozanne B: The amount of EGF receptor is elevated on squamous cell carcinomas. Cancer Cells 1:5, 1984
25. Collins SJ, Kubonishi I, Miyoshi I, Groudine MT: Altered transcription of the c-abl oncogene in K-562 and other chronic myelogenous leukemia cells. Science 225:72, 1984
26. Coussens L, Yang-Feng TL, Liao YC, Chen E, Gray A, McGrath J, Seeburg PH, Libermann TH, Schlessinger J, Francke U: Tyrosine kinase receptor with extensive homology to EGF receptor shares chromosomal location with neu oncogene. Science 230:1132, 1985
27. Crawford L: The 53,000-dalton cellular protein and its role in transformation. Int Rev Exp Pathol 25:1, 1983
28. Croce CM: Role of chromosome translocations in human neoplasia. Cell 49:155, 1987
29. Croce CM, Nowell PC: Molecular basis of human B cell neoplasia. Blood 65:1, 1985
30. Czerniak B, Herz F, Koss LG, Schlom J: ras oncogene p21 as a tumor marker in the cytodiagnosis of gastric and colonic carcinomas. Cancer 60:2432, 1987
31. Park M, Dean M, Cooper CS, Schmidt M, O'Brien SJ, Blair DG, vander Woude GF: Mechanism of *met* oncogene activation. Cell 45:895, 1986
32. DeCaprio JA, Ludlow JW, Figge J, Shew JY, Huang CM, Lee WH, Marsilio E, Paucha E, Livingston DM: SV40 Large tumor antigen forms a specific complex with the product of the retinoblastoma susceptibility gene. Cell 54:275, 1988
33. DeVos AM, Tong L, Milburn MV, Matias PM, Jancarik J, Noguchi S, Nishimura S, Miura K, Ohtsuka E, Kim SH. Three dimensional structures of an oncogene protein: Catalytic domain of human c-H ras p21. Science 239:888, 1988
34. Downward J, Yarden Y, Mayes E, Scrace G, Totty N, Stockwell P, Ullrich A, Schlessinger J, Waterfield MD: Close similarity of epidermal growth factor receptor and v-erb-B oncogene protein sequences. Nature (Lond) 37:521, 1984
35. Dreazen O, Cannani E, Gale RP: Molecular biology of chronic myelogenous leukemia. Semin Hem 25:35, 1988

36. Duesberg PH: Activated proto-oncogenes: Sufficient or necessary for cancer? Science 228:669, 1985

37. Durst M, Gissmann L, Ikenberg H, ZurHausen H: A papillomavirus DNA from a cervical carcinoma and its prevalence in cancer biopsy samples from different geographic regions. Proc Natl Acad Sci USA 80:3812, 1983

38. Durst M, Kleinheinz A, Hotz M, Gissmann L: The physical state of human papillovirus type 16 DNA in benign and malignant genital tumors. J Gen Virol 66:1515, 1985

39. Ellis RW, Lowy DR, Scolnick EM: The viral and cellular p21 (ras) gene family. In Advances in Viral Oncology, pp 107-126. New York, Raven, 1982

40. Epstein MA, Achong BG (editors): The Epstein-Barr Virus, pp 1-22. Berlin, Springer-Verlag, 1979

41. Erikson J, Finger L, Sun L, Ar-Rushidi A, Nishikura K, Minowada J, Finan J, Emanuel BS, Nowell PC, Croce CM: Deregulation of c-myc by translocation of the alpha locus of the T cell receptor in T cell leukemias. Science 232:884, 1986

42. Erikson J, Williams DL, Finan J, Nowell PC, Croce CM: Locus of the alpha-chain of the T cell receptor is split by chromosome translocation in T cell leukemias. Science 229:784, 1985

43. Farr CJ, Saiki RK, Erlich HA, McCormick F, Marshall CJ: Analysis of RAS gene mutations in acute myeloid leukemia by polymerase chain reaction and oligonucleotide probes. Proc Natl Acad Sci USA 85:1629, 1988

44. Fasano O, Aldrich T, Tamanoi F, Taparowsky E, Furth M, Wigler M: Analysis of the transforming potential of the human H-ras gene by random mutagenesis. Proc Natl Acad Sci USA 81:4008, 1984

45. Feig LA, Bast RC Jr, Kmapp RC, Cooper GM: Somatic activation of ras Ki gene in human ovarian cancer. Science 223:698, 1984

46. Feramisco JR, Clark R, Wong G, Arnheim N, Milley R, McCormick F: Transient reversion of ras oncogene-induced cell transformation by antibodies specific for amino acid 12 of ras protein. Nature 314:639, 1985

47. Ferre F, Garduno F, Peter JB: Detection of human papilloma virus types 6/11, 16 and 18 using polymerase chain reaction. Cancer Cells, in press

48. Flug F, Pelicci P-G, Bonetti F, Knowles DM II, Dalla-Favera R: T-cell receptor gene rearrangements as markers of lineage and clonality in T-cell neoplasms. Proc Natl Acad Sci USA 82:3460, 1985

49. Forrester K, Almoguera C, Han K, Grizzle WE, Perucho M: Detection of high incidence of K-ras oncogenes during human colon tumorigenesis. Nature 327:298, 1987

50. Friend SH, Bernards SR, Weinberg RA, Rapaport JM, Albert DM, Dryja TP: A human DNA segment with properties of the gene that predisposes to retinoblastoma and osteosarcoma. Nature 323:643, 1986

51. Gannon JV, Lane DP: p53 and DNA polymerase alpha compete for binding to SV40 T antigen. Nature 329:456, 1987

52. Gonda TJ, Metcalf D: Expression of myb, myc and fos proto-oncogenes during the differentiation of a murine myeloid leukemia. Nature 310:249, 1984

53. Groffen J, Stephenson JR, Heisterkamp N, deKlein A, Bartram CR, Grosveld G: Philadelphia chromosome breakpoints are clustered within a limited region, bcr, on chromosome 22. Cell 36:93, 1984

54. Guiot M-CP, Cavenee WK, Banks I, Crawford L, Arseneau J, Matlashewski G: Detection of HPV-16 early proteins in premalignant cervical lesion using monoclonal antibodies. Cancer Cells, in press

55. Hermans A, Heistercamp N, von Lindern M, Van Baals, Meijer D, van der Plas D, Wiedemann LM, Groffen J, Bootsma D, Grosveld G: Unique fusion of bcr and c-abl genes in Philadelphia chromosome positive acute lymphoblastic leukemia. Cell 51:33, 1987

56. Higuchi R, von Beroldingen CH, Sensabaugh GF, Erlich HA: DNA typing from single hairs. Nature 332:543, 1988

57. Hirai H, Kobayashi Y, Mario H, Hagiwara K, Maru Y, Omine M, Mizoguchi H, Nishida J, Takaku F: A point mutation at codon 13 of the N-ras oncogene in myelo-dysplastic syndrome. Nature 327:430, 1987

58. Hirai H, Tanaka S, Azuma M, Anraku Y, Kobayashi Y, Fujisaria M, Okabe T, Urabe A, Takaku F: Transforming genes in human leukemia cells. Blood 66:1371, 1985

59. Holtzman DA, Cook WD, Dunn AR: Isolation an sequence of a cDNA corresponding to src-related gene expressed in murine hematopoietic cells. Proc Natl Acad Sci USA 84:8325, 1987

60. Hunter T: A thousand and one protein kinases. Cell 50:823, 1987

61. Hunter T: The proteins of oncogenes. Sci Am 248:70, 1984

62. Hunts J, Ueda M, Ozawa S, Ave O, Pastan I, Shimizu N: Hyperproduction and gene amplification of the epidermoid growth factor receptor in squamous cell carcinomas. Jpn J Cancer Res (Gann) 76:663, 1985

63. Hurley JB, Simon MI, Teplow DB, Robishaw JD, Gilman AG: Homologies between signal transducing G protein and ras gene products. Science 226:860, 1984

64. Imce C, Blick M, Lee M, Pathak S, Vadhan-Raj S, Selvahayagam P, Gutterman JU, Cabanillas F: Bcl-1 gene rearrangements in B-cell lymphomas. Leukemia 2:343, 1988

65. Impraim CC, Saiki RK, Erlich HA, Teplitz RL: Analysis of DNA extracted from formalin-fixed, paraffin-embedded tissues by enzymatic amplification and hybridization with sequence specific oligonucleotides. Biochem Biophys Res Commun 142:710, 1987

66. Janssen JWG, Lyon SJ, Steenvoorden ACM, Seliger H, Bartram CR: Concurrent mutations in two different ras genes in acute myelocytic leukemia. Nucleic Acids Res 15:5669, 1987

67. Janssen JWG, Steenvoorden ACM, Lyons J, Anger B, Bohlke JU, Bos JL, Seliger H, Bartram CR: RAS gene mutations in acute and chronic myelocytic leukemias, chronic myeloproliferative disorders and myeodysplastic syndromes. Proc Natl Acad Sci USA 84:9228, 1987

68. Jenuwein T, Muller R: Structure-function analysis of fos protein: A single amino acid change activates the immortalizing potential of v-fos. Cell 48:647, 1987

69. Johnsson A, Heldin CH, Westermark B, Wasteson A: Platelet-derived growth factor: Identification of constituent polypeptide chains. Biochem Biophys Res Commun 104:66, 1982

70. Jones JF, Shurin S, Abramowsky C, Tubbs RR, Sciotto CG, Wahl R, Sands J, Gottman D, Katz BZ, Sklar J: T-cell lymphomas containing Epstein-Barr viral DNA in patients with chronic Epstein-Barr virus infections. New Engl J Med 318:733, 1988

71. Kasid U, Pfeifer A, Weichsbaum RR, Dritschilo A, Mark GE: The raf oncogene is associated with a radiation-resistant human laryngeal cancer. Science 237:1039, 1987

72. Kawasaki ES, Clark SS, Coyne MY, Smith SD, Champlin R, Witte ON, McCormick FP: Diagnosis of chronic myeloid and acute lymphocytic leukemias by detection of leukemia-specific mRNA sequences amplified in vitro. Proc Natl Acad Sci USA 85:5968, 1988

73. King CR, Kraus MH, Aaronson SA: Amplification of a novel v-erbB related gene in a human mammary carcinoma. Science 229:974, 1985

74. Klein G: The approaching era of the tumor suppressor genes. Science 238:1539, 1987

75. Klein G, Klein E: Evolution of tumors and the impact of molecular oncology. Nature (Lond) 315:190, 1985

76. Knudson AG Jr: Mutation and cancer: Statistical study of retinoblastoma. Proc Natl Acad Sci USA 68:820, 1971

77. Kok K, Osinga J, Carritt B, Davis MB, van der Hout AH, van der Veen AY, Landsvater RM, de Leij LFMH, Berendsen HH, Postmus PE, Poppema S, Buys CHCM: Deletion of a DNA sequence at the chromosomal region 3p21 in all major types of lung cancer. Nature 330:578, 1987

78. Konopka JB, Watanabe SM, Singer JW, Collins SJ, Witte ON: Cell lines and clinical isolates derived from Ph-positive chronic myelogenous leukemia patients express c-abl proteins with a common structural alteration. Proc Natl Acad Sci USA 82:1810, 1985

79. Koufos A, Hansen MF, Copeland NG, Jenkins NA, Lampkin BC, Cavenee WK: Loss of heterozygosity in three embryonal tumours suggests a common pathogenic mechanism. Nature 316:330, 1985

80. Leder P, Battey J, Lenoir G, Moulding C, Murphy W, Potter H, Stewart T, Taub R: Translocations among antibody genes in human cancer. Science 222:765, 1983

81. Lee MS, Blick MD, Pathak S, Trujillo JM, Butler J, Katz RL, McLaughlin P, Hagemeister FB, Velasquez WS, Goodacre A, Cork A, Gutterman JU, Cabanillas F: The gene located at chromosome 18 band of 21 is rearranged in uncultured diffuse as well as

follicular lymphomas. Blood 70:90, 1987

82. Levine AJ: Oncogenes of DNA tumor viruses. Cancer Res 48:493, 1988

83. Lewis WH, Michalopoulus EE, Williams DL, Minden MD, Mak TW: Breakpoints in the human T-cell antigen receptor alpha-chain locus in two T-cell leukemia patients with chromosomal translocations. Nature 317:554, 1985

84. Leyraz S, Henle W, Chahinian AP: Association of Epstein-Barr virus with thymic carcinoma. New Engl J Med 312:1296, 1985

85. Libermann TA, Nusbaum HR, Razon N, Kris R, Irit L, Soreq H, Whittle N, Waterfield MD, Ullrich A, Schlessinger J: Amplification, enhanced expression and possible rearrangement of EGF receptor gene in primary human brain tumours of glial origin. Nature 313:144, 1985

86. Liu E, Hielle B, Bishop JM: Transforming genes in chronic myelogenous leukemia. Proc Natl Acad Sci USA 85:1952, 1988

87. Lundberg C, Skoog L, Cavenee WK, Nordenskjold M: Loss of heterozygosity in human ductal breast tumors indicates a recessive mutation on chromosome 13. Proc Natl Acad Sci USA 84:2372, 1987

88. Lundy J, Grimson R, Mishriki Y, Chao S, Oravez S, Fromowitz F, Viola MV: Elevated *ras* oncogene expression correlates with lymph node metastases in breast cancer patients. J Clin Oncol 4:1321, 1986

89. Maniatis T, Fritsch EF, Sambrook J: Molecular Cloning, A Laboratory Manual. Cold Spring Harbor, Cold Spring Harbor Laboratory, 1982

90. Marth JD, Overell RW, Meier KE, Krebs EG, Perlmutter RM: Translational activation of the *lck* protooncogene. Nature 332:171, 1988

91. Masuda M, Battifora H, Yokota J, Meltzer S, Cline MJ: Specificity of proto-oncogene amplification in human malignant diseases. Mol Biol Med 4:213, 1987

92. Masuda H, Miller C, Koeffler HP, Battifora H, Cline MJ: Rearrangement of the p53 gene in human osteogenic sarcomas. Proc Natl Acad Sci USA 84:7716, 1987

93. McCormick F, Clark BFC, la Cour TF, Kjeldgaard M, Norskov-Lauritsen L, Nyborg J: A model for the tertiary structure of p21, the product of the *ras* oncogene. Science 230:78, 1985

94. McGrath JP, Capon DJ, Smith DH, Chen EY, Seeburg PH, Goeddel DV, Levinson AD: Structure and organization of the human Ki-ras proto-oncogene and a related processed pseudogene. Nature 304:501, 1983

95. McKeithan TW, Rowley JD, Shows TB, Diaz MO: Cloning of the chromosomal translocation breakpoint junction of the t(14;19) in chronic lymphocytic leukemia. Proc Natl Acad Sci USA 84:9257, 1987

96. McKeithan TW, Shima EA, Le Beau MM, Minowada J, Rowley JD, Diaz MO: Molecular cloning of the breakpoint junction of a human chromosomal 8;14 translocation involving the T cell receptor alpha chain gene and sequences in the 3' side of myc. Proc Natl Acad Sci USA 83:6636, 1986

97. Mercer WE, Avignolo C, Baserga R: Role of the p53 protein in cell proliferation as studied by microinjection of monoclonal antibodies. Mol Cell Biol 4:276, 1984

98. Merlino GT, Xu Y-H, Ishi S, Clark AJL, Semba K, Toyoshima K, Yamamoto T, Pastan I: Amplification and enhanced expression of the epidermal growth factor receptor gene in A431 human carcinoma cells. Science 224:417, 1984

99. Mitchell H, Drake M, Medley G: Prospective evaluation of risk of cervical cancer after cytological evidence of human papilloma virus infection. Lancet 1:573, 1986

100. Morse B, Rothberg PG, South VJ, Spandorfer JM, Astrin SM: Insertional mutagenesis of the *myc* locus by a LINE-1 sequence in a human breast cancer. Nature 333:87, 1988

101. Morton CC, Duby AD, Eddy RL, Shows TB, Siedman JG: Genes for beta gene of human T cell antigen receptor map to regions of chromosomal rearrangement in T cells. Science 228:582, 1985

102. Mufti GJ, Hamblin TJ, Oscier DG, Johnson S: Common ALL with pre B cell features showing (8;14) and (14;18) chromosome translocations. Blood 62:1142, 1983

103. Muleris M, Salmon RJ, Zafrani B, Girodet J, Dutrillaux B: Consistent deficiencies of chromosome 18 and of the short arm of chromosome 17 in eleven cases of human large bowel cancer: A possible recessive determinism. Ann Genet 28:206, 1985

104. Muller R, Bravo R, Burckhardt J, Curran T: Induction of *c-fos* gene and protein by growth factors precedes activation of *c-myc*. Nature 312:716, 1984

105. Muller R, Slamon DJ, Adamson ED, Tremblay JM, Muller D, Cline MJ, Verma I: Transcription of c-ras-Ki and c-fms during mouse development. Mol Cell Biol 3:1062, 1983

106. Muller WJ, Sinn E, Pattengale PK, Wallace R, Leder P: Single-step induction of mammary adenocarcinoma in transgenic mice bearing the activated c-neu oncogene. Cell 54:105, 1988

107. Murday VA, Bussey HJR, Levitt S, Jones T, Sheer D, Bodmer WF, Slack J: Clinical application of linked RFLPs in the diagnosis and management of patients with familial polyposis. The molecular diagnostics of human cancer, p 68. Cold Spring Harbor, Cold Spring Harbor Symposium, Sept 1988

108. Nagarajan L, Louie E, Tsujimoto Y, Balduzzi PC, Huebner K, Croce CM: The human *c-ros* gene (ROS) is located at chromosome region 6q16-6q22. Proc Natl Acad Sci USA 83:6568, 1986

109. Nau M, Brooks BJ Jr, Carney DN, Gazdar AF, Battley JF, Sausville EA, Minna JD: Human small-cell lung cancers show amplification and expression of the N-myc gene. Proc Natl Acad Sci USA 83:1092, 1986

110. Ngan BY, Chen-Levy Z, Weiss LM, Warnke RA, Cleary ML: Expression in non-Hodgkin's lymphoma of the *bcl*-2 protein associated with the t(14;18) chromosomal translocation. New Engl J Med 318:1638, 1988

111. Orkin SH, Goldman DS, Sallan SE: Development of homozygosity for chromosome 11p markers in Wilms' tumour. Nature 309:172, 1984

112. Ostrow RS, Manias DA, Fong WJ, Zachow KR, Faras AJ: A survey of human cancers for human papilloma virus DNA by filter hybridization. Cancer 59:429, 1987

113. Parada LF, Land H, Weinberg RA, Wolf D, Rotter V: Cooperation between encoding p53 tumor antigen and *ras* in cellular transformation. Nature 312:649, 1984

114. Pellici P-G, Knowles D.M-II, Nagrath I, Dalla Favera R: Chromosomal breakpoints and structural alterations of c-myc locus differ in endemic and sporadic forms of the disease. Proc Natl Acad Sci USA 83:2984, 1986

115. Pettenati MJ, Le Beau MM, Lemons RS, Shima EA, Kawasaki ES, Larson RA, Sherr CJ, Diaz MO, Rowley JD: Assignment of CSF-1 to 5q33.1: Evidence for clustering of genes regulating hematopoiesis and for their involvement in the deletion of the long arm of chromosome 5 in myeloid disorders. Proc Natl Acad Sci USA 84:2970, 1987

116. Pfister H, Gassenmaier A, Nurnberger F, Stuttgen G: Human papillomaviruses 5-DNA in carcinoma of an epidermodysplasia verruciformis patient infected with various human papillomavirus types. Cancer Res 43:1436, 1983

117. Piechaczyk M, Yang JQ, Blanchard JM, Jeanteur P, Marcu KB: Post transcriptional mechanisms are responsible for accumulation of truncated c-myc RNAs in murine plasma cell tumours. Cell 42:589, 1985

118. Priest JR, Robison L, McKenna RW, Lindquist LL, Warkentin PI, LeBien TW, Woods WG, Kersey JH: Philadelphia chromosome positive childhood acute lymphoblastic leukemia. Blood 56:15, 1980

119. Pulciani S, Santos E, Lauver AV, Long LK, Aaronson SA, Barbacid M: Oncogenes in solid human tumours. Nature 300:539, 1982

120. Rao VN, Papas TS, Shyam E, Reddy P: *erg* a human ets-related gene on chromosome 21: Alternative splicing, polyadenylation and translation. Science 237:635, 1987

121. Reddy E, Reynolds R, Santos E, Barbacid M: A point mutation is responsible for the acquisition of transforming properties by the T24 human bladder carcinoma oncogene. Nature 300:149, 1982

122. Reich NC, Levine AJ: Growth regulation of a cellular tumor antigen, p53 in nontransformed cells. Nature 308:199, 1984

123. Reynolds TC, Smith SD, Sklar J: Analysis of DNA surrounding the breakpoints of chromosomal translocations involving the beta T-cell receptor gene in human lymphoblastic neoplasms. Cell 50:107, 1987

124. Rodenhuis S, Bos JL, Slater RM, Behrendt H, vant Veer M, Smets LA: Absence of oncogene amplification and occasional activation of N-ras in lymphoblastic leukemia of childhood. Blood

67:1698, 1986

125. Rodenhuis S, Van de Wetering ML, Mooi WJ, Evers SG, van Zandwijk N, Bos JL: Mutational activation of the K-RAS oncogene. A possible pathogenetic factor in adenocarcinoma of the lung. N Engl J Med 317:929, 1987

126. Rous P: A sarcoma of the fowl transmissible by an agent separable from the tumor cells. J Exp Med 13:397, 1911

127. Rovinski B, Munroe D, Peacock J, Mowat M, Bernstein A, Benchimol S: Deletion of coding sequences of the cellular p53 gene in mouse leukemia: A novel mechanism of oncogene regulation. Mol Cell Biol 7:847, 1987

128. Rowley JD: Chromosomes in Cancer: From Molecules to Man. edited by Rowley JD, Ultmann JE, pp 139–159. New York, Academic, 1983

129. Saiki RK, Gelfand DH, Stoffel S, Scharf SV, Higuchi R, Horn GT, Mullis K, Erlich HA: Primer directed enzymatic amplification of DNA with a thermostable DNA polymerase. Science 239:487, 1988

130. Sangster R, Minowada J, Suciu-Foca N, Mindin M, Mak TW: Rearrangement and expression of X, B, and T-cell receptor genes in human leukemic and functional T-cell lines. J Exp Med 1631:1492, 1986

131. Scharf SJ, Horn GT, Erlich HA: Direct cloning and sequence analysis of enzymatically amplified genomic sequences. Science 233:1076, 1986

132. Schechter AL, Stern DF, Vaidyanathan L, Decker SJ, Drebin JA, Greene MI, Weinberg RA: The neu oncogene; and erb-B-related gene encoding a 185,000-M, tumor antigen. Nature 312:513, 1984

133. Schimke RT: Gene amplification in cultured animal cells. Cell 37:705, 1984

134. Schwab M, Alitalo K, Klempnauer KH, Varmus HE, Bishop JM, Gilbert F, Brodeur G, Goldstein M, Trent J: Amplified DNA with limited homology to myc cellular oncogene is shared by human neuroblastoma tumor. Nature 305:245, 1983

135. Schwarz E, Freese UK, Gissmann L, Mayer W, Roggenbuck B, Zur Hausen H: Structure and transcription of human papilloma virus sequences in cervical carcinoma cells. Nature 314:111, 1985

136. Seeger RC, Brodeur GM, Sather H, Dalton A, Siegel SE, Wong KY, Hammond D: Association of multiple copies of the N-myc oncogene with rapid progression of neuroblastomas. New Engl J Med 313:1111, 1985

137. Seizinger BR, Martuza RL, Gusella JF: Loss of genes on chromosome 22 in tumorigenesis of human acoustic neuroma. Nature 322:644, 1986

138. Semba K, Kamata N, Toyoshima K, Yamamoto T: A v-erbB related proto-oncogene, c-erbB2 is distinct from the c-erbB-1/ epidermoid growth factor gene and is amplified in a human salivary gland tumor. Proc Natl Sci USA 82:6497, 1985

139. Sherr CJ, Rettenmier CW, Sacca R, Roussel MF, Look AT, Stanley ER: The c-fms proto-oncogene product is related to the mononuclear phagocyte growth factor, CSF-1. Cell 41:665, 1985

140. Shiloh Y, Shipley J, Brodeur GM, Bruns G, Korf B, Donlon T, Schreck RR, Seeger R, Sakai K, Latt SA: Differential amplifications, assembly, and relocation of multiple DNA sequences in human neuroblastomas and neuroblastoma cell lines. Proc Natl Acad Sci USA 82:3761, 1985

141. Shimizu K, Birnbaum D, Ruley MA, Fasano O, Suard Y, Edlund L, Taparowsky E, Goldfarb M, Wigler M: Structure of the Ki-ras gene of the human lung carcinoma cell line Calu-1. Nature 304:497, 1983

142. Shtivelman E, Lifshitz B, Gale RP, Caanani E: Fused transcript of abl and bcr genes in chronic myelogenous leukemia. Nature 315:550, 1985

143. Siebenlist U, Hennighausen L, Battey J, Leder P: Chromatin structure and protein binding in the putative regulatory region of the c-myc gene in Burkitt's lymphoma. Cell 37:381, 1984

144. Sixbey JW, Nedrud JG, Raab-Traub N, Hanes RA, Pagano JS: Epstein-Barr virus replication in oropharyngeal epithelial cells. New Engl J Med 310:1225, 1984

145. Slamon DJ, Boone TC, Seeger RC, Keith DE, Chazin V, Lee HC, Souza LM: Identification and characterization of the protein encoded by the human N-myc oncogene. Science 232:768, 1986

146. Slamon DJ, Clark GM, Wong SG, Levin WJ, Ullrich A, McGuire WL: Human breast cancer correlation of relapse and survival with amplification of the HER-2/neu oncogene. Science 235:177, 1987

147. Slamon DJ, Cline MJ: Expression of cellular oncogenes during embryonic and fetal development of the mouse. Proc Natl Acad Sci USA 81:7141, 1984

148. Slamon DJ, deKernion JB, Verma IM, Cline MJ: Expression of cellular oncogenes in human malignancies. Science 224:256, 1984

149. Sobol R, Mick R, Royston F, Davey FR, Ellison RR, Newman R, Cuttner J: Clinical importance of myeloid antigen expression in adult acute lymphoblastic leukemia. New Engl J Med 316:1111, 1987

150. Solomon E, Voss R, Hall V, Bodmer WF, Jass JR, Jeffreys AJ, Lucibello FC, Patel I, Rider SH: Chromosome 5 allele loss in human colorectal carcinomas. Nature 328:616, 1987

151. Taira M, Yoshida T, Miyagawa K, Sakumoto H, Terada M, Sugimura T: cDNA sequence of human transforming gene hst and identification of the coding sequence required for transforming activity. Proc. Natl Acad Sci USA 84:2980, 1987

152. Taparowsky E, Shimizu K, Goldfarb M, Wigler M: Structure and activation of the human N-ras gene. Cell 34:581, 1983

153. Taub R, Moulding C, Battey J, Murphy W, Vasicek T, Lenoir GM, Leder P: Activation and somatic mutation of the translocated c-myc gene in Burkitt lymphoma cells. Cell 36:339, 1984

154. Tkachuk DC, Griesser H, Takihara Y, Champagne E, Minden M, Feller AC, Lennert K, Mak TW: Rearrangement of T-cell delta locus in lymphoproliferative disorders. Blood 72:353, 1988

155. Tsujimoto Y, Finger LR, Yunis J, Nowell PC, Croce CM: Cloning of the chromosome breakpoint of t(14;18) human lymphomas: Clustering around JH on chromosome 14 and near a transcriptional unit on 18. Cell 41:899, 1985

156. Tsujimoto Y, Gorham J, Cossman J, Jaffe E, Croce CM: The t(14;18) chromosome translocation involved in B-cell neoplasms results from mistakes in VDJ joining. Science 229:1390, 1985

157. Tsujimoto Y, Yunis J, Onorato-Showe L, Erikson J, Nowell PC, Croce CM: Molecular cloning of the chromosomal breakpoint of B-cell lymphomas and leukemias with the t(11;14) translocation. Science 224:1403, 1984

158. Van de Vijver MJ, Peterse JL, Mooi WJ, Wisman P, Lomans J, Dalesio O, Nusse R: Neu-protein overexpression in breast cancer: Association with comedo-type ductal carcinoma in situ and limited prognostic value in stage II cancer. New Engl J Med 319:1239, 1988

159. Varley JM, Swallow JE, Brammer WJ, Whittake JL, Walker RA: Alterations to either c-erbB-2 (neu) or c-myc proto-oncogenes in breast carcinomas correlate with poor short-term prognosis. Oncogene 1:423, 1987

160. Venter DJ, Kumar S, Tuzi NL: Overexpression of the human c-ERBB-2 oncoprotein in human breast carcinomas: Immunohistochemical assessment correlates with gene amplification. Lancet 2:69, 1987

161. Verlaan-de-Vries M, Bogaard ME, van der Elst H, van Boom JH, van der Eb AJ, Bos JL: A dot-blot screening procedure for mutated ras oncogenes using synthetic oligodeoxynucleotides. Gene 50:313, 1986

162. Viola MV, Fromowitz F, Oravez S, Debs S, Finkel G, Lundy J, Hand P, Thor A, Schlom J: Expression of ras oncogene p21 in prostate cancer. N Engl J Med 314:133, 1986

163. Vogelstein B, Fearon ER, Hamilton SR, Kern ES, Preisinger AC, Leppert M, Nakamura Y, White R, Smits AMM, Bos LJ: Genetic alterations during colorectal tumor development. New Engl J Med 319:525, 1988

164. Waterfield MD, Scrace GT, Whittle N, Strrobant P, Johnsson A, Wasteson A, Westermark B, Heldin CH, Huang JS, Deuel TF: Platelet-derived growth factor is structurally related to the putative transforming protein p28 sis of simian sarcoma virus. Nature (Lond) 304:35, 1983

165. Weichselbaum RR, Beckett M, Diamond A: Some retinoblastomas, osteosarcomas and soft tissue sarcomas may share a common etiology. Proc Natl Acad Sci USA 85:2106, 1988

166. Weinberg RA: Findng the anti-oncogene. Sci Am 259:44, 1988

167. Weinberg RA: The action of oncogenes in the cytoplasm and nucleus. Science 230:770, 1985

168. Weinberger C, Thompson CC, Ong ES, Lebo R, Gruol DJ, Evans RM: The c-erb-A gene encodes a thyroid receptor. Nature 324:641, 1986

169. Wiggs J, Nordenskjold M, Yandell D, Rapaport J, Grondin V, Janson M, Werelius B, Petersen R, Craft A, Riedel K, Liberfarb

R, Walton D, Wilson W, Dryja TP: Prediction of the risk of hereditary retinoblastoma using DNA polymorphisms within the retinoblastoma gene. New Engl J Med 318:151, 1988

170. Yancopoulos GD, Blackwell TK, Suh H, Hood L, Alt FW: Introduced T cell receptor variable region gene segments recombine in pre-B cells: Evidence that T and B cells use a common recombinase. Cell 44:251, 1986

171. Yarden Y, Kuang W-J, Yang-Feng T, Coussens L, Munemitsu S, Dull TJ, Chen E, Schlessinger J, Franke U, Ullrich A: Human proto-oncogene c-*kit*: A new cell surface receptor tyrosine. EMBO J 6:3341, 1987

172. Yokota J, Tsunetsugu-Yokota Y, Battifora H, Lefevre C, Cline MJ: Alterations of myc, myb, and ras-Ha proto-oncogenes in cancers are frequent and show clinical correlation. Science 231:261, 1986

173. Yokota J, Yamamoto T, Toyosima K, Yamamoto T, Battifora H, Cline MJ: Amplification of the c-erbB-2 oncogene in human adenocarcinomas in vivo. Lancet i:765, 1986

174. Zhou DJ, Ahuja H, Cline MJ: Proto-oncogene abnormalities in human breast cancer: c-ERBB-2 amplification does not correlate with recurrence of disease. Oncogene 4:105, 1989

175. Zhou DJ, Battifora H, Yokota J, Yamamoto T, Cline MJ: Association of multiple copies of the c-erbB-2 oncogene with spread of breast cancer. Cancer 47:6123, 1987

176. Zhou DJ, Gonzalez-Cadavid N, Ahuja H, Battifora H, Moore GE, Cline MJ: A unique pattern of proto-oncogene abnormalities in ovarian adenocarcinomas. Cancer 62:1573, 1988

177. Ziegler SF, Marth JD, Lewis DB, Perlmutter RM: Novel protein-tyrosine kinase gene (*hck*) preferentially expressed in cells of hematopoietic origin. Mol Cell Biol 7:2276, 1987

178. Zur Hausen H: Papilloma viruses in human cancer. Cancer 59:1692, 1987

Biology of Disease

Role of Inhibition of Intercellular Communication in Carcinogenesis

JAMES E. KLAUNIG AND RANDALL J. RUCH

Department of Pathology Medical College of Ohio, Toledo, Ohio

INTRODUCTION

Subsequent to the first morphologic description of the gap junction by Revel and Karnovsky in 1967 (113), a plethora of reports has appeared describing the structure, function and pathologic changes of this plasma membrane structure. The gap junction appears to serve as a conduit for the cell-to-cell exchange of low molecular weight ions and molecules between adjacent cells (intercellular communication). A number of functions have been attributed to intercellular communication including the maintenance of normal cellular homeostasis. Another function that is clearly related to the neoplastic process is the control of cellular growth (81). Yotti, Chang, and Trosko (178) and Murray and Fitzgerald (99), working independently, reported in 1979 that tumor promoting phorbol ester compounds were capable of inhibiting gap junction-mediated intercellular communication between cells in culture. These findings resulted in the hypothesis that tumor promoters stimulate cell proliferation of initiated cells by inhibiting gap junctional intercellular communication in the initiated cells (146).

STAGES OF CHEMICAL CARCINOGENESIS

The induction of cancer by chemicals appears to be a multistep process. Operationally, three stages of carcinogenesis have been defined: initiation, promotion, and progression (109). Initiation involves the induction of genetic damage by a chemical or its metabolite. If not repaired, this damage will be passed on to daughter cells.

Proliferation of initiated cells allows for the fixation of this genomic damage. Initiation is linearly dose-related and does not appear to possess a clearly defined threshold. After fixation of the DNA damage in daughter cells, initiation becomes irreversible. Promotion involves the induction of proliferation of initiated cells that allows for the "locking in" of the initiation damage as well as facilitating an environment for further mutational events in the preneoplastic initiated cells. Promotion is dose-dependent, exhibits a threshold and is reversible. The third stage, progression, is the least defined of the three steps and involves the irreversible transition from preneoplastic to neoplastic cells and from benign neoplastic lesions to malignant lesions.

The mechanisms of action of chemical carcinogens do not fall readily into the three staging categories. This has led to the classification of chemical carcinogens based upon the ability of a compound to interact with and damage the cellular genetic apparatus, that is, genotoxic and nongenotoxic (170). Genotoxic compounds damage cellular DNA through mutation and chromosome changes while nongenotoxic carcinogens appear to work through non-DNA damaging mechanisms. Most compounds that function in the promotional stage of carcinogenesis would be a subset and included in the nongenotoxic classification. Thus, some nongenotoxic carcinogens may also be tumor promoters. The mechanism by which nongenotoxic compounds exhibit their carcinogenic effect remains unresolved. However, a common property associated with their action on the target tissue is the ability to stimulate DNA synthesis and cell proliferation in the cells of the target tissue. Cytotoxic nongenotoxic carcinogens such as carbon tetrachloride and chloroform produce cell death which results in subsequent reparative hyperplasia. Other nongenotoxic compounds such as phorbol esters and the dioxin compound, 2,3,7,8-tetrachlorodibenzo-p-dioxin, possess a receptor and may induce cell division through receptor-mediated mechanisms. Agents which stimulate organelle replication may also stimulate cellular hypertrophy and hyperplasia. These would include peroxisome proliferators such as hypolipidemic drugs and environmental contaminants such as trichloroethylene and phthalate esters. Additionally, certain drugs and xenobiotics such as phenobarbital and chlorinated pesticides induce cytochrome P450 monooxygenases, proliferation of smooth endoplasmic reticulum, and hyperplasia. However, it is not clear if cellular hypertrophication stimulates cell division or if other factors are involved.

The growth stimulation produced by nongenotoxic carcinogens that function at cytotoxic doses is most likely the result of regenerative hyperplasia. However, it is less clear how other nongenotoxic carcinogens stimulate cell growth. The control and stimulation of normal cellular replication are complex interrelated processes *in vivo* that depend on humoral factors (growth factors, hormones, and nutrients), the extracellular matrix, cell-to-cell contact (contact inhibition of growth, intercellular communication through gap junctions), and cell status (differentiation status of the cell, staging of the cell cycle). Nongenotoxic carcinogens that stimulate cell growth in the absence of cell killing could affect any of these factors to alter normal cellular growth control. One common cellular effect of many nongenotoxic carcinogens is the inhibition of intercellular communication through gap junctions. Since intercellular communication may be an important component of cellular growth control, it has been hypothesized that nongenotoxic carcinogens stimulate cell replication by inhibiting intercellular communication (146).

INTERCELLULAR COMMUNICATION

GAP JUNCTION STRUCTURE AND INTERCELLULAR COMMUNICATION

Gap junctions are ubiquitous. They have been detected in animals of all invertebrate and vertebrate phyla. Similar structures, the plasmodesmata, are found in plants (51). In mammals, gap junctions have been detected in nearly all adult and embryonic tissues (82). They are not present in adult skeletal muscle or blood cells, but have been seen in skeletal myoblasts, hematopoietic tissue, and stimulated, aggregated lymphocytes (82).

Gap junctions are plasma membrane structures formed at the area of contact between two cells (Fig. 1). Gap junctions, as viewed by electron microscopy, consist of clusters of particles embedded in the plasma membrane. Each particle or connexon is tightly joined to an identical connexon within the membrane of the adjacent cell (82) (Fig. 1). Within these paired connexons, a hollow aqueous channel of approximately 1.5-2 nm in diameter in mammalian cells and 2-3 nm in diameter in insect

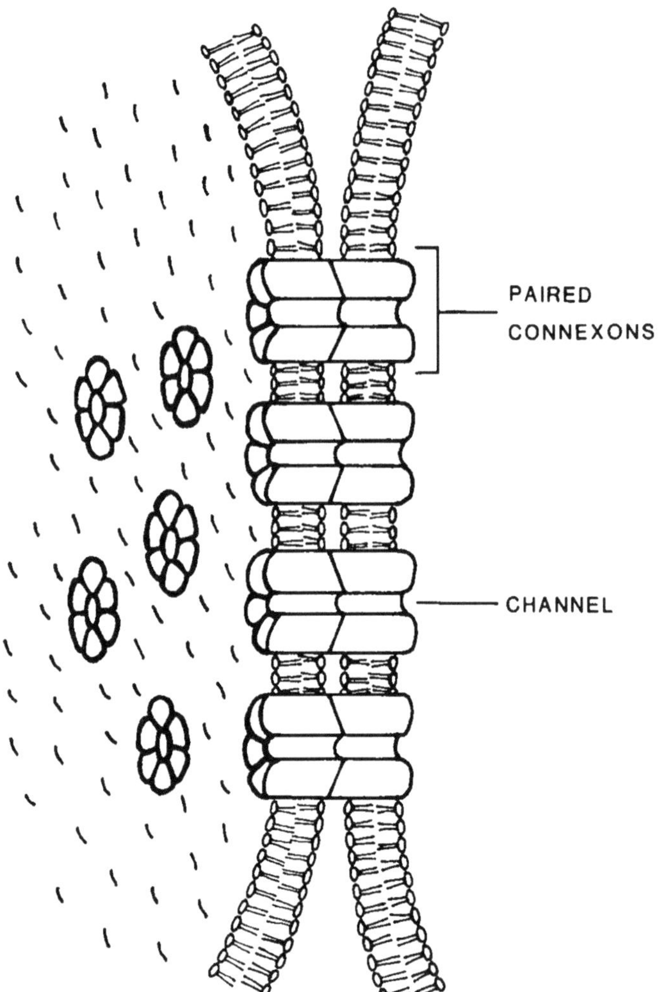

FIG. 1. Diagram of possible structure of gap junction based on morphologic and biochemical evidence. The functional units of the gap junction (the connexons) are shown forming channels between opposing plasma membranes.

cells links the cytoplasms of adjacent cells. These cell-to-cell channels permit the free diffusion of cytoplasmic ions and molecules between adjacent cells. The pore size of the mammalian gap junction is such that it excludes molecules larger than approximately 1,000 daltons while in insect gap junctions the exclusion limit is approximately 2,500 daltons (41, 131, 133). Thus, ions, nutrients, nucleotides, cyclic nucleotides, and metabolites of endogenous compounds and xenobiotics (including carcinogens (61)) are capable of passing between cells through gap junctions (82).

Gap junctions in the rat liver have been extensively studied and consist of a few to thousands of clustered connexon pairs forming large plaques (92). The average area of rat hepatocyte gap junctions is approximately 0.6 μm^2 (141) representing about 3% of the hepatocyte plasma membrane (92, 141). Meyer, Yancey, and Revel (92) have estimated that each hepatocyte forms a minimum of two gap junctions with each adjacent hepatocyte and an average of 12–14 gap junctions are seen on each hepatocyte.

How connexons are inserted into the plasma membrane, form pairs with adjacent cell connexons, and cluster into large plaques remains unknown. In the absence of gap junctions, connexons may diffuse freely in the lipid bilayer of the plasma membrane (82). Upon close apposition of the plasma membrane of two cells, the connexons may randomly interact, pair with connexons from the neighboring membrane, and open their cell-to-cell channels (82). How paired connexons form the large gap junction plaques is not clear but may be due to mutual attraction between the paired connexons (17).

The biochemical composition of gap junctions has been best characterized for liver, lens, and heart due to the abundance of the junctions in these tissues. In rodent liver, connexons are composed of six identical protein subunits of 32,000 daltons molecular weight each. This interpretation is based on X-ray diffraction, recombinant DNA, and gel electrophoresis studies of the protein (49, 71, 84, 94, 105, 181). In addition, evidence has recently been presented indicating that rodent liver gap junction connexons may be composed of two different proteins (101). It is unknown if the two types of connexons have different permeability characteristics. Lens fiber gap junctions also appear to consist of two distinct proteins of 26,000 and 70,000 daltons (38, 48, 58, 95). Meanwhile, connexons in cardiocyte gap junctions may be composed of identical protein subunits of molecular weight of 43,000 daltons (14, 87). The homology of hepatocyte, lens fiber, and cardiocyte gap junction proteins is being defined using both immunologic and biochemical approaches. Antibodies raised against rodent liver gap junction protein cross-react with gap junctions from heart, pancreas, brain, and other tissues but not lens (26, 57). Analyses of the gap junction cDNA and amino acid sequencing of the gap junction protein have demonstrated homology between liver and heart gap junctions but not lens (14, 50, 102, 114). Besides protein, lipid appears to be the only other biochemical component of gap junction plaques (56). The lipid composition of the gap junction is similar to that of nonjunctional plasma membrane (56). Cholesterol (88, 115, 116) and carbohydrates (50, 56, 164) do not appear to be present in gap junctions.

REGULATION OF GAP JUNCTION FORMATION AND PERMEABILITY

The half-life of rodent liver gap junction protein has been estimated to be 3 to 5 hours (37, 145). Intercellular communication, therefore, may be rapidly modified by treatments that affect gap junction gene expression or protein synthesis/degradation.

Intercellular communication can also be modified by protein kinases and intracellular ion concentrations. These regulatory functions may be activated by "normal" physiologic activity or upon exposure of cells to toxic agents. Gap junctions are phosphorylated by several protein kinases that may result in a modification of connexon structure and permeability. Treatment of the cells with agents that elevate cyclic AMP levels has been shown to enhance intercellular communication (25, 31, 36, 40, 66, 129, 145, 155). This effect was attributed to phosphorylation of the gap junction proteins by cyclic AMP-dependent protein kinase or to cyclic AMP enhancement of gap junction gene expression. Intercellular communication has been decreased following activation of protein kinase C by diacylglycerol or phorbol esters (35, 44, 98, 173). This may have been due to gap junction phosphorylation since protein kinase C is capable of phosphorylating gap junction proteins (143). In addition, several viral oncogene products including pp60[src] and polyoma virus middle T antigen which have protein kinase activities have been implicated in the loss of intercellular communication in cells infected with these viruses (2, 3, 6–10, 19, 119). Evidence that these latter kinases phosphorylate gap junction proteins has not been presented however.

Intercellular increases in Ca^{2+} or H^+ ions have also been implicated in regulating gap junction permeability. Increased concentrations of Ca^{2+} or H^+ may result in the loss of gap junction permeability. Increased intracellular Ca^{2+} by treatment with either the calcium ionophore, A23187, or by microinjecting Ca^{2+} resulted in the loss of intercellular communication (108, 118). The observed effects of Ca^{2+} on gap junctional intercellular communication may be mediated by calmodulin. Calmodulin binds to purified liver, lens, and heart gap junction proteins. Its binding affinity increases in the presence of Ca^{2+} (56, 106, 107). The Ca^{2+}-calmodulin complex resulting from increased Ca^{2+} concentrations may be located near the cytoplasmic openings of the gap junction channels thus, inhibiting intercellular communication by stearically hindering channel permeability (106). Others have argued that the loss of intercellular communication by Ca^{2+} elevation may be due to elevations in intracellular H^+ concentrations following Ca^{2+}/H^+ exchange (136). In rat hepatocytes, intercellular communication decreased rapidly when the cells were acidified from their normal pH of approximately 7.3 to a pH below 6.6 by CO_2 exposure (137).

CELLULAR FUNCTIONS OF GAP JUNCTION-MEDIATED INTERCELLULAR COMMUNICATION

Gap junctions are ubiquitous in the animal kingdom, thus it is likely that they have evolved to have several important cellular functions. One function of intercellular communication may be to maintain cellular homeostasis through the exchange of ions, metabolites, and water (82). However, more specific functions have been proposed for intercellular communication depending on the cell type. In electrically active cells such as neurons, cardiocytes, and smooth muscle cells, gap junctions serve as electrical synapses for the rapid conduction of action potentials (13, 55). In other cells, intercellular communication may coordinate tissue responses to hormones through the exchange of second messenger ions or molecules between hormone-stimulated and non-stimulated cells (75). In addition, gap junction mediated intercellular communication is thought to define embryonic compartments and may provide intracellular pathways for embryonic morphogens (18, 158, 171, 172).

Of more relevance to carcinogenesis, intercellular communication may be an important component of cellular growth regulation. Loewenstein (79–81) has proposed that replicative signal substances are produced periodically within cells and pass into adjacent cells through gap junctions. These signals, possibly cyclic nucleotides or ions, would activate cell division if they reached a sufficient and sustained concentration in the signal-producing cell. If the level of these chemical signals is maintained in a reduced concentration by intercellular communication, cell division would not occur in the signal-producing cell. With the inhibition of intercellular communication by either endogenously or exogenously generated treatment, the signal-producing cell would be stimulated to divide by an excess level of its own signals.

Evidence in favor of a regulatory role for intercellular communication in cell growth has recently emerged. Many cancer cells have a decreased capacity for intercellular communication and a decreased number of gap junctions (81). This loss of intercellular communication has been correlated with the degree of malignancy of the neoplasm (42, 103). Similarly, cultured tumor cells treated with growth-reducing agents showed reappearance of gap junctions and intercellular communication (40). Also, intercellular communication was rapidly lost in fibroblasts infected with temperature-sensitive mutants of Rous sarcoma virus when the cells were switched from the non-permissive to permissive temperature necessary for transformation (2, 3, 6). These cells readily regained intercellular communication when returned to the nonpermissive temperature. Additionally, the growth of cultured tumor cells was inhibited when the cells contacted normal cells and formed gap junctions with the normal cells (89). The greatest inhibition of growth in the transformed cells occurred when intercellular communication with the normal cells was greatest. Tumor cell growth inhibition was not simply due to contact with normal cells. In nontransformed, rapidly dividing tissue such as regenerating, partially hepatectomized liver, fewer gap junctions are seen at certain times of the regenerative cycle (27, 92). Finally, most nongenotoxic carcinogens that stimulate cell growth *in vivo* are capable of inhibiting intercellular communication in a variety of cell culture assays (see below). The sum of these studies suggests that intercellular communication is necessary for normal growth regulation and that cellular growth occurs when intercellular communication is decreased. However, it remains to be determined if the loss of intercellular communication in cells is a cause or consequence of the onset of cell division.

METHODS TO ASSESS INTERCELLULAR COMMUNICATION

Several methods exist to demonstrate the existence of permeable gap junctional channels between two cells (135). These methods can be broadly grouped into three categories: electrical coupling, metabolic cooperation, and fluorescent dye transfer.

Electrical Coupling. Because gap junctions have much lower resistance to current flow than the non-junctional plasma membrane, the flow of electrical current from one cell to another can be measured with the aid of microelectrodes. This method provides a rapid, repetitive, and sensitive indication of gap junction permeability.

Metabolic Cooperation. The phenomenon of metabolic cooperation involves the intercellular exchange of metabolites via gap junctions. The ability of cells to transfer metabolites in this way was first demonstrated by Subak-Sharpe, Burk, and Pitts (140) with metabolically normal cells (HGPRT+) cocultured with mutant, metabolically deficient cells (HGPRT−). When the two types of cells were cocultured in the presence of tritiated hypoxanthine, incorporation of the radiolabel was detected by autoradiography in normal cells and the few mutant cells in contact with normal cells, but not in isolated mutant cells. The incorporation of radiolabel in mutants was attributed to the passage of radioactive hypoxanthine derivatives from wild type to mutant cells. This is the so-called "kiss-of-life" method for demonstrating metabolic cooperation. A variant of this method that did not require mutant cells was presented by Pitts and Simms (111). They showed that [^{3}H]uridine passed from prelabeled "donor" cells to adjacent, nonlabeled "recipient" cells, but not to isolated recipient cells. A "kiss-of-death" method to demonstrate intercellular communication can also be utilized with HGPRT+/HGPRT− cocultures (43, 140), and is the basis of an assay to evaluate the effects of xenobiotics on metabolic cooperation in Chinese Hamster V79 cells (178). In the V79 HGPRT+/HRPRT− cocultures, 6-thioguanine was incorporated into wild type cells and mutant cells in communication with the wild type cells resulting in the death of both types of cells. Treatment with agents that blocked gap junctional intercellular communication prevented the transfer of the toxic metabolite to the mutant cells and prevented their death. These remaining mutant cells proliferated into colonies in the presence of 6-thioguanine. The number of residual colonies then indicated the ability of a compound to inhibit intercellular communication.

Fluorescent Dye Transfer. Gap junctional intercellular communication can be detected nearly instantaneously by visualizing fluorescent dye transfer between cells (dye-coupling). Usually a fluorescent dye (carboxyfluorescein or Lucifer Yellow CH) is microinjected into one cell and dye spread to adjacent cells is monitored (139). Other methods to introduce polar fluorescent dyes into cells include the use of plasma membrane permeable esters of the dyes, usually diacetate, dipropionate, or dibutyrate derivatives (47, 120, 156). Within the cell the esters are hydrolyzed to the membrane-impremeable, hydrophilic fluorescent dye by cellular esterases. Finally, scrape-loading is a recently developed method to introduce fluorescent dyes into cells (30). Confluent cell cultures can be scraped linearly across the culture plate with an instrument such as a razor blade or a rubber policeman in the presence of the dye. The cells at the scraped edge take up the dye (probably due to transient damage of their plasma membranes) which can then diffuse into adjacent cells through gap junctions.

INHIBITION OF INTERCELLULAR COMMUNICATION BY NONGENOTOXIC CARCINOGENS

As discussed above, tumor promotion involves cell division of the initiated cells (109, 170). The inhibition of intercellular communication by tumor promoters may be an important mechanism for enabling initiated cells to undergo growth.

A number of tumor promoters and nongenotoxic carcinogens have been examined for their effects of intercellular communication and nearly all are capable of inhibiting intercellular communication (Table 1). These compounds inhibited intercellular communication at noncytolethal concentrations. Early studies were performed with phorbol ester-derived skin tumor promoters such as TPA (12-O-tetradecanoylphorbol-13-acetate) in Chinese hamster embryo V79 fibroblasts and mouse HEL-37 epidermal cells (99, 178). A number of additional investigations have confirmed that TPA, other tumor-promoting phorbol esters, and mezerein inhibited intercellular communication between V79 cells (24, 27, 28, 30, 52–54, 59, 100, 110, 134, 138, 154, 161), HEL-37 cells (38–40, 44, 45), human FL cells and fibroblasts (32, 64, 97, 163), BALB/c mouse 3T3 fibroblasts (33–35, 175), NIH mouse 3T3 fibroblasts (19), C3H/10T1/2 mouse fibroblasts (15), rat liver epithelial cells (91, 96, 157), and primary cultured hepatocytes (122, 126). Several of these studies demonstrated that the ability of phorbol esters to inhibit intercellular communication correlated with their tumor promoting activity *in vivo*. The concentrations of TPA required to inhibit intercellular communi-

cation were of the order of 1 to 100 ng/ml. The studies also indicated that the maximum inhibitory effect on intercellular communication occurred after 1 to 2 hours of cell exposure to TPA (28, 31, 35, 174) although exposure times as short as 1 minute (53) and 20 minutes (38) have maximally inhibited intercellular communication in similar cells. The inhibitory effect of TPA on intercellular communication was reversible when TPA was removed. Restoration of intercellular communication occurred 2 to 12 hours after TPA removal (35, 38, 174). This recovery of intercellular communication after TPA removal was not attributed to enhanced gap junction synthesis since recovery also occurred when protein and RNA synthesis were blocked with cycloheximide and actinomycin D, respectively (174). In addition, TPA-treated cells became refractory to the inhibitory effects of the promoter on intercellular communication after prolonged exposure of 8 hours or more (28, 29, 35, 39, 91, 157, 174). Since the inhibition of intercellular communication by TPA may have been related to activation of the phorbol ester receptor, protein kinase C, the development of refractoriness in TPA-treated cells was attributed to down-regulation of the receptor (174).

TPA also decreased the number and size of gap junctions in promoter-treated cells and epidermis. TPA de-

TABLE 1. TUMOR PROMOTERS AND OTHER NONGENOTOXIC CARCINOGENS THAT INHIBIT INTERCELLULAR COMMUNICATION *IN VITRO*

Carcinogen	Cell type tested
TPA and other phorbol esters	Chinese hamster V79 fibroblasts
	Mouse epidermal HEL-37 cells
	Human FL cells and fibroblasts
	Mouse fibroblasts
	Rat liver epithelial cells
	Mouse hepatocytes
Organochlorine pesticides	Chinese hamster V79 fibroblasts
	Human fibroblasts and teratocarcinoma cells
	Rat liver epithelial cells and hepatocytes
	Mouse hepatocytes
Polyhalogenated biphenyls	Chinese hamster V79 fibroblasts
	Human teratocarcinoma cells
	Rat liver epithelial cells and hepatocytes
	Mouse hepatocytes
Phenobarbital	Chinese hamster V79 fibroblasts
	Human hepatoma cells
	Rat liver epithelial cells and hepatocytes
	Mouse hepatocytes
Unsaturated fatty acids	Chinese hamster V79 fibroblasts
Bile acids	Chinese hamster V79 fibroblasts
Anthralin	Chinese hamster V79 fibroblasts
Iodoacetate	Chinese hamster V79 fibroblasts
Peroxides	Chinese hamster V79 fibroblasts
	Human keratinocytes
	Mouse hepatocytes
Saccharin	Chinese hamster V79 fibroblasts
Retinoic acid	Chinese hamster V79 fibroblasts
	Human fibroblasts
	Rat liver epithelial cells
	Hamster kidney fibroblasts
	Hamster tracheal epithelial cells
Phthalate esters	Chinese hamster V79 fibroblasts
	Mouse hepatocytes
Nickel sulfate	Mouse fibroblasts
Butylated hydroxyanisole	Chinese hamster V79 fibroblasts
2,4-D and 2,4,5-T	Chinese hamster V79 fibroblasts

creased the incidence and size of gap junctions in V79 cells (177), chick embryo hepatocytes (60), and mouse epidermis (62, 63). The study with V79 cells is particularly interesting since the loss of gap junctions was detected after 18 hours of TPA exposure (177), a time at which other studies have indicated that these cells became refractory to the inhibition of intercellular communication by TPA (28, 29) and may have had a normal complement of gap junctions.

Several nonphorbol ester tumor promoters and nongenotoxic carcinogens also inhibited intercellular communication between cultured cells (Table 1). For example, organochlorine pesticides such as 1,1-bis(4-chlorophenyl)-2,2,2-trichloroethane (DDT), lindane, aldrin, chlordane, mirex, and kepone which are rodent liver tumor promoters and/or nongenotoxic carcinogens inhibited intercellular communication in V79 fibroblasts (72, 130, 153, 159, 160, 179), human fibroblasts (21, 22) and teratocarcinoma cells (156, 180), ARL rat liver epithelial cells and rat hepatocytes (144, 166–168), and mouse hepatocytes (122, 126). Additionally, polybrominated and polychlorinated biphenyls which are also liver tumor promoters inhibited intercellular communication between V79 cells (147, 152), human teratocarcinoma cells (65), rat liver epithelial cells and rat hepatocytes (169) and/or mouse hepatocytes (122, 126). The potent liver tumor promoter phenobarbital had no effect on V79 cell intercellular communication in one study (154) but inhibited intercellular communication in V79 cells (59, 179), human hepatoma cells (117), rat liver epithelial cells and hepatocytes (165), and mouse hepatocytes (122, 124, 126). Unsaturated fatty acids are promoters of breast carcinoma and they inhibited V79 cell intercellular communication while saturated fatty acids which may be promoters for colon carcinoma had no effect (4, 5). Oleic acid also inhibited V79 cell intercellular communication in one report (149), but was refractory in these same cells in another report (67). Similarly, bile acids are promoters of colon cancer and these agents inhibited intercellular communication between V79 cells in one study (88), but had no effect in another investigation (179). The nonphorbol ester skin tumor promoters, anthralin and iodoacetate, inhibited V79 cell intercellular communication in three studies (67, 149, 154), but were negative in two subsequent studies (132, 179). Benzoyl peroxide and other peroxides are weak skin tumor promoters and these agents inhibited V79 cell (134), human keratinocyte (74), and mouse hepatocyte intercellular communication (125). However, benzoyl peroxide was not effective in V79 cells in another report (179). Saccharin, a bladder tumor promoter, inhibited V79 cell intercellular communication in one study (148) but had no effect on these cells in another study (154) or on mouse hepatocytes (126). Retinoic acid, a weak skin tumor promoter, enhanced or inhibited intercellular communication between several types of cells depending on the concentration of the vitamin (23, 54, 96, 112, 127, 157). The peroxisome proliferator and liver tumor promoter diethylhexylphthalate inhibited V79 cell intercellular communication (85). A series of straight and branched chain phthalate monoesters were tested for their ability to inhibit mouse hepatocyte intercellular

communication and only the branched chain derivatives were effective (70). Nickel sulfate, a renal tumor promoter, inhibited intercellular communication between NIH 3T3 cells (73, 93). The tumor promoters butylated hydroxyanisole (179), 2,4-dichlorophenoxyacetic acid (2,4-D) (121), and 2,4,5-trichlorophenoxyacetic acid (2,4,5-T) (121), inhibited V79 cell intercellular communication. 2,3,7,8-Tetrachlorodibenzo-p-dioxin had no effect on intercellular communication in these cells (77) or C3H10T1/2 fibroblasts (15). Generally, the concentrations of the above nonphorbol ester tumor promoters required to inhibit intercellular communication between cultured cells were in the μM to mM range.

Phenobarbital and DDT also decreased the size of gap junctions and area of membrane occupied by these structures in rat hepatocytes after *in vivo* exposure (141). These effects were seen after 2 to 12 weeks administration of promoting doses of phenobarbital or DDT (0.05%) in the drinking water. Phenobarbital also decreased gap junction protein mRNA levels in rat liver (90).

Few studies have examined the kinetics of inhibition of intercellular communication by the nonphorbol ester tumor promoters and other nongenotoxic carcinogens and whether treated cells become refractory to the inhibitory effects of these agents on intercellular communication. A recent study by our group, however, has demonstrated that intercellular communication between mouse hepatocytes is inhibited maximally by phenobarbital after 2 hours of treatment, that the cells recover from the inhibitory effect of phenobarbital within 15 minutes after the removal of the promoter, and that these cells become refractory to the inhibitory effect after 12 hours or more exposure (124).

The inhibition of intercellular communication appears to be an effect specific to tumor promoters and nongenotoxic carcinogens and is not seen with most genotoxic carcinogens. Benzo[a]pyrene, 7,12-dimethylbenz[a]anthracene, and benz[a]anthracene, N-methyl-N'-nitrosoguanidine, and 4-nitroquinoline-1-oxide had no effect on V79 cell intercellular communication (100, 104). However, 7,12-dimethylbenz[a]-anthracene was reported to decrease gap junctions between rat lingual epithelial cells (142). Benzo[a]pyrene had no effect on ARL rat liver epithelial cell-rat hepatocyte intercellular communication (143). Similarly, dimethylnitrosamine, diethylnitrosamine, benzo[a]pyrene, and 2-acetylaminofluorene had no effect on mouse hepatocyte intercellular communication (126). Thus, the inhibition of intercellular communication appears to be a characteristic of nongenotoxic carcinogens, not genotoxic carcinogens, in most studies. However, the fact that a compound is capable of inhibiting intercellular communication does not necessarily indicate that it is a tumor promoter or nongenotoxic carcinogen. Several teratogenic agents (78), neurotoxicants (151), and a lung toxicant (125) in addition to a variety of solvents and alcohols (20) that may not be carcinogenic are also capable of inhibiting intercellular communication between cultured cells. Neither does the lack of inhibition of intercellular communication by a compound at nonlethal concentrations indicate that it does not have tumor promoting activity. *In vivo*, agents may inhibit intercellular communication and enhance carcinogenesis if administered at cytotoxic levels through the loss of cells and stimulation of regenerative hyperplasia (150). Such compounds would include hepatotoxins such as carbon tetrachloride or genotoxic carcinogens when administered at necrogenic doses. Thus, carcinogens (both genotoxic and nongenotoxic) that do not inhibit intercellular communication at noncytolethal doses may be capable of inhibiting intercellular communication and stimulating growth when administered at cytolethal concentrations.

Mechanisms of Inhibition of Intercellular Communication by Tumor Promoters and Nongenotoxic Carcinogens

How tumor promoters and nongenotoxic carcinogens inhibit intercellular communication is unknown. They may alter physiologic regulators of gap junction formation and/or permeability such as protein kinases, second messengers (Ca^{2+} and cyclic AMP), intracellular pH, and gap junction turnover (discussed above). Alternatively, these compounds may nonspecifically interact with gap junction protein or plasma membrane lipid to alter gap junction structure.

Relatively few studies have addressed the mechanisms of inhibition of intercellular communication by tumor promoters and nongenotoxic carcinogens compared to the number of reports that have merely documented the inhibitory effects of these agents. Phorbol esters such as TPA and other activators of protein kinase C, most likely function through the activation of the kinase to inhibit intercellular communication. Evidence in favor of this hypothesis is that the inhibition of intercellular communication by phorbol esters if correlated with their ability to activate protein kinase C (44). Also, the synthetic diacylglycerol, 1-oleoyl-2-acetyl-glycerol (OAG), which also activates protein kinase C, inhibited intercellular communication between BALB/c 3T3 fibroblasts (35), rat liver epithelial cells (173), HEL-37 epidermal cells (44), and V79 fibroblasts (24). How the activation of protein kinase C resulted in the inhibition of intercellular communication remains unclear, however. The kinase can phosphorylate purified gap junctions (143), but this phenomenon has not been demonstrated in intact cells. The activation of phospholipases by the kinase and release of arachidonic acid or inositol phospholipids might also be related to the inhibitory mechanism of intercellular communication. Arachidonic acid metabolism results in the production of oxygen free radicals, prostaglandins, leukotrienes, and thromboxane compounds. Several of these agents have been shown to affect intercellular communication (1, 46, 125). Similarly, inositol phospholipids, released following protein kinase C activation, may release Ca^{2+} from intracellular stores and elevate intracellular Ca^{2+} to levels inhibitory of intercellular communication. It has been shown that Ca^{2+} levels in V79 cells were elevated after treatment with TPA at concentrations that inhibited intercellular communication (83). Also, the inhibition of intercellular communication by 1-oleoyl-2-acetyl-glycerol in rat liver epithelial cells was prevented by TMB-8, an antagonist of intracellular Ca^{2+} release (173), although TMB-8 was not effective against TPA in V79 cells (54).

Similarly, Ca^{2+} may also play a role in the mechanism of inhibition of intercellular communication by organochlorine pesticides such as DDT and lindane. These agents are inhibitors of membrane Ca^{2+}-ATPases (11). These compounds may induce Ca^{2+} accumulation and inhibition of intercellular communication by poisoning the Ca^{2+} pumps. Synergistic inhibition of intercellular communication by TPA and DDT in V79 cells has been demonstrated and attributed to mechanistically different effects of these compounds on V79 cell Ca^{2+} homeostasis (160).

How other nonphorbol ester tumor promoters and nongenotoxic carcinogens inhibit intercellular communication is even less clearly defined. Compounds that are metabolized by the cytochrome P450 mixed function oxidases may stimulate oxygen free radical release from the activated oxygen-P450 complex due to uncoupling of the P450 cycle. This enhanced flux of oxygen radicals may affect intercellular communication. It has been demonstrated that the inhibition of mouse hepatocyte intercellular communication by phenobarbital, DDT, and lindane could be prevented by antioxidants (123). Intercellular communication is also inhibited by other compounds that stimulate free radical production within cells such as carbon tetrachloride (128), paraquat (125), and peroxides (74, 123, 125, 134), and by extracellular oxygen radical generating enzymes such as xanthine oxidase and glucose oxidase (123, 125). Thus, some tumor promoters may inhibit intercellular communication through a free radical mechanism.

Another mechanism by which phenobarbital and DDT inhibited mouse hepatocyte intercellular communication may be through their ability to decrease the levels of cyclic AMP in these cells (69). It was shown that intercellular communication and the levels of cyclic AMP were reduced in the hepatocytes by phenobarbital and DDT and that these effects could be prevented by simultaneous treatment with dibutyryl cyclic AMP or caffeine (69). Treatment of other types of cells with cyclic AMP agonists or inhibitors of cyclic AMP phosphodiesterase stimulated intercellular communication and gap junction formation in the absence of tumor promoters (40, 66, 155), and prevented the inhibition of intercellular communication by TPA (31, 45, 54, 64).

It has also been proposed that tumor promoters and nongenotoxic carcinogens inhibit intercellular communication through non-specific plasma membrane lipid or protein interactions (86). Although it is true that some of these compounds can interact in these ways with the plasma membrane and may inhibit intercellular communication through these effects, many of the tumor promoters that inhibit intercellular communication are lipophobic and have little protein-binding capacity (e.g., saccharin). In addition, the requirement for prolonged exposure of the cells to some agents (e.g., two or more hours exposure to phenobarbital for mouse hepatocytes) for the maximum inhibitory effect to be seen (124) suggests that some type of enzymatic or kinetic process is necessary for the loss of intercellular communication.

It is also not clear if the parent compound or a metabolite of the tumor promoter is the agent responsible for inhibiting intercellular communication. preliminary studies with phenobarbital suggest that metabolism of the promoter is required to inhibit mouse hepatocyte intercellular communication since several inhibitors of cytochrome P450 monooxygenases, prevented the inhibition of intercellular communication in these cells (162).

FUTURE DIRECTIONS

The importance of intercellular communication in the control of cellular growth needs to be more clearly defined as does the nature of any growth stimulatory or inhibitory signal(s) that pass between cells via gap junctions. Possible approaches to this problem might be to specifically inhibit intercellular communication with antibodies microinjected into cultured cells and to determine if cell division ensues. A similar approach has been undertaken with *Xenopus* embryos to demonstrate the necessity of intercellular communication for normal tadpole development (158). However, the discovery of cell division-regulating substances that pass through gap junctions might be an impossible problem since a multitude of low molecular weight messengers are produced in cells before and during cell division.

It is important to more clearly define the role of inhibited intercellular communication in the carcinogenic process. Such studies would include documenting the loss of intercellular communication during tumorigenesis as has been done for human colon carcinoma (42), and determining the sensitivities of preneoplastic cells to the inhibition of intercellular communication by tumor promoters since these cells may be more sensitive than their non-initiated counterparts. Using preneoplastic hepatocytes isolated from the rat we have shown that these preneoplastic hepatocytes have a decreased capacity for intercellular communication compared to normal hepatocytes, and an enhanced sensitivity to phenobarbital inhibition of intercellular communication (76). Beers *et al.* (12) have demonstrated decreased gap junction protein and mRNA in rat liver preneoplastic and tumor cells. In addition, other groups have reported that in *in vitro* fibroblast transformation systems, intercellular communication only occurs between normal cells or between pre-transformed cells, but not between normal and pre-transformed cells (16, 33, 175, 176). In one of these studies (175), the pre-transformed cells were more sensitive than monolayer cells to the inhibition of intercellular communication by TPA. Thus, preneoplastic cells may be incapable of communicating with normal cells and may be more sensitive to the inhibition of intercellular communication by tumor promoters. These effects may confer a growth advantage upon the preneoplastic cells.

For many types of cells such as V79 fibroblasts, there appears to be little relationship between the type of compound that inhibits intercellular communication and the *in vivo* tumor promotion target tissue of the compound (Table 1). It can also be seen in Table 1 that the V79 cell assay is sensitive to a variety of epithelial cell promoters despite the fact that the V79 cell is of mesenchymal origin. This nonspecificity may facilitate the detection of tumor promoters using V79 cells especially if the inhibition of intercellular communication is to be used as an *in vitro* assay for detecting tumor promoters. However, studies with primary cultured adult epithelial cells such as hepatocytes may be better suited to detecting strain, species and tissue specific relationships in the abilities of compounds to inhibit intercellular communication and promote neoplasia as our data indicate (68, 122, 126). In addition, studies on the mechanisms of tumor promoter inhibition of intercellular communication in fibroblastic cells may not be as relevant to the *in vivo* situation as studies with differentiated, epithelial cells. We suggest that more studies using a variety of primary cultured adult epithelial cells be undertaken. We believe that it is most important to determine the mechanisms of how tumor promoters inhibit intercellular communication. Such findings may give rise to antipromoters and to methods to re-establish intercellular communication in neoplastic tissues.

REFERENCES

1. Agrawal R, Daniel EE: Control of gap junction formation in canine trachea by arachidonic acid metabolites. Am J Physiol 250:C495, 1986
2. Atkinson MM, Anderson SK, Sheridan JD: Modification of gap junctions in cells transformed by a temperature sensitive mutant of Rous sarcoma virus. J Memb Biol 91:53, 1986
3. Atkinson MM, Menko AS, Johnson RG, Sheppard JR, Sheridan JD: Rapid and reversible reduction of junctional permeability in cells infected with a temperature-sensitive mutant of avian sarcoma virus. J Cell Biol 91:573, 1981
4. Aylsworth CF, Jones C, Trosko JE, Meites J, Welsch CW: Promotion of 7,12-dimethylbenz(a)anthracene-induced mammary tumorigenesis by high dietary fat in the rat: possible role of intercellular communication. J Natl Cancer Inst 72:637, 1984
5. Aylsworth CF Trosko JE, Welsch CW: Influence of lipids on gap junction-mediated intercellular communication between Chinese hamster cells *in vitro*. Cancer Res 46:4527, 1986
6. Azarnia, R, Loewenstein WR: Intercellular communication and the control of growth: X. Alteration of junctional permeability by the *src* gene. A study with temperature-sensitive mutant Rous sarcoma virus. J Memb Biol 82:191, 1984
7. Azarnia, R. Loewenstein WR: Intercellular communication and the control of growth: XI. Alteration of junctional permeability by the *src* gene in a revertant cell with normal cytoskeleton. J Memb Biol 82:207, 1984
8. Azarnia, R, Loewenstein WR: Intercellular communication and the control of growth: XII. Alteration of junctional permeability by Simian virus 40. Roles of the large and small T antigens. J Memb Biol 82:213, 1984
9. Azarnia R, Loewenstein WR: Polyomavirus middle T antigen down regulates junctional cell-to-cell communication. Mol Cell Biol 7:946, 1987
10. Azarnia R, Reddy S, Kmiecik TB, Shalloway D, Loewenstein WR: The cellular *src* gene product regulates junctional cell-to-cell communication. Science 239:398, 1988
11. Beeman RW: Recent advances in mode of action of insecticides. Ann Rev Entomol 2:253, 1982
12. Beer DG, Neven MJ, Paul DL, Rapp UR, Pitot HC: Expression of the c-*raf* protooncogene, -glutamyltranspeptidase, and gap junction protein in rat liver neoplasms. Cancer Res. 48:1610, 1988
13. Bennett MVL, Aljure E, Nakajima Y, Pappas GD: Electronic junctions between teleost spinal neurons: electrophysiology and ultrastructure. Science 141:262, 1963
14. Beyer EC, Paul DL, Goodenough DA: Connexin 43: A protein from rat heat homologous to a gap junction protein from liver. J Cell Biol 105:2621, 1987
15. Boreiko CJ, Abernethy DJ, Sanchez JH, Dorman BH: Effect of mouse skin tumor promoters upon [³H]uridine exchange and focus formation in cultures of C3H/10T1/2 mouse fibroblasts. Carcinogenesis 7:1095, 1986
16. Boreiko CJ, Abernethy DJ, Stedman DB: Alterations of intercellular communication associated with the transformation of C3H/

10T1/2 cells. Carcinogenesis 8:321, 1987

17. Braun J, Abney JR, Owicki JC: How a gap junction maintains its structure. Nature (London) 310:316, 1984

18. Caveney S: The role of gap junctions in development. Ann Rev Physiol 47:319, 1985

19. Chang CC, Trosko JE, Kung HJ, Bombick D, Matsumara F: Potential role of the *src* gene product in inhibition of gap-junctional communication in NIH-3T3 cells. Proc Natl Acad Sci USA 82:5360, 1985

20. Chen TH, Kavanagh TJ, Chang CC, Trosko JE: Inhibition of metabolic cooperation in Chinese hamster V79 cells by various organic solvents and simple compounds. Cell Biol Toxicol 1:155, 1984

21. Davidson JS, Baumgarten IM, Harley EH: Inhibition of intercellular junctional communication in human fibroblasts by triphenylmethane, triphenylmethylchloride, tetraphenylboron, and related compounds. Biochim Biophys Acta 847:1, 1985

22. Davidson JS, Baumgarten IM, Harley EH: Use of a new citrulline incorporation assay to investigate inhibition of intercellular communication by 1,1,1-trichloro-2,2-bis(p-chlorophenyl)ethane in human fibroblasts. Cancer Res 45:515, 1985

23. Davidson JS, Baumgarten IM, Harley EH: Effect of 12-0-tetradecanoyl-phorbol-13-acetate and retinoids on intercellular junctional communication measured with a citrulline incorporation assay. Carcinogenesis 6:645, 1985

24. Davidson JS, Baumgarten IM, Harley EH: Studies on the mechanism of phorbol ester-induced inhibition of intercellular junctional communication. Carcinogenesis 6:1353, 1985

25. DeMaziere AMGL, Scheuermann DW: Increased gap junctional area in the rat liver after administration of dibutyryl cAMP. Cell Tiss Res 239:651, 1985

26. Dermietzel R, Leibstein A, Frixen U, Jannsen-Timmen U, Traub O, Willecki K: Gap junctions in several tissues share determinants with liver gap junctions. EMBO J 3:2261, 1984

27. Dermietzel R, Yancey SB, Traub O, Willecki K, Revel JP. Major loss of the 28-KD protein of gap junction in proliferating hepatocytes. J Cell Biol 105:1925, 1987

28. Dorman BH, Boreiko CJ: Limiting factors of the V79 metabolic cooperation assay for tumor promoters. Carcinogenesis 4:873, 1983

29. Dorman BH, Butterworth BZ, Boreiko CJ: Role of intercellular communication in the promotion of C3H/10T1/2 cell transformation. Carcinogenesis 4:1109, 1983

30. El-Fouly MH, Trosko JE, Chang CC: Scrape-loading and dye transfer: a rapid and simple technique to study gap junctional intercellular communication. Exp Cell Res 168:422, 1987

31. Enomoto T, Martel N, Kanno Y, Yamasaki H: Inhibition of cell communication between Balb/C 3T3 cells by tumor promoters and protection by cAMP. J Cell Physiol 121:323, 1984

32. Enomoto T, Sasaki Y, Shiba Y, Kanno Y, Yamasaki H; Tumor promoters cause a rapid and reversible inhibition of the formation and maintenance of electrical cell coupling in culture. Proc Natl Acad Sci USA 78:5628, 1981

33. Enomoto T, Yamasaki H; Lack of intercellular communication between chemically transformed and surrounding nontransformed Balb/C 3T3 cells. Cancer Res 44:5200, 1984

34. Enomoto T, Yamasaki H: Phorbol ester-mediated inhibition of intercellular communication in Balb/C 3T3 cells: relationship to enhancement of cell transformation. Cancer Res 45:2681, 1985

35. Enomoto T, Yamasaki H; Rapid inhibition of intercellular communication between Balb/C 3T3 cells by diacylglycerol, a possible endogenous functional analogue of phorbol esters. Cancer Res 45:3706, 1985

36. Estape WE, DeMello WC: Cyclic nucleotides and calcium: their role in the control of cell communication in the heart. Cell Biol Int Rep 7:91, 1983

37. Fallon RF, Goodenough DA: Five-hour half-life of mouse liver gap-junction protein. J Cell Biol 90:521, 1981

38. Fitzgerald DJ, Knowles SE, Ballard FJ, Murray AW: Rapid and reversible inhibition of junctional communication by tumor promoters in a mouse cell line. Cancer Res 43:3614, 1983

39. Fitzgerald DJ, Murray AW: Inhibition of intercellular communication by tumor-promoting phorbol esters. Cancer Res 40:2935, 1980

40. Flagg-Newton JL, Dahl G, Loewenstein WR: Cell junction and cyclic AMP: I. Up regulation of junctional membrane permeability and junctional membrane particles by administration of cyclic nucleotide or phosphodiesterase inhibitor. J Memb Biol 63:105, 1981

41. Flagg-Newton JL, Simpson I, Loewenstein WR: Permeability of the cell-to-cell membrane channels in mammalian cell junction. Science 205:404, 1979

42. Friedman EA, Steinberg M: Disrupted communication between late-stage premalignant human colon epithelial cells by 12-0-tetradecanoylphorbol-13-acetate. Cancer Res 42:5096, 1982

43. Fujimoto WY, Subak-Sharpe JH, Seegmiller JE: Hypoxanthine-guanine phosphoribosyl transferase deficiency: chemical agents selective for mutant or normal cultured fibroblasts in mixed and heterozygote cultures. Proc Natl Acad Sci USA 68:1516, 1971

44. Gainer HSC, Murray AW: Diacylglycerol inhibits gap junctional communication in cultured epidermal cells: evidence for a role of protein kinase C. Biochem Biophys Res Commun 126:1109, 1985

45. Gainer HSC, Murray AW: The effect of cAMP on tumor promoter responses mediated by C-kinase. Exp Cell Res 166:171, 1986

46. Garfield RE, Kannan MS, Daniel EE: Gap junction formation in myometrium: control by estrogens, progesterone and prostaglandins. Am J Physiol 238:C81, 1980

47. Goodall H, Johnson MH: Use of carboxyfluorescein-diacetate to study formation of permeable channels between mouse blastomers. Nature (London) 295:524, 1982

48. Gorin MB, Yancey SB, Cline J, Revel JP, Horwitz J: The major intrinsic protein (MIP) of the bovine lens fiber membrane: characterization and structure based on cDNA cloning. Cell 39:49, 1984

49. Green CR, Harfst E, Gourdie RG, Severs NJ: Analysis of the rat liver gap junction protein: clarification of anomalies in its molecular size. Proc R Soc Lond B 233:165, 1988

50. Gros PB, Nicholson BJ, Revel JP: Comparative analysis of the gap junction protein from rat heart and liver: is there a tissue specificity of gap junctions? Cell 35:539, 1983

51. Gunning BES, Hughes JE: Age-related and origin-related control of numbers of plasmodesmata in cell walls of developing *Azolla* roots. Planta 143:181, 1978

52. Gupta RS, Singh B, Stetsko DK: Inhibition of metabolic cooperation by phorbol esters in a cell culture system based on adenosine kinase deficient mutants of V79 cells. Carcinogenesis 6:1359, 1985

53. Hartman TS, Rosen JD: The effect of some experimental parameters on the inhibition of metabolic cooperation by phorbol myristate acetate. Carcinogenesis 6:1315, 1985

54. Hartman TS, Rosen JD: The effect of antipromoters and calcium antagonists on V79 Chinese hamster lung fibroblasts exposed to phorbol myristate acetate. Carcinogenesis 7:361, 1986

55. Hepner DB, Plonsey R: Stimulation of electric interaction of cardiac cells. Biophys J 10:1057, 1970

56. Hertzberg EL, Gilula NB: Liver gap junctions and lens fiber junctions: comparative analysis and calmodulin interaction. Cold Spring Harbor Symp Quant Biol 46:639, 1982

57. Hertzberg EL, Skibbens RU: A protein homologous to the 27,000 dalton liver gap junction protein is present in a wide variety of species and tissues. Cell 39:61, 1984

58. Johnson KR, Lampe PD, Hur KC, Louis CF, Johnson RG: A lens intercellular junction protein, MP26, is a phosphoprotein. J Cell Biol 102:1334, 1986

59. Jone CM, Erickson LM, Trosko JE, Netzloff M, Chang CC: Inhibition of metabolic cooperation by the anticonvulsants, diphenylhydantoin and phenobarbital. Terat Carcinogen Mutagen 5:379, 1985

60. Jongen WMF, Sijtsma SR, Zwijsen RML, Temmink JHM: A co-cultivation system consisting of primary chick embryo hepatocytes and V79 Chinese hamster cells as a model for metabolic cooperation studies. Carcinogenesis 8:767, 1987

61. Jongen WMF, VanderLeede BJN, Chang CC, Trosko JE: The transport of reactive intermediates in a co-cultivation system: the role of intercellular communication. Carcinogenesis 8:1239, 1987

62. Kalimi GH, Sirsat SM: The relevance of gap junctions to stage I tumor promotion in mouse epidermis. Carcinogenesis 5:1671, 1984

63. Kalimi GH, Sirsat SM: Phorbol ester tumor promoter affects the mouse epidermal gap junctions. Cancer Lett 22:343, 1984

64. Kanno Y, Enomoto T, Shiba Y, Yamasaki H. Protective effect of cAMP on tumor promoter-mediated inhibition of cell-cell communication. Exp Cell Res 152:31, 1984

65. Kavanagh TJ, Chang CC, Trosko JE. Effect of various polybro-

minated biphenyls on cell-cell communication in cultured human teratocarcinoma cells. Fund Appl Toxicol 8:127, 1987

66. Kessler JA, Spray DC, Saez JC, Bennett MVL: Determination of synaptic phenotype: Insulin and cAMP independently initiate development of electronic coupling between cultured sympathetic neurons. Proc Natl Acad Sci USA 81:6235, 1984

67. Kinsella A: Elimination of metabolic cooperation and the induction of sister chromatid exchanges are not properties common to all promoting or co-carcinogenic agents. Carcinogenesis 3:499, 1982

68. Klaunig JE, Ruch RJ: Strain and species effects on the inhibition of hepatocyte intercellular communication by liver tumor promoters. Cancer Lett 36:161, 1987

69. Klaunig JE, Ruch RJ: Role of cyclic AMP in the inhibition of mouse hepatocyte intercellular communication by liver tumor promoters. Toxicol Appl Pharmacol 91:159, 1987

70. Klaunig JE, Ruch RJ, DeAngelo AB: Inhibition of mouse hepatocyte intercellular communication by phthalate monoesters. Cancer Lett 43:65, 1988

71. Kumar NM, Gilula NB: Cloning and characterization of human and rat liver cDNAs coding for a gap junction protein. J Cell Biol 103:767, 1986

72. Kurata M, Hirose K, Umeda M: Inhibition of metabolic cooperation in Chinese hamster cells by organochlorine pesticides. Gann 73:217, 1982

73. Kurokawa Y, Matsushima M, Imazawa T, Takamura N, Takahashi M, Hayashi Y: Promoting effect of metal compounds on rat renal tumorigenesis. J Am Coll Toxicol 4:321, 1985

74. Lawrence NJ, Parkinson EK, Emmerson A: Benzoyl peroxide interferes with metabolic cooperation between cultured human epidermal keratinocytes. Carcinogenesis 5:419, 1984

75. Lawrence TS, Beers WH, Gilula NB: Transmission of hormonal stimulation by cell-to-cell communication. Nature (London) 272:501, 1978

76. Lilly SG, Klaunig JE: Inhibition of intercellular communication in preneoplastic rat hepatocytes induced by the Solt-Farber model. The Toxicologist 8:194, 1988

77. Lincoln DW, Kampick SJ, Gierthy JF: 2,3,7,8-Tetrachlorodibenzo-p-dioxin (TCDD) does not inhibit intercellular communication in Chinese hamster V79 cells. Carcinogenesis 8:1817, 1987

78. Loch-Caruso R, Trosko JE: Inhibited intercellular communication as a mechanistic link between teratogenesis and carcinogenesis. CRC Crit Rev Toxicol 16:157, 1986

79. Loewenstein WR: Permeability of membrane junctions. Ann NY Acad Sci 137:441, 1966

80. Loewenstein WR: Communication through cell junctions. Implications in growth control and differentiation. Dev Biol 19 (Suppl 2):151, 1968

81. Loewenstein WR: Junctional intercellular communication and the control of growth. Biochim Biophys Acta 560:1, 1979

82. Loewenstein WR: Junctional intercellular communication: the cell-to-cell membrane channel. Physiol Rev 61:829, 1981

83. Madhukar BV, Yoneyama M, Matsumura F, Trosko JE, Tsushimoto G: Alteration of calcium transport by tumor promoters, 12-O-tetradecanoyl-phorbol-13-acetate and p,p'-dichlorodiphenyltrichloroethane, in the Chinese hamster V79 fibroblast cell line. Cancer Lett 18:251, 1983

84. Makowski L, Caspar DLD, Goodenough DA, and Phillips WC: Gap junction stuctures II. Analysis of x-ray diffraction data. J Cell Biol 74:629, 1977

85. Malcolm AR, Mills LJ, McKenna EJ. Inhibition of metabolic cooperation between Chinese hamster V79 cells by tumor promoters and other cells. Ann NY Acad Sci 407:448, 1983

86. Malcolm AR, Mills LJ, Trosko JE: Effects of ethanol, phenol, formaldehyde, and selected metabolites on metabolic cooperation between Chinese hamster V79 lung fibroblasts. In Carcinogenesis, Vol 8, edited by Mass MJ, p 305. New York, Raven Press, 1985

87. Manjunath CK, Page E. Cell biology and protein composition of cardiac gap junctions. Am J Physiol 248:H783, 1985

88. Mazet F: Filipin and digitonin studies of membrane cholesterol in frog atrial fibres with unusual gap junction configurations. J Mol Cell Cardiol 19:1121, 1987

89. Mehta PP, Bertram JS, Loewenstein WR: Growth inhibition of transformed cells correlates with their junctional communication with normal cells. Cell 44:187, 1986

90. Mesnil M, Fitzgerald DJ, Yamasaki H: Phenobarbital specifically reduces gap junction protein mRNA level in rat liver. Molec Carcinogenesis 1:79, 1988

91. Mesnil M, Montesano R, Yamasaki H: Intercellular communication of transformed and non-transformed rat liver epithelial cells. Exp Cell Res 165:391, 1986

92. Meyer DJ, Yancey SB, Revel JP: Intercellular communication in normal and regenerating rat liver: a quantitative analysis. J Cell Biol 91:505, 1981

93. Miki H, Kasprzak KS, Kenney S, Heine UI: Inhibition of intercellular communication by nickel (II): antagonistic effect of magnesium. Carcinogenesis 8:1757, 1987

94. Milks LC, Kumar NM, Houghten R, Unwin N, Gilula NB: Topology of the 32-kd liver gap junction protein determined by site-directed antibody locaizations. Embo J 7:2967, 1988

95. Miller TM, Goodenough DA: Gap junctional structures after experimental alteration of junctional channel conductance. J Cell Biol 101:1741, 1985

96. Morel-Chany E, AuJurd C, LaFarge-Frayssinet C: Effects of retinoic acid on the transformation and metabolic cooperation of rat liver cells in vitro, and on the growth of hepatoma cells in vivo. Carcinogenesis 7:653, 1986

97. Mosser DD, Bols NC: The effect of phorbols on metabolic cooperation between human fibroblasts. Carcinogenesis 3:1207, 1982

98. Muir JG, Murray AW: Mimicry of phorbol ester responses by diacylglycerols. Different effects on phosphatidylcholine biosynthesis, cell-cell communication and epidermal growth factor binding. Biochim Biophys Acta 885:176, 1986

99. Murray AW, Fitzgerald DJ: Tumor promoters inhibit metabolic cooperation in cocultures of epidermal and 3T3 cells. Biochem Biophys Res Commun 91:395, 1979

100. Newbold RF, Amos J: Inhibition of metabolic cooperation between mammalian cells in culture by tumour promoters. Carcinogenesis 2:243, 1981

101. Nicholson B, Dermietzel R, Teplow D, Traub O, Willecki K, Revel JP: Two homologous protein components of hepatic gap junctions. Nature (London) 329:732, 1987

102. Nicholson BJ, Hunkapiller MW, Grim LB, Hood LE, Revel JP: The rat liver gap junction protein: properties and partial sequence. Proc Natl Acad Sci USA 78:759, 1981

103. Nicolson G, Dulski KM, Trosko JE: Loss of intercellular junctional communication correlates with the metastatic potential in mammary adenocarcinoma cells. Proc Natl Acad Sci USA 85:473, 1988

104. Noda K, Umeda M, Ono T: Effects of various chemicals including bile acids and chemical carcinogens on the inhibition of metabolic cooperation. Gann 72:772, 1981

105. Paul DL: Molecular cloning of cDNA for rat liver gap junction protein. J Cell Biol 103:123, 1986

106. Peracchia C, Bernardini G: Gap junction structure and cell-to-cell coupling regulation: is there a calmodulin involvement? Fed Proc 43:2681, 1984

107. Peracchia C, Girsch SJ: Is the C-terminal arm of lens gap junction channel protein the channel gate? Biochem Biophys Res Commun 133:688, 1985

108. Peracchia C, Peracchia LL: Gap junction dynamics. Effects of H^+ ions. J Cell Biol 87:719, 1980

109. Pitot HC, Beer DG, Hendrich S: Multistage carcinogenesis of the rat hepatocyte. In Banbury Report 25: Nongenotoxic Mechanisms in Carcinogenesis, edited by Butterworth BE, Slaga TJ, p 41. Cold Spring Harbor, NY, Cold Spring Harbor Laboratory, 1987

110. Pitts JD, Burk RR: Mechanism of junctional communication between animal cells by phorbol ester. Cell Tissue Kinet 20:145, 1987.

111. Pitts JD, Simms JW: Permeability of junctions between animal cells. Intercellular transfer of nucleotides but not of macromolecules. Exp Cell Res 104:153 1977

112. Pitts JD, Hamilton JE, Kam E, Burk RR, Murphy JP: Retinoic acid inhibits junctional communication between animal cells. Carcinogenesis 7:1003, 1986

113. Revel JP, Karnovsky M: Hexagonal array of subunits in intercellular junctions of mouse heart and liver. J Cell Biol 33:C7, 1967.

114. Revel JP, Nicholson BJ, Yancey SB: Chemistry of gap junctions. Ann Rev Physiol 47:263, 1985

115. Risinger MA, Larsen WJ: Interaction of filipin with junctional membrane at different stages of the junctions life history. Tiss Cell 15:1, 1983.

116. Robenek H, Jung W, Gebhardt R: The topography of filipin-cholesterol complexes in the plasma membrane of cultured hepatocytes and their relation to cell junction formation. J Ultrastruct Res 78:95, 1982

117. Rolin-Limbosch S, Moens W, Szpirer C: Effects of tumor promoters on metabolic cooperation between human hepatoma cells. Carcinogenesis 7:1235, 1986

118. Rose B, Rick R: Intracellular pH, intracellular free Ca, and junctional cell-cell coupling. J Memb Biol 44:377, 1978

119. Rose B, Yada T, Loewenstein WR: Down regulation of cell-to-cell communication by the viral *src* gene is blocked by TMB-8 and recovery of communication is blocked by vanadate. J Memb Biol 94:129, 1986

120. Rotman B, Papermaster BW: Membrane properties of living mammalian cells as studied by enzymatic hydrolysis of fluorogenic esters. Proc Natl Acad Sci USA 55:134, 1966.

121. Rubinstein C, Jone C, Trosko JE, Chang CC: Inhibition of intercellular communication in cultures of Chinese hamster V79 cells by 2,4-dichlorophenoxyacetic acid and 2,4,5-trichlorophenoxyacetic acid. Fund Appl Toxicol 4:731, 1984

122. Ruch RJ, Klaunig JE: Effects of tumor promoters, genotoxic carcinogens and hepatocytotoxins on mouse hepatocyte intercellular communication. Cell Biol Toxicol 2:469, 1986

123. Ruch RJ, Klaunig JE: Antioxidant prevention of tumor promoter induced inhibition of mouse hepatocyte intercellular communication. Cancer Lett 33:137, 1986

124. Ruch RJ, Klaunig JE: Kinetics of phenobarbital inhibition of intercellular communication in mouse hepatocytes. Cancer Res 48:2519, 1988

125. Ruch RJ, Klaunig JE: Inhibition of mouse hepatocyte intercellular communication by paraquat-generated oxygen free radicals. Toxicol Appl Pharmacol 94:427, 1988

126. Ruch RJ, Klaunig JE, Pereira MA: Inhibition of intercellular communication between mouse hepatocytes by tumor promoters. Toxicol Appl Pharmacol 87:111, 1987

127. Rutten AAJJL, Jongen WMF, DeHaan LHJ, Hendriksen EGJ, Koeman JH: Effect of retinol and cigarette-smoke condensate on dye-coupled intercellular communication between hamster tracheal epithelial cells. Carcinogenesis 9:315, 1988

128. Saez JC, Bennett MVL, Spray DC: Carbon tetrachloride at hepatotoxic levels blocks reversibly gap junctions between rat hepatocytes. Science 236:967, 1987

129. Saez JC, Nairn AC, Hertzberg E, Greengard P, Bennett MVL: cAMP increases junctional conductance and stimulates phosphorylation of the 27-kDa principal gap junction polypeptide. Proc Natl Acad Sci USA 83:2473, 1986

130. Schultz NE, Ruch RJ, Klaunig JE: Mechanism of inhibition of intercellular communication by the promoters DDT, phenobarbital, and lindane in male B6C3F1 mouse hepatocytes. The Toxicologist 8:168, 1988

131. Schwarzmann G, Wiegandt H, Rose B, Zimmerman A, Ben-Haim D, Loewenstein WR: Diameter of the cell-to-cell junctional channels as probed with neutral molecules. Science 213:551, 1981

132. Si ECC, Pfeifer RW, Yim GKW: Iodoacetic acid and related sulfhydryl reagents fail to inhibit cell-cell communication: mechanisms of immunotoxicity *in vitro*. Toxicology 44:73, 1987

133. Simpson I, Rose B, Loewenstein WR: Size limit of molecules permeating the junctional membrane channels. Science 195:294, 1977

134. Slaga TJ, Klein-Szanto AJP, Triplett LL, Yotti LP, Trosko JE: Skin-tumor promoting activity of benzoyl peroxide, a widely used free radical-generating compound. Science 213:1023, 1981

135. Socolar SJ, Loewenstein WR: Methods for studying transmission through permeable cell-to-cell junctions. In Methods in Membrane Biology, Vol 10, edited by Korn E, p 121. New York, Plenum Press, 1979

136. Spray DC, Bennett MVL. Physiology and pharmacology of gap junctions. Ann Rev Physiol 47:281, 1985

137. Spray DC, Ginzberg RD, Morales EA, Gatmaitain Z, Arias IM: Electrophysiological properties of gap junctions between dissociated pairs of rat hepatocytes. J Cell Biol 103:135, 1986

138. Stedman DB, Welsch F: Effects of 6-thioguanine on communication competence and factors affecting reversibility of phorbol ester inhibition in V79 cells measured by metabolic cooperation and by dye coupling. Carcinogenesis 6:1599, 1985

139. Stewart WW: Functional connections between cells as revealed by dye-coupling with a highly fluorescent napthalimide tracer. Cell 14:741, 1978

140. Subak-Sharpe H, Burk RR, Pitts JD: Metabolic cooperation between biochemically marked mammalian cells in culture. J Cell Sci 4:353, 1969

141. Sugie S, Mori H, Takahashi M: Effect of *in vivo* exposure to the liver tumor promoters, phenobarbital or DDT, on the gap junctions of rat hepatocytes: a quantitative freeze-fracture analysis. Carcinogenesis 8:45, 1987

142. Tachikawa T, Kohno Y, Matsui Y, Yoshiki S: *In vitro* early changes in intercellular junctions by treatment with a chemical carcinogen. Carcinogenesis 7:885, 1986

143. Takeda A, Hashimoto E, Yamamura H, Shimazu T: Phosphorylation of liver gap junction protein by protein kinase C. FEBS Lett 210:169, 1987

144. Telang S, Tong C, Williams GM: Epigenetic membrane effects of a possible tumor promoting type on cultured liver cells by the non-genotoxic organochlorine pesticides chlordane and heptachlor. Carcinogenesis 3:1175, 1982

145. Traub O, Look J, Paul D, Willecki K. Cyclic adenosine monophosphate stimulates the biosynthesis and phosphorylation of the 26 kDa junction protein in cultured mouse hepatocytes. Eur J Cell Biol 43:48, 1987

146. Trosko JE, Chang CC: Role of intercellular communication in tumor promotion. In Mechanisms of Tumor Promotion. Vol IV: Cellular responses to tumor promoters, edited by Slaga TJ, p 119. Boca Raton, FL, CRC Press, Inc., 1984

147. Trosko JE, Dawson B, Chang CC: PBB inhibits metabolic cooperation in Chinese hamster cells *in vitro*: its potential as a tumor promoter. Environ Hlth Persp 37:179, 1981

148. Trosko JE, Dawson B, Yotti LP, Chang CC: Saccharin may act as a tumor promoter by inhibiting metabolic cooperation between cells. Science 285:109, 1980

149. Trosko JE, Jone C, Aylsworth C, Tsushimoto G: Elimination of metabolic cooperation is associated with the tumor promoters, oleic acid and anthralin. Carcinogenesis 3:1101, 1982

150. Trosko JE, Jone C, Chang CC: The role of tumor promoters on phenotypic alterations affecting intercellular communication and tumorigenesis. Ann NY Acad Sci 407:316, 1983

151. Trosko JE, Jone C, Chang CC: Inhibition of gap-junctional mediated intercellular communication *in vitro* by aldrin, dieldrin and toxaphen: A possible cellular mechanism for their tumor promoting and neurotoxic effects. Mol Toxicol 1:83, 1987

152. Tsushimoto G, Trosko JE, Chang CC, Aust SD: Inhibition of metabolic cooperation in Chinese hamster V79 cells in culture by various polybrominated biphenyl (PBB) congeners. Carcinogenesis 3:181, 1982

153. Tsushimoto G, Trosko JE, Chang CC, Matsumura F: Inhibition of intercellular communication by chlordecone (kepone) and mirex in Chinese hamster V79 cells *in vitro*. Toxicol Appl Pharmacol 64:550, 1982

154. Umeda M, Noda K. Ono T: Inhibition of metabolic cooperation in Chinese hamster cells by various chemicals including tumor promoters. Gann 71:614, 1980

155. Veld P, Schuit F, Pipeleers D: Gap junctions between pancreatic B-cells are modulated by cyclic AMP. Eur J Cell Biol 36:269, 1985

156. Wade MH, Trosko JE, Schindler M: A fluorescence photobleaching assay of gap junction-mediated communication between human cells. Science 232:429, 1986

157. Walder L, Lutzelschwab R: Effects of 12-0-tetradecanolylphorbol-13-acetate (TPA), retinoic acid and diazepam on intercellular communication in a monolayer of rat liver epithelial cells. Exp Cell Res 152:66, 1984

158. Warner AE, Guthrie SC, Gilula NB: Antibodies to gap-junction protein selectively disrupt junctional communication in the early amphibian embryo. Nature (London) 311:127, 1984.

159. Warngard L, Flodstrom S, Ljungquist S, Ahlborg UG: Inhibition of metabolic cooperation in Chinese hamster lung fibroblast cells (V79) in culture by various DDT-analogs. Arch Environ Contam Toxicol 14:541, 1985.

160. Warngard L, Flodstrom S, Ljungquist S, Ahlborg UG: Interaction between quercetin, TPA and DDT in the V79 metabolic cooperation assay. Carcinogenesis 8:1201, 1987

161. Warren ST, Yotti LP, Moskal JR, Chang CC, Trosko JE: Metabolic cooperation in CHO and V79 cells following treatment with a tumor promoter. Exp Cell Res 131:427, 1981

162. Weghorst CM, Klaunig JE: The role of barbiturate metabolism in the inhibition of intercellular communication between cultured hepatocytes. The Toxicologist 8:194, 1988

163. Welsch F, Stedman DB, Carol JL: Effects of a teratogen [^{3}H] uridine nucleotide transfer between human embryonal cells and gap junctions. Exp Cell Res 159:91, 1985

164. Williams EH, Kumar NM, Gilula NB: Techniques for studying the cell free synthesis of the major lens fiber polypeptide. Methods Enzymol 98:510, 1983

165. Williams GM: Classification of genotoxic and epigenetic hepatocarcinogens using liver culture assays. Ann NY Acad Sci 349:273, 1980.

166. Williams, GM: Liver carcinogenesis: the role for some chemicals of an epigenetic mechanism of liver-turmor promotion involving modification of the cell membrane. Fd Cosmet Toxicol 19:577, 1981

167. Williams GM: Epigenetic effects of liver tumor promoters and implications for health effects. Environ Hlth Persp 50:177, 1983

168. Williams GM, Telang S, Tong C: Inhibition of intercellular communication between liver cells by the liver tumor promoter 1,1,1-trichloro-2,2-bis(p-chlorophenyl)-ethane. Cancer Lett 11:339, 1981

169. Williams GM, Tong C, Telang S: Polybrominated biphenyls are nongenotoxic and produce an epigenetic membrane effect in cultured liver cells. Environ. Hlth Persp. 34:310, 1984

170. Williams GM, Weisburger JH: Chemical carcinogens. In Casarett and Doull's Toxicology, the Basic Science of Poisions, edited by Klaassen CD, Amdur MO, Doull J, p 99, New York, MacMillian Publishing Co., 1986

171. Wolpert L: Positional information and pattern formation. Curr Top Dev Biol 6:183, 1971.

172. Wolpert L: Gap junctions: Channels for communication in development. In Gap Junctions: Channels for Communication in Development, edited by Feldman J, p 83. London, Chapman and Hall, 1978

173. Yoda T, Rose B, Loewenstein WR: Diacylglycerol down regulates junctional membrane permeability. TMB-8 blocks this effect. J Memb Biol 88:217, 1985

174. Yamasaki H, Enomoto T, Martel N, Shiba Y. Kanno Y: Tumour promoter-mediated reversible inhibition of cell-cell communication (electrical coupling). Exp Cell Res 146:297, 1983

175. Yamasaki H, Enomoto T, Shiba Y, Kanno Y, Kakunaga T: Intercellular communication capacity as a possible determinant of transformation sensitivity of Balb/C 3T3 clonal cells. Cancer Res 45:637, 1985

176. Yamasaki H, Hollstein M, Mesnil M, Martel N, Aguelon AM: Selective lack of intercellular communication between transformed and nontransformed cells as a common property of chemical and oncogene transformation of Balb/C 3T3 cells. Cancer Res 47:5658, 1987.

177. Yancey SB, Edens JE, Trosko JE, Chang CC, Revel JP. Decreased incidence of gap juctions between Chinese hamster V79 cells upon exposure to the tumor promoter 12-0-tetradecanoylphorbol-13-acetate. Exp Cell Res 139:329, 1982

178. Yotti LP, Chang CC, Trosko JE: Elimination of metabolic cooperation in Chinese hamster cells by a tumor promoter. Science 206:1089, 1979

179. Zeilmaker MJ, Yamasaki H. Inhibition of junctional intercellular communication as a possible short-term test to detect tumor-promoting agents: Results with nine chemicals tested by dye transfer assay in Chinese hamster V79 cells. Cancer Res 46:6180, 1986

180. Zhong-Xiang L, Kavanagh T, Trosko JE, Chang CC: Inhibition of gap junctional intercellular communication in human teratocarcinoma cells by organochloride pesticides. Toxicol Appl Pharmacol 83:10, 1986

181. Zimmer DB, Green CR, Evans WH, Gilula NB: Topological analysis of the major protein in isolated intact rat liver gap junctions and gap junction-derived single membrane structures. J Biol Chem 262:7751, 1987.

Biology of Disease

Comparative Study of Human and Rat Mammary Tumorigenesis

JOSE RUSSO, BARRY A. GUSTERSON, ADRIANNE E. ROGERS, IRMA H. RUSSO, SEFTON R. WELLINGS, AND MATTHEW J. VAN ZWIETEN

Department of Pathology, Michigan Cancer Foundation, Detroit, Michigan; the Institute of Cancer Research, Royal Cancer Hospital, The Haddow Laboratories, Sutton, Surrey, SM2, SPXD, England; the Department of Pathology, Boston University Medical Center, Boston, Massachusetts; Friday Harbor, Washington; and the Department of Safety Assessment, Merck, Sharp and Dohme Research Laboratories, West Point, Pennsylvania 19486

Introduction
Experimentally-Induced Mammary Tumors in Rats
  Chemically-induced mammary tumorigenesis
    Endocrine influences
    Genetic influences
    Dietary influences
    Chemopreventive agents
  Radiation-induced mammary tumorigenesis
Developmental Concepts in Mammary Carcinogenesis
  Development of the rat mammary gland
  Development of the human breast
  Comparative aspects of development
Pathogenesis of Mammary Tumors
  Rat mammary tumors
  Human breast tumors
  Comparative aspects of pathogenesis
Comparison Between Human and Rat Mammary Tumors
  Histopathologic classification of mammary tumors
  Immunocytochemistry of the normal mammary gland and of its neoplasms
    Immunocytochemical Markers in the normal rat mammary gland and in its tumors
    Immunocytochemical Markers in the Normal Human Breast and Its Tumors
      Markers of myoepithelial cells
      Markers of luminal cells
      Basement membrane and breast stroma
  Criteria of malignancy
    Macroscopic criteria
    Histopathologic criteria
    Biologic criteria
Conclusions and Further Considerations

INTRODUCTION

We have learned through the study of human breast cancer that this disease is the result of a combination of factors, among them external factors such as ionizing radiation, diet, socioeconomic status and endocrinologic, familial or genetic factors. Among all of these factors, the development of breast cancer is influenced by the reproductive history of the individual; lower risk of breast cancer has been reported in women that have had an early full-term pregnancy (109, 110, 154, 162).

Very little is known, however, about the time of initiation of the carcinogenic process or what agent(s) cause it. The fact that early full-term pregnancy is protective and that a higher incidence of mammary carcinomas occurred in women exposed to ionizing radiation at ages younger than 19 (121) but not after pregnancy and lactation (158), strongly suggests that in the human female, the period between menarche and first full-term pregnancy might be critical for the initiation of breast carcinogenesis. Even though the precise site of origin of human mammary carcinomas is not known, evidence indicates that tumors originate in the terminal ductal structures most distal from the nipple (162, 198, 200). However, these pieces of information do not provide a complete picture of the pathogenesis of the disease, or of the mechanisms of interaction of the carcinogen with the target organ. Therefore, we lack effective strategies for breast cancer prevention and cure (140–143, 158, 162).

An experimental system is needed that mimics the human disease, and allows one to elucidate (a) the influence of host factors on the initiation of the neoplastic process, (b) to determine whether in the human the susceptibility of the mammary gland varies with age and reproductive history, and (c) whether it can be manipulated by treatment of the host (158). We consider that rat mammary gland carcinogenesis is the model that closely fulfills the above conditions.

This is one of the most widely studied and useful models of mammary carcinogenesis (48, 49, 82, 83, 89, 143, 144, 150–152, 174, 194, 214). Many strains of rats develop spontaneous tumors, and respond to a variety of chemical carcinogens and radiation with development of either hormone-dependent or -independent mammary tumors.

The objective of this review is to compare side by side what we know about the pathology of breast cancer in both humans and the rat model system, in order to establish a solid basis for comparison and extrapolation of knowledge from animal to human. A comparative analysis will not only further our understanding of the biology of the human disease, but will also highlight the gaps in knowledge which have to be filled.

EXPERIMENTALLY-INDUCED MAMMARY TUMORS IN RATS

CHEMICALLY-INDUCED MAMMARY TUMORIGENESIS

The two most widely used experimental systems for the study of mammary tumorigenesis are the models in which tumors are induced in the Sprague-Dawley (S-D) rat by 7,12-dimethylbenz(a)anthracene (DMBA) or in the S-D or Fischer 344 rat by *N*-methylnitrosourea (NMU). DMBA, given by gavage in a single dose of 2.5 to 20 mg induces tumors with latencies that generally range between 8 and 21 weeks with and final tumor incidences close to 100% if sufficient time elapses before necropsy (Table 1) (135). NMU, given by intravenous or subcutaneous injection in a single dose of 25 or 50 mg/kg body weight yields tumors with similar latency and incidence (Table 2) (135).

Tumor latency is, in general, inversely related to carcinogen dose, whereas both tumor incidence and number are directly related, if relatively early end points are used. For the study of modulating factors, tumor latency is often the most sensitive end point. Tumor histology is influenced by carcinogen dose. In S-D rats given a single NMU dose of 10 mg/kg body weight, 42% of tumors were malignant, whereas 86 to 94% were malignant at doses from 35 to 50 mg/kg (114). Tumor incidence, number of malignant tumors/rat and latency all showed a dose response, but number of benign tumors/rat did not (114). In comparing the two carcinogens, McCormick *et al.* (118) reported that DMBA administered at a dose of 20 mg intragastrically, and NMU given at a dose of 50 mg/

kg intravenously, induced approximately equal numbers and incidence of tumors with approximately equal latency, but a somewhat greater percentage of NMU-induced tumors were histologically malignant. There can be considerable variation in tumor incidence and latency between laboratories and between experiments in the same laboratory, as is evident from the data in Tables 1 and 2. Number of tumors per rat or per group, and number or incidence of malignant tumors are additional end points useful in analysis of data.

The susceptibility of the mammary gland to DMBA- or NMU-induced carcinogenesis is strongly age-dependent and is maximal when the carcinogens are administered to animals between the ages of approximately 45 and 60 days, that is the age of sexual maturity (70, 139). Active organogenesis and high rate of proliferation of the glandular epithelium are characteristics of that period (139, 150); DMBA activation in the gland is also high, but it may not be a significant factor, since NMU, which is similarly most effective at that age, does not require activation (38). The age-related changes in susceptibility are independent of dietary fat content; increased tumorigenesis occurs in rats fed high-fat diet at all ages tested (38). In virgin rats treated with DMBA, tumors that develop are largely carcinomas, although the proportion can be altered by carcinogen dose and dietary fat (38).

The administration of DMBA to virgin rats of different

TABLE 1. MAMMARY GLAND TUMORIGENESIS IN SD RATS FED CONTROL OR HIGH FAT DIETS AND GIVEN DMBA BY GASTRIC GAVAGE AT 50–57 DAYS OF AGE

Dietary fat[a]	DMBA (mg)	%Incidence	Mammary tumors	
			%Malignant	Latency[b]
4[d]	5	98 (21)[b]	85	15
	5	98 (21)	94	14
	20	93 (26)	54	
	2.5/100 g	88 (33)	92	13[e]
20	10	93 (25)		12
5	7.5	76 (21)		11
	7.5	84 (23)		12
5	5	33 (22)		13
25	5	60 (22)		12
5	10	68[e] (22)		10[e]
25	10	98[e] (22)		9[e]
5[d]	7.5	60 (27)	93	21
20	7.5	66 (27)	93	15
	8	88 (30)	25	14
	20	91 (43)	70	12
5	2.5	52 (32)		16
20	2.5	80 (32)		12
5	2.5	60 (32)		15
20	2.5	90 (32)		14
5	2.5	78 (12)	28	9
24	2.5	85 (12)	41	8
	12	88[e] (27)		9[e]

[a] Percentage by weight in purified diets; if value not given, rats were fed natural ingredient diets that contain, generally, 4 to 5% fat.

[b] Weeks between DMBA administration and necropsy in parentheses.

[c] Weeks between DMBA administration and detection of palpable tumor.

[d] Natural ingredient diet before and 4 to 7 days after DMBA; purified diet fed thereafter.

[e] Determined from charts or data given if not stated in publication.

TABLE 2. MAMMARY GLAND TUMORIGENESIS IN RATS FED CONTROL OR HIGH FAT DIETS AND GIVEN NMU BY INTRAVENOUS INJECTION

Rat strain[a]	Dietary fat[b]	NMU		Mammary tumors		
		Age (d)	Dose (mg/kg)	%Incidence[c]	%Malignant	Latency[d]
SD	10[e]	50	25	67 (26)	90	18
	16			77 (26)		17
	22			77 (26)		14
				60 (26)		21
F	5	35	50	40 (24)		12
		50		36 (24)		11
		90		19 (24)		13
		130		0 (24)		
	25	35		74 (24)		8
		50		79 (24)		8
		90		42 (24)		11
		130		24 (24)		20
F	5	50	50	33 (26)		18[f]
	25			80 (26)		13[f]
				34 (26)		21[f]
S-D	5			88 (26)		14[f]
	25			100 (26)		12[f]
				70 (26)		14[f]
L-E	5			31 (26)		15[f]
	25			59 (26)		15[f]
				20 (26)		22[f]
F	5[e]	50	50	66 (22)	92	17
	23			87 (22)	95	12
	5			63 (22)	90	17
	23			87 (22)	88	11
S-D		35	50×2	100 (22)	94	7[f]
		50		94 (22)	88	8[f]
		80		59 (22)	78	11[f]
		140		30 (22)	75	17[f]
		200		22 (22)	50	13[f]
		0		0 (22)	0	
S-D		50	50	100	86	9
			30	95	80	15
			10	45	42	70[f]
S-D		50	50	93 (29)	95	9
			25	80 (43)	90	18
S-D		50				
		51	50[g]	87 (21)	100	10
				89 (21)	100	10
				73 (21)	100	12

[a] S-D, Sprague-Dawley; F, Fischer 344; Long-Evans.

[b] Percentage by weight in purified diets; if value not given, rats were fed natural ingredient diets that contain, generally, 4 to 5% fat.

[c] Weeks between NMU administration and necropsy in parentheses.

[d] Weeks between NMU administration and detection of palpable tumor.

[e] Natural ingredient diet fed before and 1 to 2 days after NMU; purified diet fed thereafter.

[f] Determined from charts or data given if not stated in publication.

[g] NMU given at proestrus, estrus, diestrus, respectively.

ages induces tumors with an incidence which is directly proportional to the density of highly proliferating terminal end buds (TEBs) (150). A 100% incidence of carcinomas is obtained when DMBA is administered to rats aged 30 to 55 days, but the highest number of tumors/animal is observed when the carcinogen is given to animals when they are 40 to 46 days of age, a period when TEBs are most actively differentiating into alveolar buds (ABs). The sharp decrease in the number of TEBs observed in animals older than 55 days is also accompanied by a lower incidence of tumors as well as a lower number of tumors/animal (145, 150, 152, 158, 162).

Endocrine Influences. Mammary tumors in the rat are generally strongly hormone-dependent for both induction and growth. The influence of the endocrine system on chemically-induced carcinogenesis is of paramount importance, and the numerous studies in the field have been thoroughly reviewed by Welsch (202). Ovariectomy causes tumor regression in about 80% of DMBA-treated S-D rats fed either a control or high-fat diet (191).

Pretreatment of rats with estradiol and progesterone or completion of pregnancy and lactation before carcinogen exposure markedly reduces the susceptibility of the gland to chemical carcinogenesis (68-70, 137, 140-142, 158, 162). Pregnancy occurring early after carcinogen exposure increases tumorigenesis (69). Exposure to carcinogen at proestrus or estrus is somewhat more effective than exposure at diestrus (106, 132).

The DMBA-induced and NMU-induced mammary tumor models are useful in assessment of antiestrogen prevention of breast cancer. Treatment of rats at the time of DMBA exposure with tamoxifen and bromocriptine, to suppress the influence and secretion of estrogen and prolactin, respectively, markedly inhibits tumorigenesis and somewhat decreases the fraction of malignant tumors (202). In both models, tamoxifen and other antiestrogens given after carcinogen exposure but before tumor appearance, delayed tumor appearance until withdrawal of therapy, after which time tumors began to appear (66). A possible contribution of tamoxifen-induced anorexia to reduction of tumorigenesis has been reported (191).

An antiprogestin, mifepriston, prolonged latency of DMBA-induced tumors when given beginning immediately after DMBA administration and reduced tumor growth when given to tumor-bearing rats. The drug reduced growth of the rats by about 5%, and reduced both progesterone and estrogen receptors in the tumors but increased plasma prolactin, estradiol, and progesterone (9).

Genetic Influences. Apparently similar genetic factors control the susceptibility of different rat strains to DMBA or NMU mammary tumorigenesis; susceptibility to acetylaminofluorene tumorigenesis follows a similar pattern but has been studied less extensively. Of the commonly used strains, S-D and Wistar-Furth are the most susceptible; Fischer 344 and ACI rats show intermediate susceptibility, and Copenhagen rats are essentially completely resistant even to direct application of DMBA to the gland (90). Copenhagen rats did develop fibrosarcomas in response to parenteral DMBA (Table

TABLE 3. DMBA- OR NMU-INDUCED MAMMARY CARCINOGENESIS IN FEMALE RATS OF DIFFERENT STRAINS (Reference 106)

Carcinogen	Dose (mg)	Rat strain[a]	Mammary adenocarcinomas[b]	
			% Incidence	No./Rat
DMBA	20×1[c]	S-D	90	2.7
		W-F		2.6
		NSD		2.4
		Lew		2.3
		F		1.1
		ACI		0.4
		COP	0	0
	5×4[c]	NSD		4.0
		COP	0	0
	1×1[d]	NSD	100	
		WF	100	
		F	40	
		ACI	25	
		COP	10	
	5×1[e]	NSD	100	1.2
		COP	0	0
NMU	50[f]	NSD	100	3.0
		F		1.2
		COP	0	0
	50[g]	NSD		2.4
		COP	10	0.1
	50×2[f]	NSD		3.9
		COP	0	0
	50×3[f]	NSD		4.8
		COP	0	0

[a] SD = Sprague-Dawley; W-F = Wistar-Furth; NSD = inbred S-D; Lew = Lewis; F = Fischer 344; ACI = ACI, COP = Copenhagen. See also data in Table 2 for comparisons of S-D; F and Long-Evans rats in dietary studies.

[b] Data read from graphs if not stated in paper.

[c] Gastric gavage.

[d] Topical application to gland.

[e] Intraperitoneal injection.

[f] Per kg body weight of intravenous injection.

[g] Per kg body weight by subcutaneous injection.

3). In contrast, tumor induction by diethylstilbestrol (DES) is demonstrable in the ACI but not in the S-D strain of rats, although a co-carcinogenic effect of DES with DMBA can be shown in S-D rats (21, 137). Both malignant and benign tumors are increased by the combined treatment, but there is a relatively greater increase in benign tumors. The response to DES of target organs other than mammary gland is also different in ACI and S-D rats; the mechanisms are not known (178).

In extensive analyses comparing DMBA tumorigenesis, mammary gland growth rate, serum hormone levels, and DMBA toxicokinetics in female rats of several strains and F_1 hybrids between the strains, Isaacs (90, 91) found no major difference that correlated with susceptibility to tumorigenesis. Transplantation studies demonstrated that inherent characteristics of the gland and not of the host animal determine response to DMBA. Glands from rats from a resistant or a susceptible strain were transplanted into F_1 hybrids between the 2 strains and directly exposed to DMBA. While similar percentages of glands from the two strains developed malignant

changes (60% in resistant, 80% in susceptible), macroscopically detectable tumors developed in 70% of susceptible and only 10% of resistant glands. The result clearly suggests that genetic factors govern the progression from microscopic to macroscopic tumor rather than from normal to histologically malignant epithelium. The investigator concluded that resistant rats possess a dominant suppressor allele for the gene governing susceptibility (91).

Dietary Influences. Carcinogenesis can be modified by nutrients and other dietary constituents, by other chemicals and by endocrine alterations. Because of the great sensitivity of tumorigenesis to dietary content of fat, Tables 1 and 2 include information on the fat content of the diet fed to the test animals.

The effects of excessive fat intake on mammary tumorigenesis are: reduced tumor latency, increased tumor multiplicity and increased fraction of histologically malignant tumors (Table 4) (8, 44, 96, 133, 135). In order to yield valid results, rats fed high fat diets must be compared with rats fed diets that supply sufficient fat for normal growth and development, at least 4 to 5% fat by weight, and sufficient essential fatty acids. The control diet must be equivalent in all nutrient-to-calorie-ratios to the high fat diet. The two groups of rats must show comparable weight gain, or controls must be included to permit evaluation of caloric, as well as specific fat effects on tumorigenesis, since tumor incidence is increased with increased caloric consumption (97, 100).

Studies of the mechanisms by which fat may act have been reviewed extensively in recent publications (135, 137). No mechanism, other than increased caloric intake, has been convincingly demonstrated to contribute to, or be responsible for, the effect of fat. Reduction of caloric intake by 20% (228) 30% (15) or 40% (97, 100), even with a percentage calories from fat held at a high level, increases tumor latency and reduces incidence, number and size of tumors. However, added caloric intake and weight gain by rats fed high fat diets do not account for correlation of increased tumorigenesis with type, as well as amount, of fat (39, 45, 134, 135, 181, 206) or for results of paired-feeding studies (134).

In an examination of the effect of dietary fat content on initiation of tumors by DMBA, Clinton et al. (43) drew the following conclusions. Doubling the energy intake from fat (corn oil) from 25 to 48% of calories (from 10.5 to 24.6% by weight) for the 4 weeks between weaning and DMBA administration increased significantly mammary tumor incidence and increased the odds ratio for carcinoma by a factor of 1.6 and for any tumor by a factor of 5. Body weight and caloric intake over the 4-week period were not affected by dietary fat content, provided that the protein content was adequate for growth. This result and studies using lard in the place of corn oil (134, 135, 181) confirmed an effect of fat at initiation of tumorigenesis. After DMBA was given, all rats were fed the same diet with 24% of calories as fat, and a positive effect of caloric intake on tumor incidence was found to be independent of dietary fat content.

The high fat diets that enhance tumorigenesis do not alter significantly: (a) toxicokinetics of DMBA (104); (b)

TABLE 4. HISTOLOGY OF MAMMARY TUMORS INDUCED BY DMBA OR MNU IN FEMALE SPRAGUE-DAWLEY[a] RATS

| Carcinogen | Dose | % of Mammary tumors | | Fibroadenoma adenoma | Reference |
| | | Adenocarcinoma | | | |
		Invasive	Noninvasive		
DMBA[b]	2.5 mg	10[c]	54[c]	30[c]	Rogers et al., 1986
		13[d]	57[d]	36[d]	
	3.2 mg[e]		52[c]	48[c]	Clinton et al., 1984
			75[d]	25[d]	
	5.0 mg	6[c]	80[c]	14[c]	Rogers et al., 1986
		4[d]	87[d]	9[d]	
	5.0 mg		98	2	Welsch et al., 1988
	8.0 mg		34	66	Mcormick et al., 1985
	16.0 mg		64	26	
NMU[f]	35–50 mg/kg		86–94	6–14	McCormick et al., 1981
	20–30 mg/kg		71–80	20–29	
	10–15 mg/kg		42–59	41–58	
	50 mg/kg		94	6	Thompson and Meeker, 1983
	50 mg/kg×2		93	7	Grubbs et al., 1983
	50 mg/kg×2		97	3	Rose et al., 1980

[a] 50 to 60 days of age at carcinogen exposure, fed control, natural ingredient diet unless otherwise noted, spontaneous mammary tumors in Sprague-Dawley female rats occur in incidences of up to 90% after 18 months of age and are reported to be malignant in 22 to 50% (McCormick et al., 1981) of cases although in earlier studies fewer than 10% were reported as malignant (Young and Hallowes, 1973; Altman and Goodman, 1979).
[b] By gastric gavage.
[c] Control diet 5% fat by weight.
[d] High fat diet, 24 to 25% fat by weight.
[e] Average dose; rats were given 20 mg DMBA/kg body weight.
[f] By intravenous injection.

blood levels of prolactin, 17-β-estradiol, progesterone or luteinizing hormone or the patterns of hormone secretion through the estrous cycle (180, 207); or (c) [³H]thymidine labeling of mammary gland epithelial DNA before or after carcinogen exposure (102). Although induction of both hormone-dependent and hormone-independent tumors responds to dietary fat content (180), high fat diets do not increase the growth rate of tumors as measured by palpation (8, 135).

The factor of caloric utilization by voluntary or involuntary exercise is under investigation. Results are variable and show both increased and decreased tumorigenesis in excercised rats (14, 192). Standardization of methods with measurement of energy intake and expenditure and of body composition are needed to permit comparison and interpretation of results.

There has been interest in the effect of omega-3 fatty acids on growth and metastasis of transplanted, as well as induced, mammary tumors in rats. However, the results are not entirely consistent within or among laboratories, probably in part because acceptance of the diets by rats varies (98).

The influence of caffeine on the mammary gland is of interest because of the postulated relationships between coffee consumption and fibrocystic disease or breast cancer, although significant relationships have not been demonstrated in epidemiologic studies. Welsch *et al.* have published a series of studies that show highly variable responses to coffee and caffeine in rats and mice (203–205). In DMBA-treated, S-D rats given coffee or caffeine in drinking water before and during DMBA initiation of mammary tumorigenesis, tumor multiplicity was reduced to 38 to 67% of the value in rats given DMBA alone.

Tumor incidence and latency were not affected. The effective coffee or caffeine intakes were comparable, on a metabolic weight basis, to 13 to 14 or 26 to 28 cups of coffee/day. At the higher intake, reduced body weight may have accounted for some of the reduction of tumor number, but the lower intake did not reduce body weight gain. When coffee or caffeine was given after DMBA administration, there was no consistent effect on tumorigenesis (204). Results were the same when rats were fed a purified diet that contained 5 or 20% fat (by weight) (205). In mice given similar amounts of coffee or caffeine, DMBA-induced or murine mammary tumor virus-induced tumor multiplicity was increased but other parameters of tumorigenesis were not affected. Caffeine increased mammary gland development in mice, apparently by increasing the response to trophic hormones (203).

Epidemiologic studies strongly indicate that alcohol intake is a risk factor for breast cancer (136). The increased risk if 1.5- to 3-fold, depending upon the population studied and the amount of alcohol consumed. In DMBA or NMU-treated rats, daily doses of ethanol of 5 mg/kg body weight were associated with increased numbers of malignant tumors but no significant alteration of tumor latency or incidence (10, 69).

Chemopreventive Agents. Vitamin A and related retinoids reduce mammary tumorigenesis. The studies of retinyl acetate suppression of tumorigenesis have utilized doses that greatly exceed the vitamin A requirement, are somewhat toxic as judged by reduced weight gain and inhibit normal mammary gland growth and development, although disruption of normal estrous cycles was reported not to occur (8, 115). Retinyl esters (vitamin A)

TABLE 5. EFFECT OF DFMO ON NMU-INDUCED MAMMARY CARCINOGENESIS IN FEMALE SPRAGUE-DAWLEY RATS[a]

DFMO, % in water	Mammary gland tumors		Weight (gm)	Latency (wk)	Diet	Reference
	%Incidence	%Malignant				
1	56	82	0.2	16	Natural ingredient	188
0	100	90	2.8	7		
0.125	83	100		12	AIN	191
0	96	100		8		

[a] NMU, 50 mg/kg subcutaneously at 40 days of age.

and synthetic retinoids suppress mammary tumor development additively or synergistically with ovariectomy, inhibition of prolactin secretions, tamoxifen or selenium (120, 125). Administration of vitamin A or retinoids can be delayed for periods that range up the first appearance of tumors and still have inhibitory effects on development of additional tumors (125). In a review of published data and analysis of new data on one of the most active vitamin A analogues, N-(4-hydroxyphenyl)retinamide (4-HPR), McCormick and Moon (120) concluded that retinoid reduction of mammary carcinogenesis appeared not to be due to endocrine mechanisms, but that retinoids could enhance endocrine anticarcinogenic regimens such as ovariectomy or tamoxifen administration.

Feeding rats selenium salts at levels 30 to 50 times the requirement inhibits mammary tumorigenesis by DMBA or NMU, particularly if the rats are fed a high (20%) corn oil diet. Selenium toxicity, manifested by reduction in the rate of body weight gain is detectable at the levels fed. The toxicity may contribute to the reduction of tumorigenesis but appears not to be a major factor (85, 86).

A non-nutritive dietary component reported to reduce mammary tumorigenesis is d-limonene, a component of citrus oils (54). The antimalarial quinacrine, a phospholipase inhibitor and inhibitor of prolactin-induced mitogenesis in the mouse mammary gland, reduced tumorigenesis in rats when the carcinogen was given at a low dose (20 mg/kg) but not when it was given at the usual dose of 50 mg/kg (113). The compound was tested because it reduces production of arachidonic acid for metabolism through the cyclooxygenase and lipoxygenase pathways, and other drugs that block the same pathways inhibit low dose NMU carcinogenesis (113). The compounds are toxic and reduce body weight gain, but the occurrence and degree of reduction are not correlated with inhibition of tumorigenesis.

NMU-induced tumorigenesis was markedly delayed and reduced in rats by provision of 1% D,L-a-difluoromethylornithine (DFMO) in drinking water. A control group restricted in diet intake to 80% to match the weight reduction in DFMO-treated rats, showed a much smaller reduction in all measures of tumorigenesis, demonstrating that DFMO has a specific effect in addition to reduction of food intake and weight gain (188). Lower, less toxic doses of DFMO (0.125 to 0.5% in drinking water) were also effective in reducing NMU tumorigenesis (Table 5) (206). DFMO acts synergistically with tamoxifen or ovariectomy in reducing tumorigenesis (191).

RADIATION-INDUCED MAMMARY TUMORIGENESIS

The female breast is one of the tissues with the highest sensitivity to radiation carcinogenesis (13). Since contro-

TABLE 6. MAMMARY GLAND TUMORS IN FEMALE S-D AND WISTAR RATS EXPOSED TO RADIATION, ESTROGEN OR BOTH (Reference 25)

Rat strain	E2[a]	Treatment X-Ray[b]	Neutrons[c]	Mammary Tumors	
				%Incidence	%Carcinoma incidence
S-D	−	−	−	30	9
	+	−	−	14	5
	−	+	−	72	24
	+	+	−	50	38
	−	−	+	65	7
	+	−	+	64	35
Wistar	−	−	−	27	20
	+	−	−	42	35
	−	+	−	26	8
	+	+	−	51	45
	−	−	+	35	19
	+	−	+	68	65

[a] 17-β-estradiol, 2 mg pellet implanted at 7 weeks of age.
[b] 0.25–0.3 Gy at 8 weeks of age.
[c] 15 Mev, 0.15 Gy at 8 weeks of age.

versy exists concerning the shape of the dose-response curve, the effects of fractionated irradiation and the effect of low levels of radiation (101), animal studies are necessary to address these issues. The rat model has been widely used in this regard (194). Since the demonstration in the early 1950s that a single supralethal dose of x-rays to female Holtzman rats (a S-D stock) maintained by temporary parabiosis induced an increased number of benign and malignant mammary tumors within 6 months (55), numerous investigations of radiation-induced mammary tumorigenesis in the rat have been carried out. Sublethal doses of different types of radiation, including x-rays and neutrons, were shown to induce mammary tumor development (Table 6), often within a year, with linear dose-effect relationships for neutrons over the total dose range and for x-rays down to dose levels of 0.2 Gy (18, 24). Irradiation of animals with fractionated doses of γ-radiation has resulted in linear-quadratic dose-response curves (193). Although most studies have utilized whole-body irradiation, localized irradiation also induces mammary tumors in the rat within the irradiated field. This so-called scopal effect occurs also in women, but reportedly not in several other animal species studies, e.g., mice, dogs and guinea pigs (19, 173).

Several studies have shown that exposing rats to fractionated irradiation had no sparing or enhancing effect on mammary tumor development when compared with animals exposed to single doses. The fractions have been delivered in a variety of different protocols, for example, at 12-hour intervals for 60 days (193), semi-weekly for up to 16 weeks (170), and monthly for up to 10 months (23). In general, no increase in tumor latency, incidence or total number of mammary tumors was found, compared with animals receiving an equivalent amount of radiation given as a single dose. Some investigators (170), however, have reported an increased number of mammary carcinomas in animals receiving fractionated doses.

The hormonal status of the female rat is of paramount importance in determining the outcome of irradiation of the mammary gland. Ovariectomy completely prevents, and estrogen treatment enhances, radiation-induced mammary tumor formation (176, 194). The latency period for tumor development is shortened considerably in estrogen-treated rats; there is an increase in the number of rats with carcinomas, especially cribriform carcinomas (194), and in the number of tumors/tumor-bearing rat (176) (Table 6). Radiation and estrogens, namely 17-β-estradiol (E_2) or DES, were reported to exert either an additive (25) or synergistic effect (169, 179). The effect of E_2 administration and irradiation on mammary tumorigenesis is equal for hormone administration 1 week before, or beginning 12 weeks after irradiation (25). This additive effect of hormone administration and irradiation was not evident if the hormone was administered beginning 24 weeks after irradiation.

In studying the mechanism of the amplification of radiation-induced mammary tumorigenesis by estrogens, several investigators have pointed to the effects of estrogens on the pituitary. For example, in DES-treated ACI rats, the incidence of pituitary tumors was increased markedly as compared with non-DES-treated irradiated rats or controls (172). The development of pituitary tumors was accompanied by marked increases in plasma prolactin levels (79, 179, 213). Similarly, E_2 treatment of rats of three strains resulted in a marked increase in plasma prolactin levels which was strongly associated with the occurrence of pituitary tumors (17). The development of malignant mammary tumors after estrogen treatment in these rats appeared to be associated with the extent of increase in plasma prolactin.

Mammary carcinogenesis induced by polycyclic hydrocarbons in female rats, on the other hand, is dependent on the age and physiologic development of the mammary gland at the time of carcinogen administration. The effect of physiologic status of the rat at the time of irradiation has also been examined (80). No significant differences have been reported in mammary tumor incidence and number or type of mammary tumors produced as a result of irradiation during pregnancy, lactation, or postlactation compared with irradiation in the virginal state. The reason for the differences in physiologic influences on the inductive action of chemicals and irradiation in rat mammary gland is not clear, but it is speculated that radiation-induced changes might occur in a specific stem cell population maintained throughout the reproductive life, while chemically induced changes depend upon the number and rate of turnover of other types of mammary gland cells (80, 152).

DEVELOPMENTAL CONCEPTS IN MAMMARY CARCINOGENESIS

The mammary gland is a complex organ which from birth to senescence undergoes continuous changes under the influence of body growth on the one hand and of cyclic hormonal stimulation on the other. Under these influences, the histologic picture of the gland becomes extremely heterogeneous. Therefore, it is important to establish parameters to evaluate gland development for understanding the pathogenesis of the disease as well as the mechanism(s) of interaction between carcinogens and the target organ.

DEVELOPMENT OF THE RAT MAMMARY GLAND

The rat's mammary glands are distributed in pairs along the milk line, with one pair located in the cervical, two in the thoracic, one in the abdominal and two in the inguinal regions (7, 194). At birth, the six pairs of mammary glands consist of one or two main lactiferous ducts arising from the nipple (143, 144, 152, 214). In the mammary gland of newborn female rats, the main lacti-

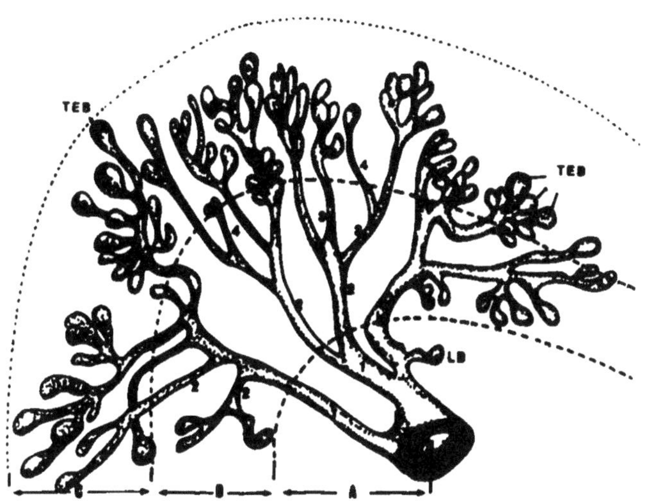

FIG. 1. Schematic representation of the third (thoracic) mammary gland of a 21-day-old female rat. The gland was divided into three zones: *A*, proximal to the nipple; *B*, medial; *C*, distal to the nipple. Branching pattern is identified sequentially as first generation or primary ducts (*1*); second generation or secondary ducts (*2*); third generation or terciary ducts (*3*); fourth generation or quartenary ducts (*4*); terminal end buds (*TEB*), lateral buds (*LB*). From: IH Russo and J Russo, Anticancer Res., 8:1247, 1988.

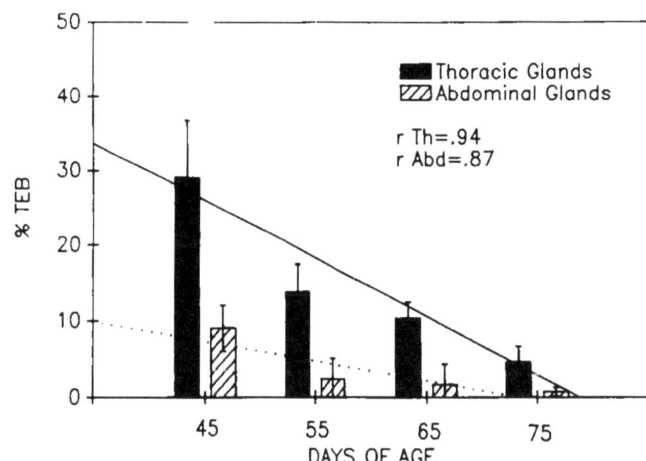

FIG. 2. Age-dependent variations in percentage of TEBs in thoracic and abdominal mammary glands of virgin rats. *r* = correlation coefficient for *Th* = thoracic and *Abd* = abdominal mammary glands. From: IH Russo and J Russo, Anticancer Res. 8:1247, 1988.

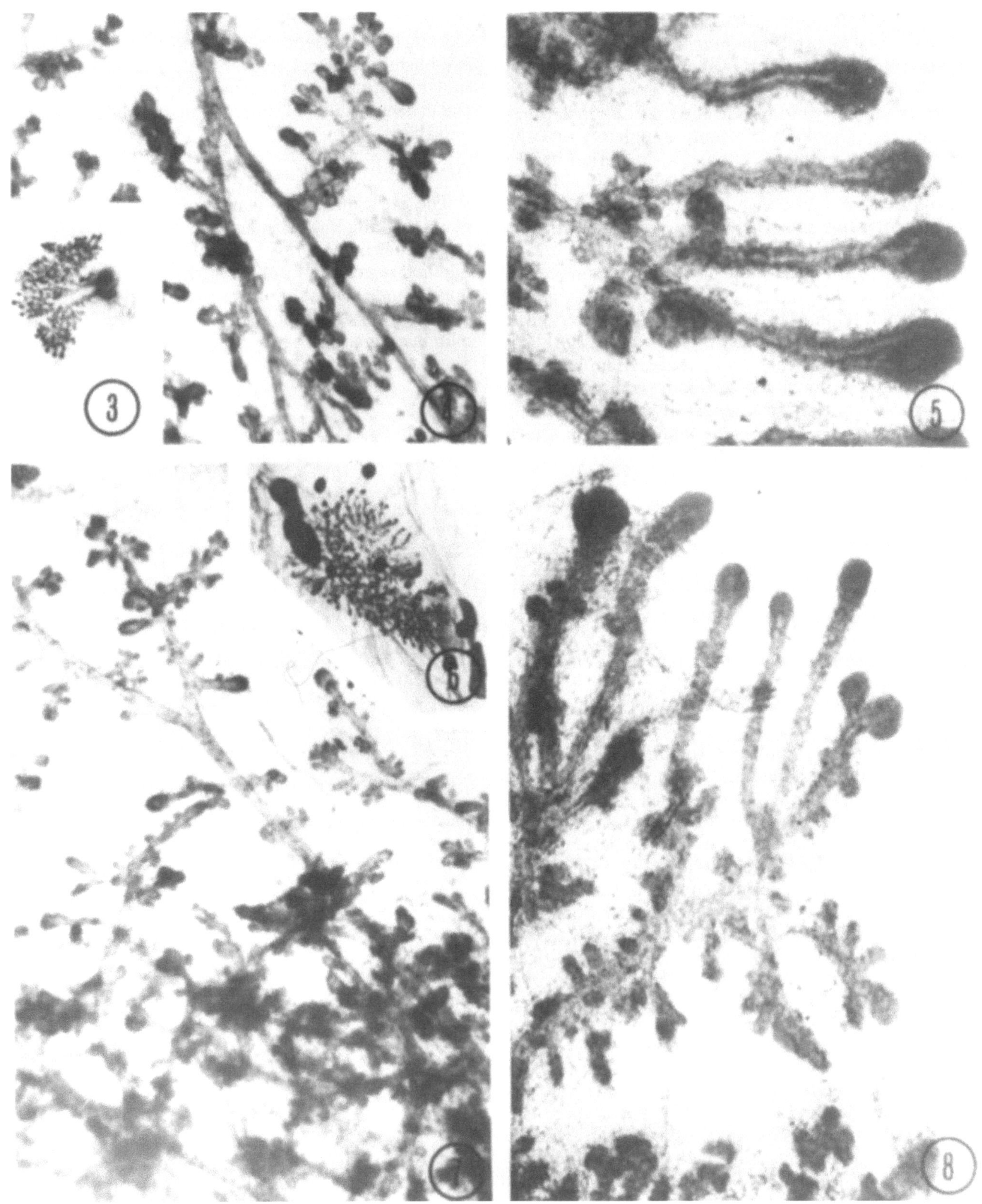

FIG. 3 to 14. From: IH Russo, M Tewari and J Russo. Integument and Mammary Glands of Laboratory Animals. Jones, T.C., Mohr, U, Hunt, RD (eds.). Springer-Verlag, Berlin, 1989.

FIG. 3. Third (thoracic) mammary gland of a 21-day-old female rat from which the diagram for Figure 1 was taken. ×3.

FIG. 4. Zone B of the thoracic mammary gland shown in Figure 3, which contains numerous lateral buds, occasional ABs and TDs. ×55.

FIG. 5. Zone C of the gland shown in Figure 3, which is almost exclusively composed of darkly stained, club-shaped TEBs. ×55.

FIG. 6. Abdominal fourth mammary gland of a 21-day-old female rat in which the mammary ducts are reaching the vicinity of the lymph node. ×3.

FIG. 7. Zone B of the gland shown in Figure 6 containing numerous lateral buds and occasional ABs. Secondary branching is abundant. ×55.

FIG. 8. Zone C of the gland shown in Figure 6. Although TEBs are bulbous and darkly stained, their average diameter is slightly smaller than those present in the thoracic gland shown in Figures 3 and 5. The ducts also contain more lateral buds. ×55.

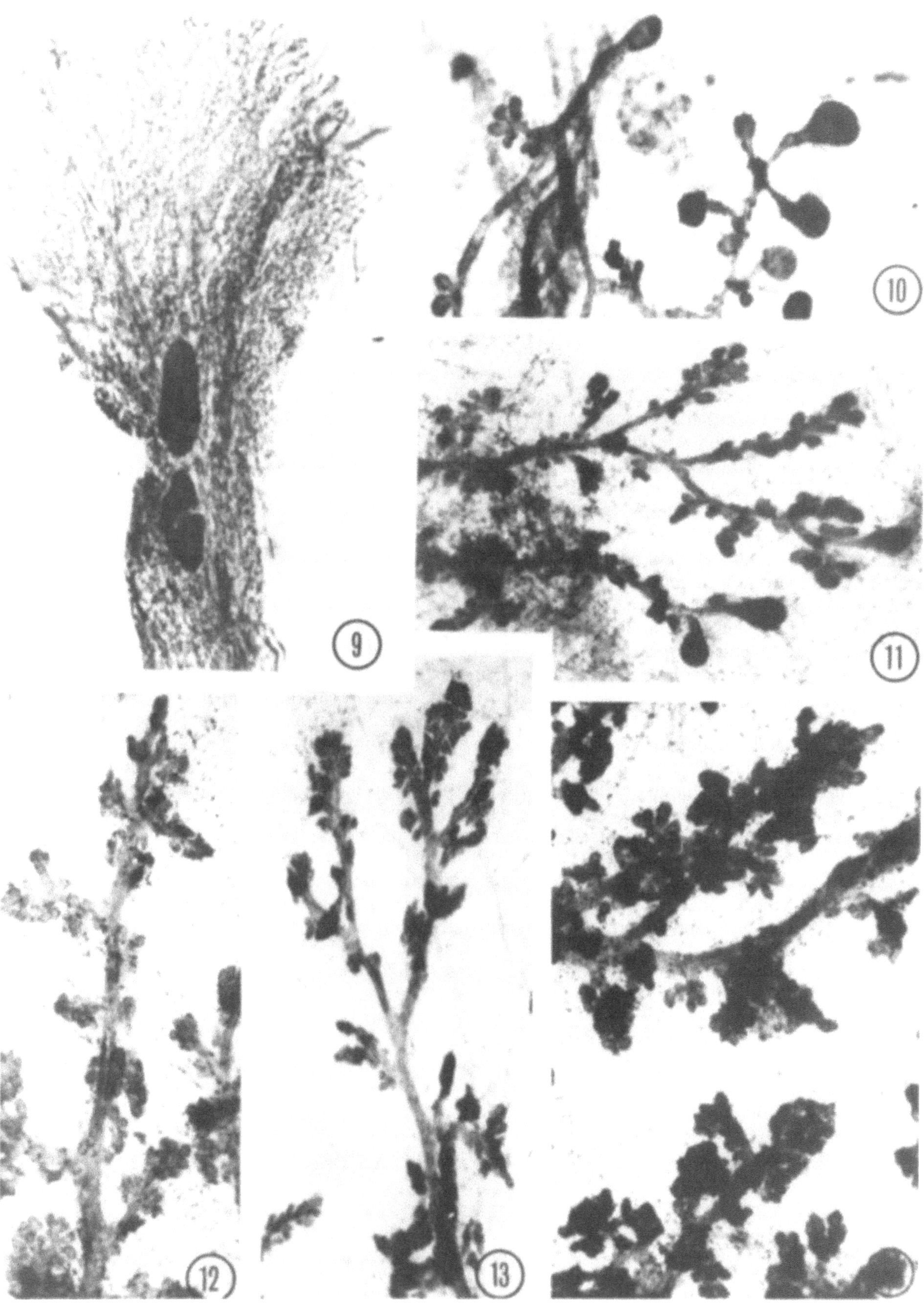

FIG. 9 to 14.

ferous duct branches into at least four or five secondary ducts, and these further branch dichotomously into a third generation of ducts.

Since the basic development of all the glands follows a uniform pattern, we have established criteria for evaluating mammary growth, development, and differentiation by dividing the mammary parenchyma into three thirds along the longitudinal axis (Fig. 1) (143). The third closest to the nipple, called zone A (Fig. 1), is composed of the main lactiferous ducts, the intermediate area called zone B, contains more abundant lateral buds; in this area is where most of the secondary ducts arise. The distal third of the gland, or zone C, contains the terminal ductal structures ending in bulbous clubs or TEBs.

Although all the mammary glands are basically composed of the three zones described above, there are differences in glandular area, as well as in the number and size of individual structures, which depend upon the location of the gland in either a cervical, thoracic, abdominal or inguinal region. Thoracic glands, mainly the third pair, are composed of more numerous and larger TEBs (Figs. 2 to 5), whereas TEBs in abdominal mammary glands are less numerous and slightly smaller than those of thoracic glands (figs. 2, and 5 to 7). There is a high correlation coefficient between aging and decreasing number of TEBs in both thoracic and abdominal glands. Gland development progresses with age by successive dichotomous or sympodial branching of new ducts, sprouting of lateral buds, elongation of existing ducts and cleavage of TEBs or lateral buds into two or more small buds called at this stage alveolar buds (ABs) (Fig. 7).

Mammary gland development is a progressive, though uneven process. Although numerous TEBs progress to ABs and these to lobules, a large number of TEBs in the virgin rat never differentiate; they become progressively smaller and finger-shaped; at this stage, these former TEBs are called terminal ducts (TDs) (Fig. 8). TDs do not undergo further morphologic changes as long as the animal remains virgin.

Between the ages of 35 and 55 days, as a consequence of progressive branching, the mammary gland occupies larger areas of the mesenchyme or mammary fat pad. The number of TEBs decreases markedly in zones A and B in all glands, but not in zone C. The reduction of TEBs becomes progressively more evident with aging (Fig. 2). There is little variation in number of ABs and lobules and in the size of lobule development in older animals in comparison with the 55-day-old ones, as long as the animals remain virgin (Figs. 9 to 14) (143, 144). Lobules in the virgin female are called lobules type 1 or virginal

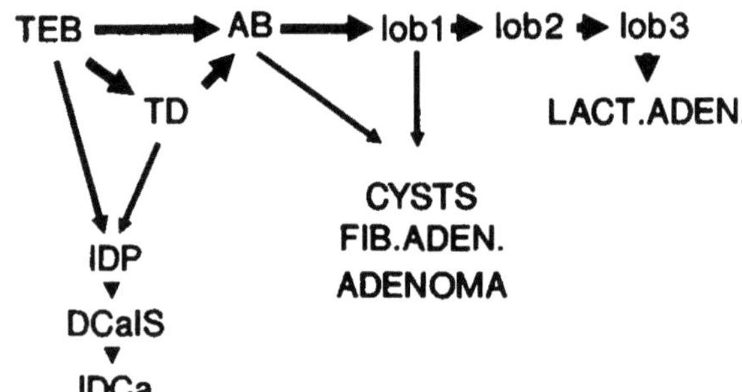

FIG. 15. Pathogenetic pathway of mammary carcinogenesis.

lobules (Fig. 15). During pregnancy and lactation, the lobules increase significantly in size and in the number of component alveoli; at this stage they are called lobules type 3. When lobules type 3 regress after lactation, they become smaller, but they remain larger than lobules type 1, and are called type 2.

DEVELOPMENT OF THE HUMAN BREAST

This review of the development of the human breast describes changes taking place in the parenchyma or ductal system of the gland during postnatal development. Changes occurring during the embryonic and fetal stages have been discussed elsewhere (149, 157).

The human breast undergoes a complete series of changes from intrauterine life to senescence. These changes can be divided into two distinct phases: the developmental or organogenetic phase and the differentiation phase.

The developmental phase includes the early stages of gland morphogenesis, from nipple epithelium to lobular formation. The development of the gland varies greatly from woman to woman, making it impossible to categorize mammary gland structure based on age (47, 50). Mammary gland development during childhood does little more than keep pace with the general growth of the body until the approach of puberty (183), when the main changes occurring in the mammary gland are initiated.

The adolescent period begins with the first signs of sexual change at puberty and terminates with sexual maturity (183). With the approach of puberty, between the ages of 10 and 12 years, the rudimentary mamma begins to show growth activity both in the glandular tissue and in the surrounding stroma. Glandular increase is due to growth and division of small bundles of primary and secondary ducts. They grow and divide partly dichotomously and partly sympodially, on a dichotomous

---

FIG. 9. Abdominal mammary gland of a 55-day-old virgin female rat showing profuse branching and extension of the mammary parenchyma beyond the lymph nodes. ×3.

FIG. 10. TEBs present in zone C of the thoracic mammary gland of a 55-day-old virgin female rat. ×55.

FIG. 11. Zone C of the abdominal mammary gland of a 55-day-old female. This zone is composed of more lateral buds and ABs. There are two TEBs which are smaller in size than those seen in the thoracic gland. ×55.

FIG. 12. Another area in the zone C of the 4th or abdominal gland of a 55-day-old virgin female rat contains almost exclusively ABs and lateral buds. ×55.

FIG. 13. Zone C of the inguinal mammary gland of a 55-day-old virgin female rat, almost exclusively composed of ABs and lateral buds. ×55.

FIG. 14. Zone B of the mammary gland of a 55-day-old virgin female rat contains primitive lobules. ×55.

basis; the distal or free end of each duct ends in a bulbous formation equivalent to the TEB described in the rat (Figs. 20 to 22) (152). Main ducts give origin to new branches (Figs. 16 to 18) (142, 189, 190). Terminal ducts or lateral buds give origin to alveolar buds (ABs), which are smaller ductules clustered around the duct forming the lobule type 1 or virginal lobule (Figs. 17 and 19). This structure represents the basic functional unit of the human breast, also called terminal ductal lobular unit (TDLU) (Table 7) (200, 201). There is a gradual condensation of the surrounding stroma to produce the adult inter- and intralobular stroma (74). Lobule formation

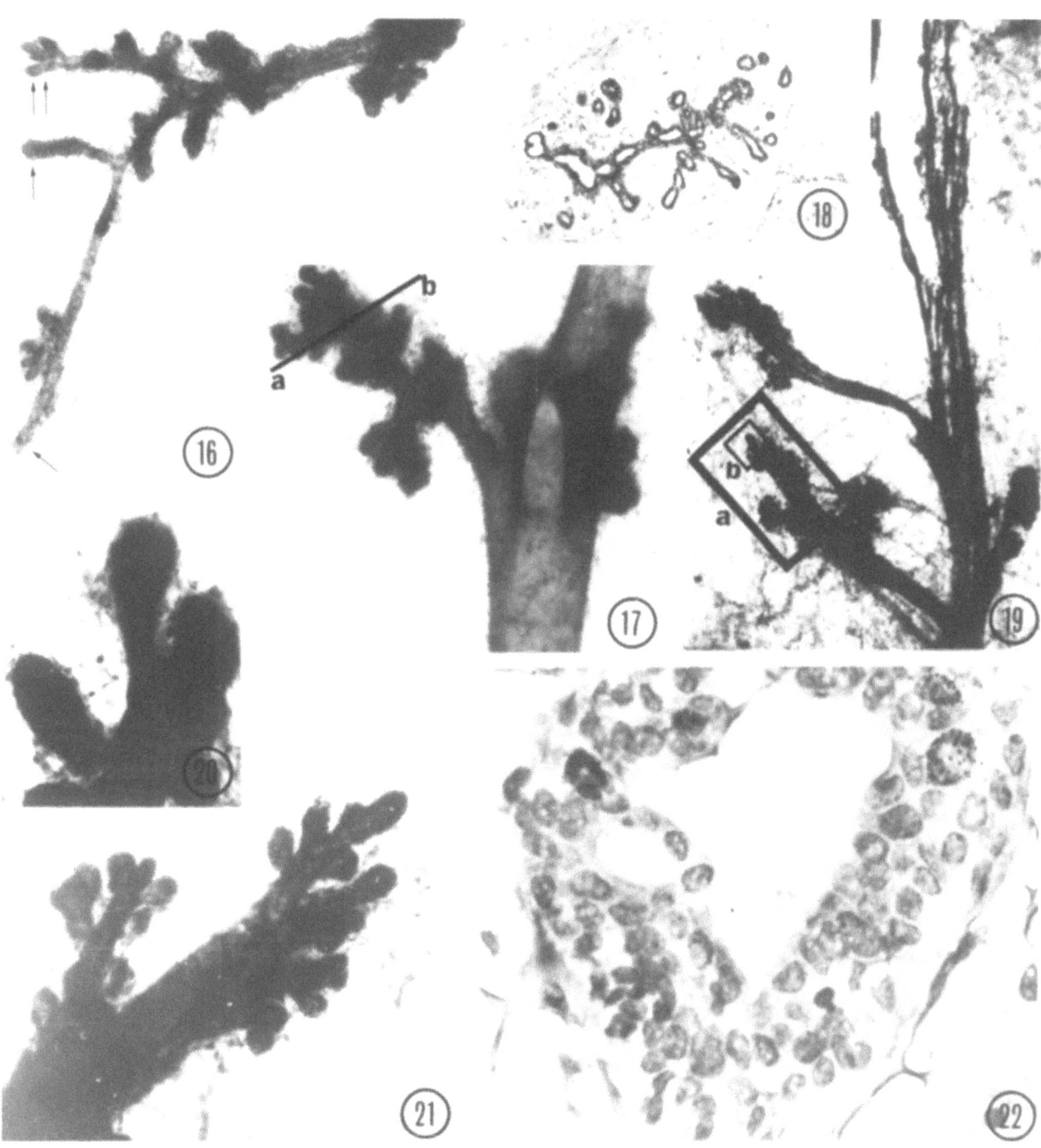

FIG. 16 to 30. Whole-mount preparation of a mammary gland of an 18-year-old nulliparous woman. Reprinted with permission from: J Russo and IH Russo (see reference 157).

FIG. 16. In Figure 16, the mammary ductal system ends in either slender TDs (*arrows*) or in type 1 lobules (*double arrows*) ×25.

FIG. 17. Another area of the same gland is shown, containing typical type 1 lobules composed of ABs. ×100.

FIG. 18. Histologic section of a lobule type 1 from Figure 17, sectioned at level *a-b* and showing a duct sprouting ABs, each one surrounded by intralobular connective tissue (H&E) ×25.

FIG. 19. The appearance of the gland is variegated, being composed of lobules type 1 (*inset a*), terminal end buds (*inset b*) ×25.

FIG. 20. Lobule type 1 (*inset b*, Fig. 19) ×100.

FIG. 21. TEB shown in Figure 19 (*inset a*) ×100.

FIG. 22. Histologic section of the TEB shown in Figure 20 (H&E) ×400.

occurs within 1 to 2 years after the onset of the first menstrual period. Full differentiation of the mammary gland is a gradual process taking many years, and if pregnancy does not supervene, is never attained. Terminal ducts (Fig. 18) and TEBs are also present in the virginal breast (Figs. 18, 20, 21, and 22).

The study of normal breast tissue of 22 adult women ranging in age from 18 to 63 years showed that in nonpregnant glands there are two identifiable types of lobules in addition to the already described type 1 (157). These are designated lobules type 2 (Figs. 23 to 26) and type 3 (Figs. 27 to 30). The transition from lobule type 1 to type 2, and of this to type 3, is a gradual process of sprouting of new ABs, which in lobules type 2 and type 3 are called ductules. They increase in number from approximately 11 in the lobule type 1 to 47 and 80 in lobules type 2 and type 3, respectively. The increase in number results in a concomitant increase in size of the lobules and a reduction in size of each individual structure. The ABs composing a lobule type 1 (Table 7), are larger, practically twice the size of the ductules composing lobules type 2 (Figs. 24 and 26), whereas the reduction in size of ductules composing lobules type 3 is less dramatic, although still significant (Table 7).

During pregnancy the breast attains its maximum development. It occurs in two distinctly dominant phases characteristic of the early and late stages of pregnancy (12, 47, 167, 195). Pregnancy is characterized by growth,

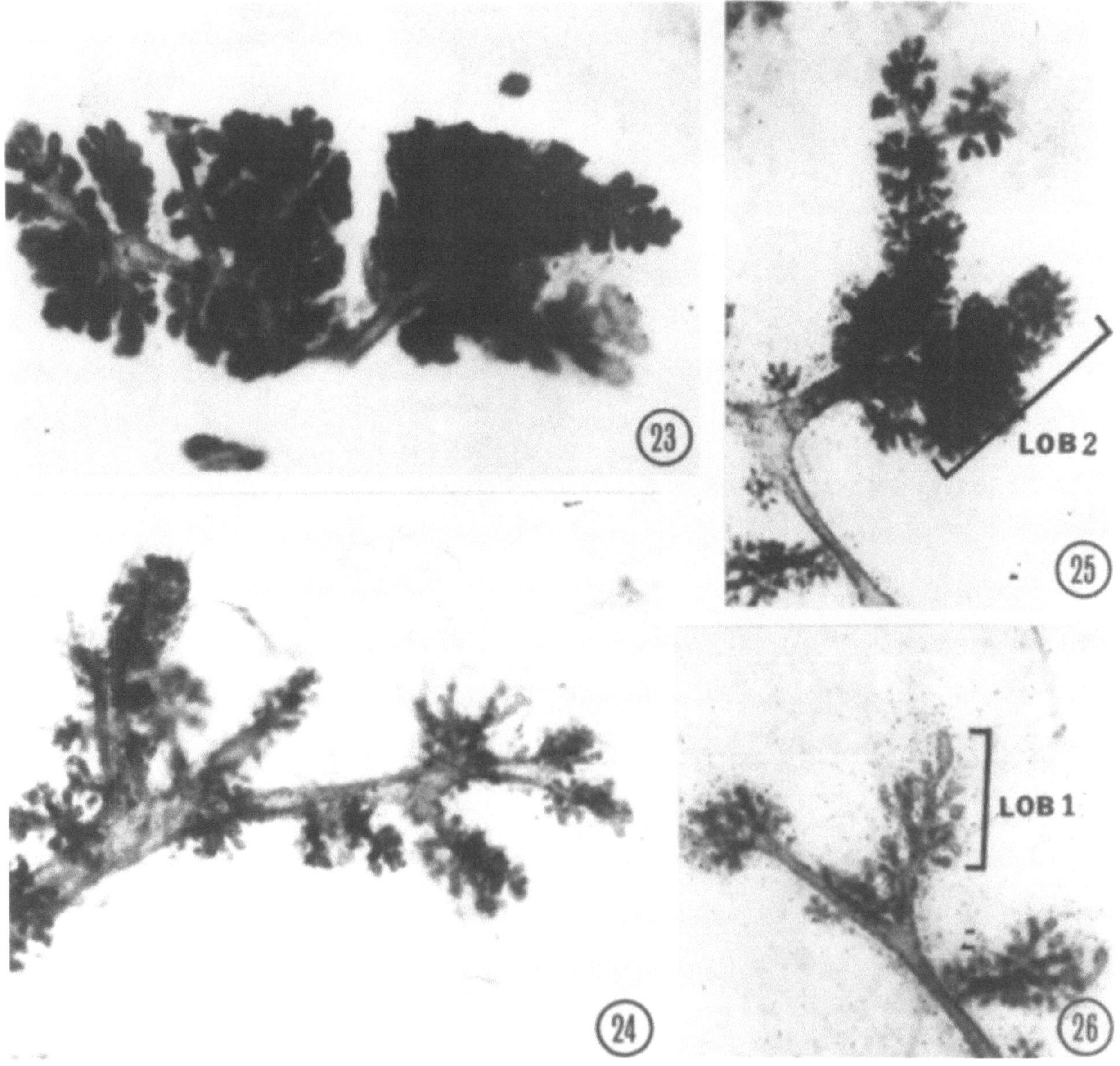

FIG. 23. Whole-mount breast tissue of a 19-year-old nulliparous woman. It is mostly composed of lobules type 1, but the increased number of ABs per lobule indicates a transitional stage of lobules type 2 (toluidine blue) ×25.

FIG. 24. Whole-mount preparation of breast tissue of a 20-year-old nulliparous woman in which lobules type 1 are present (toluidine blue) ×25.

FIG. 25. The whole-mount of the same breast tissue shown in Figure 24. Lobules type 2 (lob2) are composed of ductules, which are more abundant and smaller than the alveolar buds of type 1 lobules, which also are present (toluidine blue) ×25.

FIG. 26. Whole mount preparation of the same breast tissue shown in Figures 24 and 25. Lobules type 1 (Lob 1) are composed of alveolar buds (toluidine blue) ×25.

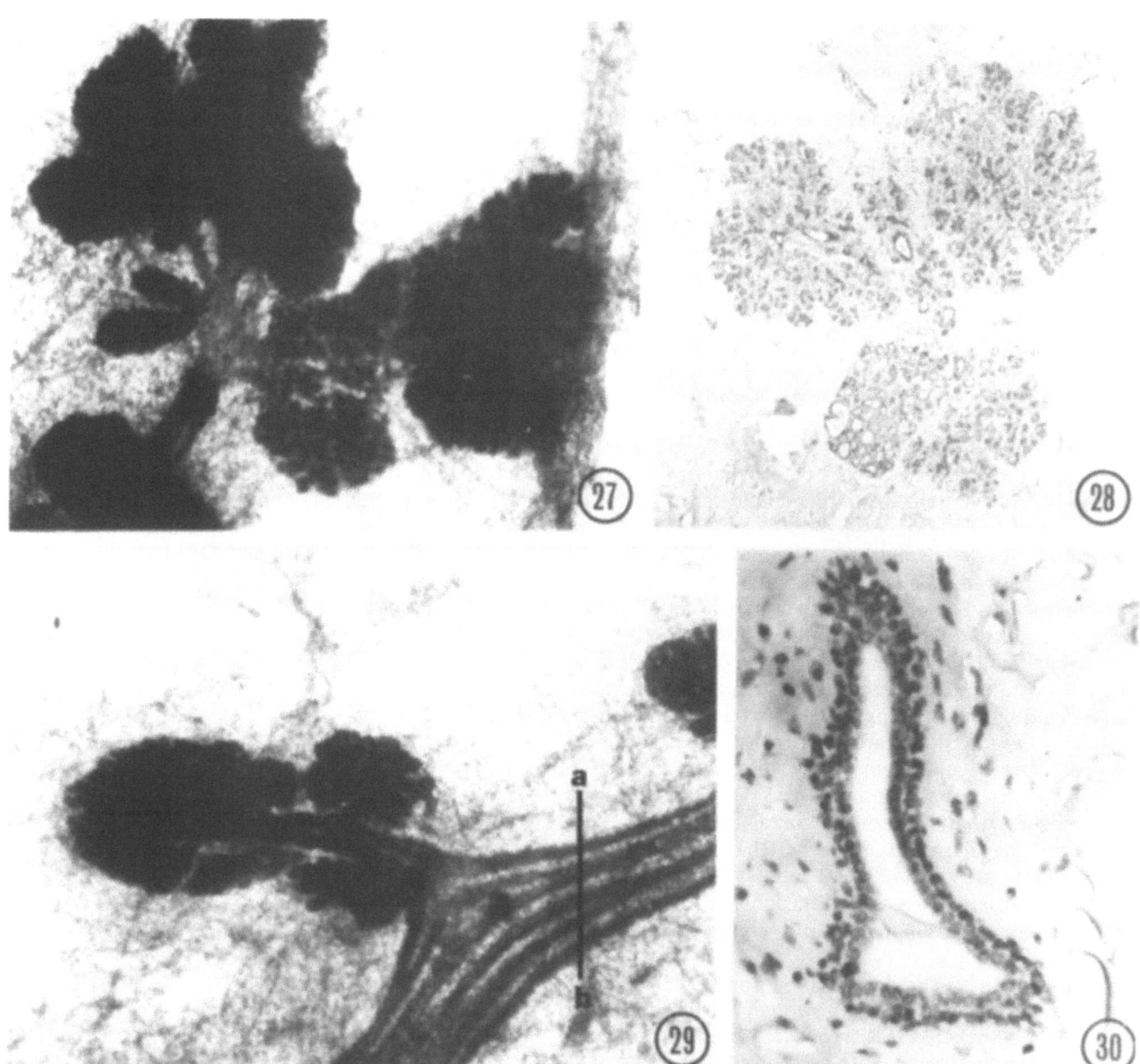

FIG. 27. Whole-mount preparation of breast tissue from a gravida 2, para 2, 30-year-old woman. The parenchyma is composed of numerous type 3 lobules. In the breast of parous women, even isolated branches like those depicted in Figure 29 are well developed. Compare with Figures 16 to 26 of a nulliparous woman.

FIG. 28. Lobules type 3 are composed of ductules that are smaller than the alveolar buds composing lobules type 1. (H & E) ×25.

FIG. 29. Isolated branch with a lobule type 3 (toluidine blue) ×25.

FIG. 30. Ductal structure. Cross-section at the level *a-b* of Figure 29. (H&E) ×160.

consisting of proliferation of the distal elements of the ductal tree, resulting in the neoformation of ductules that at this stage can be called alveoli or acini, thus developing a lobule type 3 into a lobule type 4 (Table 7). The intensity of budding and degree of lobule formation goes beyond what has been observed in the virginal breast.

In lobular formation, both development and differentiation take place simultaneously. The progressive transition of lobules type 1 to types 2, 3 and 4 requires active cell proliferation to acquire the cell mass necessary for milk secretion. This latter process implies differentiation of the mammary epithelium. The presence of lobules type 4 is the maximal expression of development and differentiation in the adult gland. The presence of lobules

type 3 may indicate that the gland has developed, but not completely differentiated, because the lobules are not secreting milk. It is important to point out that the presence of proteins that are indicative of milk secretion, such as α-lactalbumin, casein, or milk fat globule membrane protein (35–37, 144, 155), also indicates cellular differentiation of breast epithelium. However, only when all the other components of milk are coordinately synthesized within the appropriate structure, such as occurs at the end of pregnancy and during lactation, can full differentiation of the mammary gland be acknowledged. Repeated pregnancies extend lobular development.

In the absence of childbearing, the size and number of lobules decline, and only ductal structures and lobules type 1 and type 2 are observed. These lobule types, as

TABLE 7. IDENTIFICATION PROFILE OF THE DIFFERENT COMPARTMENTS OF HUMAN BREAST

Structure	Parameter[b]	Lobule 1	Lobule 2	Lobule 3	Lobule 4
Lobule	Area (mm^2)	0.048 ± 0.044	0.060 ± 0.026	0.129 ± 0.049	0.250 ± 0.060
AB/ductule/acinus[a]	Area (mm^2)	0.232×10^{-2} $\pm 0.090 \times 10^{-2}$	0.167×10^{-2} $\pm 0.035 \times 10^{-2}$	0.125×10^{-2} $\pm 0.029 \times 10^{-2}$	0.120×10^{-2} $\pm 0.050 \times 10^{-2}$
AB/ductule/acinus[a]	Number per lobule[c]	11.20 ± 6.34	47.0 ± 11.70	81.0 ± 16.6	180 ± 20.0
AB/ductule/acinus[a]	Number/mm^2 of lobule	253.8 ± 50.17	682.4 ± 169.0	560 ± 25.0	720.0 ± 150.0
AB/ductule/acinus[a]	Number cells/cross-section[d]	32.43 ± 14.07	13.14 ± 4.79	11.0 ± 2.0	10.0 ± 2.3

[a] AB/ductule/acinus: alveolar bud/ductule/acinus. The three nomenclatures used to identify the forming units of lobule are cited, with AB being used only for lobules type 1, ductule for lobules type 2 and type 3, and acini for lobules type 4.

[b] Student's t-tests were done for all possible comparisons. Lobular areas show significant differences between lobule 1 *versus* 3 and 4 and between 2,3, and 4 ($p <0.05$). Alveolar bud area differences were significant between lobules 1,2, and 3 and between 1 and 2 *versus* 3 and 4 ($p <0.001$).

[c] The number of alveolar buds per lobule was different ($p <0.01$) in all the comparisons. The number of buds per mm^2 of lobule was significant ($p <0.001$) between lobule 1 *versus* 2,3, and 4.

[d] The number of cells/cross-section was significantly different in alveolar buds of lobules 1 *versus* 2 and 3 ($p <0.01$).

From Russo *et al.* Development of the mammary gland. In The Mammary Gland, edited by Neville MC, Daniel CW, Plenum Publishing Corp, 1987.

previously indicated, are areas of epithelial proliferation; they may represent the lobular irregularities or primitive lobules that Ingleby and Gershon-Cohen (88) found in 33% of clinically normal breasts removed from women autopsied between the ages of 30 and 40.

Lobules type 1 and 2 are predominantly found in the breast of nulliparous young women, although they are also occasionally found in breast tissue of older women. Although there is a trend for type 1 lobules to predominate in nulliparous young women, type 3 lobules have been seen as the dominant type in the breast of a 13-year-old girl of unknown parity history (128 and P. Monaghan, personal communication). These observations suggest that there is no correlation between age and gland development, however, the biologic significance of the presence of these lobules in the breast of women of different ages and reproductive histories has not been elucidated completely and requires further studies.

The observation that lobules type 1 or TDLUs are also found in parous women and in women with a history of abortion suggests that this type of lobule might represent structures that have failed to respond to the influence of pregnancy and lactation (105). The meaning of this asynchronous development of the gland, even after the full stimulation of pregnancy, is not clear yet. Studies in our experimental system on the response of these structures to *in vitro* carcinogenesis suggests that they may represent an undifferentiated stage, and are, therefore, possible targets for neoplastic transformation (143, 148, 150, 152, 162, 165).

Determination of the proliferative activity of these structures by measuring the incorporation of [³H]thymidine (DNA-LI) into the mammary epithelium by the technique described by Russo and Russo (154) and Calaf *et al.* (33, 34) has shown that the DNA-LI of lobules type 2 is around 0.99 and of lobules type 3 is 0.25 (Fig. 30). These values are 5 and 20 times lower than those found in lobules type 1 and up to 60 times lower than in the terminal end bud (Fig. 31). It is important to emphasize that in the study of the proliferative activity of the mammary gland, each topographic compartment has to be analyzed individually. As it is depicted in Figure 30, there is a gradient from the TEB to the lobule type 3;

ductal structures have a proliferative activity intermediate between that of lobules type 1 and type 2. This gradient does not seem to be modified with aging, although in older women all proliferative activity is significantly reduced (122, 152, 162).

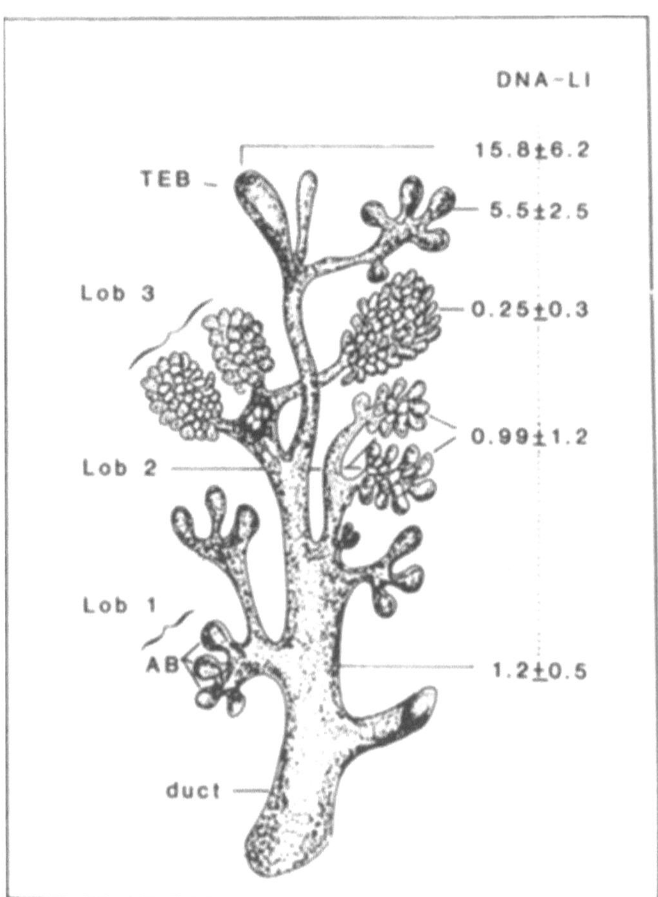

FIG. 31. Schematic representation depicting the various topographic compartments of the human mammary gland: terminal end buds (*TEB*); alveolar buds (*AB*); lobules types 1,2 and 3 (*Lob 1, Lob 2, and Lob 3*); and ducts. On the right-hand column is shown the DNA-LI of each structure (mean ± SD) of nine women ranging in age from 18 to 62 years. A gradient in proliferative activity is observed from the TEB (15.8 ± 6.2), Lob 1 (5.5 ± 2.5), Lob 2 (0.9 ± 1.2), Lob 3 (0.25 ± 0.3), and ducts (1.2 ± 0.5). From: J Russo and IH Russo (see reference 157).

COMPARATIVE ASPECTS OF DEVELOPMENT

The mammary gland differs from almost all other organs and glandular elements in the fact that during the process of development they are composed of an immature mammary parenchyma surrounded by mature stromal tissue. In other glands, on the other hand, both parenchyma and stroma develop harmoniously at the same time and in definitive space. In the mammary gland, the glandular parenchyma penetration into the surrounding tissue occurs during the prepubertal period rather slowly. By this time, the tissue surrounding the epithelium is fat, connective tissue and blood vessels which have become completely mature, whereas the gland itself remains in an embryonal state. It is during pubertal growth in both the rat and the human that the epithelial component begins to be stimulated by hormonal impulses to penetrate into the mature surrounding tissue. The concept of maturity of the stroma and of the degree of maturation of this organ and of its interaction with the parenchyma is at the present time an assumption, since very little is known at cellular and molecular level.

The postnatal development of the rat mammary gland has been thoroughly studied in the S-D strain of rats. However, it is not known whether differences in susceptibility to carcinogenesis exhibited by other strains of rats are related to variations in the pattern of gland development and branching or in relation with variations in the physiology of the animals. In the human female, the developmental pattern of the mammary gland is not completely known for the species, and no comparative studies among women of different races, genetic backgrounds or different environments are available. There are basic differences between the developmental pattern of the human and rat mammary glands. For example, in the human, the ductal structures grow along connective tissue septa, and rarely the lobular structures grow into fat tissue. In the rat, instead, there is a constant growth of ductal and lobular structures into the adjacent fat tissue. This difference must be born in mind when the influence of the parenchyma on the stroma is studied in one species or the other. Another difference that might be of importance is that in the rat there is a gradient in development from the nipple to the distal portion, which is the last to differentiate; in the human, the growth or the development is more labryinthic and a different degree of development in different portions of the breast is observed. However, this knowledge is incomplete and needs to be better assessed.

The other important different between the rat and the human is that in the rat there is in general a good correlation between gland development and age. In humans there is no good correlation between age and gland development: different degrees of glandular development are seen in women of the same age. These differences may be due to endocrinologic, genetic or socioeconomic differences, among other factors. Although some progress has been made in the assessment of degree of mammary gland development by defining different levels of lobular development as types 1, 2, 3 or 4, more needs to be done in order to understand this phenomenon.

PATHOGENESIS OF MAMMARY TUMORS

RAT MAMMARY TUMORS

Mammary gland tumors induced in rats by a single dose of DMBA, NMU or irradiation comprise a spectrum of morphology from benign, typical fibroadenomas and adenomas to papillomas with hyperplastic, atypical and dysplastic epithelium and significant stromal and myoepithelial components, to tumors that are architecturally and cytologically malignant and invade adjacent normal tissue. Metastases from even the most anaplastic tumors are low in frequency (194).

Carcinogenic initiation occurs primarily in the epithelium of TEBs (Fig. 15) while they are developing into ABs and TDs; these structures are considered to be equivalent to the terminal ductal lobular unit (TDLU) described in the human breast by Wellings *et al.* (200) (Fig. 32). Excessive epithelial proliferation and development of progressive cytologic abnormalities result from carcinogen exposure and ultimately produce tumors (158). This process can be initiated with the administration of DMBA to virgin rats (160). Its administration during the period in which TEBs are decreasing in number due to their differentiation into ABs, a process occurring when the animals are between the ages of 45 and 55 days, induces the largest number of transformed structures. Affected TEBs, instead of differentiating into ABs, become larger, and they are called intraductal proliferations. Intraductal proliferations become progressively larger and their confluence leads to the formation of carcinomas (Fig. 15) (158, 160). Tumor development does not occur as a random event in the six pairs of mammary glands. Virgin animals treated with the carcinogen develop a greater number of tumors in those glands located in the thoracic region than in glands located in the abdomino-inguinal area. These topographic differences in tumor incidence appear to be due to the asynchronous development of the thoracic mammary glands, which retain the undifferentiated TEBs for a period of time longer than mammary glands located in different topographic areas (158) (Fig. 2). However, a trend in a different direction has been observed in irradiated animals (194). Those TEBs that were already differentiated into ABs before DMBA administration do not develop carcinomas but either remain unmodified, undergo dilation, giving rise to hyperplastic lobules (Fig. 15), exhibit epithelial proliferation forming tubular adenomas, or give rise to cystic dilations. Hyperplastic lobules and cysts appear later than IDPs, the first ones being observed at 5 to 6 weeks after DMBA administration (158, 160–162). The observation that mammary carcinomas arise from undifferentiated structures of the gland, namely TEBs, whereas benign lesions, such as adenomas, cysts, and fibroadenomas arise from structures that were more differentiated at the time of carcinogen administration, indicates that the carcinogen requires an adequate structural target and the type of lesion induced is dependent upon the area of the mammary gland that the carcinogen affects. Thus, the more differentiated the structure at the time of carcinogen administration, the more benign and organized is the lesion which develops.

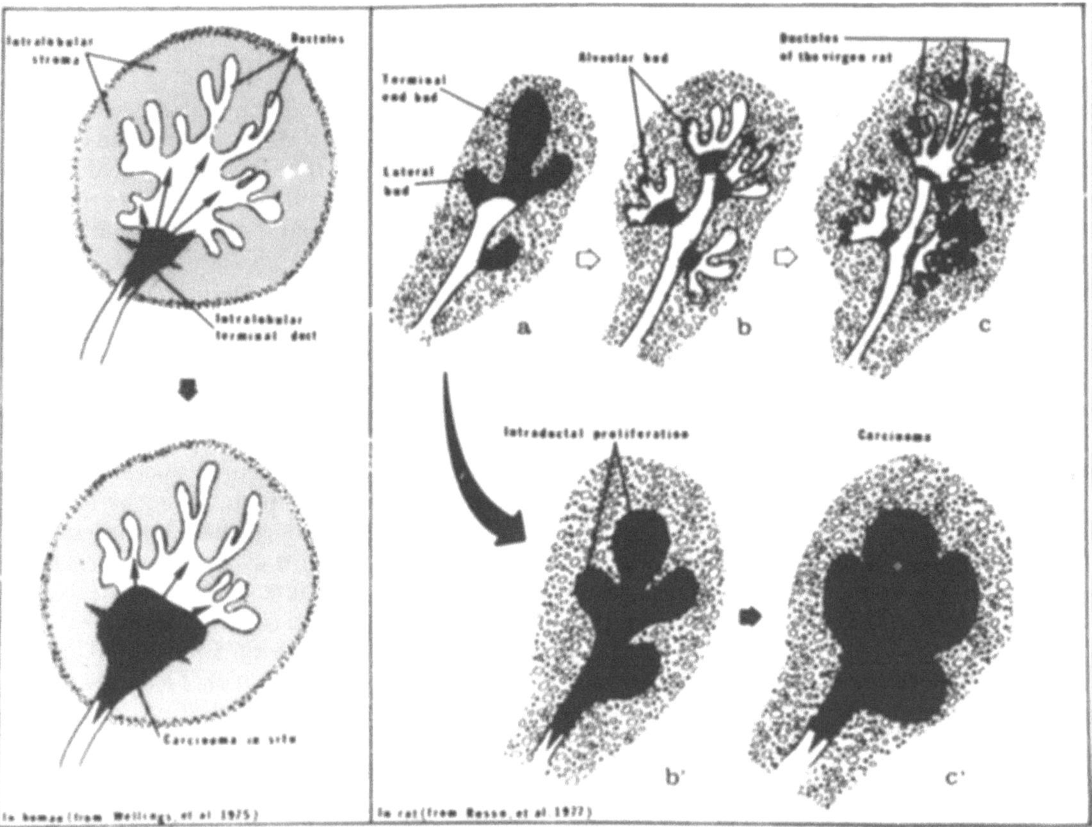

FIG. 32. Schematic representation of the site of origin of breast carcinoma in the intralobular TD and at further expansion toward the ductules and ducts (*left*). Pathogenetic pathway of mammary carcinoma in the rat. (*right*).

The high susceptibility of the TEB to neoplastic transformation is attributed to cell kinetic properties of its lining epithelium, whose rate of cell proliferation and of DNA synthetic activity (DNA-LI) are maximal at the tip, and decrease toward the ductal or proximal portion of the gland. The TEB is also characterized by having the highest growth fraction, which progressively diminishes in the more differentiated ABs and lobules (152). The high rate of cell proliferation is associated with the short length of the cell cycle (Tc), which in TEBs of young virgin rats has an average length of 11 hours, lengthening to 21 and 28 hours in TDs and ABs, respectively.

Using these cell kinetic parameters we have calculated the rate of cell loss in each one of the compartments of the mammary tree (158). Interestingly, the TEB is the structure with the highest proliferative ratio and the lowest percentage of cell loss.

DMBA is metabolized by mammary epithelial cells to polar metabolites, including epoxides (184, 186), that may be responsible for causing DNA damage. When dissociated breast epithelial cells of TEBs obtained from virgin animals and lobular cells obtained from parous animals are grown *in vitro*, they exhibit different rates of formation of polar metabolites. Cells of TEBs produce more polar and less phenolic metabolites than do lobular cells, indicating that the former, in addition to their higher proliferative activity, produce more epoxides, with a greater binding of DMBA to DNA (158, 162, 184, 185). Autoradiographic studies show that the greatest uptake of [^{3}H]DMBA occurs in the nucleus of the epithelial cells of TEBs, and the lowest uptake is observed in ABs and lobules, indicating that the highest DMBA-DNA binding is associated with the structure of the gland with the highest replicative properties (162). The ability of the cells to remove DMBA adducts from the DNA, an indication of their capability to repair the damage, is less in TEB cells than in lobular cells. This is attributed to the shorter G_1 and T_c, and not to lack of reparative enzymes (158, 184, 185).

HUMAN BREAST TUMORS

The nature and site of origin of neoplastic growth in human breast have been the subject of numerous studies based on examination of surgical and autopsy tissues. The most useful of these studies use subgross sampling of whole human breasts with histologic confirmation, allowing the identification and quantitation of essentially the entire pathologic content of each breast. On these bases it is postulated that there are four major possible sites of origin of mammary carcinomas: ducts, terminal ducts, ductules, and "acini."

The hypothesis of ductal origin (63, 105, 166, 168) is based upon the presence of presumed preneoplastic epithelial hyperplasia in ducts. The epithelial proliferations are more extensive in breasts removed for cancer than in non-malignant breasts removed at autopsy. Sandison (168) studied the histopathology of 800 autopsy breasts. Of these, 22% had epithelial hyperplasia which was ductal in 73.4%, both ductal and "acinar" (*i.e.*, ductular) in 20.4%, and "acinar" in 6.2%. Since these studies utilized only routine histology preparations (essentially 2-dimensional), clear distinctions between small ducts, terminal ducts and ductules ("acini") were not always possible, as later subgross studies have revealed.

Ductules are indicated in older works (195) as well as in recent reports (93, 94) as sites of epithelial hyperplasia which is a necessary stage for cancer development. Unfortunately, "acini" and ductules have been confused in the literature as equivalent structures. Ductules are best defined as the smallest blindly ending structure of the lobule type 1 or virginal lobule (50, 51, 157) from which a new sprouting will form the acini of the mature lobule

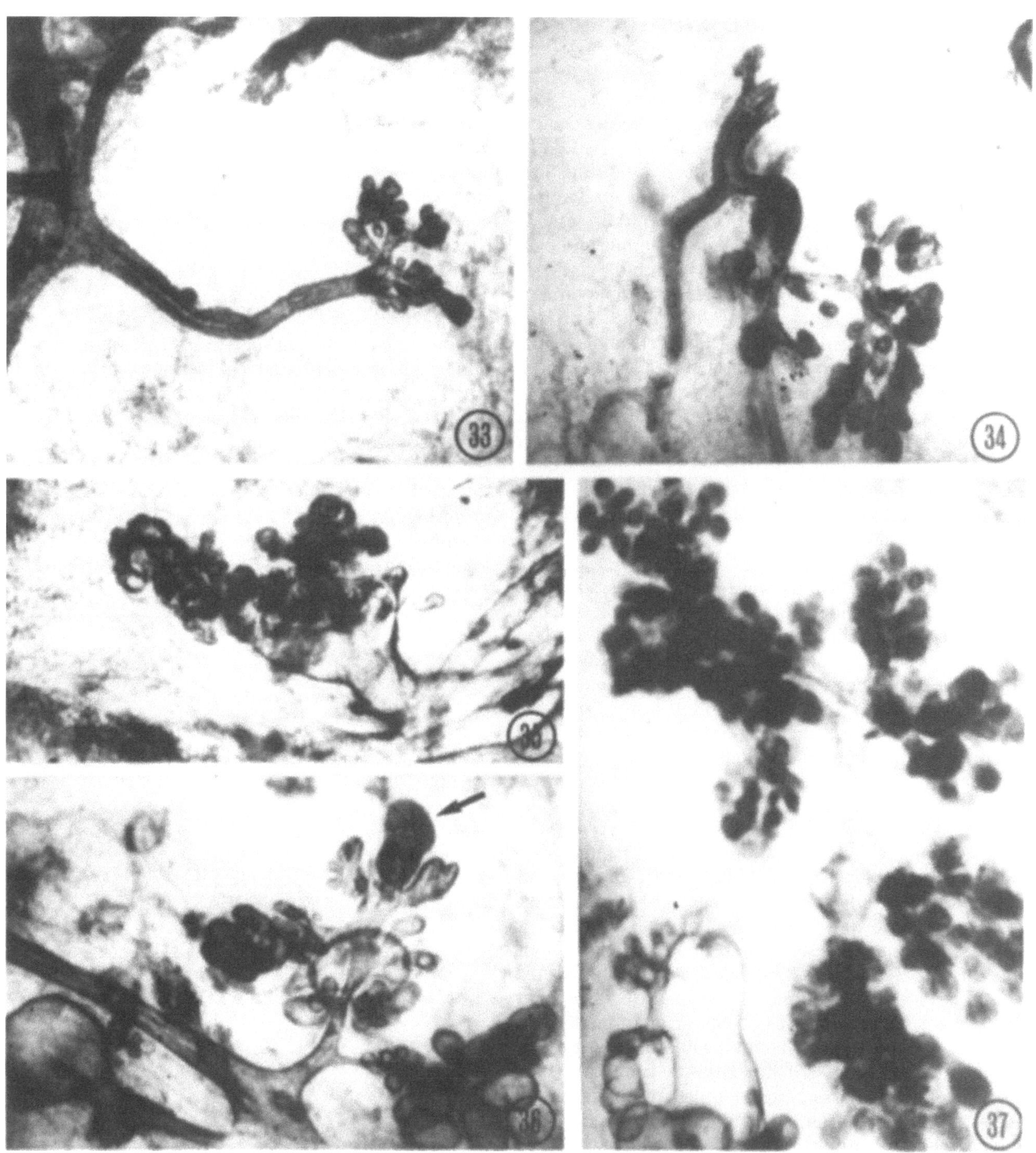

FIG. 33 to 37. Whole mount preparation of human breast tissue.

FIG. 33. Lobular structure type 1. (Hematoxylin) ×55.

FIG. 34. Carcinoma *in situ* in the TD and ductules of lobule type 1. (Hematoxylin) ×55.

FIG. 35. Severe atypical epithelial hyperplasia into lumens of dis-

tended ductules of a lobule type 1 (Hematoxylin) ×55.

FIG. 36. TEB (*arrow*) with carcinoma *in situ* and cystic structures originated from the ductules. (Hematoxylin) ×55.

FIG. 37. Lobular carcinoma *in situ* originated in lobules type 2. (Hematoxylin) ×55.

(lobules 2 and 3) and during pregnancy and lactation (lobule type 4). That breast carcinoma can originate in ductules has been indicated by several independent observations (16, 41, 42, 64, 95, 131). The TD is best regarded as having two parts (Fig. 32). The first part is closest to the nipple and is called extralobular or entering TD. This structure ends at its site of entry into the lobule at the interface of the intralobular and extralobular connective tissue. The second part of the TD is referred to as the intralobular or axial TD which is actually the sometimes poorly defined central axial space of the lobule from which the ductules arise. The ductules are truly the terminal blindly ending sacks of the mammary tree. The ductules, together with the intralobular or axial TD, and the distinctive loose intralobular connective tissue, are the three recognized constituents of the lobule (Fig. 32).

The lobule type 1 (Figs. 17, 19, 33), as previously defined in this paper, and for our present purpose essentially synonymous with TDLU, is the basic morphologic and functional microstructure of the mammary gland.

In previous studies (1, 198, 200, 201) 292 whole human breasts were studied by a subgross sampling technique with histologic confirmation. One hundred and eighty-five of these were from random autopsies (autopsy series) and 107 were from breasts that either contained a carcinoma, or were contralateral to one (cancer-associated series). The subgross method allowed the identification and quantitation of essentially the entire pathologic content of each breast. The two series are compared as to average number of lesions of each kind per breast in Table 8, which is modified and simplified from previous work cited above.

Of paramount importance were statistical data regarding the question of identity of precancerous lesions in the human breast. Different kinds of lesions in a group of breasts obtained by autopsy, cancerous ones, and those contralateral to cancer, were identified according to decade of patient's age. In classification of lesions into the main groups, modifiers such as sclerosis or dilation were not considered. Compound lesions were graded qualitatively according to the area showing the greatest pathologic and/or atypical change. Several trends were apparent: (a) In breasts from routine autopsies, atypia and ductal carcinoma in terminal ductal-lobular units were rare, as were hyperplastic TDs both with and without papillomatous proliferation at any age. (b) In cancerous breasts and those contralateral to cancer (Table 8) type 1 lobules were more frequent than in autopsy specimens after the 4th decade of age and lobules type 1 and atypia as well as foci of carcinomas of terminal ductal-lobular units were frequent (Fig. 34 to 36). Hyperplastic TDs with and without papillomatous proliferation were evident at all ages (Fig. 35). (c) Breasts from the three categories have hypersecretory lobules in any decade of life, especially in patients on digitalis, reserpine, and dilantin therapy, and in nulliparous women. Higher grade atypia in duct papillomas was rare, and the frequency of sclerosing adenosis and fibroadenoma was similar in breast cancer patients and those dying of other diseases. Apocrine cysts seldom appeared before the 4th decade in all patients but were more abundant in later decades in women with breast cancer. Hyperplastic ducts

larger than TDs occurred infrequently and represented less than 0.5% of total lesions encountered, again indicating that carcinomas do not commonly arise in larger ducts.

When all breasts were grouped irrespective of age, atypical lobules and hyperplastic TDs were more frequent in cancer breasts or in those contralateral to cancer than in breasts not so identified. The preponderance of evidence indicates that most mammary carcinomas arise from lobules type 1 (TDLU) or their precursors (Figs. 34, 35, 36). Lesions originated in lobules type 1 include at least: carcinoma *in situ*, the common infiltrating duct carcinomas, and perhaps some other kinds of infiltrating carcinomas. In contrast, it is thought that classical lobular carcinoma *in situ* may arise from the more differentiated lobules type 2 (Figs. 37, 38). In the human, the classical intraductal papillomas arise from larger ducts outside of the lobules and near to the nipple (not from the lobule themselves or their entering or axial terminal ducts).

COMPARATIVE ASPECTS OF PATHOGENESIS

The study of the pathogenesis of rat mammary carcinomas has revealed that the carcinogen acts on TEBs and TDs mainly when these structures are differentiating into ABs (Fig. 15). Transformed TEBs and TDs evolve to intraductal proliferation, carcinoma *in situ*, invasive carcinoma, and occasionally metastasize. More differentiated structures such as ABs and lobules give rise to more benign lesions such as cysts, fibroadenomas, and adenomas, and the more differentiated lobules give rise to lactating adenomas. The comparison between the rat's

TABLE 8. AVERAGE NUMBER OF SELECTED LESIONS/BREAST

Lesion	185 Random autopsy breasts	10 Cancer-associated breasts	P value for Diff. Pops. (Students t-test
Hyperplastic terminal duct	0.08	1.82	>0.999
Lobule type 1 (TDLU) with nuclear atypism	10.31	44.50	>0.999
DCIS[a] arising in lobule type 1	0.08	5.47	0.966

[a] DCIS, Ductal carcinoma *in situ*.

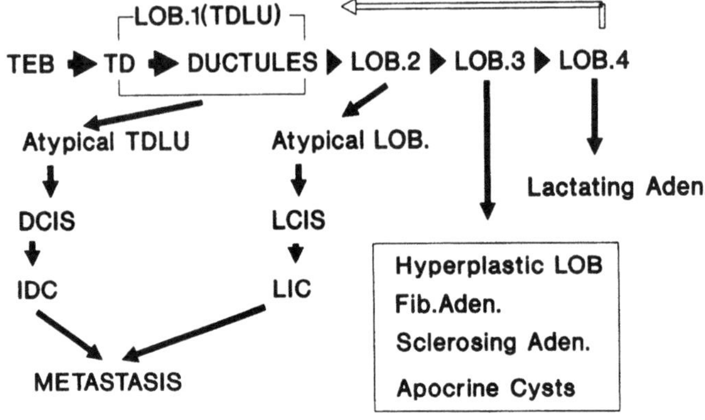

FIG. 38. Pathogenetic pathway of human breast cancer.

and the human's pathogenetic pathways of mammary carcinogenesis is only tentative, because the role of the terminal end bud in the human is not known. The TEB in the human female is a prepubertal structure and the biology and the differentiation of the structure from the prepubertal to the pubertal age needs to be studied. Most of the data collected for the study of mammary carcinogenesis are derived from observations of postpubertal breasts. In the postpubertal breast, most of the structures of the gland are mainly composed of TDs and ductules forming lobules type 1, which are the basic TDLU. As described in the previous section, the terminal ductal structures of the terminal ductal lobular unit originate preneoplastic lesions which evolve to ductal carcinoma *in situ*, progressing to invasive carcinoma and finally metastasize (Fig. 38).

The differentiation of lobules type 1 to type 2 is also important since morphologic observations suggest that lobules type 2 could be involved in the development of atypical lobules which originate lobular carcinoma *in situ* (Figs. 37 and 38) and its invasive form. Lobules type 3 present in the human breast seem to give origin to hyperplastic or hypersecretory lobules, fibroadenomas, sclerosing adenosis and apocrine cysts (Fig. 38) whereas lactating adenomas seem to originate from lobules type 4 (Fig. 38). In the rat, these more benign lesions originate from virginal and mature lobules. An important difference between the pathogenetic pathway in the rat and human is at the level of the TDLU. Such as observed in Figures 15 and 32, the TEB in the rat would be equivalent to the intralobular TD in the human, the area which is most susceptible to neoplastic growth. However, an important gap in our knowledge is the lack of observations of early carcinomas in the human breast, in order to determine whether they originate from more undifferentiated TEBs before the lobular elements have formed. Another possibility is that in humans, carcinogenesis takes place in more differentiated structures, or TDLU. More studies need to be done on the involution of the human breast, and how lobules type 3 involute to lobules type 2 or 1. The presence of lobules type 1 in the postmenopausal woman may explain the rising incidence of neoplasia in older women, however, this does not rule out the possibility that malignant transformation had occurred much earlier in life.

Chemically induced mammary carcinogenesis requires active cell replication which is maximal in the TEB. In the human breast, the highest peak of cell replication occurs in the TD during early adulthood, decreasing considerably with age (33, 34, 143, 162). This observation indicates that during early adulthood, when cell turnover is more rapid, more chances exist for a neoplastic process to be initiated. Epidemiologic findings reveal that the young woman's breast is more susceptible to ionizing radiation (121). This could be explained as a consequence of incomplete differentiation of the gland, meaning one having TDs with high replicative properties. These observations are supported by experimental data showing that the TDLU or lobule type 1 of the human female has the highest *in vitro* binding of carcinogen to DNA. When these structures are cultured and treated *in vitro* with carcinogens, they express phenotypical changes of trans-

formation that are not expressed by lobules type 2 and 3. Even though further studies are needed to confirm these preliminary data, there is strong evidence that the degree of differentiation of the mammary gland at the moment in which an etiologic agent or agents act is of extreme importance in the initiation of carcinogenesis (121, 158, 162).

COMPARISON BETWEEN HUMAN AND RAT MAMMARY TUMORS

HISTOPATHOLOGIC CLASSIFICATION OF MAMMARY TUMORS

The validity of rat mammary carcinogenesis for the study and understanding of the biology of human mammary carcinogenesis and for validating the development of strategies for breast cancer prevention and cure requires that in these two models, in addition to similarities in the basic pathogenesis and developmental concepts that: (a) the histotype of the tumors is similar; (b) that the cell types present in the rat react with similar immunocytochemical markers as do the human ones, and (c) that the biologic behavior of tumors is comparable in the two species. The objective of this section is to compare, side by side, rat and human mammary tumors.

Rat mammary tumors have been classified by several authors (67, 159, 194, 214). There is agreement that tumors appearing histologically malignant in the rat have features in common with the intraductal and infiltrating ductal carcinomas in humans, but few spontaneously metastasize (Figs. 39 to 50). This tumor type, however, constitutes a minority of the tumors developed by rats under the commonly used regimens for tumor induction. Similarly, benign fibroadenomas and adenomas (Figs. 39 to 44) that occur in rats closely resemble the human benign tumors, but constitute only a small percentage of the tumors induced in most studies. The majority of induced tumors are papillomatous with hyperplastic epithelium containing both epithelial and myoepithelial cells, and appear cytologically benign, or they may be composed of epithelial cells with varying degrees of cytologic atypia, growing in solid, papillary adenomatous patterns. In most tumors, the abnormal epithelium tends to remain rigidly confined by the adjacent stroma, and shows no clear evidence of invasion. All of these features contribute to the difficulty of making clear distinctions between benign and malignant lesions. For this reason, a consensus conference was held in Hannover, West Germany, in 1987, the result of which is the classification depicted in Table 9 (193).

In Table 9 are shown the main histological types of mammary tumors found in the rat, and it also correlates the classification of neoplastic and non-neoplastic lesions in the rat and in the human mammary glands. It is clear that most of the lesions found in the rat mammary glands have their counterpart in human pathology. However, there are specific lesions in humans, such as Paget's disease of the nipple and infiltrating ductal carcinoma, scirrhous and medullary type that have not been reported in the rat mammary gland. Lobular carcinoma, *in situ* or invasive, has not been reported in the rat.

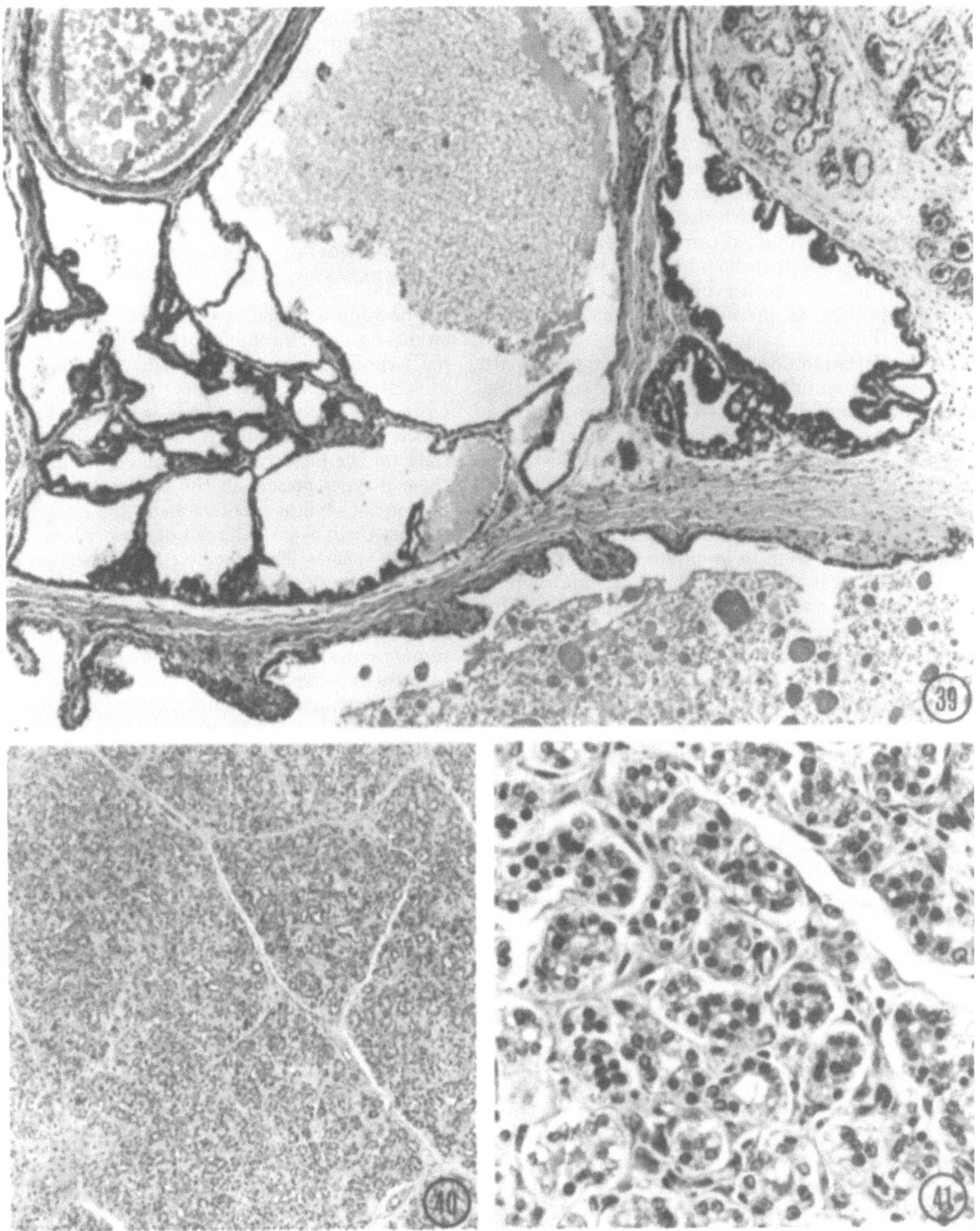

FIG. 39 to 50. Rat mammary tumors.

FIG. 39. Papillary cystadenoma of the mammary gland. Papillae lined by epithelial cells project toward a cystic cavity. The fibroconnective tissue in the papillary core is edematous (H&E) ×60.

FIG. 40. Tubular adenoma. Closely apposed alveolar or tubular structures are separated by small amount of connective tissue. (H&E) ×60.

FIG. 41. Tubular adenoma in which the tubular structures exhibit a regular contour. Individual alveoli are surrounded by a small amount of connective tissue. (H&E) ×160.

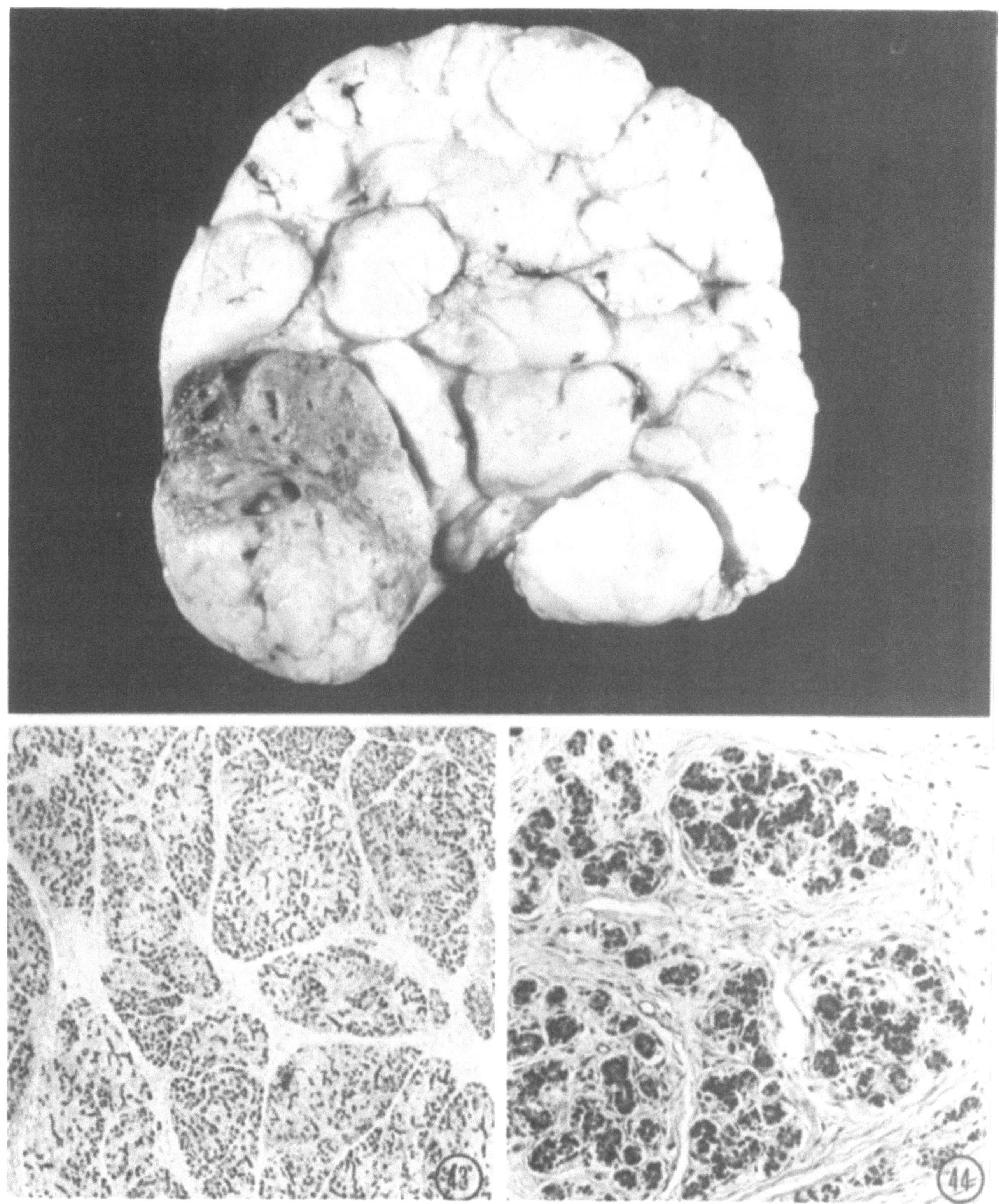

FIG. 42. Fibroadenoma.
FIG. 43. Fibroadenoma in which the desmoplastic reaction is compressing the tubular alveolar components. (H&E) ×60.

FIG. 44. Detail of the tubular elements composing the fibroadenoma shown in Figure 43. (H&E) ×160.

IMMUNOCYTOCHEMISTRY OF THE NORMAL MAMMARY GLAND AND OF ITS NEOPLASMS

The mammary gland of all mammals is a complex organ composed of a fibroconnective tissue stroma surrounding a ductular type parenchyma in which two cells types, epithelial and myoepithelial cells, are evident. The myoepithelial cells are in direct contact with the basement membrane. Each of the constituents of the breast can be identified on the basis of their ultrastructure, which is similar in rats and humans (144, 155), and by the characteristics of the antigenic profile (Table 10).

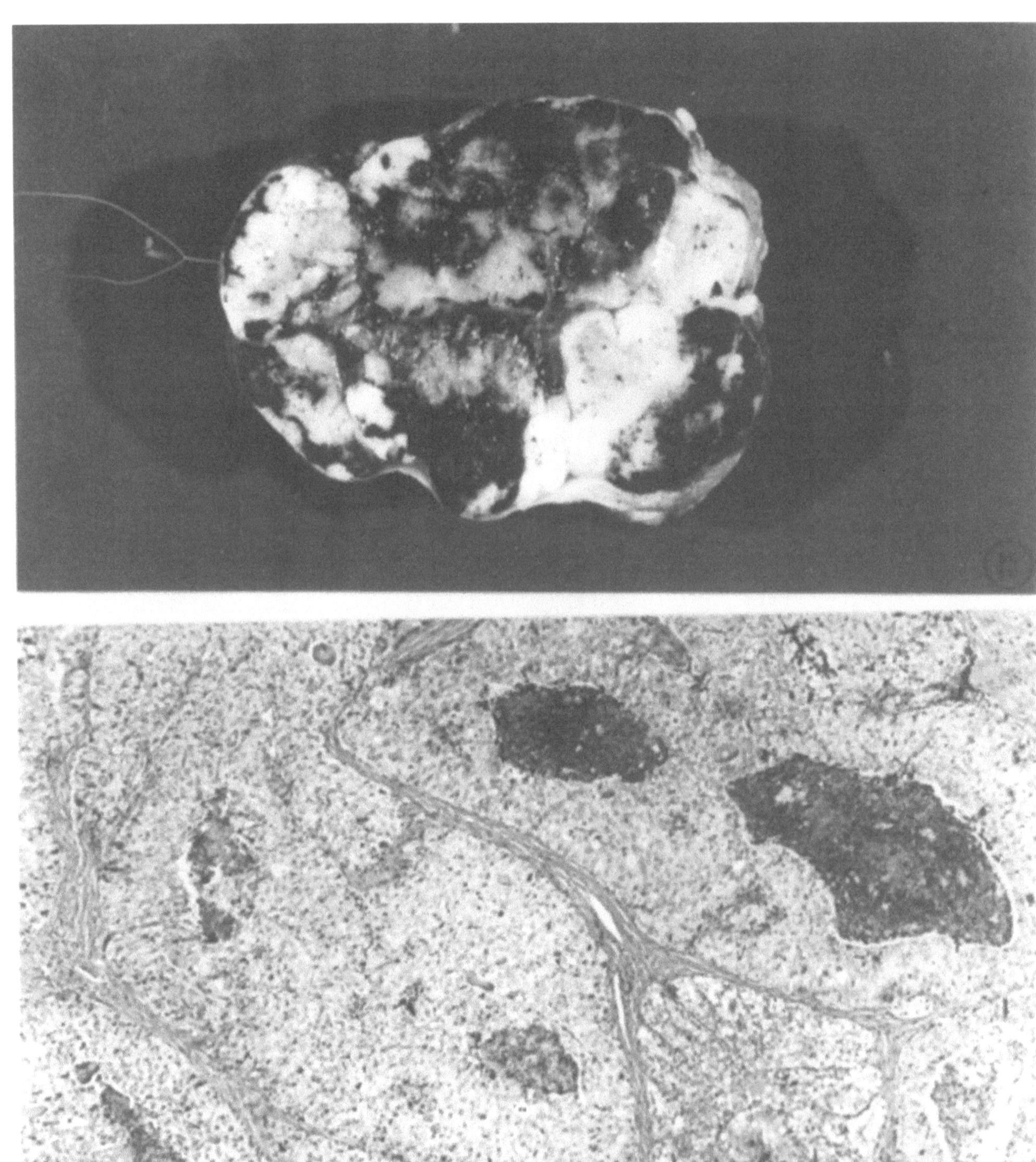

Fig. 45. Adenocarcinoma.
Fig. 46. Comedo carcinoma with cribriform pattern. (H&E) ×160.

Immunocytochemical Markers in the Normal Rat Mammary Gland and in its Tumors

The epithelial component of the mammary ductal and alveolar systems is composed of an inner luminal epithe-lial layer which is surrounded by myoepithelial cells (Figs. 51 to 54). These ducts and *alveoli* thus formed are separated from the surrounding mesenchymal cells and connective tissue by the basement membrane (Fig. 51). The luminal cell population can be stained by antibodies

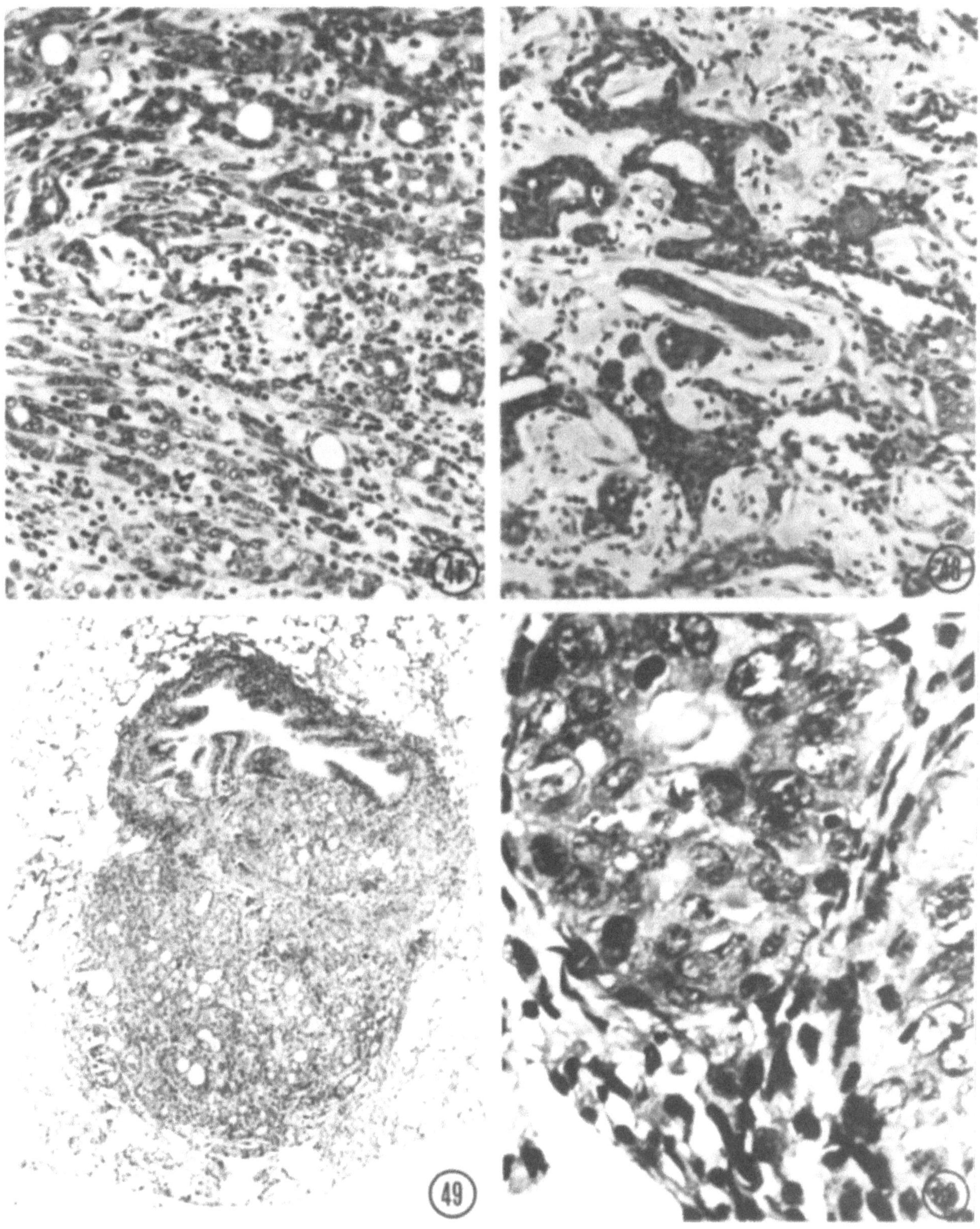

FIG. 47. Invasive cribriform carcinoma. (H&E) ×60.

FIG. 48. Invasive cribriform carcinoma with intense desmoplastic reaction. (H&E) ×60.

FIG. 49. Carcinoma cribriform type metastatic to the lung. (H&E) ×60.

FIG. 50. Detail of an infiltrating carcinoma, cribriform pattern, metastatic to the lung. (H&E) ×400.

TABLE 9. CLASSIFICATION OF NEOPLASTIC AND NON-NEOPLASTIC LESIONS OF THE RAT MAMMARY GLAND WITH COMPARISONS TO HUMAN LESIONS

Rat Lesion	Corresponding human lesion
I. Benign epithelial neoplasms:	
Adenoma (papillary, tubular, hyperplasia, lactating)	Intraductal papilloma lactating adenoma adenoma of pregnancy
II. Malignant epithelial neoplasms:	
Ductal carcinoma,	Ductal carcinoma
(a) Non-invasive:	Ductal carcinoma-*in-situ*
(1) cribriform	Cribriform
(2) comedo	Comedo
(3) solid	Solid
(4) papillary	Papillary
(b) Invasive:	Ductal carcinoma invasive
(1) cribriform	Cribiform
(2) comedo	Comedo
(3) solid	Papillary
(4) papillary	Infiltrating Ductal Carcinoma (NOS)
(5) not otherwise specified (NOS)	Scirrhous
	Medullary
	Colloid
	Others
	Lobular carcinoma
	Lobular carcinoma-in-situ
	Infiltrating lobular carcinoma
	Paget's disease of the nipple
III. Stromal Neoplasms:	
Benign	
Fibroma	Fibroma
Malignant	
Fibrosarcoma	Fibrosarcoma
IV. Epithelial-Stromal Neoplasms:	
Benign	
Fibroadenoma	Fibroadenoma cystosarcoma phylloides, benign
Malignant	
Carcinosarcoma	Carcinosarcoma cytosarcoma phylloides, malignant
V. Non-neoplastic "Lesions"	
Normal, lactating gland	Normal Lactating Gland
Lobular hyperplasia	Lobular Hyperplasia of Pregnancy Lobular Hyperplasia, Not Associated with Pregnancy
Cystic Changes	Cystic dilation of lobules
(a) ductal	Cystic dilation of ducts
(b) lobular	
Epithelial hyperplasia	Epithelial hyperplasia *without* premalignant atypia Epithelial hyperplasia *with* premalignant atypia

raised to the milk fat globule membrane (Fig. 54) and myoepithelial cells identified using antibodies directed against the cytokeratins present in these cells (Fig. 53) (197). Using antibodies specific to the individual cytokeratins it is now possible to map the distribution of these polypeptides in breast at various stages in development and in tumors. The use of the reagents as cellular markers is thus assisting in the *in vitro* as well as the *in vivo* analyses of lineage in the breast and studies on tumor histogenesis. At the present time more is known of the distribution of keratins in the human than in the rat breast, but certain generalizations can be made. Keratin 18 has been demonstrated in both rodent and human luminal cells (186). Basal (myoepithelial) cells in the rat and human have shared phenotypes with epidermal basal cells; it is thus to be predicted that as in the human, the rodent cells will contain keratins 5 and 14. Dulbecco *et al.* (52) have, on the basis of staining with anti-keratins specific for basal and luminal phenotypes in the rat, hypothesized that there is a mammary precursor stem cell which is present in the basal layer and can give rise to both luminal and myoepithelial cells (52). The outer layer of myoepithelial cells contain myofilaments that have high concentrations of actin and myosin (Fig. 52). Antibodies to these microfilaments are thus good markers of this cell population. More recently the common

TABLE 10. IMMUNOCYTOCHEMICAL MARKERS OF HUMAN AND RAT MAMMARY TISSUE

Cell type or structure	Antigen	
	Human	Rat
Myoepithelial cells	Actin	Actin
	Myosin	Myosin
	CALLA	CALLA
	gP 180	NK
	Keratin 5	NK
	Keratin 14	Keratin 14
Luminal cells	MFGM	MFGM
	Keratin 7	NK
	Keratin 8	Keratin 11
	Keratin 18	Keratin 18
	Keratin 18	NK
	Casein	Casein
	α-Lactalbumin	α-Lactalbumin
	Lactoferrin	Lactoferrin
Basement membrane	Laminin	Laminin
	Type IV	Type IV
	Fibronectin	Fibronectin
	Entactin	Entactin

acute lymphoblastic leukemia antigen (CALLA) has been described as a surface protein of the myoepithelial cells in the rat breast (74) and in the human may assist in the characterization of this cell population both *in vivo* and *in vitro* (128).

The components of the basement membrane, type IV collagen, laminin (Fig. 51), fibronectin and entactin can all be localized by using the appropriate antisera (124), while vimentin will identify the stromal cells.

In mammary gland adenomas, which are composed of acinar structures surrounded by a fragmented basement membrane (Fig. 55), the acini are lined by two layers of cells; the outer cell layer exhibits variable staining with the myoepithelial markers (Fig. 56). In carcinomas, the myoepithelial-like component is less well defined and the basement membrane becomes disorganized (130) and eventually is absent in the infiltrative component. The epithelial component of the tumors express cytokeratins (Fig. 57), therefore micrometastic deposits can be identified in lymph nodes and in the lung, using anti-cytokeratin antibodies (208).

The lumina in mammary carcinomas in general are two types: true and false (Figs. 55 to 58). True lumina are those which can be demonstrated with antibodies to the milk fat globule membrane antigen (Fig. 58) and false lumina can be demonstrated with antibodies to basement membrane components. The identification of myoepithelial-like cells is variable in these tumors, both within different areas of the same tumor and between tumors. Weak staining with the myoepithelial anti-keratin marker of a basally situated population of cells in a well differentiated area can be observed in Fig. 57. In some areas these cells are basally situated, but in the majority of the tumors these cells are difficult to identify. This is consistent with ultrastructural studies of these tumors where few myofilaments can be recognized. Strong actin stain is only observed in occasional cells but as with the keratin staining a distinct basal layer is, sometimes delineated (Fig. 56). The basement membrane at the stromal/epithelial interface of these tumors is clearly defined with an anti-laminin antibody (Fig. 55).

IMMUNOCYTOCHEMICAL MARKERS IN THE NORMAL HUMAN BREAST AND ITS TUMORS

The myoepithelial and epithelial cells of the human breast possess a large number of markers that permit their identification in both the normal organ and in neoplastic processes (Table 10).

Markers of Myoepithelial Cells. Myoepithelial cells are characterized by the presence of cytoplasmic filaments of actin and myosin (26, 27, 29, 30, 76). Actin is a contractile protein present in a variety of cells but is particularly abundant in smooth muscle and in myoepithelial cells. In the human breast, actin is present in the myoepithelial cells of the mammary parenchyma and in the pericytes surrounding the blood vessels. Actin helps in differentiating between benign and malignant epithelial proliferations of the breast, since it is present in large amounts in benign lesions but is generally absent in malignant tumors (26, 27). In lobular carcinoma *in situ*, the disappearance of myoepithelial cells observed when the process becomes invasive is detected using actin and myosin antibodies (26). Absence of reactivity with actin antibodies has been shown also to be a reliable criterion for differentiating tubular carcinoma from sclerosing adenosis. This marker is useful in those cases in which hyperplasia must be differentiated from carcinoma *in situ*. In the former, there is abundant proliferation of myoepithelial cells with a rich reaction for actin and myosin (76). This pattern is markedly altered in cases of carcinoma *in situ* (29). In keeping with their epithelial phenotype, both luminal cells and myoepithelial cells contain cytokeratin polypeptides. Keratins 5 and 14 are in the myoepithelial layer whereas keratins 7, 8, 18 and 19 are in the luminal cell population. There are slight variations in the relative distribution of these keratins in different parts of the mammary tree as recently reported (186), but in essence antibodies to keratins 8 and 18 are specific for the luminal layer and keratins 5 and 14 are excellent basal cell markers. In addition to these cytoplasmic markers CALLA is restricted to myoepithelial cells (74) as is an 180 Mol. glycoprotein which is also found as basal cells in human skin (75).

Markers of Luminal Cells. Cytokeratin pattern is apparently largely conserved after neoplastic transformation of epithelial cells (Figs. 59 and 60). Several studies have shown that neoplastic derivatives retain these characteristic cytokeratins, which can be detected with specific antibodies (2, 46, 99, 123, 127). Thus, immunocytochemical and biochemical analyses have shown that the expression of cytokeratins is maintained in epithelial cells during hyperplastic, neoplastic and metastatic process (3, 6, 59–62, 65, 123, 209, 212). The presence or absence of keratins in cells of primary or metastatic tumors, therefore, serves as an important indicator of cell of origin in lesions constituting a diagnostic problem.

Although basic tissue-specific pattern of keratins is usually preserved in tumor cells, epithelia vary considerably in the gain or loss of individual keratins during tumorigenesis (123). Ductal carcinomas of the human breast both lose and gain expression of keratins relative to those observed in the ductal epithelium of normal breast (144).

The lining epithelial surfaces of the body are protected

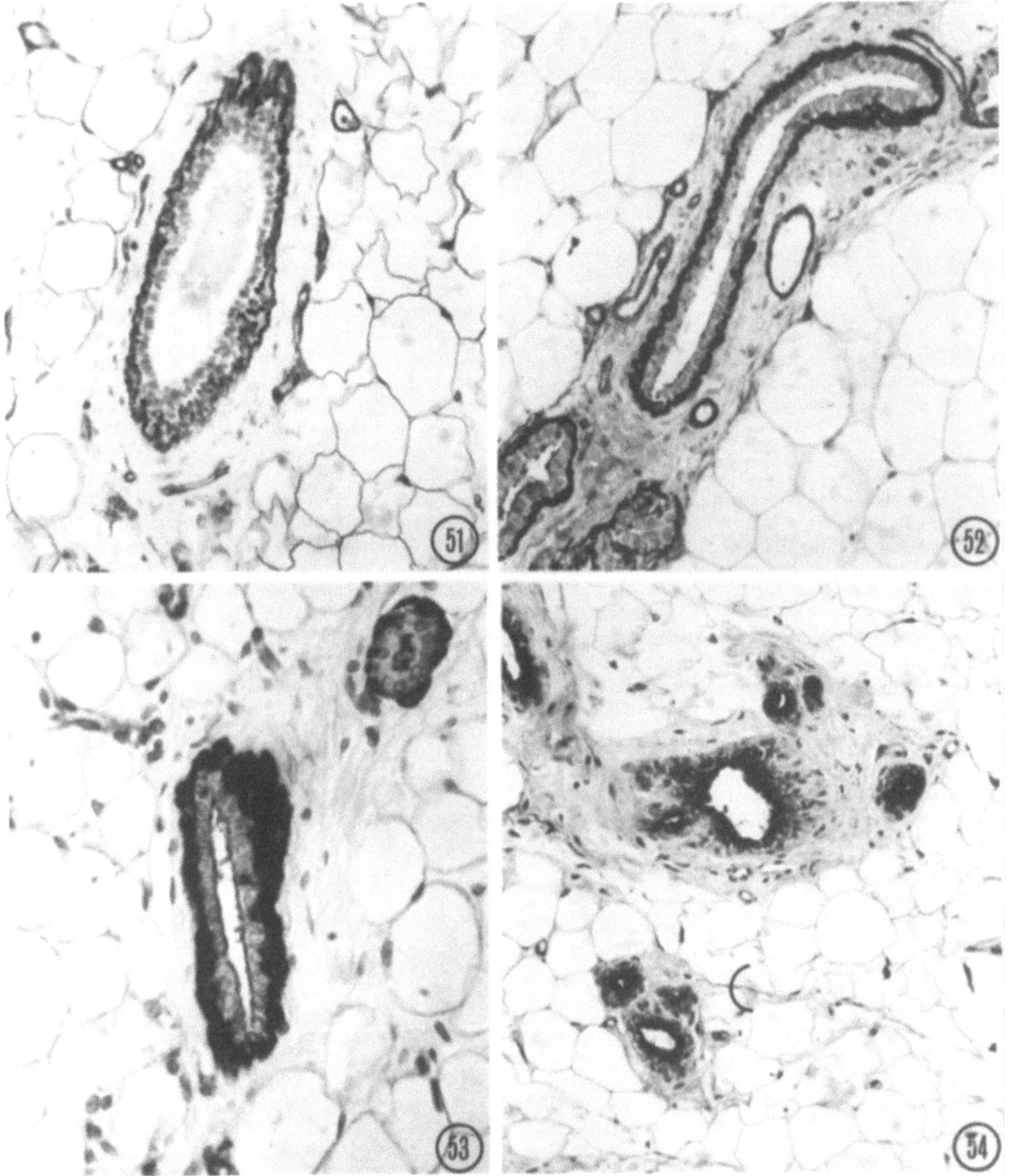

FIG. 51 to 54. Immunohistochemical staining of normal rat mammary gland.

FIG. 51. Immunohistochemical localization of laminin in the normal 50-day-old rat mammary gland. ×265.

FIG. 52. Actin is a good marker for identification of myoepithelial cells in the resting adult rat mammary gland. ×265.

FIG. 53. A polyclonal anti-keratin antibody stains myoepithelial cells. ×265.

FIG. 54. In this section of normal adult rat mammary gland the luminal surface of cells are stained with an antibody against MFGMA. ×265.

by large glycoconjugates which are referred to collectively as mucins. These molecules are highly antigenic and have similar structure and share epitopes in many areas of the body. Thus, by using breast epithelial membranes from milk (milk fat globule membrane antigen), breast carcinomas, normal breast extracts or epithelial cells from other sites in the body, a number of both monoclonal and polyclonal antibodies have been produced, which

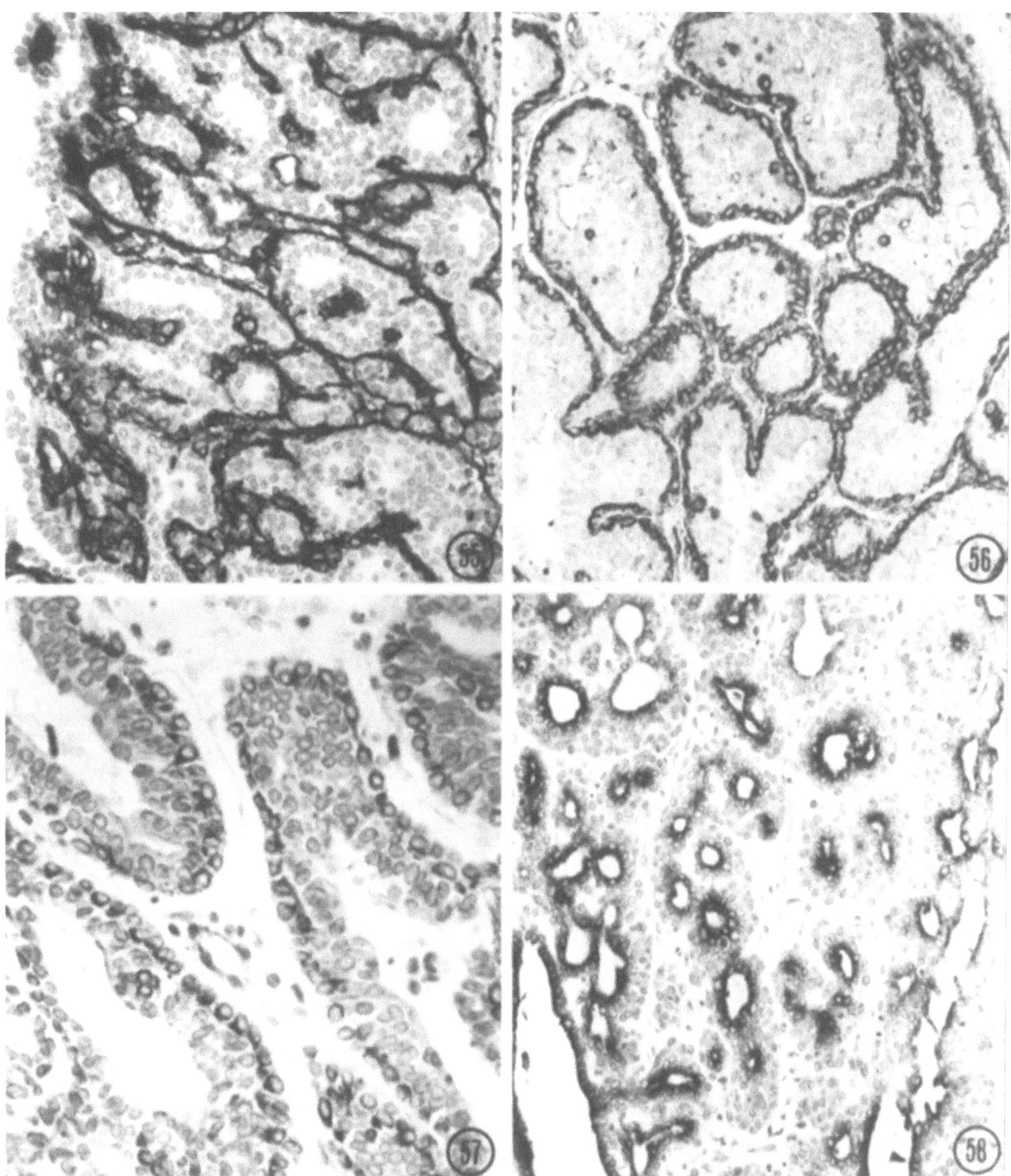

FIG. 55 to 58. Immunohistochemical staining of NMU-induced rat mammary carcinomas, cribriform type.

FIG. 55. Basement membrane at the stromal/epithelial interface defined with an anti-laminin antibody. ×265.

FIG. 56. Sections show a population of strongly actin positive cells ×265.

FIG. 57. In this section there is staining with anti-keratin marker of a basally situated population of cells in a well differentiated area. ×265.

FIG. 58. The lumina in these tumors are reacted with an anti-MFGMA. ×265.

react with the core protein or more commonly with the carbohydrate determinants on breast epithelial cells. Most of these reagents, including the now well accepted diagnostic reagent epithelial membrane antigen (77, 129, 177), HMFG1, HMFG2 (5, 32), M8, M18 (58), all react with epitopes on the same 400,000 molecular weight mucin molecule. These antibodies that define the luminal membrane in normal breast epithelium are heteroge-

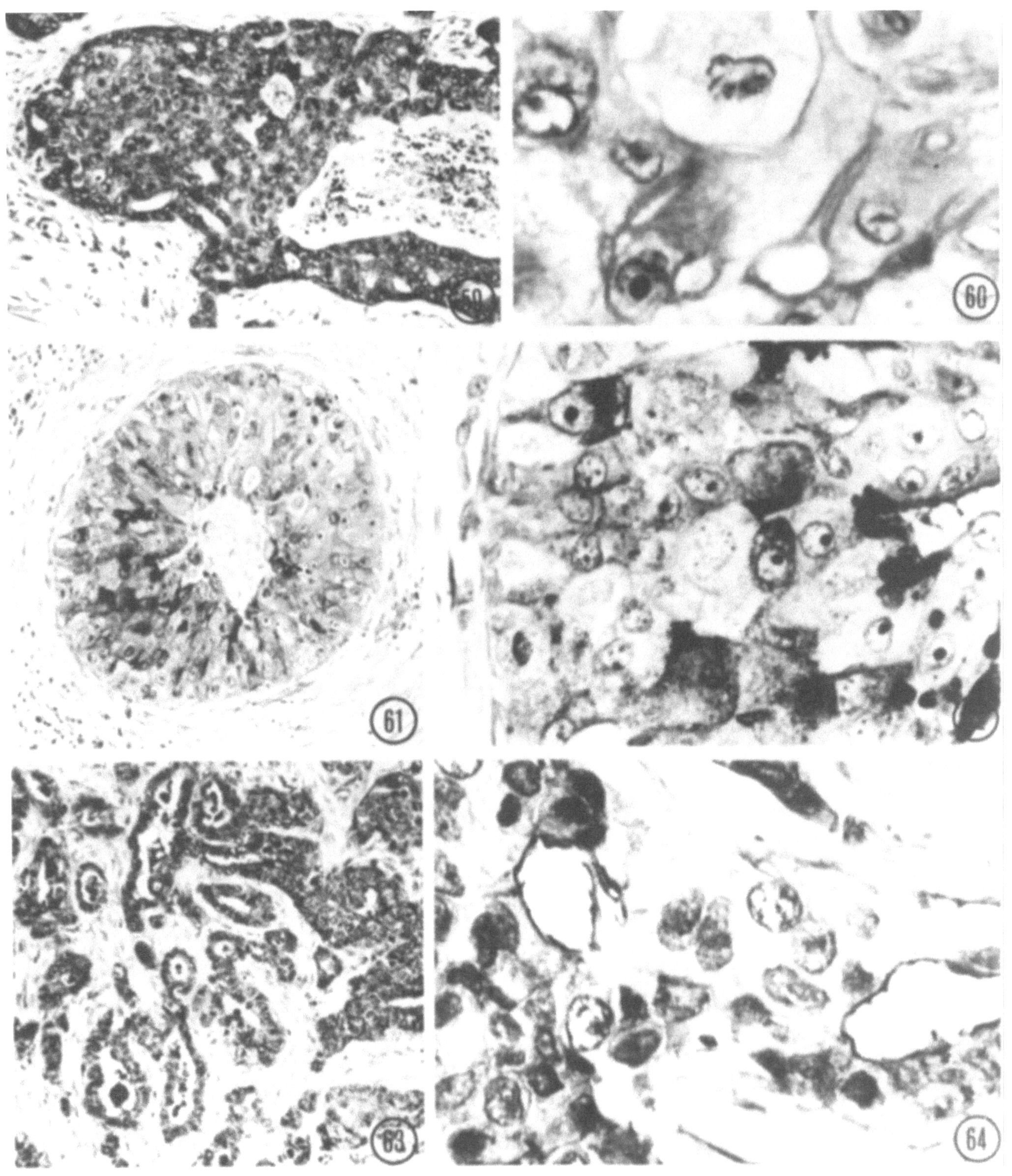

FIG. 59 to 64. Human breast carcinoma.
FIG. 59. Infiltrating ductal carcinoma reacted for keratin. ×100.
FIG. 60. High magnification of Figure 59 showing the diffuse staining of the cytoplasm. ×400.
FIG. 61. Intraductal carcinoma reacted with MC5. ×160.
FIG. 62. Intraductal carcinoma reacted with MC5, showing different degrees of reactivity. ×400.
FIG. 63. Infiltrating ductal carcinoma reacted with MC5. ×160.
FIG. 64. Infiltrating ductal carcinoma showing MC5 reactivity in the luminal surface. ×400.

neously expressed both in tumors and normal breast epithelium, the distribution probably depending upon the differential glycosylation of the protein core in different cells (Figs. 61 to 64). These reagents have a broad use as cellular markers of the luminal population and for diagnostic application (32, 35–37, 144) (Table 11).

Breast epithelium expresses a variety of gene products, including α-lactalbumin, casein, and lactoferrin (Table

TABLE 11. ANTIGENS ASSOCIATED WITH BREAST EPITHELIAL MEMBRANE

Antibody	Source of antigen
14-A-3	Milk fat globule membrane
1-10-F3	Milk fat globule membrane
MFGH-gP70	Milk fat globule membrane
HME	400,00 dalton protein (MFGM)
HMFG-1	Milk fat globule membrane
HMFG-2	Milk fat globule membrane
HMFG-(MC-5)	Defatted human milk
EMA	Milk fat globule membrane
LICR-LON-M8	Breast epithelium
LICR-LON-M18	Breast epithelium

10). α-Lactalbumin is a synthetase secreted by the differentiated mammary epithelium (28, 44), although the intensity of the reaction is variable from tumor to tumor and varies within different areas of a single positive tumor. Casein is a protein specific to the mammary epithelial cells and has been considered a marker of differentiation of cells in dysplastic and neoplastic lesions of the breast (31, 57). Casein reactivity is located along the lining surface or filling the cavity of dilated alveoli and in the apical portion of the acinar border (31), but no reactivity is apparent in atrophic or prepubertal glands. In well-differentiated carcinomas, casein has been localized in the inner border of gland-like structures. Even though casein is a breast epithelial product, the polyclonal antibody against human casein reported in the literature (31) has been shown to react also with non-breast tissues such as adnexal glands of the skin, bronchial epithelium, exocrine pancreas, endometrium in proliferative phase, and collecting tubules of the kidney (57).

Lactoferrin, an iron-binding protein found in milk and other human secretions (112), has not been used consistently in diagnostic pathology as a marker of differentiation in mammary epithelium of either normal, dysplastic, or neoplastic breast (84). Whereas the distribution of alpha-lactalbumin, casein and lactoferrin is rather constant in the normal breast, the patterns of distribution are more erratic in neoplastic cells.

Basement Membrane and Breast Stroma. Recognition of the basement membrane of the mammary gland has been accomplished using reagents against laminin and type IV collagen (76, 175) (Table 10). Early recognition of the invasive process can be achieved by using antibodies against these two components. In a recent study of 98 breast carcinomas by Charpin *et al.* (40), laminin was observed within vascular and epithelial basement membranes. Laminin displayed a continuous linear pattern in intraductal carcinomas, and is heterogeneously distributed with a discontinuous linear pattern in invasive carcinomas. Electron microscopic studies have shown laminin immunostaining in the lamina densa of basement membranes in non-neoplastic breast tissue. Laminin immunostaining frequently reveals multilayered basement membranes in tumors and abnormal multilayered basement membranes in blood vessels in the tumor stroma. Invasion in carcinoma has been reported by some investigators to be associated with a complete loss of

extracellular laminin and type IV collagen staining (10, 11, 76, 107, 108, 175).

CRITERIA OF MALIGNANCY

Whether spontaneous or carcinogen-induced rat mammary tumors are benign or malignant can be determined by applying criteria delineated in the present section. The parameters applied to the rat mammary tumor are those already developed in human pathology, such as: (a) gross examination; (b) histopathologic examination and (c) observation of the biologic behavior of the tumor. Since criteria applied to human tumors have been described in detail in the literature (138), we will outline the most applicable to the experimental model.

Gross (Macroscopic) Criteria. Rat mammary carcinomas are generally soft and fleshy with areas of necrosis and hemorrhage; they may have cysts containing blood and necrotic material (Fig. 45). Fibroadenomas are white with a rubbery and firm consistency and shell out from their capsule when sectioned (Fig. 42). However, carcinomas can be firm if they have elicited a desmoplastic response, and large benign tumors may show focal necrosis. Generally malignant tumors tend to grow faster than benign tumors.

Histopathologic Criteria. Among the histologic criteria of malignancy, the first one is the loss of the tubuloalveolar pattern of the normal mammary gland, a pattern maintained in adenomas and fibroadenomas.

Second, as in other carcinomas, the epithelial cells are larger than normal and have an increased nucleocytoplasmic ratio. The nuclear chromatin tends to be coarse, and nucleoli are prominent. The heterogeneity of the nuclear elements found in benign tumors, in which myoepithelial, dark and intermediate or clear cell types are found, is not observed in malignant lesions (162). The number of mitoses generally is higher in malignant tumors than in benign ones, but benign tumors can have significant number of mitoses.

Finally, invasion of the stroma and neighboring fat, muscle and dermis is the hallmark of malignant tumors (Fig. 47). Stromal response, as demonstrated by fibrosis and inflammatory cell infiltration, is generally more prominent in invasive malignant tumors than in noninvasive or benign lesions (Figs. 47 and 48). In some cases, because of the diffuse distribution of normal parenchymal elements, it becomes difficult to judge invasion. Sections from tumors should include adjacent, grossly normal tissue. Single lines of epithelial cells invading connective tissue should be sought at the edge of the tumor.

Biologic Criteria. The most reliable criterion of malignancy is the ability of a tumor to metastasize to distant organs, such as lymph nodes or lung (Figs. 49 and 50). Very few authors report the finding of metastases from either spontaneous or experimentally induced rat mammary tumors. This may be due to the short periods of time that tumor-bearing animals have been observed. Metastases have been reported when the study is prolonged for 2 or 3 years, essentially the whole life span of the animal (194). Because of the large size to which tumors grow and their propensity to become necrotic, it is generally not possible to hold the animals for the period needed to demonstrate metastases. The histopathologic type of a tumor does not seem to affect its metastasizing ability, since cribriform, comedo and papillary carcinomas produce metastases with similar frequency (194) (Figs. 49 and 50).

Transplantability (214) is not a reliable criterion of malignancy in rats because fibroadenomas are transplantable. The ability of neoplastic lesions to elicit angiogenesis has been postulated to be a biologic marker of malignancy but has not been extensively used (22, 111).

CONCLUSIONS AND FURTHER CONSIDERATIONS

We know that both human and rat mammary carcinogenesis are affected by similar factors, namely genetic, endocrinologic, dietary and exogenous agents such as carcinogens and/or radiation. Carcinogenic initiation in the rat occurs by a single exposure to a chemical carcinogen; it requires nulliparity, an intact endocrine system and high rate of cell proliferation. At difference with the rat, in the human we do not know what causes cancer, and when initiation takes place. Therefore, we ignore what are the biologic circumstances in operation at the time of that event.

In the search for adequate experimental models for understanding the human disease, and bearing in mind all the dissimilarities described in this review, we believe the rat mammary tumor model to be adequate for this purpose. The studies outlined above led us to conclude that a better understanding of the basic biology of the human breast, mainly its development during pubertal age, importance of the parenchyma-stroma relationship, understanding of the involution of the human breast under physiologic conditions, a more systematic approach to the study of the cellular and molecular aspects of differentiation of the breast, and finally a better understanding of the molecular endocrinology of the human breast epithelium are necessary. It suffices to say that the knowledge gained in those areas will further our understanding of the mechanisms of initiation and progression of the human disease and the clarification of not only where the lesions start, but when they occur. The understanding of the basic mechanisms of transformation of human breast epithelial cells is of pivotal importance to the comprehension of the biology of breast cancer. Supporting this claim is the realization that the knowledge gained on the pathogenesis of rat mammary carcinomas has led to definitively establishing the importance of differentiation on tumor initiation, the role of hormones and chemopreventive agents in mammary carcinogenesis and the development of strategies for breast cancer prevention. Therefore, it is expected that knowledge of this nature in the human will provide the basis for breast cancer prevention and cure.

An important consideration is that the human disease is unique and its complete understanding can be achieved only through the study of the human condition. However, the comparison of the similarities of it with rat mammary carcinogenesis is an important tool for probing hypotheses, testing new drugs for cure and prevention and for raising important questions on the influence of genetic and environmental factors. The complexity of breast cancer requires one to work hand in hand with material provided by these two sources.

Acknowledgments: We want to thank Dr. M. J. Warburton for the generous supply of antibodies for immunocytochemical reactions and to acknowledge the excellent technical assistance of Mr. Larry Tait and Ms. Vivian Powell for the skillful typing of the manuscript.

This work was supported by United States Public Health Service Grant CA38921 (to J.R.) and CA35699 awarded by the National Cancer Institute, and Grant BC-621 from the American Cancer Society (to I.H.R.), an Institutional grant from the United Foundation of Greater Detroit (to J.R.), grants from the American Institute for Cancer Research (to A.R.) and a grant from the Cancer Research Campaign of the Medical Research Council (to B.G.).

Address reprint requests to: Dr. Jose Russo, Department of Pathology, Michigan Cancer Foundation, 110 East Warren Ave., Detroit, MI 48201.

REFERENCES

1. Alpers CE, Wellings SR: The prevalence of carcinoma-in-situ in normal and cancer-associated breasts. Human Pathol 16:796, 1985
2. Altmannsberger M, Osborn M, Droese M, Weber K, Schauer A: Diagnostic value of intermediate filament antibodies in clinical cytology. Klin Wochenschr 62:114, 1984
3. Altmannsberger M, Osborn M, Holscher A, Schauer A, Weber K: The distribution of keratin type intermediate filaments in human breast cancer: an immunohistochemical study. Virchows Arch, Cell Pathol 37:277, 1981
4. Altman NH, Goodman DG: Neoplastic diseases. In *The Laboratory Rat*, vol I, Biology and Diseases, edited by Baker HJ, Lindsey JR, Weisbroth SH, Academic Press, 1979
5. Arkhie J, Taylor-Papadimitriou J, Bodmer W, Egan M, Millis R: Differentiation antigens expressed by epithelial cells in lactating breast are also detectable in breast cancers. Int J Cancer 28:23, 1981
6. Asch BB, Burstein NA, Vidrich A, Sun TT: Identification of mouse mammary epithelial cells by immunofluorescence with rabbit and guinea pig antikeratin antisera. Proc Natl Acad Sci USA 78:5643, 1981
7. Astwood EB, Geschickter CF, Rausch EO: Development of the mammary gland of the rat. Am J Anat 61:372, 1937
8. Aylsworth CF, Cullum ME, Zile MH, Welsch CW: Influence of dietary retinyl acetate on normal rat mammary gland development and on the enhancement of 7,12-dimethylbenze a anthracene-induced rat mammary tumorigenesis by high levels of dietary fat. JNCI 76:339, 1986
9. Bakker GH, Setyone-Han B, Henkelman MS, de Jong FH, Lamberts SWJ, van der Schoot P, Klijn JGM: Comparison of the actions of the antiprogestin mifepristone (RU486), the progestin megestrol acetate, the LHRH analoge buserelin, and ovariectomy in treatment of rat mammary tumors. Cancer Treatment Reports 71:1021, 1987
10. Barsky SH, Rao CN, Hyams D, Liotta LA: Characterization of laminin receptor from human breast carcinoma tissue. Breast Cancer Res Treat 4:181, 1984
11. Barsky SH, Siegal GP, Jannotta F, Liotta LA: Loss of basement membrane components by invasive tumors but not by their benign counterparts. Lab Invest 49:140, 1983
12. Bassler R: The morphology of hormone induced structural changes in the female breast. Curr Top Pathol 53:1, 1970
13. BEIR: Committee on the Biological Effects of Ionizing Radiations, National Research Council (1980) Somatic effects: Cancer. In The Effects on Populations of Exposure to Low Levels of Ionizing Radiation: Chap 5, pp 135. Washington, D.C., National Academy Press, 1980
14. Benjamin H, Storkson J, Pariza MW: Effect of voluntary exercise of mammary tumor development. FASEB J 2:1191, 1988
15. Beth M, Berger MR, Aksoy M, Schmahl D: Comparison between the effects of dietary fat level and of calorie intake on methylni-

trosourea-induced mammary carcinogenesis in female SD rats. Int J Cancer 39:737, 1987

16. Black MM, Chabon AB: In Situ Carcinoma of the breast. In Pathology Annual, edited by Sommers SC, pp 185. New York, Appleton-Century-Crofts, 1969

17. Blankenstein MA, Broerse JJ, Van Zwieten MJ, Van der Molen HJ: Prolactin concentration in plasma and susceptibility to mammary tumors in female rats from different strains treated chronically with estradiol-17β. Breast Cancer Res Treatment 4:137, 1984

18. Bond VP, Cronkite EP, Lippincott SW, Shellabarger CJ: Studies on radiation-induced mammary gland neoplasia in the rat. III. Relation of the neoplastic response to dose of total-body radiation. Radiat Res 12:276, 1960

19. Bond VP, Shellabarger CJ, Cronkite EP, Fliedner TM: Studies on radiation-induced mammary gland neoplasia in the rat. V. Induction by localized irradiation. Radiat Res 13:318, 1960

20. Bonser GM, Dossett JA, Jull JW: Human and Experimental Breast Cancer, p 175. Springfield, Ill, Charles C Thomas, 1961

21. Boylan ES, Calhoon RE: Transplacental action of diethylstibestrol on mammary carcinogenesis in female rats given one or two doses of 7,12-dimethylbenz(a)anthrancene. Cancer Res 43:4879, 1983

22. Brem SS, Jensen HM, Gullino PM: Angiogenesis as a marker of preneoplastic lesions of the human breast. Cancer 41:239, 1978

23. Broerse JJ, Hennen LA, van Zwieten MJ, Hollander CF: Dose-effect relations for mammary carcinogenesis in different rat strains after irradiation with X-rays and monoenergetic neutrons. In Biological Effects of Low-Level Radiation, p 507. Vienna, IAEA, 1983

24. Broerse JJ, Hennen LA, Solleveld HA: Actuarial analysis of the hazard for mammary carcinogenesis in different rat strains after X- and neutron irradiation. Leuk Res 10:749, 1986

25. Broerse JJ, Hennen LA, Klapwijk WM, Solleveld HA: Mammary carcinogenesis in different rat strains after irradiation and hormone administration. Int J Radiat Biol 51:1091, 1987

26. Bussolati G, Botta G, Gugliotta P: Actin-rich (myoepithelial) cells in ductal carcinoma in situ of the breast. Virchows Arch (Cell Pathol), 34:252, 1980

27. Bussolati G, Botto Micca F, Eusebi V, Betts CM: Myoepithelial cells in lobular carcinoma in situ of the breast: a parallel immunocytochemical and ultrastructural study. Ultrastruct Pathol 2:219, 1981.

28. Bussolati G, Ghiringhello B, Carlo FD, Aimone V, Voglino GF: Lactalbumin synthesis in breast cancer tissue. Lancet 2:252, 1977

29. Bussolati G, Gugliotta P, Fulcheri E: Immunohistochemistry of actin in normal and neoplastic tissues. In Advances in Immunohistochemistry, edited by DeLellis RA, p 325. New York, Masson, 1981

30. Bussolati G, Papotti M, Gugliotta P: Histology and histochemistry of cystic breast disease. In Endocrinology of Cystic Breast Disease, edited by Angeli A, Bradlow HL, Dogliotti L, pp 7 18. New York, Raven Press, 1983

31. Bussolati G, Pich A, Alfani V: Immunofluorescence detection of casein in human mammary dysplastic and neoplastic tissues. Virchows Arch (A), 365:15, 1973

32. Burchell J, Durbin H, Taylor-Papadimitriou J: Complexity of expression of antigenic determinants recognized by monoclonal antibodies HMFG-1 and HMFG-2, in normal and malignant human mammary epithelial cells. J Immunol 131:508, 1983

33. Calaf G, Martinez F, Russo IH, Russo J: Age related variations in growth kinetics of primary human breast cell cultures, Int Res Comm Syst Med Sci 10:307, 1982

34. Calaf G, Martinez F, Russo IH, Roi LD, Russo J: The influence of age on DNA-Labeling Index of human breast epithelium, Int Res Comm Syst Med Sci 10:655, 1982

35. Ceriani RL, Peterson JA, Lee JY, Moncada R, Blank EW: Characterization of cell surface antigens of normal human mammary epithelial cells with monoclonal antibodies. Somat Cell Genet 9:415, 1983

36. Ceriani RL, Sasaki M, Sussman H, William MW, Blank EW: Circulating human mammary epithelial antigens in breast cancer. Proc Natl Acad Sci USA 79:5420, 1982

37. Ceriani RL, Thompson K, Peterson JA, Abraham S: Surface differentiation antigens on human mammary epithelial cells carried on the human milk fat globules. Proc Natl Acad Sci USA 14:582, 1977

38. Chan PC, Dao TL: Effects of dietary fat on age-dependent sensitivity to mammary carcinogenesis. Cancer Letters 18:245, 1983

39. Chan PC, Ferguson KA, Dao TL: Effects of different dietary fats on mammary carcinogenesis. Cancer Res 43:1079, 1983

40. Charpin C, Lissitzki C, Jacquemier J: Immunohistochemical detection of laminin in 98 human breast carcinomas: a light and electron microscopy study. Hum Pathol 27:355, 1986

41. Cheatle GL: Desquamative and dysgenetic epithelial hyperplasia in breast: their situation and characteristics: their likeness to lesions induced by tar. Br J Surg 13:509, 1926

42. Cheatle GL, Cutler M: Tumours of the Breast: Their Pathology, Symptoms, Diagnosis, and Treatment. London, Arnold, 1931

43. Clinton SK, Alster JM, Imrey PB, Nandkumar S, Truex CR, Visek WJ: Effects of dietary protein, fat and energy intake during an initiation phase study of 7, 12-dimethylbenz[a]anthracene-induced breast cancer in rats. J Nutr 116:2290, 1986

44. Clinton SK, Imrey PB, Alster JM, Simon J, Truex CR, Visek WJ: The combined effects of dietary protein and fat on 7,12-dimethylbenz[a]-anthracene-induced breast cancer in rats. J Nutr 114:1213, 1984

45. Cohen LA, Thompson DO, Maeura Y, Choi K, Blank ME, Rose DP: Dietary fat and mammary cancer. Promoting effects of different dietary fat on N-nitrosomethylurea-induced rat mammary tumorigenesis. J Natl Cancer Inst 77:33, 1986

46. Cooper D, Schemer A, Sun TT: Classification of human epithelia and their neoplasms using monoclonal antibodies to keratins: strategies, applications and limitations. Lab Invest 52:243, 1985

47. Dabelow A: Die Milchdruse. In Handbuch der Mikroskopischen Anatomic des Menschen, Vol 3, Part 3, Haut und Sinnes Organs, edited by Bargmann W, p 277. Berlin, Springer-Verlag, 1957

48. Dao TL: The role of ovarian hormones in initiating the induction of mammary cancer in rats by polynuclear hydrocarbons. Cancer Res 22:973, 1962

49. Dao TL, Chan PC: Effect of duration of high fat intake on enhancement of mammary carcinogenesis in rats. JNCI 71:201, 1983

50. Dawson EK: A histological study of the normal mamma in relation to tumor growth. I. Early development to maturity, Edinb Med J 41:653, 1934

51. Dawson EK: Premalignant conditions in breast carcinoma. In The Morphological Precursors of Cancer, edited by Severi L, p 383. Perugia, Perugia Univ Press, 1962

52. Dulbecco R, Allen WR, Bologna M, Bowman M: Marker evolution during the development of the rat mammary gland: stem cells identified by markers and the role of myoepithelial cells. Cancer Res 46:2449, 1986

53. Edwards DP, Adams DJ, McGuire WL: Estradiol stimulate synthesis of a major intracellular protein in the human breast cancer cell line MCF-7. Breast Cancer Res Treat 1:209, 1981

54. Elegbede JA, Elson CE, Qureshi A, Tanner MA, Gould MN: Inhibition of DMBA-induced mammary cancer by the monoterpene d-limonene. Carcinogenesis 5:661, 1984

55. Finerty JC, Binhammer RT, Schneider M, Cunningham AWB: Neoplasms in rats exposed to single-dose total-body X-radiation, J Natl Cancer Inst 14:149, 1953

56. Foote FW, Stewart FW: Comparative studies of cancerous versus noncancerous breasts. Ann Surg 121:6, 1945

57. Fortt RW, Gibbs AR, Williams D: The identification of casein in human breast cancer. Histopathology 3:395, 1979

58. Foster CS, Edwards PAW, Dinsdale E, Neville AM: Monoclonal antibodies to the human mammary gland. I. Distribution of determinants in non-neoplastic mammary and extra-mammary tissues. Virchows Arch (Pathol Anat) 394:279, 1982

59. Franke WW, Mayer D, Schmid E, Denk H, Borenfreund E: Differences of expression of cytoskeletal proteins in cultured rat hepatocytes and hepatoma cells. Exp Cell Res 134:345, 1981

60. Franke WW, Schiller DJ, Moll R: Diversity of cytokeratins: differentiation specific expression of cytokeratin polypeptides in epithelial cells and tissues. J Mol Biol 153:933, 1981

61. Franke WW, Schmid E, Fruedenstin C: Intermediate filaments of the prekeratin type in myoepithelial cells. J Cell Biol 84:633, 1980

62. Franke WW, Schmid E, Osborn M, Weber K: Different interme-

diate-sized filaments distinguished by immunofluorescence microscopy. Proc Natl Acad Sci USA 75:5034, 1978

63. Gallagher HS, Martin JE: Early phases in the development of breast cancer. Cancer 24:1170, 1969

64. Geschickter CF: Pathology of mammary cancer. In Diseases of the Breast, p 412. Philadelphia, Lippincott, 1945

65. Gigi O, Gieger B, Eshhar Z: Detection of a cytokeratin determinant common to diverse epithelial cells by a broadly crossing-reacting monoclonal antibody. EMBO J 1:1429, 1982

66. Gottardis MM, Jordan VC: Antitumor actions of keoxifene and tamoxifen in the N-nitrosomethylurea-induced rat mammary carcinoma model. Cancer Res 47:4020, 1987

67. Greaves P, Faccini JM: Tumors of the mammary gland. In Rat Histopathology, p 10. Amsterdam, Elsevier, 1984

68. Grubbs CJ, Farnell DR, Hill DL, McDonough KC: Chemoprevention of N-nitroso-N-methylurea-induced mammary cancers by pretreatment with 17 β-estradiol and progesterone. J Natl Cancer Inst 4:927, 1985

69. Grubbs CJ, Hill DL, McDonough KC, Peckham JC: N-nitroso-N-methylurea-induced mammary carcinogenesis: effect of pregnancy on preneoplastic cells. J Natl Cancer Inst 71:625, 1983

70. Grubbs CJ, Juliana MM, Hill DL, Whitaker LM: Suppression by pregnancy of chemically induced preneoplastic cells of the rat mammary gland. Anticancer Res 6:2395, 1986

71. Grubbs CJ, Peckham JC, McDonough KD: Effect of ovarian hormones on the induction of 1-methyl-nitrosourea-induced mammary cancer. Carcinogenesis 4:495, 1983

72. Grubbs CJ, Peckham JC, Cato KD: Mammary carcinogenesis in rats in relation to age at time of N-nitroso-N-methylurea administration. J Natl Cancer Inst 70:209, 1983

73. Gullino PM, Pettigrew HM, Grantham FH: N-nitrosomethylurea as mammary gland carcinogen in rats. J Natl Cancer Inst 54:401, 1975

74. Gusterson BA, Monaghan P, Mahendran R, Ellis J, O'Hare MJ: Identification of myoepithelial cells in human and rat breasts by anti-common acute lymphoblastic leukemia antigen antibody A12. J Natl Cancer Inst 77:343, 1986

75. Gusterson BA, McIlhinney RAJ, Patel S, Knight J, Monaghan P, Ormerod MG: The biochemical and immunocytochemical characterization of an antigen on the membrane of basal cells of the epidermis. Differentiation 30:102, 1985

76. Gusterson BA, Warburton MJ, Mitchell D, Ellison M, Nevme AM, Rudland PS: Distribution of myoepithelial cells and basement membrane proteins in the normal breast and in benign and malignant breast diseases. Cancer Res 42:4763, 1982

77. Heyderman E, Steele K, Ormerod MG: A new antigen on the epithelial membrane: its immunoperoxidase location in normal and neoplastic tissue. J Clin Pathol 32:35, 1979

78. Hirose M, Masuda A, Inouge T, Fukushima S, Ito N: Modification by antioxidants and p,p-diaminodiphenylmethane of 7,12-dimethylbenza(a)-anthracene-induced carcinogenesis of the mammary gland and ear duct in CD rats. Carcinogenesis 7:1155, 1986

79. Holtzman S, Stone JP, Shellabarger CJ: Influence of diethylstilbestrol treatment on prolactin cells of female ACI and Sprague-Dawley rats. Cancer Res 39:779, 1979

80. Holtzman S, Stone JP, Shellabarger CJ: Radiation-induced mammary carcinogenesis in virgin, pregnant, lactating and post-lactating rats. Cancer Res 42:50, 1982

81. Horvath PM, Ip C: Synergistic effect of Vitamin E and Selenium in the Chemoprevention of mammary carcinogenesis in rats. Cancer Res 43:5335, 1983

82. Huggins C, Grand LC, Brillantes F: Critical significances of breast structure in the induction of mammary cancer in the rat. Proc Natl Acad Sci 45:1294, 1959

83. Huggins C, Yang NC: Introduction and extinction of mammary cancer. Science 137:257, 1962

84. Hurlimann J, Lichaa M, Ozello L: In vitro synthesis of immunoglobulins and other proteins by dysplastic and neoplastic human mammary tissues. Cancer Res 36:1284, 1976

85. Ip C: Interaction of vitamin C and selenium supplementation in the modification of mammary carcinogenesis in rats. J Natl Cancer Inst 77:299, 1986

86. Ip C: Selenium inhibition of chemical carcinogenesis. Fed Proc 44:2573, 1985

87. Iman A, Taylor CR, Tokes ZA: Immunohistochemical study of

the expression of human milk fat globule membrane glycoprotein 70. Cancer Res 44:2016, 1984

88. Ingleby H, Gershon-Cohen J (eds): The normal breast. In Comparative Anatomy, Pathology and Roentgenology of the Breast, p 3. Philadelphia, University of Pennsylvania Press, 1960

89. Ito N: Nitroquinolines, Carcinogenesis: A Comprehensive Survey, edited by Sugimura T, Vol 6, p 260. New York, Raven Press, 1981

90. Isaacs JT: Genetic control of resistance to chemically induced mammary adenocarcinogenesis in the rat. Cancer Res 46:3958, 1986

91. Isaacs JT: Inheritance of a genetic factor from the Copenhagen rat and the suppression of chemically induced mammary adenocarcinogenesis. Cancer Res 48:2204, 1988

92. Jensen HM, Rice J, Wellings SR: Preneoplastic lesions in the human breast. Science 191:295, 1976

93. Karpas CM, Leis HP, Oppenheim A: Relationship of fibrocystic disease to carcinoma of the breast. Ann Surg 162:1, 1965

94. Kern WH, Brooks RN: Atypical epithelial hyperplasia associated with breast cancer and fibrocystic disease. Cancer 24:688, 1969

95. Kiaer W: Relationship of Fibroadenomatosis (Chronic Mastitis) to Cancer of the Breast. p 159, Copenhagen, Munksgaard, 1954

96. King M, McCoy PB, Russo IH: Dietary fat may influence DMBA-initiated mammary gland carcinogenesis by modification of mammary gland development. In Diet Nutrition and Cancer, edited by Roe, DA, p 61. New York, Alan R. Liss, Inc., 1983

97. Klurfeld DM, Weber MM, Kirtchevsky D: Inhibition of chemically induced mammary and colon tumor promotion by caloric restriction in rats fed increased dietary fat. Cancer Res 47:2759, 1987

98. Kort WJ, Weijma IM, Bijma AM, van Schalkwijk WP, Vergroesen AJ, Westbroek DL: Omega-3 fatty acids inhibiting the growth of a transplantable rat mammary adenocarcinoma. J Natl Cancer Inst 79:593, 1987

99. Krepler R, Denk H, Weirich E, Schmid E, Franke WW: Keratin like proteins in normal and neoplastic cells of human and rat mammary gland as reveled by immunofluorescence microscopy. Differentiation 20:242, 1981

100. Kritchevesky D, Weber MM, Klurfeld DM: Dietary fat versus caloric content in initiation and promotion of 7,12-dimethylbenz(a)anthracene-induced mammary tumorigenesis in rats. Cancer Res 44:3174, 1984

101. Land CE, Boice JD, Shore RE, Norman JE, Tokunaga M: Breast cancer risk from low-dose exposures to ionizing radiation: results of parallel analysis of three exposed populations of women. J Natl Cancer Inst 65:353, 1980

102. Lee SY, Ng SF, Busby WF, Rogers AE: Mammary gland DNA synthesis in rats fed hig lard or control diets. J Nutr Growth and Cancer 4:167, 1988

103. Lee SY, Rogers AE: Dimethylbenzathracene mammary tumorigenesis in Sprague-Dawley rats fed diets differing in content of beaf tallow or rapeseed oil. Nutr Res 3:361, 1983

104. Lee SY, Walsh CT, Ng SF, Rogers AE: Toxicokinetics of 7,12-dimethylbenz(a)anthracene (DMBA) in rats fed high lard or control diets. J Nutr Growth and Cancer 3:167, 1986

105. Levin ML, Sheehe PR, Graham S, Glidewell O: Lactation and menstrual function as related to cancer of the breast. Am J Public Health 54:580, 1964

106. Lindsey WF, Das Gupta TK, Beattie CW: Influence of the estrous cycle during carcinogen exposure on nitrosomethylurea-induced rat mammary carcinoma. Cancer Res 41:3857, 1981

107. Liotta LA: Tumor invasion and metastases: role of the basement membrane. Am J Pathol 117:339, 1984

108. Liotta LA, Rao CN, Barsky SH: Tumor invasion and the extracellular matrix. Lab Invest 49:636, 1983

109. MacMahon B: Risk factors for endometrial cancer. Gynecol Oncol 2:122, 1974

110. MacMahon B, Cole P, Liu M, Lowe CR, Mirra AP, Ravinihar B, Salber EJ, Valaoras VG, Yuasa S: Age at first birth and breast cancer risk. Bulletin of WHO 34:309, 1970

111. Maiorana A, Gullino PM: Acquisition of angiogenic capacity and neoplastic transformation in the rat mammary gland. Cancer Res 38:4409–4414, 1978

112. Masson PL, Heremans JF: Studies on lactoferrin: the iron-binding protein of secretions. Prot Biol Fluids 14:115, 1966

113. McCormick DL: Anticarcinogenic activity of quinacrine in the rat

mammary gland. Carcinogenesis 9:175, 1988

114. McCormick DL, Adamowski CB, Fiks A, Moon RC: Lifetime dose-response relationships for mammary tumor induction by a single administration of n-methyl-n-nitrosurea. Cancer Res 41:1690, 1981

115. McCormick DL, Burns FJ, Albert RE: Inhibition of benzo(a)pyrene-induced mammary carcinogenesis by retinyl acetate. J Natl Cancer Inst 66:559, 1981

116. McCormick DL, Madigan MJ, Moon RC: Modulation of rat mammary carcinogenesis by indomethacin. Cancer Res 45:1803, 1985

117. McCormick DL, Major N, Moon RC: Inhibition of 7,12-dimethylbenz(a)anthracene-induced rat mammary carcinogenesis by concomitant or postcarcinogen antioxidant exposure. Cancer Res 44:2858, 1984

118. McCormick DL, Mehta RG, Thompson CA, Dinger N, Caldwell JA, Moon RC: Enhanced inhibition of mammary carcinogenesis by combined treatment with n-(4-hydroxyphenyl) retinamide and ovariectomy. Cancer Res 42:508, 1982

119. McCormick DL, Moon RC: Influence of delayed administration of retinyl acetate on mammary carcinogenesis. Cancer Res 42:2639, 1982

120. McCormick DL, Moon RC: Retinoid-tamoxifen interaction in mammary cancer chemoprevention. Carcinogenesis 7:193, 1986

121. McGregor DH, Land CE, Choi K, Tokuoka S, Liu PI, Wakabayashi I, Beebe GW: Breast cancer incidence among atomic bomb survivors, Hiroshima and Nagasaki, 1950-1969. J Natl Cancer Inst 59:799, 1977

122. Meyer SJ: Cell proliferation in normal human breast ducts, fibroadenomas, and other ductal hyperplasias as measured by tritiated thymidine, effects of menstrual phase, age and oral contraceptive hormones. Human Pathol 8:67, 1977

123. Moll RW, Franke WW, Schiller DL, Gieger B, Krepler R: The catalog of human cytokeratins: patterns of expression in normal epithelia, tumors and cultured cells. Cell 31:11, 1982

124. Monaghan P, Warburton MJ, Perushinghe N, Rudland PS: Topographical arrangement of basement membrane proteins in lactating rat mammary gland: comparison of the distribution of type IV collagen, laminin, fibronectin, and Thy-1 at the ultrastructural level. Proc Natl Acad Sci 80:3344, 1983

125. Moon RC, McCormick DL, Mehta RG: Inhibition of Carcinogenesis by Retinoids. Cancer Res 43:2469, 1983

126. Muir R: The evolution of carcinoma of the mamma. J Pathol Bacteriol 52:155, 1941

127. Nagel RB, McDaniel KM, Clark VA, Payne CM: The use of antikeratin antibodies in the diagnosis of human neoplasm. Am J Clin Pathol 79:458, 1983

128. O'Hare MJ, Ormerod MG, Monaghan P, Cooper CS, Gusterson BA: Differentiation and growth in the human breast parenchyma. Biochem Soc Transactions 17:589, 1989

129. Ormerod MG, Bussolati G, Sloane JP, Stelle K, Gugliotta P: Similarities of antisera to casein and epithelial membrane antigen. Virchows Arch [A], 397:327, 1982

130. Ormerod EJ, Warburton MJ, Gusterson B, Hughes CM, Rudland PS: Abnormal deposition of basement membrane and connective tissue components in dimethylbenzanthracene-induced rat mammary tumors: an immunocytochemical ultrastructural study. Histochem J 17:1155, 1985

131. Parks AG: The micro-anatomy of breasts. Ann R Coll Surg Engl 24:235, 1959

132. Ratko TA, Beatie CW: Estrous cycle modification of rat mammary tumor induction by a single dose of n-methyl-n-nitrosourea. Cancer Res 45:3042, 1985

133. Rogers AE, Conner B, Boulanger C, Lee S: Mammary tumorigenesis in rats fed diets high in lard: Lipids 21:275, 1986

134. Rogers AE, Conner BH, Boulanger CL, Lee SY, Carr FA, Dumouchel WH: Enhancement of 7,12-Dimethylbenz(a)anthracene mammary carcinogenesis by a high lard diet. In Dietary Fiber, edited by Vahouny GV, and Kritchevsky D, p 449, Plenum Publishing Corporation, 1985

135. Rogers AE, Lee SY: Chemically-induced mammary gland tumors in rats: modulation by dietary fat. In Dietary Fat and Cancer, edited by Ip C, Birt DF, Rogers AE, Mettlin C. p 255. New York, Alan R. Liss, Inc., NY, 1986

136. Rogers AE, Longnecker MP: Dietary and nutritional influences on cancer: a review of epidemiologic and experimental data. Lab Invest 59:729, 1988

137. Rochschild TC, Boylan ES, Calhoon RE, Vonderhaar BK: Transplacental effects of diethylstibestrol on mammary development and tumorigenesis in female ACI rats. Cancer Res 47:4508, 1987

138. Rosai J: Breast. In Ackerman's Surgical Pathology, p 1193. St Louis, The C.V. Mosby Company, 1989

139. Rose DP, Pruitt B, Stauber P, Ertur4k E, Bryan GT: Influence of dosage schedule on the biological characteristics of N-Nitrosomethylurea-induced rat mammary tumors. Cancer Res 40:235, 1980

140. Russo IH, Al-Rayess M, Russo J: Role of contraceptive agents in breast cancer prevention. Proc Biennial International Breast Cancer Research Conference, London, United Kingdom, March 24 to 28, p 87. 1985

141. Russo IH, Al-Rayess M, Sabharwal S: Effect of contraceptive agents on mammary gland structure and susceptibility to carcinogenesis. Proc Am Assoc Cancer Res 26:460, 1985

142. Russo IH, Pokorzynski T, Russo J: Contraceptives as hormone-preventative agents in mammary carcinogenesis. Proc Am Assoc Cancer Res 27:912, 1986

143. Russo IH, Russo J: Developmental stage of the rat mammary gland as determinant of its susceptibility to 7,12-dimethylbenz(a)anthracene. J Natl Cancer Inst 61:1439, 1978

144. Russo J: Immunocytochemical markers in breast cancer. In Immunocytochemistry in Tumor Diagnosis, edited by Russo J, p 207. Boston, Martinus Nijhoff Publishing, 1985

145. Russo J: Basis of cellular autonomy in susceptibility to carcinogenesis. Toxicol Pathol 11:149, 1983

146. Russo J, Calaf G, Roi L, Russo IH: Influence of age and gland topography on cell kinetics of normal human breast tissue. J Natl Cancer Inst 78:413, 1987

147. Russo J, Miller J, Russo IH: Hormonal treatment prevents DMBA-induced rat mammary carcinoma. Proc Am Assoc Cancer Res 23:348, 1982

148. Russo J, Reina D, Russo IH: Human breast differentiation susceptibility to "in vitro" transformation by chemical carcinogen. Proc Am Assoc Cancer Res 27:536, 1986

149. Russo J, Reina D, Frederick J, Russo IH: Expression of phenotypical changes by human breast epithelial cells treated with carcinogens in vitro. Cancer Res 48:2837, 1988

150. Russo J, Russo IH: DNA- labeling index and structure of the rat mammary gland as determinants of its susceptibility to carcinogenesis. J Natl Cancer Inst 61:1451, 1978

151. Russo J, Russo IH: Pregnancy interruption as a risk factor in mammary carcinogenesis. Proc Am Assoc Cancer Res 21:2700, 1980

152. Russo J, Russo IH: Influence of differentiation and cell kinetics on the susceptibility of the rat mammary gland to carcinogenesis. Cancer Res 40:2677, 1980

153. Russo J, Russo IH: Susceptibility of the mammary gland to carcinogenesis II. Pregnancy interruption as a risk factor in tumor incidence. Am J Pathol 100:497, 1980

154. Russo J, Russo IH: Is differentiation the answer in breast cancer prevention? IRCS Med Sci 10:877, 1982

155. Russo J, Russo IH: Modulation of the mammary gland's susceptibility to carcinogenesis. Proc of Am Assoc Cancer Res 29:529, 1988

156. Russo J, Russo IH: Role of differentiation on transformation of human breast epithelial cells. In Cellular and Molecular Biology of Experimental Mammary Cancer, edited by Medina D, Kidwell W, Heppner G, Anderson E, p 67. New York, Plenum Publishing Inc, 1987

157. Russo J, Russo IH: Development of the human mammary gland. Chapter 3. In The Mammary Gland Development, Regulation and Function, edited by Neville MC, Daniel C, p 67. New York, Plenum Publishing Inc., 1987

158. Russo J, Russo IH: Biological and molecular bases of mammary carcinogenesis. Lab Invest 57:112, 1987

159. Russo J, Russo IH, van Zwieten MJ, Rogers AE, Gusterson B: Classification of neoplastic and non-neoplastic lesions of the rat mammary gland. In Integument and Mammary Glands of Laboratory Animals, edited by Jones TC, Mohr U, Hunt RD, p 275. Berlin, Springer-Verlag, 1989

160. Russo J, Saby J, Isenberg WM, Russo IH: Pathogenesis of mam-

mary carcinomas induced in rats by 7,12-dimethylbenz (a) anthracene. J Natl Cancer Inst 59:435, 1977

161. Russo J, Tait L, Russo IH: Susceptibility of the rat mammary carcinogenesis III. The cell of origin of rat mammary carcinoma. Am J Pathol 43:50, 1983

162. Russo J, Tait LK, Russo IH: Differentiation of the mammary gland and susceptibility to carcinogenesis. Breast Cancer Res Treat 2:5, 1982

163. Russo J, Wells P: Na⁺K⁺-dependent ATPase as a specific marker for myoepithelial cells: ultrastructural study. Proc Electron Microsc Soc Am 33:454, 1975

164. Russo J, Wilgus G: Growth kinetics of rat mammary gland epithelial cells in culture (abstr). In Vitro 15:36, 1979

165. Russo J, Wilgus G, Russo IH: Susceptibility of the mammary gland to carcinogenesis. I. Differentiation of the mammary gland as determinant of tumor incidence and type of lesion. Am J Pathol 96:721, 1979

166. Ryan JA, Coady CJ: Ductal proliferation in breast cancer. Can J Surg 5:12, 1962

167. Salazar H, Tobon H: Morphologic changes of the mammary gland during development, pregnancy and lactation. In Lactogenic Hormones, Fetal Nutrition and Lactation, edited by Josimovich J, p 221. New York, Wiley, 1974

168. Sandison AT: An autopsy study of the adult human breast. Natl Cancer Inst Monogr 4:1, 1962

169. Segaloff A, Maxfield WS: The synergism between radiation and estrogen in the production of mammary cancer in the rat. Cancer Res 31:166, 1971

170. Shellabarger CJ, Bond BP, Aponte GE, Cronkite EP: Results of fractionation and protraction of total-body radiation on rat mammary neoplasia. Cancer Res 26:509, 1966

171. Shellabarger CJ, Machado SG, Holtzman S, Stone JP: Assessment of interaction among three carcingens on rat mammary carcinogenesis in a factorially designed experiment. J Natl Cancer Inst 79:549, 1987

172. Shellabarger CJ, Stone JP, Holtzman S: Rat differences in mammary tumor induction with estrogen and neutron radiation. J Natl Cancer Inst 61:1505, 1978

173. Shellabarger CJ: Pituitary and steroid hormones in radiation-induced mammary tumors. In Hormones and Breast Cancer, edited by Pike MC, Siiteri PK, Welsch CW, p 339. Cold Spring Harbor Laboratory, 1981

174. Shirai T, Fysh JM, Lee M-S, Vaught JB, King CM: Relationship of metabolic activation on N-hydroxy-N-acylarylamines to biological response in the liver and mammary gland of the female CD rat. Cancer Res 41:4346, 1981

175. Siegal GP, Barsky SM, Terranova VP: Stages of neoplastic transformation of human breast tissue as monitored by dissection of basement membrane components an immunoperoxidase study. Invasion Metastasis 14:54, 1981

176. Solleveld HA, van Zwieten MJ, Broerse JJ, Hollander CF: Effects of X-irradiation, ovariohysterectomy and estradiol-17β on incidence, benign/malignant ratio and multiplicity of rat mammary neoplasms—a preliminary report. Leuk Res 10:755, 1986

177. Sloane JP, Ormerod MG, Carter RL, Gusterson BA, Foster CS: An immunocytochemical study of the distribution of epithelial membrane antigen in normal and disordered squamous epithelium. Diag Histopathol 5:11, 1982

178. Stone JP, Holtzman S, Shellabarger CJ: Neoplastic responses and correlated plasma prolactin levels in diethylstilbestrol-treated ACI and Sprague-Dawley Rats. Cancer Res 39:733, 1979

179. Stone JP, Holtzman S, Shellabarger CJ: Synergistic interactions of various doses of diethylstilbestrol and X-irradiation on mammary neoplasia in female ACI rats. Cancer Res 40:3966, 1980

180. Sylvester PW, Ip C, Ip M: Effects of high dietary fat on the growth and development of ovarian-independent carcinogen-induced mammary tumors in rats. Cancer Res 46:763, 1986

181. Sylvester PW, Russell M, Ip MM, Ip C: Comparative effects of different animal and vegetable fats fed before and during carcinogen administration on mammary tumorigenesis, sexual maturation, and endocrine function in rats. Cancer Res 46:757, 1986

182. Tanaka Y, Oota K: A stereomicroscopic study of the mastopathic human breast. I. Three dimensional structures of abnormal duct evolution and their histologic entity. Virchows Arch (Pathol Anat) 349:195, 1970

183. Tanner JM (ed): The development of the reproductive system, in: Growth at Adolescence, p 28, Oxford, Blackwell Scientific, 1962

184. Tay LK, Russo J: 7,12-dimethylbenz(a)anthracene-induced DNA binding and repair synthesis in susceptible and non-susceptible mammary epithelial cells in culture. J Natl Cancer Inst 67:155, 1981

185. Tay LK, Russo J: Formation and removal of 7,12-dimethylbenz(a)-anthracene-nucleic acid adducts in rat mammary epithelial cells with different susceptibility to carcinogenesis. Carcinogenesis 2:1327, 1981

186. Taylor-Papadimitriou J, Lane EB: 1. Keratin expression in the mammary gland. In The Mammary Gland, edited by Neville MC, Daniel CW, p 181. Plenum Publishing Corporation, 1987

187. Taylor-Papadimitriou J, Peterson J, Arklie J, Burchell J, Ceriani RL, Bodmer WF: Monoclonal antibodies to epithelium specific components of the human milk fat globule membrane: production and reaction with cells in culture. Int J Cancer 28:17, 1981

188. Thompson HJ, Herbst EJ, Meeker LD, Minocha R, Ronan AM, Fite R: Effect of D,L-a-difluoromethylornithine on murine mammary carcinogenesis. Cancer Res 45:1178, 1985

189. Thompson HJ, Meeker LD: Induction of mammary gland carcinomas by the subcutaneous injection of 1-methyl-1-nitrosourea. Cancer Res 43:1628, 1985

190. Thompson HJ, Meeker LD, Herbst EJ, Ronan AM, Minocha R: Effect of concentration of D,L-a-difluoromethylornithine on murine mammary carcinogenesis. Cancer Res 45:1178, 1985

191. Thompson HJ, Ronan A: Effect of D,L-a-difluoromethyhlornithine and endocrine manipulation on the induction of mammary carcinogenesis by 1-methyl-1-nitrosourea. Carcinogenesis 57:2003, 1987

192. Thompson HJ, Ronan AM, Ritacco KA, Tagliaferro AR, Meeker LD: Effect of exercise on the induction of mammary carcinogenesis. Cancer Res 48:2720, 1988

193. van Bekkum DW, Broerse JJ, Hennen LA, Solleveld HA: The gene transfer-misrepair hypothesis of radiation carcinogenesis tested for induction of mammary tumors in rats. Leuk Res 10:761, 1986

194. van Zwieten MJ: The rat as animal model in breast cancer research. Boston, Martinus Nijhoff Publishers, 1984

195. Vorherr H: Development of the female breast. In The Breast, p 1, New York, Academic Press, 1974

196. Walker RA: The demonstration of alpha-lactabumin in human breast carcinomas. J Pathol 129:37, 1978

197. Warburton MJ, Mitchell D, Ormerod EJ, Rudland P: Distribution of myoepithelial cells and basement membrane proteins in the resting, pregnant, lactating and involuting rat mammary gland. J Histochem Cytochem 30:667, 1982

198. Wellings SR: Development of human breast cancer. I: "Advances in Cancer Research". New York, Academic Press, 31:287, 1980

199. Wellings SR, Krieger RI, Gee SJ, Lim O, Ross JH, Wiulson A, Alpers C: Disposition of toxic substances in mussels (Mytilus californianus): preliminary metabolic and histological studies. ACS Symposium Series 99:259, 1980

200. Wellings SR, Jensen MM, Martcum RG: An atlas of subgross pathology of the human breast with special reference to possible precancerous lesions. J Natl Cancer Inst 55:231, 1975

201. Wellings SR, Rice J: Preneoplastic lesions in the human breast. In Early Diagnosis of Breast Cancer. Methods and Results edited by Grundmann E, Beck L, p 910. Stuttgart and New York, Gustav Fischer Verlag, 1978

202. Welsch CW: Host factors affecting the growth of carcinogen-induced rat mammary carcinomas: a review and tribute to Charles Brenton Huggins. Cancer Res 45:3415, 1985

203. Welsch CW, DeHoog JV, O'Connor DH: Influence of caffeine consumption on carcinomatous and normal mammary gland development in mice. Cancer Res 48:2078, 1988

204. Welsch CW, DeHoog JV, O'Connor DH: Influence of caffeine and/or coffee consumption on the initiation and promotion phases of 7,12-Dimethylbenz(a)anthracene-induced rat mammary gland tumorigenesis. Cancer Res 48:2068, 1988

205. Welsch CW, DeHoog JV: Influence of caffeine consumption on 7,12-Dimethylbenz(a)anthracene-induced mammary gland tumorigenesis in female rats fed a chemically defined diet containing standard and high levels of unsaturated fat. Cancer Res 48:2074, 1988

206. Wetsel WC, Rogers AE, Newberne PM: Dietary fat and DMBA mammary carcinogenesis in rats. Cancer Detection and Prevention 4:535, 1981
207. Westel WC, Rutledge A, Rogers AE: Absence of an effect of dietary corn oil content on plasma prolactin, progesterone, and 17β-estradiol in female Sprague-Dawley rats. Cancer Res 44:1420, 1983
208. Williams JC, Gusterson B, Humphreys J, Monaghan P, Coombes RC, Rudland P, Neville AM: N-methyl-n-nitrosourea-induced rat mammary tumors. Hormone responsive but lack of spontaneous metastasis. J Natl Cancer Inst 66:147, 1981
209. Winter S, Jarasch ED, Schmid E, Franke WW, Denk H: Differences in polypeptide composition of cytokeratin filaments including tonofilaments from different epithelial tissues and cells. Eur J Cell Biol 22:371, 1980
210. Winter H, Schweizer J: Carcinoma-specific keratin polypeptide patterns in keratinizing epithelia of rodents: independence of species- and tissue-specific variations. Carcinogenesis 2:613, 1981
211. Winter H, Schweizer J, Goerttler K: Keratins as markers of malignancy in mouse epidermal tumors. Carcinogenesis 1:391, 1980
212. Wu YJ, Reinwald JG: A new small (40 kD) keratin filament protein made by some cultured human squamous cell carcinomas. Cell 25:627, 1981
213. Yokoro K, Sumi C, Ito A, Hamada K, Kanda K, Kobayashi T: Mammary carcinogenic effect of low-dose fission radiation in Wistar/Furth rats and its dependency on prolactin. J Natl Cancer Inst 64:1459, 1980
214. Young S, Hallowes RC: Tumours of the mammary gland. In Pathology of Tumors in Laboratory Animals. Vol 1, Tumours of the rat, edited by Turusov VS, IARC Sci Publ 1:31, 1973

Index

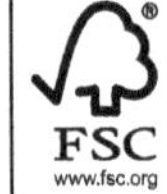

MIX
Papier aus verantwortungsvollen Quellen
Paper from responsible sources
FSC® C105338
FSC
www.fsc.org